T0202813

Lecture Notes in Artificial Intelligence   9605

Subseries of Lecture Notes in Computer Science

More information about this series at http://www.springer.com/series/1244

Andreas Holzinger (Ed.)

Machine Learning for Health Informatics

State-of-the-Art and Future Challenges

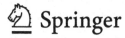
Springer

Editor
Andreas Holzinger
Institute for Medical Informatics, Statistics
   and Documentation
Medical University Graz
Graz
Austria

and

Institute of Interactive Systems
   and Data Science
Graz University of Technology
Graz
Austria

ISSN 0302-9743   ISSN 1611-3349   (electronic)
Lecture Notes in Artificial Intelligence
ISBN 978-3-319-50477-3   ISBN 978-3-319-50478-0   (eBook)
DOI 10.1007/978-3-319-50478-0

Library of Congress Control Number: 2016961250

LNCS Sublibrary: SL7 – Artificial Intelligence

This Springer imprint is published by Springer Nature
The registered company is Springer International Publishing AG
The registered company address is: Gewerbestrasse 11, 6330 Cham, Switzerland

About the Editor

Andreas Holzinger is lead of the Holzinger Group, HCI–KDD, Institute for Medical Informatics, Statistics and Documentation at the Medical University Graz, and Associate Professor of Applied Computer Science at the Faculty of Computer Science and Biomedical Engineering at Graz University of Technology. Currently, Andreas is Visiting Professor for Machine Learning in Health Informatics at the Faculty of Informatics at Vienna University of Technology. He serves as consultant for the Canadian, US, UK, Swiss, French, Italian and Dutch governments, for the German Excellence Initiative, and as national expert in the European Commission. His research interests are in supporting human intelligence with machine intelligence to help solve problems in health informatics. Andreas obtained a PhD in Cognitive Science from Graz University in 1998 and his Habilitation (second PhD) in Computer Science from Graz University of Technology in 2003. Andreas was Visiting Professor in Berlin, Innsbruck, London (twice), and Aachen. He founded the Expert Network HCI–KDD to foster a synergistic combination of methodologies of two areas that offer ideal conditions toward unraveling problems in understanding intelligence: Human–Computer Interaction (HCI) and Knowledge Discovery/Data Mining (KDD), with the goal of supporting human intelligence with machine learning. Andreas is Associate Editor of *Knowledge and Information Systems* (KAIS), Section Editor of *BMC Medical Informatics and Decision Making* (MIDM), and member of IFIP WG 12.9 Computational Intelligence: http://hci-kdd.org.

Preface

Machine learning (ML) studies algorithms that can learn from data to gain knowledge from experience and to make decisions and predictions. Health Informatics (HI) studies the effective use of probabilistic information for decision making. Consequently, to bridge these two fields is of eminent importance for improving human health and well-being.

As a matter of fact, the discipline of health is increasingly turning into a data science and health systems worldwide are confronted with big data. This may be beneficial, as algorithms that improve through experience from large data sets can be of great help here, and automatic ML (aML) approaches show impressive results. Moreover, much health data are in arbitrarily high dimensions, where manual analysis is simply impossible, hence fully automatic approaches by taking the human-out-of-the-loop make great sense.

However, sometimes we are confronted with small data sets, or rare events, where aML approaches suffer from insufficient training samples. Here interactive ML (iML) may be of help, which can be defined as algorithms that can interact with agents and can optimize their learning behavior through these interactions, where the agents can also be human. Furthermore, such a human in the loop can be beneficial in solving computationally hard problems. Particularly a doctor-in-the-loop can be helpful, e.g., in subspace clustering, protein folding, or k-anonymization, where human expertise can help reduce an exponential search space through heuristic selection of samples. Therefore, what would otherwise remain an NP-hard problem, may decrease greatly in complexity by making use of human intelligence and human intuition involved in the ML pipeline.

Intelligence is the core topic of research and Demis Hassabis from Google Deep-Mind summarizes it precisely within his mission statement: "Solve intelligence. Then solve everything else." A synergistic combination of methodologies and approaches from two areas attack the challenge of "solving intelligence" from two perspectives: Human Computer Interaction (HCI) and Knowledge Discovery and Data Mining (KDD).

Consequently, this HCI–KDD approach fosters the successful application of machine learning for health informatics, by encouraging an integrated approach, promoting a concerted cross-disciplinary effort of experts from various disciplines, including (1) data science, (2) algorithms, (3) network science, (4) topology, (5) time/entropy, (6) data visualization, and last but not least (7) privacy, data protection, safety and security.

Hence, the mission of the HCI–KDD expert network is to bring together professionals from diverse areas with various backgrounds and different views, but who share a common vision: "solving intelligence," following the HCI–KDD motto "Science is to test crazy ideas – engineering is to bring those ideas into business."

The HCI–KDD expert network organizes special sessions, the first took place in Graz (Austria), the second in Macau (China), the third in Maribor (Slovenia), the fourth in Regensburg (Germany), the fifth in Lisbon (Portugal), the sixth in Warsaw (Poland), the seventh in Banff (Canada), the eight in London (UK), the ninth in Salzburg (Austria), and the tenth is planned to take place in Reggio di Calabria (Italy) in summer 2017.

Volume 9605 of the *Lecture Notes in Computer Science* series is a state-of-the-art survey (SOTA) and an output of the international HCI–KDD expert network. The volume features 22 carefully selected and peer-reviewed chapters on hot topics in ML for HI. Each chapter discuss open problems and future challenges in order to stimulate further research and international progress in this field.

To acknowledge here all those who contributed to the efforts and stimulating discussions would be impossible. Many people contributed to the development of this volume, either directly or indirectly, and it would be simply impossible to list all of them, so let me thank my international, national, and local colleagues, my family and friends for all their nurturing and positive encouragement. Last but not least I thank the Springer management team and the Springer production team for their smooth support; a cordial thank you to all!

October 2016   Andreas Holzinger

Organization

Scientific Committee: HCI–KDD Expert Network

I am grateful for the support of all members of the expert network HCI–KDD, http://hci-kdd.org/international-expert-network

MED = medical doctor ("doctor-in-the-loop"); IND = industry member; ESR = early-stage researcher, e.g., PhD student); 1 = data science; 2 = ML; 3 = graphs/network science; 4 = topology; 5 = entropy; 6 = visualization; 7 = privacy, data protection, safety and security.

Rakesh Agrawal, Microsoft Search Labs, Mountain View, California, USA
IND (1, 2, 7) <Data mining, Web search, privacy>

Beatrice Alex, Institute for Language, Cognition and Computation, School of Informatics, University of Edinburgh, UK
(1) <text mining, information extraction, NLP, computational linguistics>

Amin Anjomshoaa, SENSEable City Laboratory, MIT – Massachusetts Institute of Technology, Cambridge, MA, USA
(1, 2) <Semantic Web, cloud computing, linked open data>

Matthieu d'Aquin, Knowledge Media Institute, The Open University, Milton Keynes, UK
(1) <Semantic Web, ontologies, linked open data, knowledge representation>

Joel P. Arrais, Centre for Informatics and Systems, University of Coimbra, Portugal
(1, 2) <Bioinformatics, biomedical informatics, computational biology>

John A. Atkinson-Abutridy, Department of Computer Science, Universidad de Concepcion, Chile
(1, 2) <Artificial intelligence, NLP, text Mining>

Chloe-Agathe Azencott, Centre for Computational Biology (CBIO), Mines Paris Tech, France
ESR (1, 2, 3) <Machine Learning, Computational Biology, Personalized Health>

Alexandra Balahur, European Commission Joint Research Centre, Ispra, Italy
(1, 2) <Artificial Intelligence, NLP, computational linguistics>

Peter Bak, IBM Haifa Research Lab, Mount Carmel, Israel
IND (6) <information visualization, visual analytics, spatiotemporal data analysis>

Robert Baumgartner, Lixto Web Information Extraction, Vienna, Austria
IND (1, 2) Web information extraction

Smaranda Belciug, Department of Computer Science, Faculty of Mathematics and Computer Science, University of Craiova, Romania
(2) <Artificial intelligence, genetic algorithms, data mining, statistics, neural networks>

Andreas Bender, Unilever Centre for Molecular Science Informatics, Cambridge, UK
IND (3) <Cheminformatics, drug design, chemogenomics>

Mounir Ben Ayed, Research Group Intelligent Machines, Ecole Nationale d'Ingenieurs de Sfax, Tunisia
(1, 2) <Decision support systems, data mining, HCI, KDD>

Elisa Bertino, Department of Computer Science, Purdue University, West Lafayette, USA
(1, 7) <database systems, computer security, data privacy>

Chris Biemann, Language Technology Group, FB Informatik, Technische Universität Darmstadt, Germany
(1, 2) <information retrieval, natural language processing, computational linguistics, cognitive computing>

Miroslaw Bober, Department of Electronic Engineering, University of Surrey, Guildford, UK
(2, 6) <Computer vision, machine learning, multimedia>

Rainer Boehme, Security and Privacy Lab, Institute of Computer Science, Innsbruck University, Austria
(7) <privacy, information security, digital forensics, privacy-enhancing technology>

Matt-Mouley Bouamrane, Institute of Health and Wellbeing, University of Strathclyde, Glasgow, UK
(1, 6) <eHealth, health informatics, knowledge engineering, decision support systems, HCI>

Francesco Buccafurri, Security and Social Networks Group, Università Mediterranea di Reggio Calabria, Italy
(1, 3, 7) <Social Networks, Information security and privacy, artificial intelligence>

Andre Calero-Valdez, RWTH Aachen University, Aachen, Germany
ESR (3, 6) <Networks, Scientometrics, information visualization, HCI>

Mirko Cesarini, Department of Statistics and Quantitative Methods, Università di Milano Bicocca, Milan, Italy
(1, 2) <data quality, data analysis, data integration, business intelligence, information systems>

Polo Chau, School of Computational Science and Engineering, College of Computing, Georgia Tech, Atlanta, USA
(2, 3, 6) <data mining, fraud detection, visualization, HCI>

Chaomei Chen, College of Information Science and Technology, Drexel University, Philadelphia, USA
(6) <information visualization, visual analytics, scientometrics>

Elizabeth S. Chen, Center for Biomedical Informatics, Brown University, Providence, RI, USA
(1) <Biomedical informatics, electronic health records, standards, NLP, data mining>

Veronika Cheplygina, Biomedical Imaging Group, Erasmus Medical Center, Rotterdam, The Netherlands
ESR (1, 2) <machine learning, pattern recognition, medical image analysis, computer aided diagnosis>

Nitesh V. Chawla, Data, Inference, Analytics and Learning Lab, University of Notre Dame, IN, USA
(1, 2, 3) <Data mining, machine learning, network science, healthcare analytics>

Anni R. Coden, IBM T.J. Watson Research Center Hawthorne, NY, USA
IND (1, 2) <machine learning, text and image analytics>

Matthias Dehmer, University for Health and Medical Informatics Tyrol, Innsbruck, Austria
(2, 3, 4, 5) <Systems biology, bioinformatics, complex networks>

Alexiei Dingli, Intelligent Systems Technologies Research Group, University of Malta, Valletta, Malta
(1, 2) <Artificial intelligence, semantic Web, mobile technology>

Tomasz Donarowicz, Institute of Mathematics and Computer Science, Wroclaw University of Technology, Poland
(4, 5) entropy, topological entropy

Mike Duerr-Specht, Emergency Doctor, Duke University Hospital, Durham, North Carolina, USA
MED emergency doctor

Max J. Egenhofer, Center for Geographic Information and Analysis, University of Maine, Orono, ME, USA
(3, 4) <spatial informatics, spatial reasoning, geographic information systems>

Kapetanios Epaminondas, Computer Science and Software Engineering Department, University of Westminster, London, UK
(1, 2) <Knowledge engineering, ontologies, semantic computing, NLP>

Massimo Ferri, Department of Mathematics, University of Bologna, Italy
(3, 4) <computational topology, persistent homology>

Sara Johansson Fernstad, Computer Science and Digital Technologies, Northumbria University, Newcastle, UK
(6) <Visualization, Visual Analytics, Biological Visualization>

Ana Fred, Communication Theory and Pattern Recognition Group, IST – Technical University of Lisbon, Portugal
(2) <Pattern recognition, machine learning, biometrics, signal processing, biomedical applications>

Bogdan Gabrys, Smart Tech Research Centre, Computational Intelligence Group, Bournemouth University, UK
(2) <Computational intelligence, data science, complex adaptive systems, machine learning, predictive analytics>

Hugo Gamboa, PLUX Wireless Biosensors, and Universidade Nova de Lisboa, Portugal
IND (1, 2) <machine learning, signal processing, instrumentation>

Aryya Gangopadhyay, UMBC Center of Cybersecurity, University of Maryland, Baltimore County, USA
(1, 2, 7) <Health IT, data mining, privacy>

Panagiotis Germanakos, Department of Computer Science, University of Cyprus, Cyprus
(2, 6) <Computational intelligence, adaptive cognitive systems, user modeling, HCI>

Marie Gustafsson Friberger, Computer Science Department, Malmö University, Sweden
(1) <linked data, open data, semantic Web technologies, medical informatics>

Randy Goebel, Centre for Machine Learning, Department of Computer Science, University of Alberta, Edmonton, Canada
(1, 2, 6) <machine learning, data mining, NLP, data visualization, visual analytics>

Bart Goethals, Advanced Database Research and Modelling, University of Antwerp, Belgium
(1, 2) <data mining, machine learning, big data analytics, data science>

Venu Govindaraju, Department of Computer Science and Engineering, University at Buffalo, Amherst, NY, USA
(1, 2) <Machine learning, biometrics, language technologies>

Leo Grady, Heart Flow Inc., Redwood, California, USA
IND (3, 6) <graph theory, medical imaging, computer vision>

Michael Granitzer, Media Computer Science, University of Passau, Germany
(1, 6) <Information retrieval, NLP, visual analytics>

Dimitrios Gunopulos, Knowledge Discovery in Databases Lab, Department of Informatics, University of Athens, Greece
(1, 2) <Data mining, data management, big data, Web mining, sensor networks>

Siegfried Handschuh, Insight Centre for Data Analytics, NUI Galway, Ireland
(1,2) <Semantic Web, linked data, artificial intelligence, NLP>

Helwig Hauser, Visualization Group, University of Bergen, Norway
(6) <visualization>

Julian Heinrich, Biodata Visualization team, CSIRO, Australia
(6) <Visualization, parallel coordinates, bioinformatics>

Kristina Hettne, BioSemantics group, Department of Human Genetics, Leiden University Medical Center, The Netherlands
(1) <Text mining, Semantic Web, Bioinformatics, Cheminformatics>

Rainer Hofmann-Wellenhof, Division of General Dermatology, Graz University Hospital, Austria
MED – Dermato-Oncologist

Andreas Hotho, Data Mining and Information Retrieval Group, University of Würzburg, Germany
(1, 2) <Data science, data mining, information retrieval, Semantic Web mining>

Jun Luke Huan, Computational Knowledge Discovery Lab, University of Kansas, Lawrence, USA
(1, 2) <machine learning, data mining, data science, big data, bioinformatics>

Anthony Hunter, Intelligent Systems Group, Department of Computer Science, UCL University College London, UK
(1, 2) <knowledge representation, reasoning, argumentation, inconsistency>

Beatriz De La Iglesia, Knowledge Discovery and Data Mining Group, Computing Sciences, University of East Anglia, UK
(2) <artificial intelligence, data mining, optimization, business intelligence, health informatics>

Kalervo Jaervelin, School of Information Science, University of Tampere, Finland
(1) information retrieval, evaluation, interactive information retrieval

Igor Jurisica, IBM Life Sciences Discovery Centre, and Princess Margaret Cancer Centre, Toronto, Canada
IND (1, 2, 6) <machine learning, knowledge discovery, bioinformatics, visualization, cancer informatics>

Andreas Kerren, ISOVIS Group, Department of Computer Science, Linnaeus University, Växjö, Sweden
(3, 6) <graph drawing, visualization, visual analytics>

Jiri Klema, Department of Cybernetics, Faculty of Electrical Engineering, Czech Technical University, Prague, Czech Republic
(1, 2) <machine learning, data mining, bioinformatics>

Peter Kieseberg, SBA Research gGmbH – Secure Business Austria, Vienna, Austria
ESR (7) <data security, safety, privacy, IT security, forensics>

Negar Kiyavash, Department of Industrial and Enterprise Systems, University of Illinois at Urbana-Champaign, USA
(1, 2, 5) <machine learning, statistical signal processing, information theory>

Gudrun Klinker, Computer Aided Medical Procedures and Augmented Reality, Technische Universität Munich, Germany
(6) <augmented reality, virtual reality, 3D user interfaces, HCI>

Lubos Klucar, Bioinformatics Lab, Institute of Molecular Biology, Slovak Academy of Sciences, Bratislava, Slovakia
(1, 3) biological data bases, protein network science, protein function prediction bioinformatics

David Koslicki, Mathematics Department, Oregon State University, Corvallis, USA
(3, 4, 5) <mathematical biology, genomics, metagenomics, entropy, compressive sensing>

Patti Kostkova, eHealth Research Centre, Department of Computer Science, University College London, UK
(1) <digital health, semantic Web, serious games, epidemic intelligence>

Damjan Krstajic, Research Centre for Cheminformatics, Belgrade, Serbia
(2) <statistical learning, applied statistics>

Natsuhiko Kumasaka, Center for Genomic Medicine (CGM), RIKEN, Tokyo, Japan
(1, 2, 6) <Bayesian Gaussian mixture model, statistics, data visualization, graphic design>

Robert S. Laramee, Data Visualization Group, Department of Computer Science, Swansea University, UK
(6) <visualization>

Nada Lavrac, Department of Knowledge Technologies, Joszef Stefan Institute, Ljubljana, Slovenia
(1, 2) <machine learning, data mining>

Sangkyun Lee, Artificial Intelligence Unit, Dortmund University, Germany
ESR (1, 2) <machine learning, large scale numerical optimization, statistical data analysis>

Matthijs van Leeuwen, Machine Learning Group, KU Leuven, Heverlee, Belgium
(2, 6) <exploratory data mining, pattern mining, interactive data exploration>

Alexander Lex, Visualzation Design Lab, University of Utah, USA
(6) <visualization, bioinformatics>

Chunping Li, School of Software, Tsinghua University, China
(1, 2) machine learning, artificial intelligence, data mining, automated reasoning

Haibin Ling, Center for Data Analytics and Biomedical Informatics, Temple University, Philadelphia, USA
(6, 7) <computer vision, medical image analysis, privacy, HCI>

Luca Longo, Knowledge and Data Engineering Group, Trinity College Dublin, Ireland
ESR (1, 2, 6) <Knowledge representation, artificial intelligence, decision making, HCI>

Lenka Lhotska, Department of Cybernetics, Faculty of Electrical Engineering, Czech Technical University of Prague, Czech Republic
(1, 2) <artificial intelligence, biomedical engineering>

Andras Lukacs, Institute of Mathematics, Hungarian Academy of Sciences and Eoetvos University, Budapest, Hungary
(1, 3) <data mining, network science, combinatorics, graph theory>

Avi Ma'ayan, Systems Biology Center, Mount Sinai Hospital, New York, USA
(3) <network science, computational biology, bioinformatics, systems pharmacoglogy>

Ljiljana Majnaric-Trtica, Department of Family Medicine, Medical School, University of Osijek, Croatia
MED – family doctor, specialist in general/family medicine

Vincenzo Manca, Dipartimento di Informatica, University of Verona, Italy
(1, 2, 5) <Bioinformatics, computational systems biology, natural computing, discrete mathematics>

Ernestina Menasalvas, Data Mining Group, Polytechnic University of Madrid, Spain
(1, 2) <big data, predictive analytics, data mining>

Yoan Miche, Nokia Bell Labs, Helsinki, Finland
IND – (2, 7) <machine learning, Network Security, Steganography, Malware/Anomaly Detection>

Martin Middendorf, Institut für Informatik, Fakultät für Mathematik und Informatik, University of Leipzig, Germany
(1, 2, 3, 5) evolutionary algorithms, bioinformatics, combinatorial optimization

Silvia Miksch, Centre of Visual Analytics Science and Technology, Vienna University of Technology, Vienna, Austria
(6) <visualization, visual analytics, interaction methods, time, temporal reasoning>

Antonio Moreno-Ribas, Intelligent Technologies for Advanced Knowledge Acquisition, University Rovira i Virgili, Tarragona, Spain
(1, 2) <artificial intelligence, ontologies, multi-agent systems, semantics, decision making>

Katharina Morik, Fakultät Informatik, Lehrstuhl für Künstliche Intelligenz, Technische Universität Dortmund, Germany
(1, 2) <machine learning, data mining, big data, ubiquitous knowledge discovery, industry 4.0>

Abbe Mowshowitz, Department of Computer Science, The City College of New York, USA
(3, 5) <network science, graph theory, entropy>

Marian Mrozek, Computational Mathematics, Institute of Computer Science, Jagiellonian University, Krakow, Poland
(4) <computational topology, homology, topological dynamics, morse theory>

Zoran Obradovic, Data Analytics and Biomedical Informatics Center, Temple University, Philadelphia, PA, USA
(1, 2) <machine learning, artificial intelligence, data mining, bioinformatics>

Daniel E. O'leary, School of Business, University of Southern California, Los Angeles, USA
(1, 2) <artificial intelligence, knowledge management, decision support, information systems>

Patricia Ordonez-Rozo, Department of Computer Science, University of Puerto Rico Rio Piedras, San Juan, Puerto Rico
(1, 2, 6) <health informatics, machine learning, data mining, visual analytics>

Vasile Palade, School of Computing, Electronics and Mathematics, Coventry University, UK
(2) <machine learning>

Jan Paralic, Department of Cybernetics and Artificial Intelligence, Technical University of Kosice, Slovakia
(1, 2) <data mining, text mining, knowledge management, big data>

Valerio Pascucci, Scientific Computing and Imaging Institute, University of Utah, USA
(2, 4, 6) <data analysis, topological methods for image segmentation, visualization>

Gabriella Pasi, Laboratorio di Information Retrieval, Università di Milano Bicocca, Milan, Italy
(1) <information retrieval, information filtering, fuzzy logic>

Armando J. Pinho, Departamento de Electrónica, Telecomunicações e Informática, University of Aveiro, Portugal
(2, 5) <knowledge discovery, machine learning, bioinformatics, entropy>

Pavel Pilarczyk, Edelsbrunner Group, Institute of Science and Technology Austria, Klosterneuburg, Austria
(1, 4) data mining, algebraic topology, homology theory, persistent homology

Margit Pohl, Human-Computer Interaction Group, Vienna University of Technology, Vienna, Austria
(6) HCI, information visualization

Massimiliano Pontil, Centre for Computational Statistics and Machine Learning, UCL London, UK
(2, 3) <machine learning, artificial intelligence, learning theory, statistics, applied mathematics>

Raul Rabadan, Biomedical Informatics, Columbia University, New York, USA
(3, 4, 5) <network science, computational topology, entropy, biology, graph theory, evolution>

Heri Ramampiaro, Data and Information Management Group, Norwegian University of Science and Technology, Trondheim, Norway
(1) <information retrieval, text mining, data management>

Dietrich Rebholz, European Bioinformatics Institute, Cambridge and University of Zurich, Switzerland
MED (1) <semantic Web, biomedical informatics, information representation>

Chandan K. Reddy, Data Mining and Knowledge Discovery Lab, Wayne State University, USA
(2) machine learning, health informatics

Gerhard Rigoll, Lehrstuhl Mensch-Maschine Kommunikation, Technische Universität München, Germany
(1, 2, 6) machine learning, pattern recognition, usability engineering, multimodal fusion, HCI

Jianhua Ruan, Computational Biology, Department of Computer Science, University of Texas, San Antonio, USA
(1) <bioinformatics, computational biology, big data>

Lior Rokach, Department of Information Systems Engineering, Ben-Gurion University of the Negev, Beer-Sheva, Israel
(1, 2, 7) <machine learning, data science, machine learning, recommender systems, forecasting, cyber security>

Carsten Roecker, Fraunhofer IOSB-INA and Ostwestfalen-Lippe University of Applied Sciences, Germany
(6) <HCI, smart environments, smart health, ambient assisted living>

Timo Ropinski, Visual Computing Research Group, Ulm University, Germany
(6) <visusalization, volume rendering, scientific visualization, visual computing>

Giuseppe Santucci, Dipartimento di Informatica e Sistemistica, La Sapienza, University of Rome, Italy
(6) <visual analytics>

Pierangela Samarati, Dipartimento die Informatica, University of Milan, Crema, Italy
(7) <privacy, data security, secure cloud computing, trust management>

Reinhold Scherer, Graz BCI Lab, Institute of Neural Engineering, Graz University of Technology, Austria
(1) <brain-computer interfacing, statistical signal processing, rehabilitation engineering>

Michele Sebag, Laboratoire de Recherche en Informatique, CNRS, Universite Paris Sud, France
(2) <machine learning>

Paola Sebastiani, Department of Biostatistics, School of Public Health, Boston University, USA
(2) <Bayesian statistics, statistical genetics, statistical genomicspertise, biostatistics>

Christin Seifert, Media Computer Science, University of Passau, Germany
(1, 6) <visualization, visual analytics, knowledge discovery>

Christian Claus Schiller, Nuclear Medicine and Endocrinology, St Vincent's Hospital, Linz, Austria
MED – Endocrinologist

Tanja Schultz, Cognitive Systems Lab, Karlsruhe Institute of Technology, Germany
(1, 6) <speech recognition, biosignals, brain-computer interfaces, human-machine interfaces>

Bracha Shapira, Department of Information Systems Engineering, Ben-Gurion University of the Negev, Eilet, Israel
(1, 2, 7) <recommender systems, data mining, privacy, cyber security, personalization>

Yongtang Shi, Center for Combinatorics, Nankai University, China
(3, 5) <graph theory, discrete mathematics, combinatorial optimization, complex systems, mathematical chemistry>

Arno Siebes, Algorithmic Data Analysis, Artificial Intelligence, Universiteit Utrecht, The Netherlands
(1, 2) artificial intelligence, machine learning, algorithmic data analysis, biomedical data

Andrzej Skowron, Group of Mathematical Logic, Institute of Mathematics, University of Warsaw, Poland
(1, 2) <artificial intelligence, approximate reasoning, rough sets, data mining, adaptive systems>

Neil R. Smalheiser, College of Medicine, Department of Psychiatry, University of Illinois at Chicago, USA
MED (1) neuroscience, RNA biology, synaptic plasticity, pathogenesis of neuropsychiatric disorders, medical informatics

Rainer Spang, Statistical Bioinformatics Department, Institute of Functional Genomics, University of Regensburg, Germany
(1) <bioinformatics, biostatistics, tumor biology>

Jessica Staddon, Google Research and Computer Science Department NC State University, Raleigh, USA
IND (1, 2, 6, 7) <data mining, HCI, privacy, security>

Irena Spasic, Health Informatics, School of Computer Science and Informatics, Cardiff University, UK
(1, 2, 3) <ontologies, text mining, NLP, health informatics, bioinformatics>

Jerzy Stefanowski, Institute of Computing Science, Poznan University of Technology, Poland
(1, 2) <machine learning, data mining, rule induction, ensembles, data streams>

Gregor Stiglic, Stanford Center for Biomedical Informatics, Stanford School of Medicine, Stanford, USA
(1, 2) <machine learning, data mining, healthcare analytics, bioinformatics>

Marc Streit, Institute of Computer Graphics, Johannes-Kepler University Linz, Austria
(6) <visualization, visual analytics, biological data visualization>

Dimitar Trajanov, Department of Computer Science, Cyril and Methodius University, Skopje, Republic of Macedonia
(1, 2, 3) <semantic Web, health data, parallel computing, linked open data>

Catagaj Turkay, Department of Computer Science, City University London, UK
(6) <interactive visual analysis, visual analytics, biological data visualization>

A Min Tjoa, Information and Software Engineering Group, Vienna University of Technology, Austria
(1, 7) <data bases, security, semantic Web, risk analysis, personal information management>

Olof Torgersson, Applied Information Technology, Chalmers University of Technology, Gothenburg, Sweden
(6) <interaction design, medical informatics, intelligent user interfaces, declarative programming>

Shusaku Tsumoto, Department of Medical Informatics, Faculty of Medicine, Shimane University, Japan
MED (1, 2) neurology, medical informatics, risk mining, decision support, big data analytics health

Nikolaus Veit-Rubin, Department of Gynecology and Obstetrics, University Hospital Geneva, Switzerland
MED – Operative Gynecologist

Karin Verspoor, Health and Life Sciences, National Information and Communications Technology Australia, Victoria, Australia
(1, 2) <biomedical NLP, computational linguistics, text mining, bioinformatics, computational biology>

Jean-Philippe Vert, Cancer computational genomics and bioinformatics, Mines ParisTech, Paris, France
(2) <machine learning, computational biology>

Daniel Weiskopf, Visualization and Interactive Systems Institute, Universität Stuttgart, Germany
(6) <visualization, visual analytics, computer graphics>

Edgar Weippl, SBA Research – Secure Business Austria, Vienna, Austria
IND (7) <information security>

Raffael Wiemker, Philips Research Hamburg, Germany
IND (6) <medical image analysis and visualization>

Pak Chung Wong, Pacific Northwest Laboratory, Washington, USA
(1, 6) <visual analytics, data visualization, extreme scale data analytics, high performance computing>

William Bl Wong, HCI, Computing and Multimedia Department, Middlesex University London, UK
(6) <HCI, visual analytics, cognitive systems engineering>

Kai Xu, Visual Analytics, Computing and Multimedia Department, Middlesex University London, UK
(6) <HCI, information visualization, visual analytics, bioinformatics>

Jieping Ye, Center for Evolutionary Medicine and Informatics, Arizona State University, USA
(2) <machine learning, data mining, biomedical informatics>

Pinar Yildirim, Department of Computer Engineering, Okan University, Istanbul, Turkey
(2) <machine learning, medical informatics, biomedical data mining>

Martina Ziefle, e-Health Group, RWTH Aachen University, Germany
(6) <HCI, technology acceptance, smart health, user diversity>

Elena Zheleva, University of Maryland Institute for Advanced Computer Studies, College Park, USA
(1, 2, 3, 7) <machine learning, data mining, network analysis, privacy>

Ning Zhong, Knowledge Information Systems Laboratory, Maebashi Institute of Technology, Japan
(1, 2) machine learning, brain informatics, Web intelligence, intelligent information systems, big data

Xuezhong Zhou, School of Computer and Information Technology, Beijing Jiaotong University, China
(1, 2, 3) <data mining, complex networks, medical informatics>

Contents

Machine Learning for Health Informatics

Andreas Holzinger[1,2(✉)]

[1] Holzinger Group, HCI-KDD, Institute for Medical Informatics,
Statistics and Documentation, Medical University Graz, Graz, Austria
a.holzinger@hci-kdd.org
[2] Institute for Information Systems and Computer Media,
Graz University of Technology, Graz, Austria

Abstract. Machine Learning (ML) studies algorithms which can learn from data to gain knowledge from experience and to make decisions and predictions. Health Informatics (HI) studies the effective use of probabilistic information for decision making. The combination of both has greatest potential to rise quality, efficacy and efficiency of treatment and care. Health systems worldwide are confronted with "big data" in high dimensions, where the inclusion of a human is impossible and automatic ML (aML) show impressive results. However, sometimes we are confronted with complex data, "little data", or rare events, where aML-approaches suffer of insufficient training samples. Here interactive ML (iML) may be of help, particularly with a *doctor-in-the-loop*, e.g. in subspace clustering, k-Anonymization, protein folding and protein design. However, successful application of ML for HI needs an *integrated* approach, fostering a concerted effort of four areas: (1) data science, (2) algorithms (with focus on networks and topology (structure), and entropy (time), (3) data visualization, and last but not least (4) privacy, data protection, safety & security.

Keywords: Machine learning · Health informatics

1 Introduction and Motivation

Since the early days of Machine Learning (ML) in the 1950ies [1] the goal was to learn from data, to gain knowledge from experience and to make predictions. The field accelerated by the introduction of *statistical learning theory* in the late 1960ies; although it was at that time a purely theoretical analysis of the problem of *function estimation* from a given collection of data [2]. With the introduction of new statistical learning algorithms (e.g. support vector machine [3]) statistical learning theory became more and more interesting as a tool for developing algorithms of practical use for the estimation of multidimensional functions [4].

Today, ML is the most growing subfield in computer science and Health Informatics (HI) is the greatest application challenge [5,6]. This is not surprising, because in the health domain we are confronted with probabilistic, uncertain,

© Springer International Publishing AG 2016
A. Holzinger (Ed.): ML for Health Informatics, LNAI 9605, pp. 1–24, 2016.
DOI: 10.1007/978-3-319-50478-0_1

unknown, incomplete, heterogenous, noisy, dirty, unwanted and missing data sets which endangers the modelling of artifacts. Moreover, in the biomedical world we are confronted with a further problem: time. Whilst most computational approaches assume homogeneity in time, people and processes in the health domain are not homogenous in time and cannot be forecasted, sometimes it can happen the completely unexpected. That makes automatic solutions in this domain difficult, yet sometimes impossible.

A grand challenge in HI is to discover relevant *structural* patterns and/or *temporal* patterns ("knowledge") in such data, which are often hidden and not accessible to the human expert but would be urgently needed for better decision support. Another problem is that most of the data sets in HI are weakly-structured and non-standardized [7], and most data is in dimensions much higher than 3, and despite human experts are excellent at pattern recognition in dimensions of ≤ 3, high dimensional data sets make manual analysis difficult, yet often impossible.

The adoption of data-intensive methods can be found throughout various branches of health, leading e.g. to more evidence-based decision-making and to help to go towards personalized medicine [8]: A grand goal of future biomedicine is to tailor decisions, practices and therapies to the individual patient. Whilst personalized medicine is the ultimate goal, stratified medicine has been the current approach, which aims to select the best therapy for groups of patients who share common biological characteristics. Here, ML approaches are indispensable, for example *causal inference trees (CIT)* and aggregated grouping, seeking strategies for deploying such stratified approaches. Deeper insight of personalized treatment can be gained by studying the personal treatment effects with *ensemble CITs* [9]. Here the increasing amount of heterogenous data sets, in particular "-omics" data, for example from genomics, proteomics, metabolomics, etc. [10] make traditional data analysis problematic and optimization of knowledge discovery tools imperative [11,12]. On the other hand, many large data sets are indeed large collections of small data sets. This is particularly the case in personalized medicine where there might be a large amount of data, but there is still a relatively small amount of data for each patient available [13]. Consequently, in order to customize predictions for each individual it is necessary to build a model for each patient along with the inherent uncertainties, and to couple these models together in a hierarchy so that information can be "borrowed" from other similar patients. This is called *model personalization*, and is naturally implemented by using hierarchical Bayesian approaches including e.g. hierarchical Dirichlet processes [14] or Bayesian multi-task learning [15].

This variety of problems in the application of ML for HI requires a synergistic combination of various methodological approaches which are combined in the HCI-KDD approach, which is described in Sect. 3. In Sect. 4 an example curriculum is briefly discussed and Sect. 5 provides an outlook to three future challenges.

2   Glossary and Key Terms

automatic Machine Learning (aML) in bringing the human-out-of-the-loop is the grand goal of ML and works well in many cases with "big data" [16].

Big Data is a buzz word to indicate the flood of data today; however, large data sets are necessary for aML approaches to learn effectively, the problem is rather in "dirty data" and sometimes we have large collections of "little data".

Cognitive Science mainly deals with questions of human intelligence, problem solving and decision making and is manifested to a large extent in the field of Human–Computer Interaction (HCI) [17].

Computer Science today has a large focus on machine learning algorithms and these are manifested to a large part in the field of Knowledge Discovery/Data Mining (KDD). *Deep Learning* allows models consisting of multiple layers to learn representations of data with multiple levels of abstraction, e.g. in speech recognition, visual object recognition, object detection, genomics etc. [6].

Dimensionality of data is high, when the number of features p is larger than the number of observations n by magnitudes. A good example for high dimensional data is gene expression study data [18].

Entropy quantifies the expected value of information contained in data and can be used as a measure of uncertainty, hence it is of tremendous importance for HI with many applications to discover e.g. anomalies in data [19].

Health has been defined by the World Health Organization (WHO) in 1946 as *"a state of complete physical, mental, and social well-being"* and is undeniably one of the most important aspects concerning every human [20].

Health Informatics is concerned with the use of computational intelligence for the management of processes relevant for human health and well-being, ranging from the collective to the individual [21].

interactive Machine Learning (iML) in bringing the human-in-the-loop is necessary if we have small amounts of data ("little data"), rare events or deal with complex problems [22,23].

Knowledge Discovery (KDD) includes exploratory analysis and modeling of data and the organized process to identify valid, novel, useful and understandable patterns from these data sets [24].

Topological Data Mining uses algebraic geometry to recover parameters of mixtures of high-dimensional Gaussian distributions [25].

Visualization can be defined as transforming the symbolic into the geometric and the graphical presentation of information, with the goal of providing the viewer with a qualitative understanding of the information contents [12,26].

3   The HCI-KDD Approach

The original idea of the HCI-KDD approach [8,27,28] is in combining aspects of the best of two worlds: Human–Computer Interaction (HCI), with emphasis on cognitive science, particularly dealing with *human intelligence*, and Knowledge Discovery/Data Mining (KDD), with emphasis on machine learning, particularly dealing with *computational intelligence* [29].

Cognitive science (CS) studies the principles of human learning from data to understand intelligence. The Motto of Demis Hassabis from Google Deepmind is *"Solve intelligence - then solve everything else"* [30]. Our natural surrounding is in $\mathbb{R}^3$ and humans are excellent in perceiving patterns out of data sets with dimensions of ≤ 3. In fact, it is amazing how humans extract so much knowledge from so little data [31] which is a perfect motivator for the concept of iML.

The problem in HI is that we are challenged with data of arbitrarily high dimensions [7,18,32]. Within such data, relevant *structural* patterns and/or *temporal* patterns ("knowledge") are hidden, difficult to extract, hence not accessible to a human. A grand challenge is to bring the results from high dimensions into the lower dimension, where the health experts are working on 2D surfaces on different devices (from tablet to large wall-displays), which can represent data only in $\mathbb{R}^2$.

Machine Learning (ML) studies the principles of computational learning from data to understand intelligence [5]. Computational learning has been of general interest for a very long time, but we are far away from solving intelligence: facts are not knowledge and descriptions are not insight. A good example is the famous book by Nobel prize winner Eric Kandel *"Principles of Neural Science"* [33] which doubled in volume every decade - effectively, our goal should be to make this book shorter!

HCI and KDD did not harmonize in the past. HCI had its focus on specific experimental paradigms, embedded deeply in Cognitive *Science*; and aimed to be cognitively/neutrally plausible. KDD had its focus on computational learning problems and tried to optimize in the range of 1% because it was embedded in Computer *Engineering*, and aimed to have working systems to solve practical problems - whether mimicking the human brain or not.

Consequently, a concerted effort of both worlds and a comprehensive understanding of the data ecosystem along with a multi-disciplinary skill-set, encompassing seven specializations: (1) data science, (2) algorithms, (3) network science, (4) graphs/topology, (5) time/entropy, (6) data visualization and visual analytics, and (7) privacy, data protection, safety and security can be highly beneficial for solving the aforementioned problems (Fig.1).

3.1   Research Track 1 DAT: Data Preprocessing, Integration, Fusion

Understanding the data ecosystem is of eminent importance in HI. Considering the context in which the data is produced, we can determine between four large data pools: (1) Biomedical research data (e.g. clinical trial data, -omics data [10]), e.g. from genomic sequencing technologies (Next Generation Sequencing,

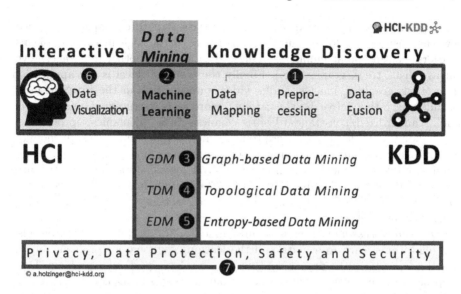

Fig. 1. The big picture of the HCI-KDD approach: The horizontal process chain (blue box) encompasses the whole machine learning pipeline from physical aspects of raw data, to human aspects of data visualization; while the vertical topics (green box) include important aspects of structure (graphs/networks), space (computational topology) and time (entropy); privacy, data protection, safety and security are mandatory topics within the health domain and provide kind of a base compartment (Color figure online) (Image taken from hci-kdd.org)

NGS etc.), microarrays, transcriptomic technologies, proteomic and metabolomic technologies, etc., which all plays important roles for biomarker discovery and drug design [34,35]. (2) Clinical data (e.g. patient records, clinicians documentations, medical terminologies (e.g. ICD, SNOMED-CT), medical surveys, laboratory tests, clinical and physiological parameters, ECG, EEG etc.), (3) Health business data (e.g. costs, utilization, management data, logistics, accounting, billing, resource planning, prediction etc.), and (4) private patient data, produced by various customers and stakeholders outside the clinical context (e.g., wellness data, Ambient Assisted Living data, sport data, insurance data, etc.) [36]. The US Department of Health and Human Services (HHS) created a taxonomy of health data with the following dimensions [37]: (1) Demographics and socio-economic Data: age, race, sex, education, etc. (2) Health Status Data: Health status of the patient, e.g., morbidities, problems, complaints, disabilities, diagnoses, symptoms, etc. (3) Health Resources Data: Characteristics and capacity of the health system, etc. (4) Healthcare Utilization Data: Characteristics(e.g., time, duration, tests, procedures, treatment) about medical care visits like discharge, stay, use of healthcare services, etc. (5) Healthcare Financing and Expenditure Data: Costs, charges, insurance status, etc. (6) Healthcare Outcomes of current and past prevention, treatments, etc. (7) Other data: -omics data, environmental exposures, etc.

Technically, there exist various levels of data structures [38] from physical level as basic indissoluble unit (bit, Shannon) to the logical level (Booleans, integers, floating-point numbers, strings, etc.) and conceptual (abstract) Level (arrays, lists, trees, graphs, etc.). Finally the technical level is the application data (text, graphics, images, audio, video, multimedia) an the Hospital Level includes narrative ("free text") patient record data (structured/unstructured and standardized/non-standardized), -omics data (genomics, proteomics, metabolomics, lipidomics, transcriptomics, microbiomics, fluxomics, phenomics, cytomics, connectomics, environomics, exposomics, exonomics, foodomics, toponomics, etc.), numerical measurements (physiological data, lab results, vital signs, etc.), recorded signals (ECG, EEG, EOG, etc.), Images (standard X-ray, MR, CT, PET, SPECT, microscopy, confocal laserscans, ultrasound imaging, molecular imaging, etc.)

Data preprocessing is often a required first step for machine learning because ML algorithms learn from data and the learning outcome for problem solving heavily depends on the proper data needed to solve a particular problem. Data preprocessing, however, inflicts a heavy danger, e.g. during the preprocessing data can be inadvertently modified, e.g. "interesting" data may be removed. Consequently, for discovery purposes it would be wise to have a look at the original raw data first.

Data integration is a hot topic generally and in health informatics specifically and solutions can bridge the gap between clinical and biomedical research [39]. This is becoming even more important due to the increasing amounts of heterogeneous, complex patient related data sets, resulting from various sources including picture archiving and communication systems (PACS) and radiological information systems (RIS), hospital information systems (HIS), laboratory information systems (LIS), physiological and clinical data repositories, and all sorts of -omics data from laboratories, using samples from Biobanks. The latter include large collections of DNA sequence data, proteomic and metabolic data; resulting from sophisticated high-throughput analytical technologies. Along with classical patient records, containing large amounts of unstructured and semi-structured information, integration efforts incorporate enormous problems, but at the same time offers new possibilities for translational research. However, before starting any data integration or machine learning task, it is necessary to get a deep understanding of the underlying physics of the available data. In this paper we provide an overview about the modern data landscape in a clinical and biomedical research domain, with a focus on typical clinical/biomedical research, imaging and -omics data-sources, and the structure, quality and size of the produced patient related health information.

Whilst data integration is on combining data from different sources and providing users with a unified view on these data (e.g. combining research results from different bioinformatics repositories), *data fusion* is matching various data sets which represent one and the same object into a single, consistent, and clean representation [40]; in health informatics these unified views are particularly important in high-dimensions, e.g. for integrating heterogeneous descriptions of the same set of genes [41]. The main expectation is that fused data is more informative than the original inputs.

Capturing all information describing a biological system is the implicit objective of all -omics methods, however, genomics, transcriptomics, proteomics, metabolomics, etc. need to be combined to approach this goal: valuable information can be obtained using various analytical techniques such as nuclear magnetic resonance, liquid chromatography, or gas chromatography coupled to mass spectrometry. Each method has inherent advantages and disadvantages, but are complementary in terms of biological information, consequently combining multiple data sets, provided by different analytical platforms is of utmost importance. For each platform, the relevant information is extracted in the first step. The obtained latent variables are then fused and further analyzed. The influence of the original variables is then calculated back and interpreted. There is plenty of open future research to include all possible sources of information [42].

3.2 Research Track 2 ML: Machine Learning Algorithms

There are uncountable future challenges in the design, development, experimentation and evaluation of ML algorithms generally and in the application to health informatics specifically. The ultimate goal ever since is to develop algorithms which can *automatically* learn from data, hence can improve with experience over time *without any human-in-the-loop*. Most colleagues from the ML community are concentrating on automatic Machine Learning (aML), with the grand goal of excluding humans, hence to make it fully automatic and best practice real-world examples can be found in speech processing [43], recommender systems [44], or autonomous vehicles [45], just to mention a few.

However, the application of such aML approaches in the complex health domain seems elusive in the near future and a good example are Gaussian processes, where aML approaches (e.g. standard kernel machines) struggle on function extrapolation problems which are trivial for human learners. Consequently, *interactive ML-approaches,* by integrating a *human-into-the-loop* (e.g. a human kernel [46]), thereby making use of human cognitive abilities, is a promising approach for solving problems in the complex health domain. iML can be defined as algorithms that can interact with *both computational agents and human agents* and can optimize their learning behaviour through these interactions [22]. In Active Learning such agents are referred to as oracles [47].

iML-approaches can be of particular interest to solve problems, where we are lacking big data sets, deal with complex data and/or rare events, where traditional learning algorithms suffer due to insufficient training samples. Here the doctor-in-the-loop can help, where human expertise and long-term experience can assist in solving problems which otherwise would remain NP-hard; examples include subspace clustering [48], protein folding [49], or privacy preserving ML, which is an important issue, fostered by anonymization, in which a record is released only if it is indistinguishable from k other entities in the data, but where k-anonymity is highly dependent on spatial locality in order to effectively implement the technique in a statistically robust way. In high dimensionalities data becomes sparse, hence the concept of spatial locality is not easy to define. Consequently, it becomes difficult to anonymize the data without an unacceptably high amount of information loss [50] - here iML could be of help.

Despite these apparent findings, so far there is little quantitative evidence on effectiveness and efficiency of iML-algorithms. Moreover, there is practically no evidence, how such interaction may really optimize such algorithms. Even though such "natural" intelligent agents are present in large numbers on our world and are studied by cognitive scientists for quite a while [51]. One possible explanation for the dominance of aML-approaches could be, that these are much better to evaluate and therefore are more rapidly publishable. In iML approaches methodically correct evaluations are not only much more difficult and time-consuming, but also very difficult or even impossible to replicate, due to the fact that human agents are subjective, individual and therefore can not be copied - in contrast to data, algorithms and computational agents. Robustness of iML is an open question.

3.3   Research Track 3 GDM Graph-Based Data Mining

Graph-Theory [52] provides powerful tools to map data structures and to find novel connections between single data objects [53,54]. The inferred graphs can be further analyzed by using graph-theoretical, statistical and machine learning techniques [55]. A mapping of already existing and in medical practice approved *knowledge spaces* as a conceptual graph (as e.g. demonstrated in [56]) and a subsequent visual and graph-theoretical analysis can bring novel insights on hidden patterns in the data, which exactly is the goal of knowledge discovery. Another benefit of a graph-based data structure is in the applicability of methods from network topology and network analysis and data mining, e.g. small-world phenomenon [57,58], and cluster analysis [59,60]. However, the first question is "How to get a graph?", or simpler "How to get point sets?", because point cloud data sets (PCD) are used as primitives for such approaches. The answer to this question is not trivial (see [61]), apart from "naturally available" point clouds, e.g. from laser scanners, protein structures [62], or text mapped into a set of points (vectors) in $\mathbb{R}^n$. Sticking on the last example, graphs are intuitively more informative as example words/phrase representations [63], and graphs are the best studied data structures in computer science, with a strong relation to logical languages [64]. The beginning of graph-based data mining approaches was two decades ago, some pioneering work include [65–67]. According to [64] there are five theoretical bases of graph-based data mining approaches such as (1) subgraph categories, (2) subgraph isomorphism, (3) graph invariants, (4) mining measures and (5) solution methods. Furthermore, there are five groups of different graph-theoretical approaches for data mining such as (1) greedy search based approach, (2) inductive logic programming based approach, (3) inductive database based approach, (4) mathematical graph theory based approach and (5) kernel function based approach [68]. However, the main disadvantage of graph-theoretical text mining is the computational complexity of the graph representation, consequently the goal of future research in the field of graph-theoretical approaches for text mining is to develop efficient graph mining algorithms which implement effective search strategies and data structures [63].

In [69] a graph-theoretical approach for text mining is used to extract relation information between terms in "free-text" electronic health care records that are semantically or syntactically related. Another field of application is the text analysis of web and social media for detecting influenza-like illnesses [70].

Moreover there can be content-rich relationship networks among biological concepts, genes, proteins and drugs developed with topological text data mining like shown in [71]. According to [72] network medicine describes the clinical application field of topological text mining due to addressing the complexity of human diseases with molecular and phenotypic network maps.

3.4   Research Track 4 TDM Topological Data Mining

Closely related to graph-based methods are topological data mining methods; for both we need point cloud data sets - or at least distances - as input. A set of such primitives forms a space, and if we have finite sets equipped with proximity or similarity measure functions $sim_q \colon S^{q+1} \to [0, 1]$, which measure how "close" or "similar" $(q + 1)$-tuples of elements of S are, we speak about a *topological space*. A value of 0 means totally different objects, while 1 corresponds to equivalent items. Interesting are manifolds, which can be seen as a topological space, which is locally homeomorphic (that means it has a continuous function with an inverse function) to a real n-dimensional space. In other words: X is a d-manifold if every point of X has a neighborhood homeomorphic to $\mathbb{B}^d$; with boundary if every point has a neighborhood homeomorphic to $\mathbb{B}$ or $\mathbb{B}^d_+$ [73].

A topological space may be viewed as an abstraction of a metric space, and similarly, manifolds generalize the connectivity of d-dimensional Euclidean spaces $\mathbb{B}^d$ by being locally similar, but globally different. A d-dimensional chart at $p \in X$ is a homeomorphism $\phi : U \to \mathbb{R}^d$ onto an open subset of $\mathbb{R}^d$, where U is a neighborhood of p and open is defined using the metric. A d-dimensional manifold (d-manifold) is a topological space X with a d-dimensional chart at every point $x \in X$ [74].

For us also interesting are simplicial complexes ("simplicials") which are spaces described in a very particular way, the basis is in Homology. The reason is that it is not possible to represent surfaces precisely in a computer system due to limited computational storage; thus, surfaces are sampled and represented with triangulations. Such a triangulation is called a simplicial complex, and is a combinatorial space that can represent a space. With such simplicial complexes, the topology of a space from its geometry can be separated. Zomorodian [74] compares it with the separation of syntax and semantics in logic.

The two most popular techniques are *homology* and *persistence*. The connectivity of a space is determined by its cycles of different dimensions. These cycles are organized into groups, called homology groups. Given a reasonably explicit description of a space, the homology groups can be computed with linear algebra. Homology groups have a relatively strong discriminative power and a clear meaning, while having low computational cost. In the study of persistent homology the invariants are in the form of persistence diagrams or barcodes [75]. For us it is important to extract significant features, and thus these methods are useful, since they provide robust and general feature definitions with emphasis on global information, e.g. Alpha Shapes [76]. A recent example for topological data mining is given by [77]: Topological text mining, which builds on the well-known vector space model, which is a standard approach in text mining [78]: a collection of text documents (corpus) is mapped into points (=vectors) in $\mathbb{R}^n$. Moreover, each word can be mapped into so-called term vectors, resulting in a very high dimensional vector space. If there are n words extracted from all the documents then each document is mapped to a point (*term vector*) in $\mathbb{R}^n$ with coordinates corresponding to the weights. This way the whole corpus can be transformed into a point cloud data set. Instead of the Euclidean metric the use of a similarity (proximity) measure is sometimes more convenient; the *cosine similarity measure* is a typical example: the cosine of the angle between two vectors (points in the cloud) reflects how "similar" the underlying weighted combinations of keywords are. Amongst the many different text mining methods (for a recent overview refer to [79]); topological approaches are promising, but need a lot of further research. One of the main tasks of applied topology is to find and analyse higher dimensional topological structures in lower dimensional spaces (e.g. point cloud from vector space model as discussed in [80]). A common way to describe topological spaces is to first create simplicial complexes, because a simplicial complex structure on a topological space is an expression of the space as a union of simplices such as points, intervals, triangles, and higher dimensional analogues. Simplicial complexes provide an easy combinatorial way to define certain topological spaces [81]. A simplical complex K is defined as a finite collection of simplices such that $\sigma \in K$ and τ, which is a face of σ, implies $\tau \in K$, and $\sigma, \sigma' \in K$ implies $\sigma \cap \sigma'$ can either be a face of both σ and σ' or empty [82]. One way to create a simplical complex is to examine all subsets of points, and if any subsets of points are close enough, a p-simplex (e.g. line) is added to the complex with those points as vertices. For instance, a Vietoris-Rips complex of diameter ϵ is defined as $VR(\epsilon) = \sigma|diam(\sigma) \leq \epsilon$, where $diam(\epsilon)$ is defined as the largest distance between two points in σ [82]. A common way a analyse the topological structure is to use persistent homology, which identifies cluster, holes and voids therein. It is assumed that more robust topological structures are the one which persist with increasing ϵ. For detailed information about persistent homology, see [82–84].

3.5   Research Track 5 EDM Entropy-Based Data Mining

Information Entropy can be used as a measure of *uncertainty in data*. To date, there have emerged many different types of entropy methods with a large number of different purposes and applications; here we mention only a few: *Graph Entropy* was described by [85] to measure structural information content of graphs, and a different definition, more focused on problems in information and coding theory, was introduced by Körner in [86]. Graph entropy is often used for the characterization of the structure of graph-based systems, e.g. in mathematical biochemistry, but also for any complex network [87]. In these applications the entropy of a graph is interpreted as its structural information content and serves as a complexity measure, and such a measure is associated with an equivalence relation defined on a finite graph; by application of Shannons Eq. 2.4 in [88] with the probability distribution we get a numerical value that serves as an index of the structural feature captured by the equivalence relation.

Topological Entropy (TopEn), was introduced by [89] with the purpose to introduce the notion of entropy as an invariant for continuous mappings: Let (X, T) be a topological dynamical system, i.e., let X be a nonempty compact Hausdorff space and $T : X \rightarrow X$ a continuous map; the TopEn is a nonnegative number which measures the complexity of the system [90].

Hornero et al. [91] performed a complexity analysis of intracranial pressure dynamics during periods of severe intracranial hypertension. For that purpose they analyzed eleven episodes of intracranial hypertension from seven patients. They measured the changes in the intracranial pressure complexity by applying ApEn, as patients progressed from a state of normal intracranial pressure to intracranial hypertension, and found that a decreased complexity of intracranial pressure coincides with periods of intracranial hypertension in brain injury. Their approach is of particular interest to us, because they proposed classification based on ApEn tendencies instead of absolute values.

Pincus et al. took in [92] heart rate recordings of 45 healthy infants with recordings of an infant one week after an aborted sudden infant death syndrom (SIDS) episode. They then calculated the ApEn of these recordings and found a significant smaller value for the aborted SIDS infant compared to the healthy ones.

3.6   Research Track 6 DAV Data Visualization

Visualization is a very important method of transforming the symbolic into the geometric, offers opportunities for discovering knowledge in data and fosters insight into data [26]. There are endless examples for the importance of visualization in health, e.g. Otasek et al. [12] present a work on Visual Data Mining (VDM), which is supported by interactive and scalable network visualization and analysis. Otasek et al. emphasize that knowledge discovery within complex data sets involves many workflows, including accurately representing many formats of source data, merging heterogeneous and distributed data sources, complex database searching, integrating results from multiple computational and mathematical analyses, and effectively visualizing properties and results. Mueller et al. [93] demonstrate the successful application of data Glyphs in a disease analyser for the analysis of big medical data sets with automatic validation of the data mapping, selection of subgroups within histograms and a visual comparison of the value distributions. A good example for the catenation of visualization with ML is clustering: Clustering is a descriptive task to identify homogeneous groups of data objects based on the dimensions (i.e. values of the attributes). Clustering methods are often subject to other systems, for example to reduce the possibilities of recommender systems (e.g. Tag-recommender on Youtube videos [94]); for example clustering of large high-dimensional gene expression data sets has widespread application in -omics [95]. Unfortunately, the underlying structure of these natural data sets is often fuzzy, and the computational identification of data clusters generally requires (human) expert knowledge about cluster number and geometry. The high-dimensionality of data is a huge problem in health informatics general and in ML in particular, and the curse of dimensionality is a critical factor for clustering: With increasing dimensionality the volume of the space increases so fast that the available data becomes sparse, hence it becomes impossible to find reliable clusters; also the concept of distance becomes less precise as the number of dimensions grows, since the distance between any two points in a given data set converges; moreover, different clusters might be found in different sub spaces, so a global filtering of attributes is also not sufficient. Given that large number of attributes, it is likely that some attributes are correlated, therefore clusters might exist in arbitrarily oriented affinity sub spaces. Moreover, high-dimensional data likely includes *irrelevant* features, which may obscure to find the relevant ones, thus increases the danger of modeling artifacts. The problem is that we are confronted with subjective similarity functions; the most simplest example is the grouping of cars in a showroom: a technician will most likely group the cars differently than a mother of three kids (cylinder capacity versus storage capacity). This subspace clustering problem is hard, because for the grouping very different characteristics can be used: highly subjective and context specific. What is recognized as comfort for end-users of individual systems, can be applied in scientific research for the interactive exploration of high-dimensional data sets [96]. Consequently, iML-approaches can be beneficial to support finding solutions in hard biomedical problems [48]. Actually, humans are quite good in comparison for the determination of similarities and dissimilarities - described by nonlinear multidimensional scaling (MDS) models [97]. MDS models represent similarity relations between entities as a geometric model that consists of a set of points within a metric space. The output of an MDS routine is a geometric model of the data, with each object of the data set represented as a point in n-dimensional space.

3.7   Research Track 7 DAP Privacy

Privacy aware machine learning and privacy preserving machine learning is an important issue [98,99], fostered by anonymization concepts, in which a record is released only if it is indistinguishable from k other entities in the data. k-anonymity is highly dependent on spatial locality in order to effectively implement the technique in a statistically robust way and in high dimensions data becomes sparse, hence the concept of spatial locality is not easy to define. Consequently, it becomes difficult to anonymize the data without an unacceptably high amount of information loss [50]. Consequently, the problem of k-Anonymization is on the one hand NP-hard, on the other hand the quality of the result obtained can be measured at the given factors (k-Anonymity, l-diversity, t-closeness, delta-presence), but not with regard to the actual security of the data, i.e. the re-identification through an attacker. For this purpose certain assumptions about the background knowledge of the hypothetical enemy must be made. With regard to the particular demographic and cultural clinical environment this is best done by a human agent. Thus, the problem of (k-)Anonymization represents a natural application domain for iML.

4   Example Curriculum

Most universities offer excellent courses on machine learning, neural networks, data mining, and visualization, so a course on ML for HI should be complementary and follow a research-based teaching (RBT) style, showing the students state-of-the-art science and engineering example from biomedicine and the life sciences for discussing the underlying concepts, theories, paradigms, models, methods and tools on practical cases and examples (Fig. 2). For practical reasons the exercises can be done with Python [100], which is to date still the

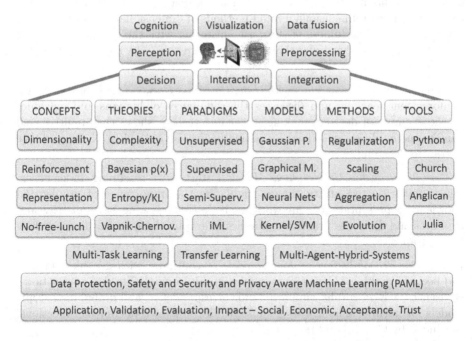

Fig. 2. The top level view of the contents of the Machine Learning for Health Informatics course at Vienna University of Technology, developed by A. Holzinger. Besides from focusing on practical examples from biology, biomedicine, clinical medicine and healthcare, issues including privacy, safety, security, data protection, validation, evaluation, social and economic impact, acceptance and trust are important parts of this course

most used ML-tool worldwide, and probabilistic programming [101] should be fostered (with at least a short touch on, e.g., Anglican, Church, or PyMC). The course 183.A83 at Vienna University of Technology (http://hci-kdd.org/machine-learning-for-health-informatics-course/) is consisting of twelve lectures plus practicals for a one-semester course on Master level with the following contents:

Lecture 01: Introduction and Overview of ML and HI explains the HCI-KDD approach, shows the complexity of the application area health informatics, demonstrates what aML can do and shows the limitations of aML, and the usefulness iML with a human-in-the-loop on practical examples and outlines some future challenges.

Lecture 02: Fundamentals of Data and Information discusses the underlying physics of data and biomedical data sources, taxonomy of data, data structures, data integration, data fusion, and a clinical view on data, information and knowledge; focuses then on probabilistic information, information theory, cross-entropy, mutual information and Kullback-Leibler Divergence.

Lecture 03: Dimensionality Reduction and Subspace Clustering provides an introduction into classification vs. clustering, feature spaces, feature engineering, discusses the curse of dimensionality and methods of dimensionality reduction, and demonstrates the usefulness of subspace clustering with the expert-in-the-loop; finally discusses the hard question "what is interesting?" by showing projection pursuit.

Lecture 04: Human Learning vs. Machine Learning: Decision Making starts with reinforcement learning and discusses the differences of humans and machines on the example of decision making under uncertainty, shows then multi-armed bandits and applications in health and finally gives an outlook on the importance of transfer learning.

Lecture 05: Probabilistic Graphical Models I starts with reasoning under uncertainty and expected utility theory, highlights the importance of graphs and knowledge representation in network medicine, shows some basic metrics and measures and discusses practical examples of graphical model learning and how to get graphs.

Lecture 06: Probabilistic Graphical Models II continues with graphical models and decision making, shows factor graphs, graph isomorphism and applications, Bayes nets, ML on graphs, similarity and correspondence, and probabilistic topic models for natural language to get insight into unknown document collections, concluded by Graph bandits.

Lecture 07: Evolutionary Computing for HI I poses medical decision making as search problem and shows evolutionary principles (Lamarck, Darwin, Baldwin, Mendel) and applications of evolutionary computing with the special case of genetic algorithms and k-armed bandits and genetic algorithms (global optimization problem).

Lecture 08: Evolutionary Computing for HI II continues with examples from medical applications for EA, discusses natural computing concepts and their usefulness in principle, focuses then on Ant Colony Optimization and the traveling salesman problem with motivation on protein folding, simulated annealing, and the human-in-the-loop, and finalizes with multi-agents and neuro evolution.

Lecture 09: Towards Open Data Sets: Privacy Aware Machine Learning motivates privacy, data protection safety and security and discusses anonymization methods (k-Anonymization, l-diversity, t-closeness, delta-presence, pertubative approaches, differentially private kernel learning, etc.), and how iML can help anonymization.

Lecture 10: Active Learning, Multi-Task Learning and Transfer Learning discusses the principles of active learning, preference learning, active preference learning with an excursion on PAC-learning, and programming by feedback, highlights some problems of the human-in-the-loop and continues with MTL and TL, where humans are still better than machines.

Lecture 11: Machine Learning from Text focuses on natural language understanding and the problems involved, and highlights word vectors for sentiment analysis (continous bag-of-words model, skip-gram model, global vectors for word embedding) with giving an outline on neural probabilistic language models and alternative models.

Lecture 12: Discrete Multi-Agent Systems on the topic of stochastic simulation of tumor kinetics and key problems for cancer research, tumor growth modeling, cellular potts model, tumor growth visualization and towards using open tumor growth data for machine learning in the international context [102].

5 Future Challenges

Much future research has to be done, particularly in the fields of Multi-Task Learning and Transfer Learning to go towards Multi-Agent-Hybrid Systems as applications of the iML-approach.

5.1 Future Challenge 1: Multi-task Learning

Multi-task learning (MTL) aims to improve the prediction performance by learning a problem together with multiple, different but related other problems through shared parameters or a shared representation. The underlying principle is *bias learning* based on probable approximately correct learning (PAC learning) [103]. To find such a bias is still the hardest problem in any ML task and essential for the initial choice of an appropriate hypothesis space, which must be large enough to contain a solution, and small enough to ensure a good generalization from a small number of data sets. Existing methods of bias generally require the input of a human-expert-in-the-loop in the form of heuristics and domain knowledge to ensure the selection of an appropriate set of features, as such features are key to learning and understanding. However, such methods are limited by the accuracy and reliability of the expert s knowledge (robustness of the human) and also by the extent to which that knowledge can be transferred to new tasks (see next subsection). Baxter (2000) [104] introduced a model of bias learning which builds on the PAC learning model which concludes that learning multiple related tasks reduces the sampling burden required for good generalization and bias that is learnt on sufficiently many training tasks is likely to be good for learning novel tasks drawn from the same environment (the problem of transfer learning to new environments is discussed in the next subsection). A practical example is *regularized MTL* [105], which is based on the minimization of regularization functionals similar to Support Vector Machines (SVMs), that have been successfully used in the past for singletask learning. The regularized MTL approach allows to model the relation between tasks in terms of a novel kernel function that uses a taskcoupling parameter and largely outperforms singletask learning using SVMs. However, multi-task SVMs are inherently restricted by the fact that SVMs require each class to be addressed explicitly with its own weight vector. In a multi-task setting this requires the different learning tasks to share the *same set of classes*. An alternative formulation for MTL is an extension of the large margin nearest neighbor algorithm (LMNN) [106]. Instead of relying on separating hyper-planes, its decision function is based on the nearest neighbor rule which inherently extends to many classes and becomes a natural fit for MTL. This approach outperforms state-of-the-art MTL classifiers, however, much open research challenges remain open in this area [107].

5.2 Future Challenge 2: Transfer Learning

A huge problem in ML is the phenomenon of *catastrophic forgetting*, i.e. when learned one task and transferred to another task the ML algorithm "forgets" how to perform the learned task. This is a well-known problem which affects ML-systems and was first described in the context of connectionist networks [108]; whereas natural cognitive systems rarely completely disrupt or erase previously learned information, i.e. natural cognitive systems do not forget "catastrophically" [109]. Consequently the challenge is to discover how to avoid the problem of catastrophic forgetting, which is a current hot topic [110].

According to Pan & Yang (2010) [111] a major assumption in many ML algorithms is, that both the training data and future (unknown) data must be in the same feature space and required to have the same distribution. In many real-world applications, particularly in the health domain, this is not the case: Sometimes we have a classification task in one domain of interest, but we only have sufficient training data in another domain of interest, where the latter data may be in a completely different feature space or follows a different data distribution. In such cases transfer learning would greatly improve the performance of learning by avoiding much expensive data-labeling efforts, however, much open questions remain for future research [112].

5.3   Future Challenge 3: Multi-agent-Hybrid Systems

Multi-Agent-Systems (MAS) are collections of many agents interacting with each other. They can either share a common goal (for example an ant colony, bird flock, or fish swarm etc.), or they can pursue their own interests (for example as in an open-market economy). MAS can be traditionally characterized by the facts that (a) each agent has incomplete information and/or capabilities for solving a problem, (b) agents are autonomous, so there is no global system control; (c) data is decentralized; and (d) computation is asynchronous [113]. For the health domain of particular interest is the *consensus problem*, which formed the foundation for distributed computing [114]. The roots are in the study of (human) experts in group consensus problems: Consider a group of humans who must act together as a team and each individual has a subjective probability distribution for the unknown value of some parameter; a model which describes how the group reaches agreement by pooling their individual opinions was described by DeGroot (1974) [115] and was used decades later for the aggregation of information with uncertainty obtained from multiple sensors [116] and medical experts [117]. On this basis Olfati-Saber et al. (2007) [118] presented a theoretical framework for analysis of consensus algorithms for networked multi-agent systems with fixed or dynamic topology and directed information flow. In complex real-world problems, e.g., for the epidemiological and ecological analysis of infectious diseases, standard models based on differential equations very rapidly become unmanageable due to too many parameters, and here MAS can also be very helpful [119]. Moreover, collaborative multi-agent reinforcement learning has a lot of research potential for machine learning [120].

6   Conclusion

There are uncountable future challenges in ML generally and in the application of ML to health informatics specifically. The ultimate goal is to design and develop algorithms which can *automatically* learn from data, hence can improve with experience over time *without any human-in-the-loop*. However, the application of such aML approaches in the complex health domain seems elusive in the near future and a good example are Gaussian processes, where aML approaches (e.g. standard kernel machines) struggle on function extrapolation problems which are trivial for human learners. Consequently, iML-approaches, by integrating a human-into-the-loop (e.g. a human kernel [46]), thereby making use of human cognitive abilities, seems to be a promising approach. iML-approaches can be of particular interest to solve problems in HI, where we are lacking big data sets, deal with complex data and/or rare events, where traditional learning algorithms suffer due to insufficient training samples. Here the doctor-in-the-loopcan help, where human expertise and long-term experience can assist in solving problems which otherwise would remain NP-hard. A cross-domain integration and appraisal of different fields provides an atmosphere to foster different perspectives and opinions and is an ideal think-tank and incubator to foster novel ideas and a fresh look on different methodologies to put these ideas into Business.

Acknowledgments. I am very grateful for fruitful discussions with members of the HCI-KDD network and I thank my Institutes both at Graz University of Technology and the Medical University of Graz, my colleagues and my students for the enjoyable academic freedom, the inspiring intellectual environment, and the opportunity to follow my personal motto: Science is to test crazy ideas - Engineering is to put these ideas into Business. Last but not least, I thank all students of my course LV 185.A83 (http:// hci-kdd.org/machine-learning-for-health-informatics-course), at Vienna University of Technology for their kind interest and motivating feedback.

References

1. Samuel, A.L.: Some studies in machine learning using the game of checkers. IBM J. Res. Dev. **3**, 210–229 (1959)
2. Vapnik, V.N.: An overview of statistical learning theory. IEEE Trans. Neural Netw. **10**, 988–999 (1999)
3. Boser, B.E., Guyon, I.M., Vapnik, V.N.: A training algorithm for optimal margin classifiers. In: Proceedings of the Fifth Annual Workshop on Computational Learning Theory COLT, pp. 144–152. ACM (1992)
4. Hastie, T., Tibshirani, R., Friedman, J.: The Elements of Statistical Learning: Data Mining, Inference, and Prediction, 2nd edn. Springer, New York (2009)
5. Jordan, M.I., Mitchell, T.M.: Machine learning: trends, perspectives, and prospects. Science **349**, 255–260 (2015)
6. LeCun, Y., Bengio, Y., Hinton, G.: Deep learning. Nature **521**, 436–444 (2015)
7. Holzinger, A., Dehmer, M., Jurisica, I.: Knowledge discovery and interactive data mining in bioinformatics - state-of-the-art, future challenges and research directions. BMC Bioinform. **15**, I1 (2014)
8. Holzinger, A.: Trends in interactive knowledge discovery for personalized medicine: cognitive science meets machine learning. IEEE Intell. Inform. Bull. **15**, 6–14 (2014)
9. Su, X., Kang, J., Fan, J., Levine, R.A., Yan, X.: Facilitating score and causal inference trees for large observational studies. J. Mach. Learn. Res. **13**, 2955–2994 (2012)
10. Huppertz, B., Holzinger, A.: Biobanks a source of large biological data sets: open problems and future challenges. In: Holzinger, A., Jurisica, I. (eds.) Knowledge Discovery and Data Mining. LNCS, vol. 8401, pp. 317–330. Springer, Heidelberg (2014)
11. Mattmann, C.A.: Computing: a vision for data science. Nature **493**, 473–475 (2013)
12. Otasek, D., Pastrello, C., Holzinger, A., Jurisica, I.: Visual data mining: effective exploration of the biological universe. In: Holzinger, A., Jurisica, I. (eds.) Knowledge Discovery and Data Mining. LNCS, vol. 8401, pp. 19–33. Springer, Heidelberg (2014)
13. Ghahramani, Z.: Probabilistic machine learning and artificial intelligence. Nature **521**, 452–459 (2015)
14. Teh, Y.W., Jordan, M.I., Beal, M.J., Blei, D.M.: Hierarchical Dirichlet processes. J. Am. Stat. Assoc. **101**, 1566–1581 (2006)
15. Houlsby, N., Huszar, F., Ghahramani, Z., Hernndez-lobato, J.M.: Collaborative gaussian processes for preference learning. In: Pereira, F., Burges, C., Bottou, L., Weinberger, K. (eds.) Advances in Neural Information Processing Systems (NIPS 2012), pp. 2096–2104 (2012)
16. Shahriari, B., Swersky, K., Wang, Z., Adams, R.P., de Freitas, N.: Taking the human out of the loop: a review of bayesian optimization. Proc. IEEE **104**, 148–175 (2016)

17. Clark, A.: Whatever next? Predictive brains, situated agents, and the future of cognitive science. Behav. Brain Sci. **36**, 181–204 (2013)
18. Lee, S., Holzinger, A.: Knowledge discovery from complex high dimensional data. In: Michaelis, S., Piatkowski, N., Stolpe, M. (eds.) Solving Large Scale Learning Tasks. Challenges and Algorithms. LNCS (LNAI), vol. 9580, pp. 148–167. Springer, Heidelberg (2016). doi:10.1007/978-3-319-41706-6_7
19. Mayer, C., Bachler, M., Holzinger, A., Stein, P., Wassertheurer, S.: The effect of threshold values and weighting factors on the association between entropy measures and mortality after myocardial infarction in the cardiac arrhythmia suppression trial. Entropy **18**, 1–15 (2016)
20. Jadad, A.R., OGrady, L.: How should health be defined? Br. Med. J. **337**, a2900 (2008)
21. Parry, D.: Health informatics. In: Kasabov, N. (ed.) Springer Handbook of Bio-/Neuro-informatics, pp. 555–564. Springer, Heidelberg (2014)
22. Holzinger, A.: Interactive machine learning for health informatics: when do we need the human-in-the-loop? Brain Inform. (BRIN) **3**, 119–131 (2016)
23. Holzinger, A., Plass, M., Holzinger, K., Crişan, G.C., Pintea, C.-M., Palade, V.: Towards interactive Machine Learning (iML): applying ant colony algorithms to solve the traveling salesman problem with the human-in-the-loop approach. In: Buccafurri, F., Holzinger, A., Kieseberg, P., Tjoa, A.M., Weippl, E. (eds.) CD-ARES 2016. LNCS, vol. 9817, pp. 81–95. Springer, Heidelberg (2016). doi:10.1007/978-3-319-45507-5_6
24. Fayyad, U., Piatetsky-Shapiro, G., Smyth, P.: From data mining to knowledge discovery in databases. AI Mag. **17**, 37–54 (1996)
25. Holzinger, A.: On topological data mining. In: Holzinger, A., Jurisica, I. (eds.) Knowledge Discovery and Data Mining. LNCS, vol. 8401, pp. 331–356. Springer, Heidelberg (2014)
26. Ward, M., Grinstein, G., Keim, D.: Interactive Data Visualization: Foundations, Techniques, and Applications. AK Peters Ltd., Natick (2010)
27. Holzinger, A.: On knowledge discovery and interactive intelligent visualization of biomedical data - challenges in human computer interaction & biomedical informatics. In: Helfert, M., Fancalanci, C., Filipe, J. (eds.) DATA 2012, International Conference on Data Technologies and Applications, pp. 5–16 (2012)
28. Holzinger, A.: Human-computer interaction and knowledge discovery (HCI-KDD): what is the benefit of bringing those two fields to work together? In: Cuzzocrea, A., Kittl, C., Simos, D.E., Weippl, E., Xu, L. (eds.) CD-ARES 2013. LNCS, vol. 8127, pp. 319–328. Springer, Heidelberg (2013). doi:10.1007/978-3-642-40511-2_22
29. Holzinger, A., Jurisica, I.: Knowledge discovery and data mining in biomedical informatics: the future is in integrative, interactive machine learning solutions. In: Holzinger, A., Jurisica, I. (eds.) Knowledge Discovery and Data Mining. LNCS, vol. 8401, pp. 1–18. Springer, Heidelberg (2014)
30. Mnih, V., Kavukcuoglu, K., Silver, D., Rusu, A.A., Veness, J., Bellemare, M.G., Graves, A., Riedmiller, M., Fidjeland, A.K., Ostrovski, G., Petersen, S., Beattie, C., Sadik, A., Antonoglou, I., King, H., Kumaran, D., Wierstra, D., Legg, S., Hassabis, D.: Human-level control through deep reinforcement learning. Nature **518**, 529–533 (2015)
31. Tenenbaum, J.B., Kemp, C., Griffiths, T.L., Goodman, N.D.: How to grow a mind: statistics, structure, and abstraction. Science **331**, 1279–1285 (2011)
32. Burges, C.J.: Dimension reduction: a guided tour. Found. Trends Mach. Learn. **2**, 275–365 (2010)

33. Kandel, E.R., Schwartz, J.H., Jessell, T.M., Siegelbaum, S.A., Hudspeth, A.: Principles of Neural Science, 5th edn. McGraw-Hill, New York (2012). (1760 pages)
34. McDermott, J.E., Wang, J., Mitchell, H., Webb-Robertson, B.J., Hafen, R., Ramey, J., Rodland, K.D.: Challenges in biomarker discovery: combining expert insights with statistical analysis of complex omics data. Expert Opin. Med. Diagn. **7**, 37–51 (2013)
35. Swan, A.L., Mobasheri, A., Allaway, D., Liddell, S., Bacardit, J.: Application of machine learning to proteomics data: classification and biomarker identification in postgenomics biology. Omics- J. Integr. Biol. **17**, 595–610 (2013)
36. Manyika, J., Chui, M., Brown, B., Bughin, J., Dobbs, R., Roxburgh, C., Byers, A.H.: Big Data: The Next Frontier for Innovation, Competition, and Productivity. McKinsey Report, May 2011 (available online)
37. Goolsby, A.W., Olsen, L., McGinnis, M., Grossmann, C.: Clincial data as the basic staple of health learning - creating and protecting a public good. National Institute of Health (2010)
38. Holzinger, A.: Lecture 2 fundamentals of data, information, and knowledge. In: Biomedical Informatics: Discovering Knowledge in Big Data, pp. 57–107. Springer, Cham (2014)
39. Jeanquartier, F., Jean-Quartier, C., Schreck, T., Cemernek, D., Holzinger, A.: Integrating open data on cancer in support to tumor growth analysis. In: Renda, M.E., Bursa, M., Holzinger, A., Khuri, S. (eds.) ITBAM 2016. LNCS, vol. 9832, pp. 49–66. Springer, Heidelberg (2016). doi:10.1007/978-3-319-43949-5_4
40. Bleiholder, J., Naumann, F.: Data fusion. ACM Comput. Surv. (CSUR) **41**, 1–41 (2008)
41. Lafon, S., Keller, Y., Coifman, R.R.: Data fusion and multicue data matching by diffusion maps. IEEE Trans. Pattern Anal. Mach. Intell. **28**, 1784–1797 (2006)
42. Blanchet, L., Smolinska, A.: Data fusion in metabolomics and proteomics for biomarker discovery. In: Jung, K. (ed.) Statistical Analysis in Proteomics, pp. 209–223. Springer, New York (2016)
43. Bellegarda, J.R., Monz, C.: State of the art in statistical methods for language and speech processing. Comput. Speech Lang. **35**, 163–184 (2016)
44. Ricci, F., Rokach, L., Shapira, B.: Recommender systems: introduction and challenges. In: Ricci, F., Rokach, L., Shapira, B. (eds.) Recommender Systems Handbook, pp. 1–34. Springer, New York (2015)
45. Spinrad, N.: Google car takes the test. Nature **514**, 528 (2014)
46. Wilson, A.G., Dann, C., Lucas, C.G., Xing, E.P.: The human kernel. arXiv preprint arXiv:1510.07389 (2015)
47. Settles, B.: From theories to queries: active learning in practice. In: Guyon, I., Cawley, G., Dror, G., Lemaire, V., Statnikov, A. (eds.) Active Learning and Experimental Design Workshop 2010, vol. 16, pp. 1–18. JMLR Proceedings, Sardinia (2011)
48. Hund, M., Sturm, W., Schreck, T., Ullrich, T., Keim, D., Majnaric, L., Holzinger, A.: Analysis of patient groups and immunization results based on subspace clustering. In: Guo, Y., Friston, K., Aldo, F., Hill, S., Peng, H. (eds.) BIH 2015. LNCS (LNAI), vol. 9250, pp. 358–368. Springer, Heidelberg (2015). doi:10.1007/978-3-319-23344-4_35
49. Lathrop, R.H.: The protein threading problem with sequence amino-acid interaction preferences is np-complete. Protein Eng. **7**, 1059–1068 (1994)
50. Aggarwal, C.C.: On k-anonymity and the curse of dimensionality. In: Proceedings of the 31st International Conference on Very Large Data Bases VLDB, pp. 901–909 (2005)

51. Gigerenzer, G., Gaissmaier, W.: Heuristic decision making. Annu. Rev. Psychol. **62**, 451–482 (2011)
52. Harary, F.: Structural Models. An Introduction to the Theory of Directed Graphs. Wiley, New York (1965)
53. Strogatz, S.: Exploring complex networks. Nature **410**, 268–276 (2001)
54. Dorogovtsev, S., Mendes, J.: Evolution of Networks: From Biological Nets to the Internet and WWW. Oxford University Press, New York (2003)
55. Dehmer, M., Emmert-Streib, F., Pickl, S., Holzinger, A. (eds.): Big Data of Complex Networks. CRC Press Taylor & Francis Group, Boca Raton, London, New York (2016)
56. Holzinger, A., Ofner, B., Dehmer, M.: Multi-touch graph-based interaction for knowledge discovery on mobile devices: state-of-the-art and future challenges. In: Holzinger, A., Jurisica, I. (eds.) Knowledge Discovery and Data Mining. LNCS, vol. 8401, pp. 241–254. Springer, Heidelberg (2014)
57. Barabasi, A.L., Albert, R.: Emergence of scaling in random networks. Science **286**, 509–512 (1999)
58. Kleinberg, J.: Navigation in a small world. Nature **406**, 845 (2000)
59. Koontz, W., Narendra, P., Fukunaga, K.: A graph-theoretic approach to nonparametric cluster analysis. IEEE Trans. Comput. **100**, 936–944 (1976)
60. Wittkop, T., Emig, D., Truss, A., Albrecht, M., Boecker, S., Baumbach, J.: Comprehensive cluster analysis with transitivity clustering. Nat. Protoc. **6**, 285–295 (2011)
61. Holzinger, A., Malle, B., Bloice, M., Wiltgen, M., Ferri, M., Stanganelli, I., Hofmann-Wellenhof, R.: On the generation of point cloud data sets: the first step in the knowledge discovery process. In: Holzinger, A., Jurisica, I. (eds.) Knowledge Discovery and Data Mining. LNCS, vol. 8401, pp. 57–80. Springer, Heidelberg (2014)
62. Canutescu, A.A., Shelenkov, A.A., Dunbrack, R.L.: A graph-theory algorithm for rapid protein side-chain prediction. Protein Sci. **12**, 2001–2014 (2003)
63. Jiang, C., Coenen, F., Sanderson, R., Zito, M.: Text classification using graph mining-based feature extraction. Knowl. Based Syst. **23**, 302–308 (2010)
64. Washio, T., Motoda, H.: State of the art of graph-based data mining. ACM SIGKDD Explor. Newsl. **5**, 59 (2003)
65. Cook, D.J., Holder, L.B.: Substructure discovery using minimum description length and background knowledge. J. Artif. Int. Res. **1**, 231–255 (1994)
66. Yoshida, K., Motoda, H., Indurkhya, N.: Graph-based induction as a unified learning framework. Appl. Intell. **4**, 297–316 (1994)
67. Dehaspe, L., Toivonen, H.: Discovery of frequent DATALOG patterns. Data Min. Knowl. Discov. **3**, 7–36 (1999)
68. Windridge, D., Bober, M.: A kernel-based framework for medical big-data analytics. In: Holzinger, A., Jurisica, I. (eds.) Knowledge Discovery and Data Mining. LNCS, vol. 8401, pp. 196–207. Springer, Heidelberg (2014)
69. Zhou, X., Han, H., Chankai, I., Prestrud, A., Brooks, A.: Approaches to text mining for clinical medical records. In: Proceedings of the 2006 ACM Symposium on Applied Computing - SAC 2006, New York, USA, p. 235. ACM, New York (2006)
70. Corley, C.D., Cook, D.J., Mikler, A.R., Singh, K.P.: Text and structural data mining of influenza mentions in Web and social media. Int. J. Environ. Res. Public Health **7**, 596–615 (2010)
71. Chen, H., Sharp, B.M.: Content-rich biological network constructed by mining PubMed abstracts. BMC Bioinform. **5**, 147 (2004)

72. Barabási, A., Gulbahce, N., Loscalzo, J.: Network medicine: a network-based approach to human disease. Nat. Rev. Genet. **12**, 56–68 (2011)
73. Cannon, J.W.: The recognition problem: what is a topological manifold? Bull. Am. Math. Soc. **84**, 832–866 (1978)
74. Zomorodian, A.: Computational topology. In: Atallah, M., Blanton, M. (eds.) Algorithms and Theory of Computation Handbook. Applied Algorithms and Data Structures Series, vol. 2, 2nd edn, pp. 1–31. Chapman and Hall/CRC, Boca Raton (2010). doi:10.1201/9781584888215-c3
75. Epstein, C., Carlsson, G., Edelsbrunner, H.: Topological data analysis. Inverse Prob. **27**, 120–201 (2011)
76. Edelsbrunner, H., Mucke, E.P.: 3-dimensional alpha-shapes. ACM Trans. Graph. **13**, 43–72 (1994)
77. Wagner, H., Dlotko, P.: Towards topological analysis of high-dimensional feature spaces. Comput. Vis. Image Underst. **121**, 21–26 (2014)
78. Kobayashi, M., Aono, M.: Vector space models for search and cluster mining. In: Berry, M.W. (ed.) Survey of Text Mining: Clustering, Classification, and Retrieval, pp. 103–122. Springer, New York (2004)
79. Holzinger, A., Schantl, J., Schroettner, M., Seifert, C., Verspoor, K.: Biomedical text mining: open problems and future challenges. In: Holzinger, A., Jurisica, I. (eds.) Knowledge Discovery and Data Mining. LNCS, vol. 8401, pp. 271–300. Springer, Heidelberg (2014)
80. Wagner, H., Dłotko, P., Mrozek, M.: Computational topology in text mining. In: Ferri, M., Frosini, P., Landi, C., Cerri, A., Fabio, B. (eds.) CTIC 2012. LNCS, vol. 7309, pp. 68–78. Springer, Heidelberg (2012). doi:10.1007/978-3-642-30238-1_8
81. Carlsson, G.: Topology and data. Bull. Am. Math. Soc. **46**, 255–308 (2009)
82. Zhu, X.: Persistent homology: an introduction and a new text representation for natural language processing. In: Rossi, F. (ed.) IJCAI. IJCAI/AAAI (2013)
83. Cerri, A., Fabio, B.D., Ferri, M., Frosini, P., Landi, C.: Betti numbers in multi-dimensional persistent homology are stable functions. Math. Methods Appl. Sci. **36**, 1543–1557 (2013)
84. Bubenik, P., Kim, P.T.: A statistical approach to persistent homology. Homology Homotopy Appl. **9**, 337–362 (2007)
85. Mowshowitz, A.: Entropy and the complexity of graphs: I. An index of the relative complexity of a graph. Bull. Math. Biophys. **30**, 175–204 (1968)
86. Körner, J.: Coding of an information source having ambiguous alphabet and the entropy of graphs. In: 6th Prague Conference on Information Theory, pp. 411–425 (1973)
87. Holzinger, A., Ofner, B., Stocker, C., Calero Valdez, A., Schaar, A.K., Ziefle, M., Dehmer, M.: On graph entropy measures for knowledge discovery from publication network data. In: Cuzzocrea, A., Kittl, C., Simos, D.E., Weippl, E., Xu, L. (eds.) CD-ARES 2013. LNCS, vol. 8127, pp. 354–362. Springer, Heidelberg (2013). doi:10.1007/978-3-642-40511-2_25
88. Dehmer, M.: Information theory of networks. Symmetry **3**, 767–779 (2011)
89. Adler, R.L., Konheim, A.G., McAndrew, M.H.: Topological entropy. Trans. Am. Math. Soc. **114**, 309–319 (1965)
90. Adler, R., Downarowicz, T., Misiurewicz, M.: Topological entropy. Scholarpedia **3**, 2200 (2008)
91. Hornero, R., Aboy, M., Abasolo, D., McNames, J., Wakeland, W., Goldstein, B.: Complex analysis of intracranial hypertension using approximate entropy. Crit. Care Med. **34**, 87–95 (2006)

92. Pincus, S.M.: Approximate entropy as a measure of system complexity. Proc. Natl. Acad. Sci. **88**, 2297–2301 (1991)

93. Mueller, H., Reihs, R., Zatloukal, K., Holzinger, A.: Analysis of biomedical data with multilevel glyphs. BMC Bioinform. **15**, S5 (2014)

94. Toderici, G., Aradhye, H., Paca, M., Sbaiz, L., Yagnik, J.: Finding meaning on youtube: tag recommendation and category discovery. In: IEEE Conference on Computer Vision and Pattern Recognition (CVPR 2010), pp. 3447–3454. IEEE (2010)

95. Sturm, W., Schreck, T., Holzinger, A., Ullrich, T.: Discovering medical knowledge using visual analytics a survey on methods for systems biology and omics data. In: Bühler, K., Linsen, L., John, N.W. (eds.) Eurographics Workshop on Visual Computing for Biology and Medicine, Eurographics EG, pp. 71–81 (2015)

96. Müller, E., Assent, I., Krieger, R., Jansen, T., Seidl, T.: Morpheus: interactive exploration of subspace clustering. In: Proceedings of the 14th ACM SIGKDD International Conference on Knowledge Discovery and Data Mining KDD 2008, pp. 1089–1092. ACM (2008)

97. Shepard, R.N.: The analysis of proximities: multidimensional scaling with an unknown distance function. Psychometrika **27**, 125–140 (1962)

98. Duchi, J.C., Jordan, M.I., Wainwright, M.J.: Privacy aware learning. J. ACM (JACM) **61**, 38 (2014)

99. Malle, B., Kieseberg, P., Weippl, E., Holzinger, A.: The right to be forgotten: towards machine learning on perturbed knowledge bases. In: Buccafurri, F., Holzinger, A., Kieseberg, P., Tjoa, A.M., Weippl, E. (eds.) CD-ARES 2016. LNCS, vol. 9817, pp. 251–266. Springer, Heidelberg (2016). doi:10.1007/978-3-319-45507-5_17

100. Bloice, M.D., Holzinger, A.: A tutorial on machine learning and data science tools with python. In: Holzinger, A. (ed.) ML for Health Informatics. LNCS (LNAI), vol. 9605, pp. 435–480. Springer, Heidelberg (2016)

101. Gordon, A.D., Henzinger, T.A., Nori, A.V., Rajamani, S.K.: Probabilistic programming. In: Proceedings of the on Future of Software Engineering, pp. 167–181. ACM (2014)

102. Jeanquartier, F., Jean-Quartier, C., Kotlyar, M., Tokar, T., Hauschild, A.C., Jurisica, I., Holzinger, A.: Machine learning for in silico modeling of tumor growth. In: Holzinger, A. (ed.) ML for Health Informatics. LNCS (LNAI), vol. 9605, pp. 415–434. Springer, Heidelberg (2016)

103. Valiant, L.G.: A theory of the learnable. Commun. ACM **27**, 1134–1142 (1984)

104. Baxter, J.: A model of inductive bias learning. J. Artif. Intell. Res. **12**, 149–198 (2000)

105. Evgeniou, T., Pontil, M.: Regularized multi-task learning. In: Proceedings of the Tenth ACM SIGKDD International Conference on Knowledge Discovery and Data Mining, pp. 109–117. ACM (2004)

106. Weinberger, K.Q., Saul, L.K.: Distance metric learning for large margin nearest neighbor classification. J. Mach. Learn. Res. **10**, 207–244 (2009)

107. Parameswaran, S., Weinberger, K.Q.: Large margin multi-task metric learning. In: Lafferty, J., Williams, C., Shawe-Taylor, J., Zemel, R., Culotta, A. (eds.) Advances in Neural Information Processing Systems (NIPS 2010), vol. 23, pp. 1867–1875 (2010)

108. McCloskey, M., Cohen, N.J.: Catastrophic interference in connectionist networks: the sequential learning problem. In: Bower, G.H. (ed.) The Psychology of Learning and Motivation, vol. 24, pp. 109–164. Academic Press, San Diego (1989)

109. French, R.M.: Catastrophic forgetting in connectionist networks. Trends Cogn. Sci. **3**, 128–135 (1999)

110. Goodfellow, I.J., Mirza, M., Xiao, D., Courville, A., Bengio, Y.: An empirical investigation of catastrophic forgeting in gradient-based neural networks arXiv:1312.6211v3 (2015)

111. Pan, S.J., Yang, Q.A.: A survey on transfer learning. IEEE Trans. Knowl. Data Eng. **22**, 1345–1359 (2010)

112. Taylor, M.E., Stone, P.: Transfer learning for reinforcement learning domains: a survey. J. Mach. Learn. Res. **10**, 1633–1685 (2009)

113. Sycara, K.P.: Multiagent systems. AI Mag. **19**, 79 (1998)

114. Lynch, N.A.: Distributed Algorithms. Morgan Kaufmann, San Francisco (1996)

115. DeGroot, M.H.: Reaching a consensus. J. Am. Stat. Assoc. **69**, 118–121 (1974)

116. Benediktsson, J.A., Swain, P.H.: Consensus theoretic classification methods. IEEE Trans. Syst. Man Cybern. **22**, 688–704 (1992)

117. Weller, S.C., Mann, N.C.: Assessing rater performance without a gold standard using consensus theory. Med. Decis. Making **17**, 71–79 (1997)

118. Olfati-Saber, R., Fax, J.A., Murray, R.M.: Consensus and cooperation in networked multi-agent systems. Proc. IEEE **95**, 215–233 (2007)

119. Roche, B., Guegan, J.F., Bousquet, F.: Multi-agent systems in epidemiology: a first step for computational biology in the study of vector-borne disease transmission. BMC Bioinform. **9**, 435 (2008)

120. Kok, J.R., Vlassis, N.: Collaborative multiagent reinforcement learning by payoff propagation. J. Mach. Learn. Res. **7**, 1789–1828 (2006)

Bagging Soft Decision Trees

Olcay Taner Yıldız[1]([✉]), Ozan İrsoy[2], and Ethem Alpaydın[3]

[1] Department of Computer Engineering, Işık University, Şile, 34398 İstanbul, Turkey
olcaytaner@isikun.edu.tr
[2] Department of Computer Science, Cornell University, Ithaca, NY 14853-7501, USA
oirsoy@cs.cornell.edu
[3] Department of Computer Engineering, Boğaziçi University,
Bebek, 34730 İstanbul, Turkey
alpaydin@boun.edu.tr

Abstract. The decision tree is one of the earliest predictive models in machine learning. In the soft decision tree, based on the hierarchical mixture of experts model, internal binary nodes take soft decisions and choose both children with probabilities given by a sigmoid gating function. Hence for an input, all the paths to all the leaves are traversed and all those leaves contribute to the final decision but with different probabilities, as given by the gating values on the path. Tree induction is incremental and the tree grows when needed by replacing leaves with subtrees and the parameters of the newly-added nodes are learned using gradient-descent. We have previously shown that such soft trees generalize better than hard trees; here, we propose to bag such soft decision trees for higher accuracy. On 27 two-class classification data sets (ten of which are from the medical domain), and 26 regression data sets, we show that the bagged soft trees generalize better than single soft trees and bagged hard trees. This contribution falls in the scope of research track 2 listed in the editorial, namely, machine learning algorithms.

Keywords: Decision trees · Regression trees · Regularization · Bagging

1 Introduction

Trees are frequently used in computer science to decrease search complexity from linear to log time. In machine learning too, decision trees are frequently used and unlike other non-parametric methods such as the k-nearest neighbor where an input test pattern needs to be compared with all the training patterns, the decision tree uses a sequence of tests at internal decision nodes to quickly find the leaf corresponding to the region of interest. In classification, a leaf carries the class label and in regression, it carries a constant which is the numeric regression value [1,2].

In the canonical *hard* binary decision tree, each decision node applies a test and depending on the outcome, one of the branches is taken. This process is repeated recursively starting from the root node until a leaf node is hit at which point the class label or the numeric regression value stored at the leaf constitutes

© Springer International Publishing AG 2016
A. Holzinger (Ed.): ML for Health Informatics, LNAI 9605, pp. 25–36, 2016.
DOI: 10.1007/978-3-319-50478-0_2

the output. In the hard decision tree, therefore, a single path from the root to one of the leaves is traversed and the output is given by the value stored in that particular leaf.

There are different decision tree architectures depending on the way decision is made at a node: The most typical is the *univariate tree* where the test uses a single input attribute and compares it against a threshold value [2]. In the *multivariate linear tree*, the test defines a linear discriminant in the d-dimensional space [3,4]. In the *multivariate nonlinear tree*, the test can use a nonlinear discriminant—for example, a multilayer perceptron [5]. In the *omnivariate tree*, the test can use any of the above, chosen by a statistical model selection procedure [6].

So from a geometrical point of view, in the d-dimensional input space, each univariate split defines a boundary that is orthogonal to one of the axes; a multivariate linear split defines a hyperplane of arbitrary orientation, and a multivariate nonlinear split can define a nonlinear boundary.

In the hierarchical mixture of experts, Jordan and Jacobs [7] replace each expert with a complete system of mixture of experts in a recursive manner. Though it can also be viewed as an ensemble method, this architecture defines a soft decision tree where gating networks act as decision nodes. The soft gating function in a binary decision node chooses both children, but with probabilities (that sum up to 1). Hence, the node merges the decision of its left and right subtrees unlike a hard decision node that chooses one of them.

This implies that in a soft tree for a test input, we are traversing all the paths to all the leaves and all those leaves contribute to the final decision, but with different probabilities, as specified by the gating values on each path. In our proposed extension [8], the tree structure is not fixed but is trained incrementally one subtree at a time, where the parameters of the node and the leaf values are learned using gradient-descent.

Because the soft decision tree is multivariate and uses all input attributes in all nodes, it may have high variance on small data sets. As a variance reduction procedure, in this paper, we use bagging [9] which has been used successfully to combine hard decision trees in many applications; in our case of soft decision trees too, the use of bagging corresponds to averaging over soft trees trained with different data splits and initial parameter values in gradient-descent, and hence leads to a more robust estimate.

This paper is organized as follows: In Sect. 3, we review the soft decision tree model and its training algorithm. We discuss bagging soft decision trees in Sect. 4. We give our experimental results in Sect. 5 and conclude in Sect. 6.

Our work on extensions of decision trees falls in the scope of research track 2 of the editorial, namely machine learning algorithms.

2   Glossary and Key Terms

Bagging is an ensemble method where from a single training set, we draw multiple training sets using bootstrapping, with each of these sets we train a different model, and then combine their predictions, for example, using voting.

Bootstrapping is a resampling method where we randomly draw from a set *with replacement.*

Decision tree is a hierarchical model composed of decision nodes applied to the input and leaves that contain class labels.

Ensemble contains multiple trained models that are trained separately. In bagging, each of these models is trained on a slightly different data sets and hence may fail on slightly different cases, so accuracy can be increased by combining these multiple predictions.

Multivariate model uses all of the input attributes in making a decision whereas a univariate model uses only one of the input attributes.

Soft decision is different from a hard decision in that if there are m outcomes, in a hard decision we choose one of the m and ignore the remaining $m - 1$; in a soft decision, we choose all m but with different probabilities–these probabilities sum up to 1.

3 Soft Decision Trees

3.1 The Model

As opposed to the hard decision node which directs instances to one of its children depending on the outcome of the test at node m, $g_m(\boldsymbol{x})$, a soft decision node directs instances to all its children with probabilities calculated by a *gating function* $g_m(\boldsymbol{x})$ [7]. Without loss of generality, let us consider a *binary node* where we have left and right children:

$$F_m(\boldsymbol{x}) = F_m^L(\boldsymbol{x})g_m(\boldsymbol{x}) + F_m^R(\boldsymbol{x})(1 - g_m(\boldsymbol{x})) \qquad (1)$$

This is a recursive definition where $F_m^L(\boldsymbol{x})$ for example corresponds to the value returned by the subtree whose root is the left child of node m. Recursion ends when the subtree is just a leaf, in which case the value stored in the leaf is returned.

In the case of a hard tree, the *hard* decision node returns $g_m(\boldsymbol{x}) \in \{0, 1\}$, whereas in a soft tree, $g_m(\boldsymbol{x}) \in [0, 1]$, as given by the *sigmoid function*:

$$g_m(\boldsymbol{x}) = \frac{1}{1 + \exp[-(\boldsymbol{w}_m^T \boldsymbol{x} + \boldsymbol{w}_{m0})]} \qquad (2)$$

Separating the regions of responsibility of the left and right children can be seen as two-class classification problem and from that perspective, the gating model implements a discriminative (logistic linear) model estimating the posterior probability of the left child: $P(L|\boldsymbol{x}) \equiv g_m(\boldsymbol{x})$ and $P(R|\boldsymbol{x}) \equiv 1 - g_m(\boldsymbol{x})$.

In a hard tree, because $g_m(\boldsymbol{x})$ returns 0 or 1, in Eq. (1), the node copies the value of its left or right child, whereas in a soft tree because $g_m(\boldsymbol{x})$ returns a value between 0 and 1, the node returns a weighted average of its two children.

This allows a smooth transition at the decision boundary, leads to a smoother fit and hence better generalization. Because the tree is traversed recursively, Eq. (1) is defined recursively and as a result, all the paths to all the leaves are traversed and at the root node, we get a weighted average of all the leaves where the weight of each leaf is given by the product of the gating values on the path to each leaf.

Incidentally, this model can easily be generalized to m-ary nodes where each node has $m > 2$ children, by replacing Eq. (1) with a convex combination of the values of the m children and the sigmoid of Eq. (2) by the softmax.

3.2   Training

Learning the soft decision tree is incremental and recursive, as with the hard decision tree [8]. The algorithm starts with one node and fits a leaf. Then, as long as there is improvement, it replaces the leaf by a subtree of a node and its two children leaves. This involves optimizing the gating parameters at the node and the values of its children leaves.

The error function is cross-entropy for classification and square loss for regression (In classification, the final output should be a probability and that is why for a two-class task, the final output at root is filtered through a sigmoid):

$$
E = \begin{cases}
\sum_t (r^{(t)} - y^{(t)})^2 & \text{Regression} \\
\sum_t r^{(t)} \log y^{(t)} + (1 - r^{(t)}) \log(1 - y^{(t)}) & \text{Classification}
\end{cases}
\tag{3}
$$

At each growth step, node m, which was previously a leaf is replaced by a decision node and its two children leaves. The gating parameters $(\boldsymbol{w}_m)$ of the decision node and the numeric leaf values of the children nodes (z_m^L, z_m^R) are set to small random values initially and are then updated using gradient-descent:

$$
\Delta w_{mi} = -\eta \frac{\partial E}{\partial w_{mi}} = \eta(r - y)[F_m^L(\boldsymbol{x}) - F_m^R(\boldsymbol{x})]\alpha_m g_m(\boldsymbol{x})(1 - g_m(\boldsymbol{x}))x_i
$$

$$
\Delta z_m^L = -\eta \frac{\partial E}{\partial z_m^L} = \eta(r - y)\alpha_m g_m(\boldsymbol{x})
$$

$$
\Delta z_m^R = -\eta \frac{\partial E}{\partial z_m^R} = \eta(r - y)\alpha_m(1 - g_m(\boldsymbol{x}))
$$

where η is the learning factor,

$$
\alpha_m = \prod_{n=m, p=n.parent}^{n \neq root} \delta_{n,p.left} g_p(\boldsymbol{x}) + \delta_{n,p.right}(1 - g_p(\boldsymbol{x}))
$$

and $\delta_{i,j}$ is the Kronecker delta.

Note that only the three nodes of the last added subtree (current decision node and the leaf values of its children) are updated and all the other nodes are fixed. But since soft trees use a soft gating function, all the data points have an effect on these parameters, whereas in a hard tree, only those data points that fall in the partition of the current node have an effect. Any input instance should pass through all the intermediate decision nodes until it reaches the added node and its leaves and the error should be discounted by all the gating values along the way to find the "back-propagated error" for that instance (denoted by α above). This value is then used to update the gating parameters and the leaf values.

In the hierarchical mixture of experts [7], the tree structure is fixed and the whole tree is learned using gradient-descent or expectation-maximization, whereas in our case, the tree is built incrementally, one subtree at a time. One recent work by Ruta and Li [10] is the fuzzy regression tree which is different from our work in several aspects. First, their splits are defined over kernel responses, hence, are univariate (one-dimensional), whereas our gating functions are multivariate and defined directly over the input space. Second, they apply an exhaustive search to learn the parameters (as in the hard univariate tree, which is possible because the splits use a single dimension) whereas we use gradient-descent.

For cases where the input dimensionality is high, we have previously proposed to use L_1 and L_2-norm regularization where we add a model complexity term to the usual misfit error of Eq. (3) to get an augmented error [11]:

$$E' = E + \lambda \begin{cases} \displaystyle\sum_{i=0}^{d} |w_{mi}| & L_1\text{-norm} \\ \displaystyle\sum_{i=0}^{d} w_{mi}^2 & L_2\text{-norm} \end{cases}$$

and then we use the partial derivative of the augmented error in gradient-descent. λ trades off data misfit and model complexity. w_{mi} are the gating parameters of all nodes m in the tree for all attributes $i = 1, \ldots, d$.

Especially as we go down the tree, we localize in parts of the input space where certain dimensions may not be necessary or when certain dimensions are highly correlated; at the same time, as we go down the tree, we have fewer data that reach there; so, regularization helps.

4   Bagging Soft Decision Trees

Bagging, short for bootstrap aggregating, was introduced by Breiman [9]. The idea is to generate a set of training data from an initial data by bootstrapping, that is, drawing with replacement, then train a predictor on each training data, and then combine their predictions. Because drawing is done with replacement, certain instances may be drawn more than once, and certain instances not at all.

Different training data will differ slightly and the resulting trained predictors can be seen as noisy estimates to the ideal discriminant; combining them removes noise and leads to a smooth estimator with low variance, and hence better generalization [12].

Decision trees are frequently used in bagging and here we use soft decision trees to see if we also have the advantage due to bagging when we combine soft trees. The soft decision tree has multivariate splits and risks overfitting when the input dimensionality is high and data set is small; hence averaging by combination will have a regularizing effect.

Additional to the randomness due to data, there is also the randomness due to the initialization of parameters before gradient-descent; averaging over trees will also average this randomness out. A single soft tree may overfit due to noisy instances in the data or a bad initialization, but we expect the majority of the models to converge to good trees and hence by combining their predictions, we get an improved overall estimate.

Figure 1 shows the pseudocode of the algorithm BaggedSoftTree that creates B soft trees for a data set $\mathcal{X}$ containing N instances. For each, first we build a bootstrap sample $\mathcal{D}_i$ of size N by drawing with replacement from the original $\mathcal{X}$ (Line 2). Because the new set also contains N instances and drawing is done with replacement, the new set may contain certain instances multiple times and certain instances may not appear at all. Therefore, $\mathcal{D}_i$ will be similar to $\mathcal{X}$ but also slightly different. Then on each $\mathcal{D}_i$, we learn a soft tree $\mathcal{T}_i$ (Line 3).

These trees will be similar but also slightly different due to the randomness in training, both due to their sampled data and also the initialization of parameters. As the last step, for any new given test data, we combine the predictions of these soft trees using a committee-based procedure, such as voting.

BaggedSoftTree($\mathcal{X}$, B)
1 **for** $i = 1$ to B
2      $\mathcal{D}_i$ = BootStrap($\mathcal{X}$)
3      $\mathcal{T}_i$ = LearnSoftTree($\mathcal{D}_i$)
4 **end for**
5 Return prediction by aggregating classifiers $\mathcal{T}_i$

Fig. 1. The pseudocode of the algorithm that creates bagged soft trees consisting of B soft trees for a data set $\mathcal{X}$.

5   Experiments

5.1   Setup

We compare single and bagged soft decision trees with single and bagged hard decision trees on classification and regression data sets. Our methodology is as follows: We first separate one-third of the data set as the test set over which we evaluate the final performance. With the remaining two-thirds, we apply 5×2-fold cross-validation, i.e. we randomly separate the data into two stratified parts five times, and for each time, we interchange the roles of the parts as training set and validation set, which gives a total of 10 folds for each data set.

In bagging, we train and combine 100 models. In combining the output of the 100 trees to get the overall output, in regression we use the median of the 100 predictions, and in classification we take a vote over the 100 class predictions.

We compare soft and hard trees, single and bagged, in terms of their error on the left-out test set. We give a table where for each data set separately we show the average and standard deviation error for all compared tree algorithms. To compare the overall performance on all data sets, we use Nemenyi's test in terms of average ranks on all data sets and check for statistically significant difference [13]: On each data set, we rank the methods in terms of their average error so the first one gets the rank of 1, the second rank 2, and so on. Then we calculate the average rank of each method and Nemenyi's test tells us how much difference between ranks in significant.

5.2   Classification Data Sets

We compare the soft tree (Soft) with C4.5 tree (Hard), linear discriminant tree (Ldt) (which is a multivariate hard tree) [4], and the bagged versions of Soft, Hard, and Ldt trees (Soft$_B$, Hard$_B$, Ldt$_B$) on 27 two-class classification data sets from the UCI repository [14].

Ten of these classification data sets are from the medical domain: *Breast* is a breast cancer database obtained from the University of Wisconsin Hospitals, Madison, *Haberman* contains cases from a study on the survival of patients who had undergone surgery for breast cancer, *Heart* is a database concerning heart disease diagnosis, *Parkinsons* is composed of a range of biomedical voice measurements from 31 people, 23 with Parkinson's disease, *Pima* contains patients with diabetes who are females at least 21 years old of Pima Indian heritage, *Promoters* contains E. coli promoter gene sequences (DNA) with associated imperfect domain theory, *Spect* describes diagnosing of cardiac Single Proton Emission Computed Tomography (SPECT) images. *Acceptors* and *Donors* are splice site detection data sets and the trained models should distinguish 'GT' and 'AG' sites occurring in the DNA sequence that function as splice sites and those that do not [15]. *Polyadenylation* datasets contains polyadenylation signals in human sequences [16].

Table 1 shows the average and standard deviation of test errors of Hard, Ldt, Soft, Hard$_B$, Ldt$_B$, and Soft$_B$ on the separate data sets, where we see that bagged soft tree most of the time has the smallest error. Figure 2 shows the result of post-hoc Nemenyi's test applied on the average ranks of these algorithms in terms of their error on all data sets.

We see that the bagged soft tree has the lowest average rank (slightly above 1) and is significantly better than all other tree variants. The bagged versions of Ldt and Hard are only as good as a single soft tree. The single soft tree is significantly more accurate than single Ldt or hard tree. Ldt is also multivariate but uses hard splits; the fact that the soft tree (bagged or single) is more accurate than Ldt shows that it is the softness of the split that leads to higher accuracy rather than whether the split is uni or multivariate.

Table 1. On two-class classification data sets, the average and standard deviation of test errors of Hard, Ldt, Soft, and their bagged versions, $Hard_B$, Ldt_B, and $Soft_B$.

Dataset	Hard	Ldt	Soft	$Hard_B$	Ldt_B	$Soft_B$
acceptors	16.1 ± 2.0	9.6 ± 0.8	8.7 ± 0.7	18.2 ± 0.1	8.7 ± 0.5	8.1 ± 0.5
artificial	1.1 ± 1.8	1.5 ± 1.9	1.1 ± 1.8	1.1 ± 1.8	0.7 ± 1.6	0.7 ± 1.6
breast	6.7 ± 1.1	4.9 ± 0.6	3.5 ± 0.7	4.7 ± 0.8	4.7 ± 0.7	3.1 ± 0.4
bupa	38.6 ± 4.1	39.1 ± 3.4	39.7 ± 4.2	35.4 ± 3.6	38.2 ± 2.3	36.5 ± 2.7
donors	7.7 ± 0.4	5.4 ± 0.3	5.7 ± 0.4	7.2 ± 0.4	5.4 ± 0.2	5.3 ± 0.3
german	29.9 ± 0.0	25.8 ± 2.0	24.0 ± 3.0	29.9 ± 0.0	27.0 ± 2.8	23.2 ± 0.8
haberman	26.6 ± 0.3	27.2 ± 1.5	25.9 ± 1.8	26.5 ± 0.0	26.5 ± 0.0	24.7 ± 1.6
heart	28.3 ± 4.7	18.4 ± 2.3	19.7 ± 3.4	24.7 ± 6.0	18.4 ± 2.2	15.7 ± 1.3
hepatitis	22.1 ± 4.4	20.4 ± 2.9	20.2 ± 2.4	20.8 ± 1.2	20.2 ± 1.6	18.7 ± 2.4
ironosphere	13.1 ± 1.9	12.3 ± 2.2	11.5 ± 2.0	9.4 ± 3.2	12.4 ± 1.9	11.6 ± 1.3
krvskp	1.2 ± 0.4	4.5 ± 0.7	1.8 ± 0.6	1.2 ± 0.5	4.7 ± 0.7	1.8 ± 0.2
magic	17.5 ± 0.6	16.9 ± 0.1	14.7 ± 0.5	16.4 ± 0.3	16.7 ± 0.2	13.9 ± 0.1
monks	12.8 ± 7.8	23.8 ± 8.2	0.0 ± 0.0	11.9 ± 4.6	24.0 ± 2.0	0.0 ± 0.0
mushroom	0.0 ± 0.1	1.8 ± 0.5	0.1 ± 0.0	0.1 ± 0.1	0.9 ± 0.2	0.1 ± 0.1
musk2	5.5 ± 0.6	6.4 ± 0.3	4.3 ± 0.7	5.3 ± 0.1	6.3 ± 0.2	3.8 ± 0.3
parkinsons	13.8 ± 2.3	13.5 ± 2.5	14.3 ± 2.7	14.0 ± 3.1	14.8 ± 4.1	10.9 ± 0.9
pima	27.9 ± 3.4	23.1 ± 1.4	24.9 ± 2.0	24.2 ± 1.2	22.6 ± 1.0	23.6 ± 1.0
polyaden	30.5 ± 1.3	22.6 ± 0.6	22.9 ± 0.5	29.2 ± 0.5	22.4 ± 0.4	22.1 ± 0.3
promoters	26.1 ± 9.9	34.4 ± 9.4	15.3 ± 6.7	14.7 ± 9.7	31.7 ± 5.9	10.8 ± 4.0
ringnorm	12.2 ± 1.1	22.8 ± 0.3	9.9 ± 1.7	7.2 ± 0.7	22.7 ± 0.3	5.1 ± 0.3
satellite47	15.4 ± 1.5	16.7 ± 1.4	12.4 ± 1.4	12.2 ± 0.5	16.7 ± 0.6	11.5 ± 0.6
spambase	9.9 ± 0.7	10.1 ± 0.7	7.5 ± 0.5	8.1 ± 0.4	9.8 ± 0.4	7.2 ± 0.3
spect	19.1 ± 2.8	20.1 ± 2.4	19.6 ± 2.4	20.4 ± 2.1	21.1 ± 0.0	17.4 ± 3.3
tictactoe	23.8 ± 2.2	31.9 ± 2.4	1.8 ± 0.3	22.1 ± 2.5	29.4 ± 1.0	1.6 ± 0.0
titanic	21.8 ± 0.5	22.4 ± 0.4	21.5 ± 0.2	22.1 ± 0.0	22.7 ± 0.2	21.5 ± 0.2
twonorm	17.0 ± 0.7	2.0 ± 0.1	2.1 ± 0.2	4.8 ± 0.7	2.0 ± 0.1	2.0 ± 0.1
vote	5.2 ± 0.7	6.7 ± 2.6	5.1 ± 0.9	4.9 ± 0.2	6.4 ± 1.1	4.6 ± 0.6

5.3   Regression Data Sets

We also compare soft regression trees (Soft) with the univariate regression tree (Hard) and their bagged versions, $Soft_B$ and $Hard_B$, on 26 regression data sets [17].

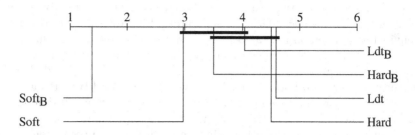

Fig. 2. On two-class classification data sets, the result of Nemenyi's test applied on the ranks of Hard, Ldt, Soft, $Hard_B$, Ldt_B, and $Soft_B$ in terms of error. Indicated points are the average ranks and a thick underline implies no significant difference.

Table 2. On the regression data sets, the average and standard deviation of errors of Hard and Soft trees and their bagged versions, $Hard_B$, and $Soft_B$.

Dataset	Hard	Soft	$Hard_B$	$Soft_B$
abalone	0.53 ± 0.01	0.41 ± 0.01	0.50 ± 0.02	0.41 ± 0.01
add10	0.24 ± 0.01	0.08 ± 0.01	0.19 ± 0.00	0.05 ± 0.00
bank32fh	0.50 ± 0.01	0.40 ± 0.01	0.46 ± 0.01	0.40 ± 0.01
bank32fm	0.12 ± 0.00	0.04 ± 0.00	0.10 ± 0.00	0.04 ± 0.00
bank32nh	0.59 ± 0.01	0.45 ± 0.01	0.56 ± 0.01	0.43 ± 0.00
bank32nm	0.41 ± 0.02	0.20 ± 0.00	0.34 ± 0.01	0.19 ± 0.00
bank8fh	0.30 ± 0.01	0.26 ± 0.01	0.28 ± 0.01	0.26 ± 0.01
bank8fm	0.08 ± 0.00	0.04 ± 0.00	0.08 ± 0.01	0.04 ± 0.00
bank8nh	0.69 ± 0.02	0.56 ± 0.02	0.65 ± 0.02	0.56 ± 0.02
bank8nm	0.37 ± 0.03	0.12 ± 0.01	0.35 ± 0.02	0.10 ± 0.01
boston	0.34 ± 0.09	0.23 ± 0.03	0.27 ± 0.05	0.24 ± 0.02
comp	0.03 ± 0.00	0.02 ± 0.00	0.08 ± 0.00	0.02 ± 0.00
concrete	0.93 ± 0.05	0.23 ± 0.02	0.67 ± 0.03	0.22 ± 0.01
kin32fh	0.73 ± 0.03	0.32 ± 0.01	0.64 ± 0.01	0.32 ± 0.01
kin32fm	0.61 ± 0.02	0.08 ± 0.00	0.51 ± 0.01	0.07 ± 0.00
kin32nh	0.94 ± 0.02	0.75 ± 0.03	0.92 ± 0.03	0.75 ± 0.02
kin32nm	0.90 ± 0.01	0.62 ± 0.03	0.87 ± 0.01	0.60 ± 0.01
kin8fh	0.54 ± 0.02	0.26 ± 0.00	0.42 ± 0.02	0.26 ± 0.00
kin8fm	0.32 ± 0.01	0.03 ± 0.00	0.22 ± 0.01	0.03 ± 0.00
puma8fh	0.42 ± 0.01	0.38 ± 0.01	0.39 ± 0.01	0.38 ± 0.01
puma8nh	0.40 ± 0.02	0.36 ± 0.01	0.37 ± 0.01	0.35 ± 0.01
puma8fm	0.07 ± 0.00	0.05 ± 0.00	0.08 ± 0.00	0.05 ± 0.00
puma8nm	0.06 ± 0.01	0.05 ± 0.00	0.08 ± 0.00	0.04 ± 0.00
puma32fh	0.59 ± 0.01	0.59 ± 0.01	0.59 ± 0.01	0.59 ± 0.01
puma32fm	0.04 ± 0.00	0.07 ± 0.01	0.08 ± 0.01	0.06 ± 0.00
puma32nh	0.39 ± 0.01	0.43 ± 0.02	0.36 ± 0.01	0.41 ± 0.01

Table 2 shows the average and standard deviation of errors of Hard, Soft, Hard$_B$, and Soft$_B$ on each data set separately. Figure 3 shows the result of Nemenyi's test applied on the ranks of the error rates of these algorithms.

We see again that the bagged soft tree has the lowest rank; the bagged soft tree is significantly more accurate than the single soft tree and they are significantly better than both the hard tree and bagged hard tree. Bagging the hard tree leads to some improvement in terms of average rank but the difference is not significant here. Note that this does not mean bagging hard trees is useless, it is only with respect to the others that the difference between them seems insignificant—single and bagged hard trees rank mostly in 3rd and 4th ranks.

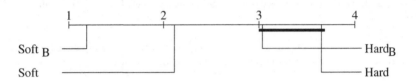

Fig. 3. On the regression data sets, the result of Nemenyi's test applied on the ranks of errors of Hard and Soft trees and their bagged versions, Hard$_B$, and Soft$_B$.

6   Conclusions and Future Outlook

The soft tree has several advantages: First, it provides a continuous fit whereas the hard tree has a discontinuous response at the leaf boundaries. This enables the soft tree to have smoother fits and hence lower bias around the split boundaries. Second, the linear gating function enables the soft tree to make oblique splits in contrast to the axis-orthogonal splits made by the univariate hard tree.

In our previous experiments [8], we see that these two properties improve accuracy and also reduce the number of nodes required to solve a regression or a classification problem. Soft trees seem especially suited to regression problems where the gating function allows a smooth interpolation between the children of a node.

Here, we build on top of the soft decision tree model and show how its accuracy can be further improved by bagging. We see that on both classification and regression problems, we get significant improvement in terms of accuracy by bagging soft decision trees.

Bagging averages over both the randomness in sampling of data and the randomness in the initialization of parameters (before gradient-descent) and this leads to a smoother fit and better generalization.

Bagging is only one way to build an ensemble. We previously worked on methods for training and pruning an ensemble [12] and combining them to construct uncorrelated metaclassifiers [18] and these ensemble construction approaches can also use soft decision trees as the base learner.

Another possible future direction is in combining multiple sources: In some applications, there are multiple views or representations associated with each instance that complement each other and one possible future work is to train different soft trees with different views and then combine their predictions.

Even with a single representation, different soft trees can use different randomly chosen subsets of the features [19] and we can have soft random decision forests—these are possible future research directions.

Acknowledgments. This work is partially supported by Boğaziçi University Research Funds with Grant Number 14A01P4.

References

1. Breiman, L., Friedman, J.H., Olshen, R.A., Stone, C.J.: Classification and Regression Trees. John Wiley and Sons, New York (1984)
2. Quinlan, J.R.: C4.5: Programs for Machine Learning. Morgan Kaufmann, San Meteo (1993)
3. Murthy, S.K., Kasif, S., Salzberg, S.: A system for induction of oblique decision trees. J. Artif. Intell. Res. **2**, 1–32 (1994)
4. Yıldız, O.T., Alpaydın, E.: Linear discriminant trees. Int. J. Pattern Recogn. Artif. Intell. **19**(3), 323–353 (2005)
5. Guo, H., Gelfand, S.B.: Classification trees with neural network feature extraction. IEEE Trans. Neural Netw. **3**, 923–933 (1992)
6. Yıldız, O.T., Alpaydın, E.: Omnivariate decision trees. IEEE Trans. Neural Netw. **12**(6), 1539–1546 (2001)
7. Jordan, M.I., Jacobs, R.A.: Hierarchical mixtures of experts and the EM algorithm. Neural Comput. **6**, 181–214 (1994)
8. İrsoy, O., Yıldız, O.T., Alpaydın, E.: Soft decision trees. In: Proceedings of the International Conference on Pattern Recognition, Tsukuba, Japan, pp. 1819–1822 (2012)
9. Breiman, L.: Bagging predictors. Mach. Learn. **26**, 123–140 (1996)
10. Ruta, A., Li, Y.: Learning pairwise image similarities for multi-classification using kernel regression trees. Pattern Recogn. **45**, 1396–1408 (2011)
11. Yıldız, O.T., Alpaydın, E.: Regularizing soft decision trees. In: Proceedings of the International Conference on Computer and Information Sciences, Paris, France (2013)
12. Ulaş, A., Semerci, M., Yıldız, O.T., Alpaydın, E.: Incremental construction of classifier and discriminant ensembles. Inf. Sci. **179**, 1298–1318 (2009)
13. Demsar, J.: Statistical comparisons of classifiers over multiple data sets. J. Mach. Learn. Res. **7**, 1–30 (2006)
14. Blake, C., Merz, C.: UCI repository of machine learning databases (2000)
15. Kulp, D., Haussler, D., Reese, M.G., Eeckman, F.H.: A generalized hidden markov model for the recognition of human genes in dna. In: International Conference on Intelligent Systems for Molecular Biology (1996)
16. Liu, L., Han, H., Li, J., Wong, L.: An in-silico method for prediction of polyadenylation signals in human sequences. In: International Conference on Genome Informatics (2003)

17. Rasmussen, C.E., Neal, R.M., Hinton, G., van Camp, D., Revow, M., Ghahramani, Z., Kustra, R., Tibshirani, R.: Delve data for evaluating learning in valid experiments (1996)
18. Ulaş, A., Yıldız, O.T., Alpaydın, E.: Eigenclassifiers for combining correlated classifiers. Inf. Sci. **187**, 109–120 (2012)
19. Ho, T.K.: The random subspace method for constructing decision forests. IEEE Trans. Pattern Anal. Mach. Intell. **20**, 832–844 (1998)

Grammars for Discrete Dynamics

Vincenzo Manca[✉]

Department of Computer Science, and Center for BioMedical Computing,
University of Verona, Verona, Italy
`vincenzo.manca@univr.it`

Abstract. The paper reviews a new perspective to discover and compute discrete dynamics, which is based on MP grammars. They are a particular type of multiset rewriting grammars, introduced in 2004 for modeling metabolic systems, which express dynamics in terms of finite difference equations. MP regression algorithms, providing the best MP grammar reproducing a given time series of observed states, were introduced since 2008. Applications of these grammars to the analysis of biological dynamics were developed, and their flexibility to model complex and uncertain phenomena was apparent in the last years. In this paper we recall the main features of this modeling framework, by stressing their peculiarity to afford complex situations, where classical continuous methods cannot be applied or are computationally prohibitive. Moreover, the computational universality of MP grammars of a very simple type is shown, and one of the most relevant cases of MP biological models is shortly presented.

Keywords: Discrete dynamics · Dynamics inverse problem · MP grammar · MP regression · Metabolic computing · Machine Learning · Biomedical informatics

1 Introduction

If we consider the emergence of computability, since the years around 1930, and its relationship with classical mathematical concept of algorithm, we easily realize that, from an initial logical mathematical kernel of concepts (related to famous Hilbert's program), the notion of computation continued to enlarge its perspectives, by including technical and conceptual aspects, where information, inference, and uncertainty become essential notions of any computation engine, in a wide sense, or shortly, *(informational) machine*. In fact, the initial idea underlying the Leibnitz-Hilbert research line, aimed at discovering a universal *calculus ratiocinator*, almost contemporarily, found the limitative Gödel result, and strictly related to it, Turing's computational universality. Therefore, machines able to run any possible algorithm exist, but they cannot deduce all the theorems of powerful theories (*e.g.* including all arithmetic truths).

However, the following research in computer science, made widely available complex computational tools of increasing efficiency, and determined a rich integration of results and knowledge from different fields such as cybernetics, artificial intelligence (solution spaces and algorithms for exploring them), numerical

© Springer International Publishing AG 2016
A. Holzinger (Ed.): ML for Health Informatics, LNAI 9605, pp. 37–58, 2016.
DOI: 10.1007/978-3-319-50478-0_3

analysis, optimization, statistics (see [1] for a more detailed analysis of the field). This situation radically changed the terms of "Leibnitz's dream", passing from the goal of discovering machines that deduce the truths of rich mathematical theories, to machines that can help us to infer theories that explain the data collected from a given phenomenon. This is the essence of Machine Learning (ML) and the reason of its centrality in the historical development of computer science, along the tracks of its founders, Wiener, Shannon, Turing, and von Neumann.

From a technical point of view, a common aspect to many "inferential" approaches are the so called inverse problems, which also played a central role in many mathematical fields. In general terms, the objective of these problems is not that of finding particular solutions satisfying some constraints, but conversely, discovering constraints that underly to data collected in a given context. Let us provide a basic example, a Chomsky grammar generates a set of strings, by means a suitable process of string manipulation. Therefore, in this case, an inverse problem arises when a set of strings is given and a grammar is required that is able, possibly within an error threshold, to generate the given strings. In this sense the MP theory, which we are going to introduce, provides methods for automatically, and approximately, solving a wide class of inverse problems (especially, from biological contexts), discovering some dynamical laws that rule an observed dynamics. For this reason, statistics, optimization, and numerical analysis are implicitly internalized in the MP regression algorithms, which yield the inferential motor of MP theory. This perspective motivates the pertinence of MP theory to the wider field of Machine Learning.

MP grammars are discrete dynamical systems arisen in the context of membrane computing [2]. They introduce a deterministic perspective where multiset rewriting rules are equipped with state functions that determine the quantities of transformed elements. The attribute MP comes from the initial context suggesting MP grammars, focused on expressing metabolic processes in the context of P systems (multiset rewriting rules distributed in compartments) introduced by Păun [3–6]. Applications in modeling biological systems were developed in the last years [7–16], as well as, methods of MP regression, were defined, in order to determine MP grammars able to generate observed time series of given phenomena (MP-Dynamics Inverse Problems, shortly MP-DIP). Very often, such kind of inverse process, unravels possible MP grammars, underlying real systems that make evident hidden mechanisms inherent to deep internal logics. MP regression algorithms use a wide spectrum of techniques, from algebraic manipulation and Least Square Evaluation, to statistical methods, and to genetic algorithms, by obtaining, in many cases, high levels of accuracy in the solutions [2,7,11,13,17–25]. A great number of concepts and algorithms developed within MP theory were implemented in public software platforms equipped with examples and technical documentation [26,27] (see also some related links: http://mptheory.scienze.univr.it/, http://mplab.sci.univr.it/plugins/mpgs/index.html, http://mplab.sci.univr.it/, http://www.cbmc.it/software/Software.php).

2 Glossary

2.1 Multiset:

Is a set of elements each considered with a positive integer occurrence multiplicity. If we generalize the usual brace set-theoretic notation, then $\{a, a, b, b, b, c\}$ denotes a multiset with two occurrences of a, three occurrences of b, and one occurrence of c. In the notation above, the order of occurrence of a, b, c is not relevant, but only the number of times they occur. Other equivalent notions are very often used in literature. A molecule is a multiset of atoms. Many basic chemical laws are easy consequences of this definition of molecule.

2.2 MP Variable

Is an entity assuming values, in a given set, in dependence on some contexts. Very often contexts are instants of time.

2.3 MP State

Are the current values assumed by some variables (w. r. t. state is considered).

2.4 MP Grammar

Is a set of rules of type "left-side" $\rightarrow$ "right-side" : "regulator". Right and left sides are multisets of variables, and regulator is a function defined on the states of some variables. At any step, each rule decreases the current values of each left variable instance and increases the current value of each right variable instance. The amount of increase/decrease, called flux, is the value that the regulator assumes in the current state of its variables.

2.5 MP Graph

Is a representation of an MP grammar by means of a two level graph (nodes, multi-edges, and inter-edges), where edges connect a set of source nodes to a set target nodes, and inter-edges connect a set of source nodes to only one target node (sets of nodes may be empty) (Fig. 1).

2.6 Time Series

Is a sequence of states. The states of this sequence are assumed to be located along a discrete and oriented line of time. Starting from an initial state, by iteratively applying all the rules of an MP grammar, we get a time series of states.

2.7   Discrete Dynamical System

Is a set S of states and a function δ from S to S [28]. From an initial state, by applying iteratively the function δ, a time series is generated. Therefore an MP grammar is a particular kind of Discrete Dynamical System.

2.8   Discrete Dynamics Inverse Problem

Is the search for an MP grammar that generates a given time series.

3   State of the Art

3.1   MP Grammars

An MP grammar G is a discrete dynamical system based on a set X of variables, and a state space constituted by the assignments of values to variables X. Let $\mathbb{N}$ be the set of natural numbers. Assuming variables in some order, if X is a finite set of $n \in \mathbb{N}$ variables, the set of possible *states* of G coincides with the set $\mathbb{R}^n$ of real vectors of dimension n. A dynamics function δ_G is associated to G that provides a **next state function**, which changes the variable values, according to an increase-decrease variations specified by all the rules (if a variable does not occur in a rule, its value remains unchanged). Namely, a reading of "MP" is the basic Minus-Plus mechanism of the rules of an MP grammar. A formal definition follows.

Definition 1. *An* MP grammar G *is given by a structure [11]:*

$$G = (X, R, \Phi)$$

where:

1. X *is a finite set of real* variables;
2. R *is a finite set of* rules *(usually we denote by n is the number of variables and m the number of rules). Each rule $r \in R$ is expressed by $\alpha_r \to \beta_r$ with α_r, β_r multisets over X (a multiset over X is functions assigning a natural number, called* multiplicity, *to every $x \in X$). Therefore, $\alpha_r(x)$ and $\beta_r(y)$ denote the multiplicities of x and y in α_r and in β_r, respectively;*
3. $\Phi = \{\varphi_r \mid r \in R\}$ *is the set of* regulators, *or flux functions*

$$\varphi_r : \mathbb{R}^n \to \mathbb{R}$$

from states of variables to real numbers. A regulator φ_r associates to any state $s \in \mathbb{R}^n$ a positive or null value $u = \varphi_r(s)$, called "flux", that establishes an updating of the current state of variables, by decreasing any variable x occurring in α_r by the value $u \cdot \alpha_r(x)$, and by increasing any variable y occurring in β_r by the value $u \cdot \beta_r(y)$.

A variation function $\Delta_G(s)_x$ is associated to every variable $x \in X$ of G, such that:

$$\Delta_G(s)_x = \sum_{r \in R} (\beta_r(x) - \alpha_r(x)) \varphi_r(s).$$

and

$$\Delta_G(s) = (\Delta_G(s)_x)_{x \in X}^T$$

(superscript T denotes transposition, so that $\Delta_G(s)$ is viewed a column vector).

The dynamics δ_G of G is given by (subscript G is omitted when it is implicitly understood):

$$\delta_G(s) = s + \Delta_G(s)$$

When an initial state s_0 is given, then an MP grammar G, starting from it, generates a time series of states $(\delta_G^i(s_0))_{i \geq 0}$, by iteratively applying the dynamics function δ.   □

An MP grammar is completely defined by its rules and regulators (variables are those occurring in the rules). When variables are equipped with measurement units (related to their interpretation), and a time duration is associated to each step, the MP grammar is more properly called an *MP system*.

It is easy to show that the dynamics of an MP grammar can be naturally expressed by a system of (first-order) recurrent equations, synthetically represented in matrix notation (see [11] for details). In fact, rules define the following matrix, called *rule stoichiometric matrix*.

$$\mathbb{A} = (\beta_r(x) - \alpha_r(x))_{x \in X, r \in R}.$$

If fluxes are given by vector $U(s)$ (superscript T stands for transposition):

$$U(s) = (\varphi_r(s))_{r \in R}^T$$

and the vector of variable variations $\Delta(s)$ is given by:

$$\Delta(s) = (\Delta_x(s))_{x \in X}^T$$

then, the system of variable variations can be expressed by ($\times$ is the usual matrix product):

$$\Delta(s) = \mathbb{A} \times U(s).$$

This formulation of MP grammar dynamics, introduced in [17], is called *EMA* (Equational Metabolic Algorithm) and allows us to generate a sequence of states from any given initial state.

Example 1. It is easy to verify that the following MP grammar generates, as values of variable x, the Fibonacci sequence, starting from the initial state $x = 1$, $y = 0$ ($\emptyset$ denotes the empty multiset of variables).

$$\emptyset \to y \ : \ x \tag{1}$$
$$y \to x \ : \ y \tag{2}$$

$(x = 1, y = 0) \Rightarrow (x = 1, y = 1) \Rightarrow (x = 2, y = 1) \Rightarrow (x = 3, y = 2) \Rightarrow (x = 5, y = 3) \ldots$

Example 2. The following grammar provides a predator-prey dynamics.

$$\begin{aligned} \emptyset \to x \;\; &: \;\; 0.061 \cdot x + 0.931 \\ x \to y \;\; &: \;\; 0.067 \cdot x + 0.15 \cdot y \\ y \to \emptyset \;\; &: \;\; 0.154 \cdot y + 0.403, \end{aligned} \tag{3}$$

Matrix A below is the *stoichiometric matrix* of MP grammar in Example 2.

$$\mathbb{A} = \begin{pmatrix} 1 & -1 & 0 \\ 0 & 1 & -1 \end{pmatrix} \tag{4}$$

MP grammars have an intrinsic versatility in describing oscillatory phenomena [11, 14].

The schema of MP grammars given in Example 2, called *bicatalyticus* [11], has an input rule r_1 and an output rule r_3 (incrementing and decrementing the variable x and y, respectively). Both rules are regulated by the same variable that they change (a sort of *autocatalysis*), while the transformation rule r_2 from x to y is regulated by both variables (*bicatalysis*). An MP grammar of this type provides a simple model for predator-prey dynamics firstly modeled in differential terms by Lotka and Volterra [29]. The model assumes a simple schema ruling the growth of the two populations x, y (preys and predators): preys grow by eating nutrients taken from the environment (according to some reproduction factor) and die by predation, while predators grows by eating preys and naturally die (according to some death factor). When predators increase then preys are more abundantly eaten and therefore they decrease. But prey decrease results in a minor food for predators which start to decrease (by providing a consequent increase of preys). This means that the increase of predators produces, after a while, their decrease (and symmetrically, a corresponding inverse oscillation happens for preys) (Fig. 2).

Example 3. The following grammar, obtained by using MP regression (see next subsection), provides sine and cosine dynamics with linear regulators ($x = 0$, $y = 1$ is the initial state). It was proved in [30] that this is exactly the grammar deduced from the classical analytical and geometric definitions of sine and cosine functions. In other words, the MP regression algorithm, which we will introduce in the next section, is able to discover the logic implied by deep mathematical properties of circular functions.

$$\begin{aligned} r_1 : \emptyset \to x \;\; &: \;\; k_1 \cdot x \\ r_2 : x \to y \;\; &: \;\; k_2 \cdot (x + y) \\ r_3 : y \to \emptyset \;\; &: \;\; k_3 \cdot y \end{aligned} \tag{5}$$

where $k_1 = 0.000999499833375$, $k_2 = 0.000999999833333$ and $k_3 = 0.001000499833291$ (the coefficient estimates are truncated to the 15th decimal

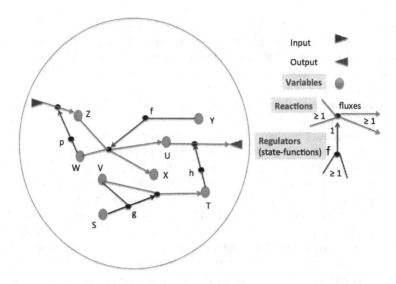

Fig. 1. The structure of MP graphs.

digits, according to the accuracy of the computer architecture used during the computation). MP grammar (5) provides a very precise sine/cosine oscillator, with maximum absolute error of order 10^{-14}.

A natural way of expressing MP grammars by means of graphs, called MP graphs, was introduced in [31]. In an MP graph rules (or reactions) are multi-edges connecting variables nodes (sources) to other variable nodes (targets) entering and exiting, respectively, from a rule node. Moreover a regulation inter-edge goes from some variable nodes, called tuners, to a rule node, for indicating the variable nodes regulating the rule, according to a function, called *regulator*, which is put as label of the regulation inter-edge. Input and output nodes are considered in correspondence to rules with left and right parts consisting of the empty multi-set. From this representation, an interesting interplay results among the notions of membrane, object, and variable. In fact objects can be

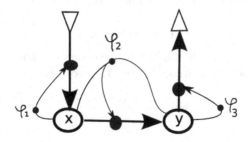

Fig. 2. The MP graph of the prey-predator grammar.

considered as membranes including all the same type of matter, where the quantity corresponds to the multiplicity (if matter are tokens) or to some measure associated to the object. But at same time, membranes are particular objects, and variables are membranes when the (positive) value assumed by them, are seen as the quantities of matter that they include.

Dynamics inverse problems were the beginning of modern science aimed at discovering the motion laws of planets around the sun. In general, a typical problem of mechanics is the determination of motion laws: from the observed motion to the underlying equations deduced from the knowledge of the forces acting on bodies. The approach we will outline here is similar, but here the forces as "causes of motion changes" are not assumed. Rather, we are interested in inferring a possible (approximate) internal logic regulating how (instead that why) changes of variables are cooperatively organized in a given system. This of course is a solution less precise and less explicative than the classical approach (usually based on ordinary differential equations). However, very often, in very complex systems with poor information about the causes acting in a system, it is the only possibility that can be realistically investigated. In the context of MP theory, a DIP can be formulated in the following way. *Given a time series* $S = (s_i)_{i=0,1,...t}$ *of observed states (equally spaced in time), find the MP grammar able to generate S within a given approximation threshold.* In formal terms this means to solve, with the best approximation, the following equation where G is the unknown value:

$$\left(\delta_G^i(s_0)\right)_{i=0,1,...t} = S.$$

General and specific cases of DIP were intensively investigated, in the context of the MP theory, in the last ten years (see [11] for a detailed account, and [14–16, 25–27, 32] for new developments and applications to biological modeling).

3.2   MP Regression

Let us suppose that we observe some time series of states. Very often the time series related to an inverse dynamics problem is not sampled at regular time intervals. In this case a preprocessing phase is appropriate for determining an interpolation curve fitting the observed values along the observation points, by obtaining a time series uniformly spaced in time:

$$(s[i]|i \leq t \in \mathbb{N})$$

then, we can read the equation EMA by reversing the known values with the unknown ones. In fact, by writing the variation vector:

$$s[i+1] - s[i] = \Delta[i]$$

and, assuming n variables and m rules, then we get the following system (see [7]), where fluxes $U[i]$ are the unknown values:

$$\mathbb{A} \times U[i] = \Delta[i]. \qquad (6)$$

For the determination of the regulators that provide the best approximate solution of Eq. (6), we apply a procedure we call *stoichiometric expansion* (see [19, 22, 23]).

Given a positive integer t, let us assume that the regulators we are searching for can be expressed as linear combinations of some basic regressors

$$g_1, g_2, \ldots, g_d$$

which usually include constants, powers, and products of variables, plus some basic functions which are considered suitable in the specific cases under investigation:

$$\varphi_1 = c_{1,1} g_1 + c_{1,2} g_2 + \ldots + c_{1,d} g_d \qquad (7)$$
$$\varphi_2 = c_{2,1} g_1 + c_{2,2} g_2 + \ldots + c_{2,d} g_d$$
$$\ldots = \ldots \ldots \ldots \ldots$$
$$\varphi_m = c_{m,1} g_1 + c_{m,2} g_2 + \ldots + c_{m,d} g_d.$$

Equation (7) can be written, in matrix notation, in the following way, where $U[i]$ is the column vector of regulators evaluated at state s_i, $\mathbb{G}[i]$ the column vector of regressors evaluated at the same state, and $\mathbb{C}$ is the matrix $m \times d$ of the unknown coefficients of regressors:

$$U[i] = \mathbb{C} \times \mathbb{G}[i]. \qquad (8)$$

Substituting the right member of Eq. (8) in Eq. (6), we obtain the following system of equations ($\mathbb{A}$ is the stoichiometric matrix):

$$\mathbb{A} \times \mathbb{C} \times \mathbb{G}[i] = \Delta[i]. \qquad (9)$$

Now, if we consider t systems of type (9), for $1 \le i \le t$, and if n is the number of variables, we obtain nt equations with md unknown coefficients of $\mathbb{C}$. If $nt > md$ and the system has maximum rank, then we can apply a Least Square Evaluation which provides the coefficients that minimize the errors between left and right sides of the equations. These coefficients provide the regulator representations that we are searching for.

By elaborating on Eq. (9) it is proved that matrix $\mathbb{C}$ is given by the following equation (see [11, 23]), where the stoichiometric expansion is joint to the Least Square Approximation method and $\otimes$ denotes the Kronecker product defined in Table 1, and $vec(\mathbb{C})$ is matrix $\mathbb{C}$ after the vectorization operation, where all the colums of $\mathbb{C}$ are concatenated in a single column vector.

Theorem 1. *The coefficients of regressors that best approximate regulators are given by the following equation:*

$$vec(\mathbb{C}) = \left((\mathbb{A} \otimes \mathbb{G})^T \times (\mathbb{A} \otimes \mathbb{G}) \right)^{-1} \times (\mathbb{A} \otimes \mathbb{G})^T \times vec(\mathbb{D}). \qquad (10)$$

Table 1. Kronecker product of two real matrix A, B of dimension $n \times m$ and $t \times d$ respectively, having dimension $nt \times md$, and constituted by nm blocks $B_{i,j}$, such that, if $A = (a_{i,j} \mid 1 \le i \le n,\ 1 \le j \le m)$, then $(A \otimes B)_{i,j} = a_{i,j}B$ (all the elements of B are multiplied by $a_{i,j}$).

$$
A \otimes B = \begin{pmatrix}
a_{1,1}B & a_{1,1}B & \dots & a_{1,m}B \\
a_{2,1}B & a_{2,2}B & \dots & a_{2,mn}B \\
\dots & \dots & \dots & \dots \\
a_{n,1}B & a_{n,2}B & \dots & a_{n,m}B.
\end{pmatrix} \quad (11)
$$

3.3   Algorithms of MP Regression

MP regression can be realized with different kinds of algorithms. The first method of regression was based on a kind of inductive method, where the system EMA for computing the dynamics is extended in a kind of system, called OLGA, determining the fluxes of each step [17,33]. From the fluxes for a number of steps, regulators can be approximated. The weak point of this method is that it relies on the evaluation of the initial values of fluxes. This evaluation, in general, is not easy to be obtained, therefore errors in the initial values of fluxes can determine a bad evaluation of regulators. However, this was the initial algorithm from which the following ones emerged. Other two methods overcome the limitation of OLGA by means of a direct evaluation of regressors by using some initial functions called regressors. LGSS is an algorithm [11,19,22,23] based on the stoichiometric expansion that applies methods of statistical regression, by using a stepwise methodology. In fact, stoichiometric expansion is a powerful method to get regulators, by Least Square Estimation, but it is efficient only if the right regressors are provided as input. Therefore stepwise strategy is a mechanism devoted to the best choice of regressors that have to be given as input of the stoichiometric expansion. The main idea of stepwise is to start by a small set of regulators (for example constant and linear functions), then step by step a new regressor (from a fixed set of possible functions) is added to be evaluated (together with those of the previous step) and its addition is performed only if it improves the dynamics approximation. Moreover, after an addition of a new regressor another trial is executed, by trying to remove one regressor from the previous set (apart the last one inserted), in the case this removal could meliorate the dynamics approximation. The evaluations of insertion and deletion are based on classical statistical tests (related to Fischer distribution and variance analysis). Another MP regression method, MP-GenSynth, also uses the stoichiometric expansion, but tries to obtain the best regressors for this expansion, by using a genetic algorithm approach [24–26], that is, by replacing statistics by an evolutionary strategy. Specific mechanisms are used for the tuning of the evolutionary process and for improving the adaptability and the robustness of the method. Both LGSS and MP-GenSynth were developed in public domain platforms available in the sites mentioned in the introduction. It is whorthwile to remark that LGSS is a multi-platform software including several components for comparing and integrating MP regressions with classical methods of regression (ordinary differential equations, non linear optimization methods, graphical tools, components for random generations, and so on).

3.4 Input-Output and Positive MP Grammars

Any MP grammar has an equivalent grammar (providing the same dynamics) where rules have an input or output form (with the empty multiset $\emptyset$ on the right or on the left of the rule) [11]. Equivalence is intended in dynamical terms, that is, two MP grammars are (dynamically) equivalent, with respect a set of variables common to the two grammars, when these variables change in the same way in the two MP grammars.

The following theorem holds.

Theorem 2. *Any MP grammar can be equivalently represented in terms of input-output rules. Moreover, any system of (first order) recurrent equations can be expressed in terms of some MP grammar with input-output rules.*

Proof. In fact, any rule $\alpha \rightarrow \beta : \varphi$ that is not an input-output rule can be transformed into the set of rules $x \rightarrow \emptyset : \varphi$ (output rule) for every $x \in \alpha$, and $\emptyset \rightarrow y : \varphi$ (input rule) for every $y \in \beta$. Of course the effect of applying $\alpha \rightarrow \beta : \varphi$ is the same of applying all these input-output rules.

Conversely, Any system of (first order) recurrent equations (where values of variables at step $n+1$ depend on values of variables at step n) can be expressed by a system of equations, for $j = 1, 2, \ldots, n$:

$$\Delta_j(s) = P_{1,j}(s) + \ldots + P_{k,j}(s) - Q_{1,j}(s) \ldots - Q_{h,j}(s)$$

then we can consider n variables $x_1, \ldots, x_j, \ldots x_n$ with rules $\emptyset \rightarrow x_j : P_{i,j}$ for $i = 1, 2, \ldots k$ and $j = 1, 2, \ldots n$; and rules $x_j \rightarrow \emptyset : Q_{i,j}$ for $i = 1, 2, \ldots h$. $\square$

For example, Fig. 3 shows the MP graph of an MP input-output grammar equivalent to that given in Fig. 2, where in the input-output grammar $\varphi_2 = \varphi_3$ is equal to φ_2 of the previous grammar, while φ_4 of the input-output grammar is equal to φ_3 of the previous grammar.

The notion of input-output can be applied not only to the rules, but also to the variables. An *external variable* (called *parameter* in [11]) is a variable of an input rule without flux, therefore, a time series of values is assumed to be associated to it, in order to compute the dynamics of the grammar. Variables are called *internal* if they are not external. An MP grammar with external variables is also called *open*. It is not a generator of time series, but a function transforming the time series of its external variables into the time series of its internal variables.

An MP grammar is *non-cooperative* when in it each rule has at most one left variable, and it is *monic* when this variable occurs at most with multiplicity one. The following lemma can be proved in a similar way as the previous theorem [11].

Lemma 1. *For any MP grammar there exists a monic MP grammar that is dynamically equivalent to it.*

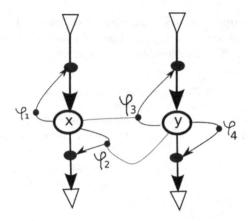

Fig. 3. The MP graph of a prey-predator input-output grammar.

An MP grammar is **positive** when, starting from a state where all variables are positive, then in all the following states variables and fluxes are always positive. Given an MP grammar G a positive grammar G', called the **positively controlled grammar associated to** G, is defined in the following manner. The grammar G' has the same variables and the same rules as G. Moreover, a regulator φ' is defined in G' in correspondence to each regulator φ of G in the following way. Let $s(x)$ be the value of variable x in the state s, and let $\varphi^+(s) = max\{\varphi(s), 0\}$. If we denote by $\Phi^-(x)$ the regulators of rules decreasing the variable x, then regulators φ' are defined from the regulators of G by requiring, for any variable x and for any state s, and for every $\varphi \in \Phi^-(x)$, that:

$$\varphi'(s) = 0 \quad \text{if} \quad \sum_{\varphi \in \Phi^-(x)} \varphi^+(s) > s(x) \tag{12}$$

$$\varphi'(s) = \varphi^+(s) \qquad \textbf{otherwise.} \tag{13}$$

A class of positive MP grammars, called **reactive MP grammars**, can be defined, by means of reaction weight functions and variable inertia functions. Namely, if we restrict to the case of monic grammars, this means that in any state s, for each rule r of type $x \to y$, the regulator is given by:

$$\varphi_r(s) = f_r(s) / \left(\sum_{l \in R^-(x)} f_l(s) + h_x(s) \right)$$

where $R^-(x)$ is the set of rules consuming x, f are the reaction weight functions (indexed by the rule symbols) and h_x is the inertia function of variable x (for input rules, regulators coincide with their reaction weight functions). The following theorem is proved in [11].

Theorem 3. *For any positive MP grammar there exists a dynamically equivalent reactive MP grammar and vice versa.*

3.5 MP Computability

In this section, we extend previous results (see [34, 35]) by showing that the class of positively controlled MP grammars is *computational universal*, and moreover, a particular simple form for regulators ensures the computational universality.

Let us consider a definition of register machine which is a variant of the Minsky's model given in [36]. It is a construct:

$$M = (\mathbb{R}, \mathbb{I}, \mathbb{O}, \mathbb{P})$$

where $\mathbb{R}$ is a set $\{R_1, ..., R_n\}$ of registers, $\mathbb{I} \subseteq \mathbb{R}$ is the set of input registers, while $\mathbb{O} \subseteq \mathbb{R}$ is the set of output registers. $\mathbb{P}$ is a program, that is, a sequence of instructions $I_1, ..., I_m$ of the following types:

- Increment of register R, denoted with $Inc(R)$.
- Decrement of register R, denoted with $Dec(R)$.
- Go-to instruction I_k if register $R_j = 0$, denoted with $Jnz(R_j, l_k)$.
- *Halt*, stopping the computation.

A computation of M is obtained by putting positive integers in the input registers (all the other registers implicitly contain zero) and by executing the instructions of the program in the order they are, apart the go-to instructions that specify as next instruction to execute one which possibly is not the following one in the sequential order. When the Halt instruction is executed, the results of the computation are the numbers put in the output registers.

For example the sum of two numbers greater than zero, which are put in registers R_1 and R_2, is given by the content of register R_1 at the end of the computation of the following program:

$1 : Inc(R_1)$
$2 : Dec(R_2)$
$3 : Jnz(R_2, 1)$
$4 : Halt$

Theorem 4. *For any Register Machine M there exists a monic positive MP grammar G_M equivalent to M.*

Proof. Given a register machine M with a program of m instruction, we consider an MP grammar G_M with an instruction variable for each instruction I_h of M, plus an extra instruction variable H, and a register variable for each register R_j of M (register variables are denoted in the same way registers are denoted in M). All register variables are initialized with the same values that the registers have in M, and all instruction variables are zero. If M has the program consisting of instruction $I_1, I_2, \ldots, I_m$, then G_M has the set of rules R_M translating into MP rules the program of M, according the following procedure.

Transtation Algorithm from Register Machines to MP Positive Grammars

1. $R_M := \{\emptyset \to I_1 : 1\}$
2. **for** $h = 1$ **to** m **do**
3. **begin**
4. **if** $I_h = Halt$ **then** add to R_M the rule $I_h \to H : I_h$
5. **if** $I_h = Inc(R_j)$ **then** add to R_M the rules $\emptyset \to R_j : I_h$ and $I_h \to I_{h+1} : I_h$
6. **if** $I_h = Dec(R_j)$ **then** add to R_M the rule $R_j \to \emptyset : I_h$ and $I_h \to I_{h+1} : I_h$
7. **if** $I_h = Jnz(R_j, k)$ **then** add to R_M the rules specified below.
8. **end**

The translation of $Halt, Inc, Dec$ is very clear. In order to translate $Jnz(R_j, k)$, which is the more complex instruction to translate, we follow a step-by-step method. First, we assume that (the content of) register R_j is either 0 or 1. In this case $I_h = Jnz(R_j, k)$ is translated by the two following rules (where exponent $+$ is in the sense of Eq. (13)):

1. $I_h \to I_k : (R_j)^+$
2. $I_h \to I_{h+1} : (R_j + I_h)^+$

In fact, if $R_j = 0$ the first rule does not change its variables and the second rule applies that produces $I_{h+1} = 1$. Otherwise, if $R_j = 1$ the first rule is active and the second one is blocked by the control of positivity because its flux is 2, but $I_h = 1$.

If R_j can contain any null or positive value, the idea of the translation above needs to be realized in a more complex way, and some auxiliary variables have to be introduced: H_j, L_h, F_h, F_{h+1}, and these MP rules are added to our translation of the register program (for simplicity sake, in fluxes of rules symbol $()^+$ is omitted, but implicitly intended).

1. $R_j \to H_j : I_h$
2. $I_h \to L_h : I_h$
3. $L_h \to F_k : H_j$
4. $L_h \to F_{h+1} : L_h + H_j$
5. $H_j \to R_j : F_k$
6. $H_j \to R_j : F_{h+1}$
7. $F_k \to I_k : F_k$
8. $F_{h+1} \to I_{h+1} : F_{h+1}$

Here, (if $R_j > 0$), the value 1 from I_h and 1 from R_j are moved, with the same flux, to the auxiliary variables H_j, L_h respectively. In this manner, the same strategy of the translation above can be applied to these copy variables, by means of the rules (3) and (4). Then, the original value of register R_j (that possibly was decremented) has to be restored, by means of the rules (5) and (6). In conclusion, the values of copy variables have to be transferred to the original ones, by means of the rules (7) and (8). In this manner, any register machine program is translated into a set of MP rules.

However, we want go a step further, by giving a translation where the MP rules are regulated by single variables. To this end, rule (4) is replaced by other rules, where sum of variables does not appear. Namely, an auxiliary variable K_h is added, such that, rules (4) and (5) put in K_h the sum of H_j and L_h, and rule (4) of the translation above is replaced by rule (6) of the new translation. The overall translation becomes as follows:

1. $R_j \rightarrow H_j : I_h$
2. $I_h \rightarrow L_h : I_h$
3. $L_h \rightarrow F_k : H_j$
4. $H_j \rightarrow K_h : H_j$
5. $L_h \rightarrow K_h : L_h$
6. $L_h \rightarrow F_{h+1} : K_h$
7. $H_j \rightarrow R_j : F_k$
8. $H_j \rightarrow R_j : F_{h+1}$
9. $F_k \rightarrow I_k : F_k$
10. $F_{h+1} \rightarrow I_{h+1} : F_{h+1}$.

Now, let us consider the dynamics of G_M, starting from the initial state ($I_1 = 1$, the remaining instruction variables are set equal to zero), and with the register variables having as values the contents that the corresponding registers in M. According to the rules given in G_M, we can easily verify that in G_M, register variables change according to the program of machine M, and the dynamics of G_M halts in the configuration that corresponds to the halting configuration of the machine M (with the same contents of registers). It is easy to verify that the obtained MP grammar is positive, because, when rules consuming a variable are more than one, we can check that only one of them has a flux different from zero.   □

The last part of the proof of previous theorem provides the following general result ensuring the computational universality for an extremely simple class of MP grammars (Fig. 4).

Theorem 5. *For any Register Machine M there exists a monic positive MP grammar G_M (dynamically) equivalent to M where regulators are single variables.*

A result given in [11], which is related to the MP grammars as computing devices, shows that in an MP representation of an algorithm, the notion of program, as sequence of instructions, it completely replaced by a graph. In fact when some input tokens are placed in some input membranes, then the computation flux is determined by the topology of the MP graph. This implies, that, as far as, efficient realizations of MP graphs are available, they become a sort of "universal computational circuits". This possibility suggest to investigate about possible physical implementations of computational MP graphs (based on photon movements?) (Fig. 5).

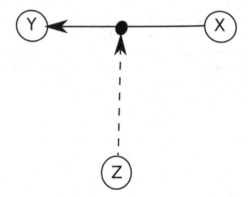

Fig. 4. The basic module of a (monic) MP grammar where regulators are single variables (the analogy with an electronic valve is clearly apparent).

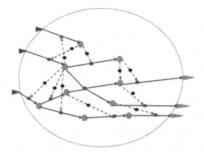

Fig. 5. The MP graph of an MP grammar variable regulated. Inputs are on the left and outputs on the right. The whole graph consists of a networks of ternary modules: left and right variables of an MP monic rule with a variable regulating the rule.

A second aspect of MP computing (or metabolic computing) is related to the natural representation of circular functions by means of MP grammar [18,30]. In this way computing with (approximate) real numbers can be done in the same framework used for integer based computations. Moreover, according to Fourier representation by trigonometric series, we could reformulate, in terms of MP grammars, DFT Discrete Fourier Transforms and investigate about the possible advantages of applying MP grammars to this field.

3.6 Complex Oscillations

MP grammars providing exact periodical dynamics, such as those of circular functions, can be defined by means of simple rules [18]. However, it is really surprising that when we apply MP regression to time series of sine and cosine functions, we get essentially regulators that are implied by the classical definitions of these functions, according to their geometrical or analytical characterization

[30]. This is strong proof the capacity of MP regression of discovering the MP logic responsible of an observed dynamics.

In [11,14,32] analyses of MP grammars with oscillating behaviors were developed. Oscillations are a key features of biological phenomena. At end of Chap. 3 in [11] it is argued that this aspect is intrinsically related to the open membrane organization of life, and to the natural orientation of chemical reactions. MP grammars allow us to express in rigorous terms this aspect and to investigate on some important features of oscillations. For example, a precise definition of oscillating system shows that this concept has to be carefully distinguished from the notion of periodic system. In fact, the oscillator Vega, an MP grammar defined in [11], is surely oscillating in a very wide interval, but it is shown in [14] that it is never passes twice on the same point of its state space, and that complex MP oscillators can be obtained by MP grammars where rules are organized in *overlapping cycles* (chains of rules sharing variables, of kind depicted in Fig. 6), where the more is the number of these cycles, the more is complex the resulting oscillatory dynamics.

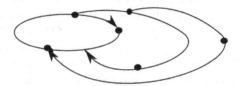

Fig. 6. An example of overlapping cycles in the structure of an MP grammar.

Elaborating on this idea of overlapping cycles, it was possible to design MP grammars exhibiting chaotic dynamics. Moreover, in [32] it is shown that when MP regression is applied to time series of chaotic MP dynamics, the regulators responsible of chaos generation are completely recognized, even when chaos seems to hide any pattern of dynamical regularity.

3.7   Biological Applications

An interesting application of MP grammars is presented in [16]. Here we started from the time series of gene expressions of a cancer cell under an effect E that inhibits the cancer growth factor HER2. After standard procedures of error filtering and data normalization, the expression time series were selected that show a behavior clearly correlated to the inhibitory effect E. This means that genes having time series that are constant in time, or with a chaotic shape, are considered to be scarcely related to E. Therefore, only about one thousand genes having time series with "regular" shapes were selected. Then we clustered these curves in eight types: linear-quick-up, linear-slow-up, linear-quick-down, linear-slow-down, parabolic-up, parabolic-down, cubic-up-down, cubic-down-up. Consequently, genes were grouped in eight clusters: C1, C2, C3, C4, C5, C6, C7, C8, to which an average curve was associated, and which constituted the variables of a dynamical system under investigation. By means of the LGSS algorithm, MP grammars over these variables were searched for generating the related curves. The LGSS algorithm was applied with a set of regressors constituted by simple monomials over the variables. At end, we got a number of possible MP grammars. One of them had the most reasonable set of regulation maps, according to the literature about gene regulatory networks (Fig. 7). We know that the cancer cell presents a resistance to the inhibition of the HER2 factor. Can our MP grammar tell us something about this resistance phenomenon? A deduction, coming from the obtained grammar, concerns with clusters with cubic behavior C7, C8. In fact, from the MP grammar we obtained, with a very easy translation, a regulation networks among clusters. In this network it appears clearly that the HER2 factor promotes C7, while inhibits C8. However, their curves expressions behave in conflict with this HER2 effect. We interpreted this phenomenon as related to the observed resistance. In fact, a possible explanation of the discordance of behaviors of C7 an C8, with respect to HER2 effect, could be the chain of regulation influences in the network. Namely, it transforms the effect of a linear regulation at the beginning of the chain into a non-linear effect at the end of it (this is a typical situation occurring in MP grammars). Based on this intuition, the genes in the clusters C1 and C3 (regulating clusters that regulate C7 and C8) were analyzed. The investigations about genes of clusters C1 and C3 allowed physicians to discover genes whose inhibition determine the disappearing of resistance, by finding an unknown role of gene E2F2 in breast cancer gene regulations. This is a proof that conceptual analyses based on MP grammars can reveal deep interactions having important roles in the observed dynamics. In Table 2 other examples of MP-modeling are listed, with the corresponding references.

Table 2. MP models obtained by MP Regression.

Belousov-Zhabotinsky, Prigogine's Brusselator (BZ)	[37,38]
Lotka-Volterra, Predator-Prey dynamics (LV)	[29,39,40]
Susceptible-Infected-Recovered Epidemics (SIR)	[38,41]
Early Amphybian Mitotic Cycle (AMC)	[20,42,43]
Drosophila Circadian Rythms (DCR)	[38]
Non Photochemical Quenching in Photosynthesis (NPQ)	[44]
Minimal Diabetes Mellitus (MDM)	[15,21]
Bi-catalytic Synthetic Oscillator	[17]
Synthetic Oscillators	[14,18]
Gene Expression Dynamics	[15,16]

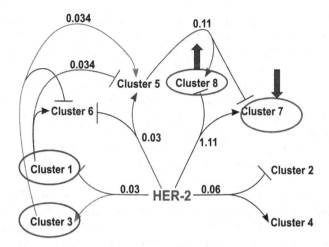

Fig. 7. The gene expression network represented by the eight-variables MP grammar deduced in [16]. Arrows denote promotion, while bars denote inhibition. The dynamics is obtained during inhibition of the cancer growth factor HER2. Full arrows indicate the expected behaviors, which contradicts the observed one.

4   Open Problems

This paper presents a new perspective of considering recurrent equations. Usually, their investigation is aimed at finding analytical methods to solve them or to determine properties of their dynamics [45]. On the contrary, here we do not cope with their solutions, because their intrinsic algorithmic (iterative) nature provides a direct computation of their dynamics. Of course, in this computation the dynamics at step n can be computed only after computing it in the steps preceding n, but this is not a real limitation if the computation is performed automatically and with a good approximation.

Using MP grammars, recurrent equations are constructed by assigning regulators to MP rules. In this perspective, regulators replace forces that in classical mechanics are the causes of observed motions. In fact, regulators may be related to a big number of unknown forces, very difficult to individuate and to discriminate. Therefore, regulators express abstract entities of rational and compact reconstruction of the internal logic underlying an observed dynamics. When the complexity and the indetermination of systems do not allow us other ways of analysis, this could be an important chance to the comprehension of phenomena.

We would like to stress that MP regression automatically calculates not only the values of the coefficients, *but also the form of regulators as linear combinations of some primitive functions.*

Some open problems naturally arise in the context of MP grammars, some of them were partially addressed [11], but systemic solutions deserve a further research and probably new ideas and methods. Some of them are listed below.

Problem 1. Given a system with thousands variables, how to simplify it in order to obtain a reduced system that, at same time, retains many important dynamical aspects of the original one, so that discovering MP grammars for the reduced system provides a useful knowledge about the investigated system?

Problem 2. When an MP Regression Algorithm is applied, according to different values of its parameters, many possible solutions can be found. How to systematically evaluate the solutions in order to choose the best one for a given kind of dynamics inverse problem?

Problem 3. MP Regression algorithms based on different methods have been developed. How to integrate them in order to improve the adequacy and of the results?

Problem 4. In the context of biological dynamics, when an MP grammar is found by means of MP regression, we get a sort of "abstract rule" associated to an observed dynamics. How to "read" this rule in a significant biological way? For example, if our variables represent quantities of proteins produced inside a cell, can the MP rules to be linked to specific mechanisms of gene, or gene complexes, activations? If only in some cases this could be successfully obtained, an important achievement would be reached toward the reasons determining specific forms of biological regulations.

5   Future Outlook

As we claimed in the introduction, MP theory shares many aspects that are crucial in problems addressed by Machine Learning. Therefore it seems natural to search for integrative approaches which could bring benefits to both two fields. This kind of cross-fertilization could be a sure advantage for biomedical applications. In fact, computational models of pathological processes are a topic of increasing interest in all the situations where personalized medical approaches are required in the medical challenges of the next future.

References

1. Holzinger, A.: Editorial integrative machine learning for health. In: Machine Learning for Health Informatics. Springer (2016)
2. Manca, V., Bianco, L., Fontana, F.: Evolution and oscillation in P systems: applications to biological phenomena. In: Mauri, G., Păun, G., Pérez-Jiménez, M.J., Rozenberg, G., Salomaa, A. (eds.) WMC 2004. LNCS, vol. 3365, pp. 63–84. Springer, Heidelberg (2005). doi:10.1007/978-3-540-31837-8_4
3. Gh, P.: Membrane Computing: An Introduction. Springer, Heidelberg (2002)
4. Ciobanu, G., Perez-Jimenez, M.J., Păun, G.: Applications of Membrane Computing. Spinger, Heidelberg (2006)
5. Păun, G., Rozenberg, G., Salomaa, A.: Oxford Handbook of Membrane Computing. Oxford University Press, New York (2010)
6. Frisco, P., Gheorghe, M., Pérez-Jiménez, M.J. (eds.): Applications of Membrane Computing in Systems and Synthetic Biology. Springer, Switzerland (2014)

7. Manca, V.: Fundamentals of metabolic P systems. In: The Oxford Handbook of Membrane Computing, pp. 475–498. Oxford University Press (2009)
8. Manca, V.: From P to MP systems. In: Păun, G., Pérez-Jiménez, M.J., Riscos-Núñez, A., Rozenberg, G., Salomaa, A. (eds.) WMC 2009. LNCS, vol. 5957, pp. 74–94. Springer, Heidelberg (2010). doi:10.1007/978-3-642-11467-0_7
9. Manca, V.: Metabolic P systems. In: Scholarpedia, vol. 5(3), pp. 9273 (2010). http://www.scholarpedia.org/
10. Manca, V.: An outline of MP modeling framework. In: Csuhaj-Varjú, E., Gheorghe, M., Rozenberg, G., Salomaa, A., Vaszil, G. (eds.) CMC 2012. LNCS, vol. 7762, pp. 47–55. Springer, Heidelberg (2013). doi:10.1007/978-3-642-36751-9_4
11. Manca, V.: Infobiotics: Information in Biotic Systems. Springer, Heidelberg (2013)
12. Manca, V., Castellini, A., Franco, G., Marchetti, L., Pagliarini, R.: Metabolic P systems: a discrete model for biological dynamics. Chin. J. Electron. **22**, 717–723 (2013)
13. Marchetti, L., Manca, V.: A methodology based on MP theory for gene expression analysis. In: Gheorghe, M., Păun, G., Rozenberg, G., Salomaa, A., Verlan, S. (eds.) CMC 2011. LNCS, vol. 7184, pp. 300–313. Springer, Heidelberg (2012). doi:10.1007/978-3-642-28024-5_20
14. Manca, V.: Algorithmic models of biochemical dynamics: Mp grammars synthetizing complex oscillators. Int. J. Nanotechnol. Mol. Comput. **3**, 24–37 (2013)
15. Marchetti, L., Manca, V., Pagliarini, R., Bollig-Fischer, A.: MP modelling for systems biology: two case studies. In: Frisco, P., Gheorghe, M., Pérez-Jiménez, M.J. (eds.) Applications of Membrane Computing in Systems and Synthetic Biology. ECC, vol. 7, pp. 223–245. Springer, Heidelberg (2014). doi:10.1007/978-3-319-03191-0_7
16. Bollig-Fischer, A., Marchetti, L., Mitrea, C., Wu, J., Kruger, A., Manca, V., Draghici, S.: Modeling time-dependent transcription effects of her2 oncogene and discovery of a role for e2f2 in breast cancer cell-matrix adhesion. Bioinformatics **30**, 3036–3043 (2014)
17. Manca, V.: The metabolic algorithm for P systems: principles and applications. Theoret. Comput. Sci. **404**, 142–155 (2008)
18. Manca, V., Marchetti, L.: Metabolic approximation of real periodical functions. J. Logic Algebraic Program. **79**, 363–373 (2010)
19. Manca, V., Marchetti, L.: Log-gain stoichiometric stepwise regression for MP systems. Int. J. Found. Comput. Sci. **22**, 97–106 (2011)
20. Manca, V., Marchetti, L.: Goldbeter's mitotic oscillator entirely modeled by MP systems. In: Gheorghe, M., Hinze, T., Păun, G., Rozenberg, G., Salomaa, A. (eds.) CMC 2010. LNCS, vol. 6501, pp. 273–284. Springer, Heidelberg (2010). doi:10.1007/978-3-642-18123-8_22
21. Manca, V., Marchettii, L., Pagliarini, R.: MP modelling of glucose-insulin interactions in the intravenous glucose tolerance test. Int. J. Natural Comput. Res. **3**, 13–24 (2011)
22. Manca, V., Marchetti, L.: Solving dynamical inverse problems by means of metabolic p systems. Biosystems **109**, 78–86 (2012)
23. Manca, V., Marchetti, L.: An algebraic formulation of inverse problems in mp dynamics. Int. J. Comput. Math. **90**, 845–856 (2013)
24. Castellini, A., Zucchelli, M., Busato, M., Manca, V.: From time series to biological network regulations. Mol. Biosyst. **9**(1), 225–233 (2013)
25. Castellini, A., Zucchelli, M., Busato, M., Manca, V.: From time series to biological network regulations: an evolutionary approach. Mol. Biosyst. **9**, 225–233 (2013)

26. Castellini, A., Paltrinieri, D., Manca, V.: Mp-geneticsynth: Inferring biological network regulations from time series. Bioinformatics **31**, 785–787 (2015)
27. Marchetti, L., Manca, V.: Mptheory Java library: a multi-platform Java library for systems biology based on the metabolic P theory. Bioinformatics **31**, 1328–1330 (2015)
28. Brin, M., Stuck, G.: Introduction to Dynamical Systems. Cambridge University Press, Cambridge (2002)
29. Fontana, F., Manca, V.: Predator-prey dynamics in P systems ruled by metabolic algorithm. BioSystems **91**, 545–557 (2008)
30. Manca, V., Marchetti, L.: Recurrent solutions to dynamics inverse problems: a validation of MP regression. J. Appl. Comput. Math. **3**, 1–8 (2014)
31. Manca, V., Bianco, L.: Biological networks in metabolic p systems. BioSystems **372**, 165–182 (2008)
32. Manca, V., Marchetti, L., Zelinka, I.: On the inference of deterministic chaos: evolutionary algorithm and metabolic P system approaches. In: 2014 IEEE Congress on Evolutionary Computation (CEC), pp. 1483–1488. IEEE, Beijing (2014)
33. Manca, V.: Log-gain principles for metabolic P systems. In: Condon, A., Harel, D., Kok, J.N., Salomaa, A., Winfree, E. (eds.) Algorithmic Bioprocesses, pp. 585–605. Springer, Heidelberg (2009)
34. Manca, V., Lombardo, R.: Computing with Multi-membranes. In: Gheorghe, M., Păun, G., Rozenberg, G., Salomaa, A., Verlan, S. (eds.) CMC 2011. LNCS, vol. 7184, pp. 282–299. Springer, Heidelberg (2012). doi:10.1007/978-3-642-28024-5_19
35. Gracini–Guiraldelli, R.H., Manca, V.: Automatic translation of MP$^+$V systems to register machines. In: Rozenberg, G., Salomaa, A., Sempere, J.M., Zandron, C. (eds.) CMC 2015. LNCS, vol. 9504, pp. 185–199. Springer, Heidelberg (2015). doi:10.1007/978-3-319-28475-0_13
36. Minsky, M.L.: Computation: Finite and Infinite Machines. Prentice Hall, Englewood Cliffs (1967)
37. Hilborn, R.C.: Chaos and Nonlinear Dynamics. Oxford University Press, New York (2000)
38. Bianco, L., Fontana, F., Franco, G., Manca, V.: P systems for biological dynamics. In: Ciobanu, G., et al. (eds.) Applications of P Systems, Vol. 3, N. 1, pp. 5–23. Springer, Heidelberg (2006)
39. Lotka, A.J.: Analytical note on certain rhythmic relations in organic systems. Proc. Natl. Acad. Sci. U.S. **6**, 410–415 (1920)
40. Volterra, V.: Fluctuations in the abundance of a species considered mathematically. Nature **118**, 558–60 (1926)
41. Lambert, J.D.: Computational Methods in Ordinary Differential Equations. Wiley, New York (1973)
42. Goldbeter, A.: Biochemical Oscillations and Cellular Rhythms: The Molecular Bases of Periodic and Chaotic Behaviour. Cambridge University Press, Cambridge (1996)
43. Bonnici, V.: Computational approaches to cellular rhythms. Nature **420**, 238–245 (2002)
44. Manca, V., Pagliarini, R., Zorzan, S.: A photosynthetic process modelled by a metabolic p system. Nat. Comput. **8**, 847–864 (2009)
45. Luenberger, D.G.: Introduction to Dynamic Systems. Wiley, New York (1979)

Empowering Bridging Term Discovery
for Cross-Domain Literature Mining
in the TextFlows Platform

Matic Perovšek[1,2]([✉]), Matjaž Juršič[1,2], Bojan Cestnik[1,3], and Nada Lavrač[1,2,4]

[1] Jožef Stefan Institute, Ljubljana, Slovenia
matic.perovsek@ijs.si
[2] Jožef Stefan International Postgraduate School, Ljubljana, Slovenia
[3] Temida d.o.o, Ljubljana, Slovenia
[4] University of Nova Gorica, Nova Gorica, Slovenia

Abstract. Given its immense growth, scientific literature can be explored to reveal new discoveries, based on yet uncovered relations between knowledge from different, relatively isolated fields of research specialization. This chapter proposes a bisociation-based text mining approach, which shows to be effective for cross-domain knowledge discovery. The proposed cross-domain literature mining functionality, including text acquisition, text preprocessing, and bisociative cross-domain literature mining facilities, is made publicly available within a new browser-based workflow execution engine TextFlows, which supports visual construction and execution of text mining and natural language processing (NLP) workflows. To support bisociative cross-domain literature mining, the TextFlows platform includes implementations of several elementary and ensemble heuristics that guide the expert in the process of exploring new cross-context bridging terms. We have extended the TextFlows platform with several components, which—together with document exploration and visualization features of the CrossBee human-computer interface—make it a powerful, user-friendly text analysis tool for exploratory cross-domain knowledge discovery. Another novelty of the developed technology is the enabled use of controlled vocabularies to improve bridging term extraction. The potential of the developed functionality was showcased in two medical benchmark domains.

Keywords: Literature mining · Literature-based discovery · Cross-context linking terms · Creativity support tools · Human-computer interaction · Workflows

1 Introduction

Understanding complex phenomena and solving difficult problems often requires knowledge from different domains to be combined and cross-domain associations to be taken into account. These kinds of context crossing associations, called *bisociations* [1], are often needed for creative, innovative discoveries.

© Springer International Publishing AG 2016
A. Holzinger (Ed.): ML for Health Informatics, LNAI 9605, pp. 59–98, 2016.
DOI: 10.1007/978-3-319-50478-0_4

Bisociative knowledge discovery is a challenging task motivated by a trend of over-specialization in research and development, which usually results in deep— but relatively isolated—knowledge islands. Scientific literature too often remains closed and cited only in professional sub-communities. In addition, the information that is related across different contexts is difficult to identify using associative approaches, like the standard association rule learning [2] known from the data mining and machine learning literature. Therefore, the ability of literature mining methods and software tools to support the experts in their knowledge discovery processes—especially in searching for yet unexplored connections between different domains—is becoming increasingly important. Cross-domain literature mining is closely related to bisociative knowledge discovery as defined in [3]. Assuming two different domains of interest, a crucial step in cross-domain knowledge discovery is the identification of interesting bridging terms (B-terms), appearing in both literatures, which carry the potential of revealing the links connecting the two domains.

This chapter presents a powerful approach to literature based cross-context knowledge discovery that supports the process of bridging term extraction. The developed methodology helps the experts in searching for hidden links that connect seemingly unrelated domains. The main novelty of the presented approach is the combination of document acquisition and text preprocessing facilities with a new facility for term extraction through ensemble-based ranking of terms according to their bisociative potential, which may contribute to novel cross-domain discoveries. The proposed methodology is implemented in a web-based text mining platform TextFlows[1]. To this end, the TextFlows platform was connected to the human-computer interface of system CrossBee [4,5]. In the methodology presented in this chapter, the CrossBee web application—which we originally developed as an off-the-shelf solution for finding bisociations bridging two domains—is used as a user interface to facilitate bridging term discovery through sophisticated document visualization and exploration. This work proposes a further extension of the methodology by facilitating the use of controlled vocabularies, enhancing the heuristics capability to rank the actual B-terms at the top of the ranked term list. With all these features, the TextFlows platform, which now includes the reusable text analytics workflows combined with the CrossBee document exploration interface, has become a publicly available creativity support tool (CST), supporting creative discovery of new cross-domain hypotheses.

The chapter is organized as follows. Section 2 provides a brief glossary of key terms that will facilitate a common understanding of the main topics presented here. Section 3 presents the state-of-the-art in the area of literature-based discovery. Section 4 illustrates the problem of bridging term ranking and B-term exploration through a use case scenario, followed by an overview of the methodology. Section 5 comprises the core contribution of this chapter. The TextFlows

---

[1] Our new text mining platform, named TextFlows, is publicly available for use at http://textflows.org. The source code (open sourced under the MIT Licence) is available at https://github.com/xflows/textflows. Detailed installation instructions are provided with the source code.

platform, acting as the enabling technology for implementing the developed cross-domain link discovery approach, is described in Sect. 5.1. The elementary and ensemble heuristics used in bridging term discovery are described in Sect. 5.2. Section 5.3 presents details of document acquisition, text preprocessing and literature based discovery workflows implemented in TextFlows. Controlled vocabulary extension of the methodology is presented in Sect. 5.4. Evaluation of the developed methodology on two medical benchmark problems is provided in Sect. 6, Finally, Sect. 7 concludes with a summary of most important features of the presented approach and some directions for further work.

2   Glossary

Bisociation: the combination of knowledge from seemingly unrelated domains into novel cross-domain knowledge.

Bridging term: a term common to two disjoint domains, which is a candidate for the discovery of new knowledge or for formulation of new hypotheses, acting as a "bridge" between the two domains.

Literature-based discovery: using academic literature to find previously uncovered connections in existing domain knowledge.

Outlier detection: finding irregular or unusual data instances (documents in the case of literature mining) that do not conform to the expected distribution.

3   State-of-the-Art

According to Koestler [1], bisociative thinking occurs when a problem, idea, event or situation is perceived simultaneously in two or more "matrices of though" or domains. When two matrices of thought interact with each other, the result is either their fusion in a novel intellectual synthesis or their confrontation in a new aesthetic experience. He regarded many different mental phenomena that are based on comparison (such as analogies, metaphors, jokes, identification, anthropomorphism, and so on) as special cases of bisociation. More recently, this work was followed by the researchers interested in so-called bisociative knowledge discovery [6], where—according to Berthold—two concepts are bisociated if there is no direct, obvious evidence linking them and if one has to cross different domains to find the link, where a new link must provide some novel insight into the problem addressed.

In the area of literature based discovery (LBD), Swanson [7] and Smalheiser [8] developed an approach to assist the user in literature based discovery by detecting interesting cross domain terms with a goal to discover unknown relations between previously unrelated concepts. The online system ARROW-SMITH [8] takes as input two sets of titles of scientific papers from disjoint domains A and C and lists terms that are common to A and C; the resulting bridging terms (B-terms) are further investigated by the user for their potential to generate new scientific hypotheses. They defined the so-called *closed discovery process*, where domains A and C are specified by the expert at the beginning of the discovery process.

Inspired by this early work, literature mining approaches were further developed and successfully applied to different problems, such as finding associations between genes and diseases [9], diseases and chemicals [10], and others. [11] describe several quality-oriented web-based tools for the analysis of biomedical literature, which include the analysis of terms (biomedical entities such as disease, drugs, genes, proteins and organs) and provide concepts associated with a given term. A recent approach by Kastrin et al. [12] is complementary to the other LBD approaches, in that it uses different similarity measures (such as common neighbors, Jaccard index, and preferential attachment) for link prediction of implicit relationships in the Semantic MEDLINE network.

Early work by Swanson has shown that databases such as PubMed can serve as a rich source of yet hidden relations between usually unrelated topics, potentially leading to novel insights and discoveries. By studying two separate literatures—the literature on migraine headache and the articles on magnesium—[13] discovered "Eleven neglected connections", all of them supportive for the hypothesis that magnesium deficiency might cause migraine headache. Swanson's literature mining results have been later confirmed by laboratory and clinical investigations. This well-known example has become a gold standard in the literature mining field and has been used as a benchmark in several studies, including those presented in [14–16] as well as in our own past work [17,18]. Research in literature mining, conducted by Petrič et al. [17,18], suggests that bridging terms are more frequent in documents that are in some sense different from the majority of documents in a given domain. For example, [18] have shown that such documents, considered outlier documents of their own domain, contain a substantially larger amount of bridging-linking terms than the normal, non-outlier documents.

The experimental data used to test the methodology proposed in this work are papers from the combined migraine-magnesium domain, studied extensively by Swanson and his followers, as well as the combined autism-calcineurin domain pair explored in [17,19].

Our contribution in this chapter follows two lines of our past research. First, it continues the work on cross-domain document exploration in [17,18], which explore outlier documents as means for literature based discovery. Note that the problem of finding outliers has been extensively studied also by another researcher [20] and has an immense use in many real-world applications. Second, and most importantly, the chapter continues our work on cross-domain bisociation exploration with CrossBee [5], which is most closely related to the work described here. CrossBee is an off-the-shelf solution for finding bisociative terms bridging two domains, which—as will be shown—can be used as the default user interface to the methodology presented in this chapter. Given that the CrossBee user interface is an actual ingredient of the technology developed in this work, its user interface is described in some more detail than other LBD systems mentioned in this section.

The CrossBee HCI functionality includes the following facilities: (a) *Performance evaluation* that can be used to measure the quality of results, e.g., through plotting ROC curves when the actual bridging terms are known in advance. (b) *Marking of high-ranked terms* by emphasizing them, thus making them easier to spot throughout the application. (c) *B-term emphasis* can be used to mark the terms predefined as B-terms by the user. (d) *Domain separation* colors all the documents from the same domain with the same color, making an obvious distinction between the documents from the two domains. (e) *User interface customization* enables the user to decrease or increase the intensity of the following features: high-ranked term emphasis, B-term emphasis and domain separation; this facility was introduced to enable the user to set the intensity of these features, given that in cooperation with the experts we discovered that some of them like the emphasizing features while others do not.

Note that the CrossBee web interface was designed for end-users who are not computer scientists or data miners and who prefer using the system by following a fixed sequence of predefined methodological steps. However, for a more sophisticated user of developer, the weakness of CrossBee is the lack of possibility to experiment with different settings as well as the lack of possibility to extend the methodology with new ideas and then compare or evaluate the developed approaches. As another weakness, the CrossBee web application does not offer a downloadable library and documentation distribution or extensive help. These weaknesses were among the incentives for our new developments, resulting in the TextFlows platform and its elaborate mechanisms for detecting and exploring bisociative links between the selected domains of interest.

4   Methodology Overview

In cross-domain knowledge discovery, estimating which of the terms have a high potential for interesting discoveries is a challenging research question. It is especially important for cross-context scientific discovery such as understanding complex medical phenomena or finding new drugs for yet not fully understood illnesses.

In our approach we focus on the closed discovery process, where two disjointed domains A and C are specified at the beginning of the discovery process and the main goal is to find bridging terms (see Fig. 1) which support validation of the novel hypothesized connection between the two domains. Given this motivation, the main functionality of the presented approach is bridging term (B-term) discovery, implemented through ensemble based term ranking, where an ensemble heuristic composed of six elementary heuristics was constructed for term evaluation.

To ensure the best user experience in the process of bridging term discovery we have combined the visual programming interface of the TextFlows workflow construction and execution platform with the bridging term exploration system CrossBee; CrossBee provides a user interface for term and document visualization that additionally supports the expert in finding relevant documents and exploration of the top-ranked bisociative terms.

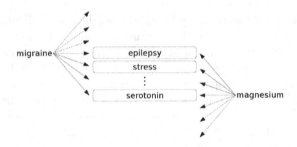

Fig. 1. Bridging term discovery when exploring migraine and magnesium document corpora, with B-terms as identified in [13] in the middle.

4.1 Methodology Illustration

The ensemble based term ranking methodology (using the final ensemble heuristic) is illustrated in Fig. 2.

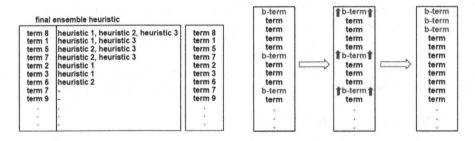

Fig. 2. Term ranking approach: first, ensemble heuristics vote for terms, next, terms are sorted according to their potential B-term (as shown on left). Consequently, bridging terms with the highest bridging term potential should receive the highest scores (as shown on the right side).

The user starts the bridging term discovery process in TextFlows by either constructing a new workflow for cross-domain discovery or by opening an existing workflow (such as the workflow shown in Fig. 4 of Sect. 4.2). In the first case, the user is required to input either a PubMed query or a file with documents from the two domains, where each line contains a document with exactly three tab-separated entries: (a) document identifier, (b) domain acronym, and (c) the document text. The user is able to tailor the preprocessing steps to his own needs by simply altering the workflow using the TextFlows visual programming user interface, which enables simple addition, connection and removal of components from the workflow canvas. In this way, the user can also modify the ensemble of elementary heuristics, outlier documents identified by external outlier detection software, the already known bisociative terms (B-terms), and others. When the user runs the workflows (by clicking the run button) the system starts with the process of text preprocessing, followed by the computation of elementary heuristics, the ensemble bisociation scores and term ranking.

After performing the calculation of bisociative potentials for every term in the vocabulary in TextFlows, the user is directed to the user-friendly tool Cross-Bee where one can efficiently investigate cross-domain links pointed out by the ensemble-based ranking methodology. CrossBee's document focused exploration empowers the user to filter and order the documents by various criteria, including detailed document view that provides a more detailed presentation of a single document including various term statistics. Methodology performance analysis supports the evaluation of the methodology by providing various data which can be used to measure the quality of the results, e.g., data for plotting the ROC curves. High-ranked term emphasis marks the terms according to their bisociation score calculated by the ensemble heuristic. When using this feature all high-ranked terms are emphasized throughout the whole application thus making them easier to spot (see different font sizes in Fig. 3). B-term emphasis marks the terms defined as B-terms by the user (yellow terms in Fig. 3). Domain separation is a simple but effective option which colors all the documents from the same domain with the same color, making an obvious distinction between the documents from the two domains (different colors in Fig. 3). User interface customization enables the user to decrease or increase the intensity of the following features: high-ranked term emphasis, B-term emphasis and domain separation.

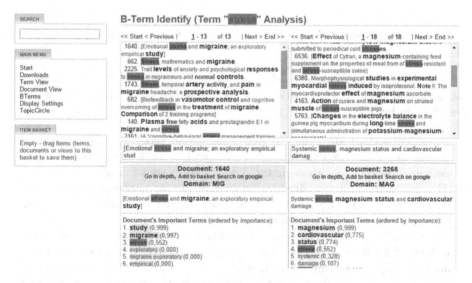

Fig. 3. One of the useful features of the CrossBee interface is the side-by-side view of documents from the two domains under investigation. The analysis of the "stress" term from the migraine-magnesium domain is shown. The presented view enables efficient comparison of two documents, the left one from the migraine domain and the right one from the magnesium domain. (Color figure online)

4.2   Methodology Outline

This section describes how the complex methodology was developed as a work-flow in the TextFlows platform, by presenting the entire pipeline of natural language processing (NLP) and literature based discovery (LBD) components. The top-level overview of the methodology, shown in Fig. 4, consists of the following steps: document acquisition, document preprocessing, heuristics specification, candidate B-term extraction, heuristic terms scores calculation, and visualization and exploration. An additional ingredient shown in Fig. 4—methodology evaluation—is not directly part of the methodology, however it is an important step of the developed approach.

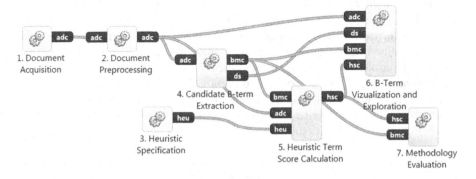

Fig. 4. Methodological steps of the cross-domain literature mining process.

Top-level procedural explanation of the workflow shown in Fig. 4 is given below, while detailed explanations of individual steps of the workflow are described in Sect. 5.3.

1. Document acquisition is the first step of the methodology. Its goal is to acquire documents of the two domains, label them with domain labels and pack both domains together into the annotated document corpus format.
2. The document preprocessing step is responsible for applying standard text preprocessing to the document corpus. The main parts are tokenization, stopword tagging, and token stemming/lemmatization.
3. The heuristic specification step enables detailed specification of the heuristics to be used for B-term ranking. The user specifies one or more heuristics, which are to be applied to evaluate the B-term candidates. Note that each individual heuristic can be composed of other heuristics, therefore an arbitrary complex list of heuristics can be composed in this step.
4. The candidate B-term extraction step takes care of extracting the terms which are later scored by the specified heuristics. There are various parameters which control which kind of terms are extracted from the documents (e.g., the maximal number of tokens to be joined together as a term, minimal term

corpus frequency, and similar). The outputs are the *BoW Dataset* (i.e. the documents in the standard Bag-of-Words (BoW) vector format) and a *Bow Model Constructor*. The latter stores the list of all candidate B-terms along with the information about the input documents from annotated document corpus as well as the exact data how each document was parsed. This data is needed e.g., by the CrossBee web application when displaying the documents since it needs to be able to exactly locate specific words inside a document, in order to color or emphasize such words.

5. Heuristic term score calculation is the most important step of the methodology. It takes the list of extracted B-term candidates and the list of specified heuristics and calculates a heuristic score for each candidate term for each heuristic. The heuristics calculation is optimized so that common information used by different heuristics is calculated only once. The output is structurally still a list of heuristics, however now each of them contains a bisociation score for each candidate B-term.

6. Visualization and exploration is the final step of the methodology. It has three main functionalities. It can either take the heuristically scored terms, rank the terms, and output the terms in the form of a table, or it can take the heuristically scored terms along with the parsed document corpus and send them both to the CrossBee web application for advanced visualization and exploration. Besides improved bridging concept identification and ranking, CrossBee also provides various content presentations which further speed up the process of bisociation exploration. These presentations include e.g., side-by-side document inspection (see Fig. 3), emphasizing of interesting text fragments, and uncovering similar documents.

7. Methodology evaluation was introduces as an additional step, which can be used during the development of the methodology. Its purpose is to calculate and visualize various metrics that were used to assess the quality of the methodology. Requirement to use these facilities is to allow the actual (predefined) B-terms of the domain of investigation to act as gold standard B-terms available for evaluating the quality of B-term extraction and ranking.

Evaluation of the methodology was actually performed on two problems: the standard migraine-magnesium problem well-known in LBD, and a more recent autism-calcineurin literature mining problem. The evaluation of the methodology (its results are presented in detail in Sect. 6) provides evidence that the users empowered with the CrossBee functionality of term ranking and visualization are able to perform the crucial actions in cross-domain discovery more effectively than with conventional text mining tools.

Note that the described pipeline represents an actual executable workflow implemented in the online cloud-based workflow composition and execution environment TextFlows. The entire workflow, whose components are explained in detail in Sect. 5.3, is available for public reuse[2].

---

[2] http://textflows.org/workflow/486/.

5   Methodology Implementation

After presenting the main functionality of the TextFlows platform, this section presents the core mechanism of bisociative term detection, i.e., the designed heuristics and the workflows implementing the methodology in TextFlows. The section concludes by presenting the methodology empowered by using a controlled vocabulary in the search for bridging term.

5.1   The TextFlows Platform

We developed the TextFlows platform[3] as an open-source, web-based text mining platform that supports the construction and execution of text mining and natural language processing workflows. TextFlows was designed as a cloud-based web application that can be accessed and controlled from anywhere while the processing is performed in a cloud of computing nodes. TextFlows differs from comparable text mining platforms by its design that allows that during runtime the TextFlows platform resides on a server (or on a cluster of machines) while its graphical user interface that allows workflow construction is served as a web application accessible from any modern web browser. Furthermore, the platform's distinguishing feature is the ease of sharing and publicizing workflows constructed in TextFlows, together with an ever growing roster of reusable workflow components and entire workflows. As completed workflows, data, and results can also be made public by the author of the workflow, the platform was used to serve as an integration platform for development of various components supporting the literature based cross-domain discovery process, and for construction and evaluation of workflows, implementing the methodology proposed in Sect. 4.2.

Following a modular design, workflow components in TextFlows are organized into packages which allows for easier distributed development. The TextFlows packages implement several text mining algorithms from LATINO[4][22], NLTK [23] and scikit-learn [24] libraries. Moreover, TextFlows is easily extensible by adding new packages and workflow components. Workflow components of several types allow graphical user interaction during run-time, and visualization of results by implementing views in JavaScript, HTML or any other format that can be rendered in a web browser (e.g., Flash, Java Applet).

Below we explain the concept of workflows in more detail, describe the key text mining concepts of TextFlows and present the newly implemented package with workflow components supporting literature based discovery.

---

[3] Our platform TextFlows is a fork of data mining platform ClowdFlows [21], adapted to text mining and enriched with text analytics and natural language processing algorithms. As a fork of ClowdFlows, it benefits from its service-oriented architecture, which allows the user to utilize arbitrary web-services as workflow components. In addition to the new functionality, its novelty is a common text representation structure and the development of 'hubs' for algorithm execution.

[4] LATINO (Link Analysis and Text Mining Toolbox) is open-source—mostly under the LGPL license—and is available at https://github.com/LatinoLib/LATINO/.

Workflows. Executable graphical representations of complex procedures can be represented as workflows. The workflow model is the main component of the TextFlows platform and consists of an abstract representation of workflows and workflow components. The graphical user interface used for constructing workflows follows a visual programming paradigm which simplifies the representation of complex procedures into a spatial arrangement of building blocks. The most basic unit component in a TextFlows workflow is a processing component, which is represented as a widget in the graphical representation. Considering its inputs and parameters, every such component performs a task and stores the results on its outputs. Different processing components are linked via connections through which data is transferred from a widget's output to another widget's input. An alternative widget input for a widget are parameters, which the user enters into the widgets text fields. The graphical user interface implements an easy-to-use way of arranging widgets on a canvas to form a graphical representation of a complex procedure.

Workflows in TextFlows are processed and stored on remote servers from where they can be accessed from anywhere, requiring only an internet connection. By default each workflow can only be accessed by its author, although the user can also choose to make it publicly available. The TextFlows platform generates a specific URL for each workflow that has been saved as public. The users can then simply share their workflows by publishing the corresponding URL. Whenever a public workflow is accessed by another user, a copy of the workflow is created on the fly and added to his private workflow repository. The workflow is copied with all the data to ensure the experiments can be repeated. This enables the user to tailor the workflow to his needs without modifying the original workflow.

Key Text Mining Concepts in TextFlows. The key concepts in text mining are a corpus or a document collection, a single document, and document features [25]. Below we describe the model of corpora, documents and annotations on documents in TextFlows, which are the fundamental parts of our methodology. When designing TextFlows, the emphasis was on providing common representations which are passed among the majority of widgets:

Annotated corpus. A document collection is any grouping of text documents to be used for text analytics purposes. In TextFlows the Python[5] class that represents a corpus of documents is called *AnnotatedDocumentCorpus (ADC)*. An ADC instance contains the collection of documents and its meta-data such as the authors, creation date, facts and notes about the dataset, etc. Features are stored in a simple key-value Python dictionary, where keys are strings and the values can store any Python object.

Annotated document. A single textual data unit within a collection—a document—is represented by the *AnnotatedDocument* class. An *AnnotatedDocument* instance may vary in size from a single sentence to a whole book. As with

---

[5] https://www.python.org/.

ADC, *AnnotatedDocument* instances also contain meta-data, such as author, date of publication, document length, assigned keywords, etc.

Annotation. Instances of the *Annotation* class are used to mark parts of the document, e.g., words, terms or sentences. Each *Annotation* instance has two pointers, one to the start and one to the end of the annotated stretch in the document text. These instances also have a type attribute used for grouping annotations of similar nature and contain key-value dictionaries of features, used by taggers to annotate parts of document with specific tags, e.g., annotations of type "token" that have a feature named "StopWord" with value "true", represent stop words in the document.

The Widget Repository. The following paragraphs present a subset of the TextFlows repository of widgets, which will be used in the workflows that implement the methodology proposed in Sect. 4.2.

Corpus and vocabulary acquisition. Document acquisition is usually the first step of every text mining methodology. TextFlows employs widgets which enable loading document corpora, labeling of documents with domain labels and converting them into the ADC structure. Document corpora can be loaded from files, where the dataset can be either a single text file, with each line representing a separate document, or a zip of files in which a document is represented as a file. Also supported is the upload of Word (.doc or .docx) and PDF files. Together with the text of the document the files may optionally contain document meta-data.

Corpus manipulation and visualization. TextFlows implements several widgets for manipulation of ADC data objects. These widgets allow the user to add new features, extract existing features from the document corpus, split document corpora (by either specifying conditions or by indices), merge different corpora, etc. A special widget in the platform is the *Document Corpus Viewer* widget, which visualizes the ADC data objects (note that TextFlows design emphasizes the importance of the ADC common document corpus representation which is passed among the majority of widgets). The interactive *Document Corpus Viewer* widget allows the user to check the results of individual widgets by visualizing the ADC data object from their outputs.

Text preprocessing. Preprocessing is a very important part of any form of knowledge extraction from text documents. Its main task is the transformation of unstructured data from text documents into a predefined well-structured data representation by extracting a high quality feature vector for every document in a given document corpus.

Our implementation employs the LATINO[6] [22], scikit-learn [24] and NLTK[7] [23] software libraries for its text preprocessing (and other processing) needs. These libraries *inter alia* contain the majority of elementary text preprocessing procedures as well as a large number of advanced procedures which support the conversion of a document corpus into a table of instances, thus converting every document into a table row representation of an instance.

The TextFlows preprocessing techniques are based on standard text mining concepts [25] and are implemented as separate categories. Every category possesses a unique hub widget, which has the task of applying a preprocessing technique from its category to the ADC data object. Every such widget is library independent, meaning that it can execute objects from either LATINO, NTLK or scikit-learn libraries. A standard collection of preprocessing techniques implemented in TextFlows includes: tokenization, stopword removal, Part-of-speech (PoS) tagging, as well as stemming and lemmatization.

In the data mining modeling phase (i.e. document classification or heuristic calculation), each document from the ADC structure needs to be represented as a set of document features it contains. In TextFlows the *Construct BoW Dataset and BoW Model Constructor* widget takes as an input an ADC data object and generates a sparse BoW model dataset (which can then be handed e.g. to a classifier). The widget takes as an input also several user defined parameters, which are taken into account when building the feature dataset. Besides the sparse BoW model dataset this widget also outputs a *BowModelConstructor* instance. This additional object contains settings which allow repetition of the feature construction steps on another document corpus. These settings include the input parameters, as well as the learned term weights and vocabulary.

Literature based discovery. This category of widgets supports the literature based discovery process. The package contains several widgets which specify different elementary heuristics. As will be described in Sect. 5.2, the basic heuristics are grouped into one of four categories: frequency-based, TF-IDF-based, similarity-based, outlier-based. Each category is represented by its own widget and the user is able to manually select its elementary heuristics through an interactive dialog. The literature based discovery package also contains several widgets which specify operations between elementary widgets, such as minimum, maximum, sum, norm, etc.

The library also contains two widgets which support the specification of ensemble heuristics, which will be described in Sect. 5.2: *Ensemble Heuristic Vote* and *Ensemble Average Position* widget. The first defines an ensemble voting heuristic (it calculates term votes according to Eq. 1 of Sect. 5.2), while the latter specifies an ensemble that calculates normalized sum of term position scores of the inputted heuristics (see Eq. 2 of Sect. 5.2).

---

[6] LATINO (Link Analysis and Text Mining Toolbox library) is open-source— mostly under the LGPL license—and is available at https://github.com/LatinoLib/ LATINO/.
[7] Natural Language Toolkit.

The most important widget from this package is the *Calculate Term Heuristic Scores* widget which takes as an input several heuristics specifications and performs the actual calculations. The decision for such an approach—having one widget which calculates all the heuristics—is that several elementary heuristics require the same intermediate results. These results can be cached and calculated only once, which results in faster computation. To this end, the TextFlows platform uses Compressed Sparse Row (CSR) matrices[8] to be able to store the matrix of features in memory and also to speed up algebraic operations on vectors and matrices.[9]

Literature based discovery package also contains the *Explore in CrossBee* widget which exports the final ranking results and the annotated document corpus into web application CrossBee, which offers manual exploration of terms and documents. Also, the *Rank Terms* widget can be used to display the ranked terms in the form of a table along with their respective scores.

5.2 Implemented Heuristics for Bridging Term Discovery

This section presents different groups of elementary and ensemble heuristics, which are used for B-term ranking in the core step of the proposed methodology, i.e. in the heuristic term score calculation step.

The heuristics are defined as functions that numerically evaluate the term quality by assigning it bisociation score to a term (measuring the potential that a term is actually a B-term). For the definition of an appropriate set of heuristics, we define a set of special (mainly statistical) properties of terms, which aim at distinguishing B-terms from regular terms; thus, these heuristics can also be viewed as advanced term statistics. All heuristics operate on the data retrieved from the documents in text preprocessing. Ranking all the terms using the scores calculated by an ideal heuristic should result in ranking all the B-terms at the top of a ranked list. This is an ideal scenario, which is not realistic; however, ranking by heuristic scores should at least increase the proportion of B-terms at the top of the ranked term list. Formally, a heuristic is a function with two inputs, i.e. a set of domain labeled documents D and a term t appearing in these documents, and one output, i.e. a score that represents the term's bisociation potential.

We will use the following notation: to state that the term's bisociation score b is equal to the result of a heuristic named *heurX*, we can denote it as $b = heurX(D, t)$. However, since the set of input documents is static when dealing with a concrete dataset, we can—for the sake of simplicity—omit the set of input

---

[8] Compressed Sparse Row (CSR) matrices are implemented in the scipy.sparse package http://docs.scipy.org/doc/scipy/reference/sparse.html.

[9] The *Calculate Term Heuristic Scores* widget also takes as input the *BowModelContructor* object and the *AnnotatedDocumentCorpus*. The parse settings from the *BowModelConstructor* object are used to construct Compressed Sparse Row (CSR) matrices, which represents the BoW model. TextFlows uses mathematical libraries numpy and scipy to efficiently perform the heuristics calculations.

documents from a heuristic notation and use only $b = heurX(t)$. Whenever we need to explicitly specify the set of documents to which the function is applied (never needed for a heuristic, but sometimes needed for auxiliary functions used in the formula for the heuristic), we write it as $funcX_D(t)$. For specifying the function's input document set, we have two options: either use D_u that stands for the (union) set of all the documents from all the domains, or use $D_n : n \in \{1..N\}$, which stands for the set of documents from the given domain n. In general, the following statement holds: $D_u = \cup_{n=1}^{N} D_n$, where N is the number of domains. In the most common scenario, when there are exactly two distinct domains, we also use the notation D_A for D_1 and D_C for D_2, similarly to Swanson's notation of symbols A and C as representatives of the initial and the target domain in the closed discovery setting, mentioned in Sect. 3.

Base Heuristics. We divide the heuristics into different sets for easier explanation; however, most of the described heuristics work fundamentally in a similar way—they all manipulate solely the data present in term and document vectors and derive the terms bisociation score. The exceptions to this are the outlier-based heuristics, which first evaluate outlier documents and only later use the information from the term vectors for B-term evaluation.

We can thus define four sets of base heuristics: frequency based, TF-IDF based, outlier based and similarity based heuristics. In following sections we describe each set in more detail.[10]

Frequency-based heuristics. We first define two auxiliary functions:

- $countTerm_D(t)$: counts the number of occurrences of term t in a document set D (called term frequency in TF-IDF related contexts),
- $countDoc_D(t)$: counts the number of documents in which term t appears in document set D (called document frequency in TF-IDF related contexts).

We define the following base heuristics:

- $freqTerm(t) = countTerm_{D_u}(t)$: term frequency in the two domains,
- $freqDoc(t) = countDoc_{D_u}(t)$: document frequency in the two domains,
- $freqRatio(t) = \frac{countTerm_{D_u}(t)}{countDoc_{D_u}(t)}$: term to document frequency ratio,
- $freqDomnRatioMin(t) = \min(\frac{countTerm_{D_1}(t)}{countTerm_{D_2}(t)}, \frac{countTerm_{D_2}(t)}{countTerm_{D_1}(t)})$: minimum of term frequencies ratio of the two domains,
- $freqDomnProd(t) = countTerm_{D_1}(t) \cdot countTerm_{D_2}(t)$: product of term frequencies of the two domains,
- $freqDomnProdRel(t) = \frac{countTerm_{D_1}(t) \cdot f countTerm_{D_2}(t)}{countTerm_{D_u}(t)}$: product of term frequencies of the two domains relative to the term frequency in all domains.

---

[10] Due to a large number of heuristics and auxiliary functions, we use the so called camel casing multi-word naming scheme for easier distinction; names are formed by word concatenation and capitalization of all non first words (e.g., *freqProdRel* and *tfidfProduct*).

TF-IDF-based heuristics. TF-IDF is a standard measure of term's importance in a document, which is used heavily in text mining research [26]. In the following heuristics definitions, we use the following auxiliary functions:

- $tfidf_d(t)$ stands for TF-IDF weight of term t in document d,
- $tfidf_D(t)$ represents TF-IDF weight of term t in the centroid vector of all documents d, $d \in D$, where the centroid vector is defined as an average of all document vectors and thus presents an average document of document collection D.

Heuristics based on TF-IDF are listed below:

- $tfidfSum(t) = \sum_{d \in D_u} tfidf_d(t)$: sum of all TF-IDF weights of term t in the two domains; this heuristic is analogous to freqTerm(t),
- $tfidfAvg(t) = \frac{\sum_{d \in D_u} tfidf_d(t)}{freqDoc_{D_u}(t)}$: average TF-IDF weights of term t across all domains,
- $tfidfDomnProd(t) = tfidf_{D_1}(t) \cdot tfidf_{D_2}(t)$: product of TF-IDF weights of term t in the two domains,
- $tfidfDomnSum(t) = tfidf_{D_1}(t) + tfidf_{D_2}(t)$: sum of term TF-IDF weights of term t in the two domains.

Similarity-based heuristics. Another approach to construct a relevant heuristic measure is to use the cosine similarity measure that is frequently used in text mining to compute the similarity of documents. We start by creating a representational BoW model as a document space and by converting terms into BoW document vectors. Next, we get the centroid vectors for both domains in the document space representation. Finally, we apply TF-IDF weighting on top of all the newly constructed vectors and centroids. We define the following auxiliary function:

- $simCos_D(t)$: calculates the cosine similarity of the document vector of term t and the document vector of a centroid of documents $d \in D$.

The base heuristics are the following:

- $simAvgTerm(t) = simCos_{D_u}(t)$: similarity of term t to an average term, i.e. the distance from the center of the cluster of all terms,
- $simDomnProd(t) = simCos_{D_1}(t) \cdot simCos_{D_2}(t)$: product of similarity of term t to the centroids of the two domains,
- $simDomnRatioMin(t) = \min(\frac{simCos_{D_1}(t)}{simCos_{D_2}(t)}, \frac{simCos_{D_2}(t)}{simCos_{D_1}(t)})$: minimum of term's frequency ratios of the two domains.

Outlier-based heuristics. Outlier detection is an established area of data mining [20]. Conceptually, an outlier is an unexpected event, entity or—in our case—an irregular document. We are especially interested in outlier documents since they frequently embody new information that is often hard to explain in the context of existing knowledge. Moreover, in data mining, an outlier is occasionally a primary object of study as it can potentially lead to the discovery of new knowledge. These assumptions are well aligned with the bisociation potential that we wish to optimize, thus, we have constructed several heuristics that harvest the information possibly residing in outlier documents.

We concentrate on a specific type of outliers, i.e. domain outliers, which are the documents that tend to be more similar to the documents of the opposite domain than to those of their own domain. The techniques that we use to detect outlier documents [18] is based on using classification algorithms to detect outlier documents. First we train a classification model for each domain and afterwards classify all the documents using the trained classifier. The documents that are misclassified—according to their domain of origin—are declared as outlier documents, since according to the classification model they do not belong to their domain of origin.

We defined three different outlier sets of documents based on three classification algorithms utilized. These outlier sets are:

- D_{CS}: documents misclassified by the Centroid Similarity (CS) classifier,
- D_{RF}: documents misclassified by the Random Forest (RF) classifier,
- D_{SVM}: documents misclassified by the Support Vector Machine (SVM) classifier.

Centroid similarity is a basic classifier model implemented in our system. It classifies each document to the domain whose centroid's TF-IDF vector is the most similar to the document's TF-IDF vector. The description of the other two classification models is beyond the scope of this chapter, as we used external procedures to retrieve these outlier document sets; a detailed description is provided by [18].

For each outlier set we defined two heuristics: the first counts the frequency of a term in an outlier set and the second computes the relative frequency of a term in an outlier set compared to the relative frequency of a term in the whole dataset. The resulting heuristics are listed below:

- $outFreqCS(t) = countTerm_{D_{CS}}(t)$: frequency of term t in the CS outlier set,
- $outFreqRF(t) = countTerm_{D_{RF}}(t)$: frequency of term t in the RF outlier set,
- $outFreqSVM(t) = countTerm_{D_{SVM}}(t)$: frequency of term t in the SVM outlier set,
- $outFreqSum(t) = countTerm_{D_{CS}}(t) + countTerm_{D_{RF}}(t) + countTerm_{D_{SVM}}(t)$: sum of frequencies of term t in all three outlier sets,
- $outFreqRelCS(t) = \frac{countTerm_{D_{CS}}(t)}{countTerm_{D_u}(t)}$: relative frequency of term t in the CS outlier set,
- $outFreqRelRF(t) = \frac{countTerm_{D_{RF}}(t)}{countTerm_{D_u}(t)}$: relative frequency of term t in the RF outlier set,
- $outFreqRelSVM(t) = \frac{countTerm_{D_{SVM}}(t)}{countTerm_{D_u}(t)}$: relative frequency of term t in the SVM outlier set,
- $outFreqRelSum(t) = \frac{countTerm_{D_{CS}}(t)+countTerm_{D_{RF}}(t)+countTerm_{D_{SVM}}(t)}{countTerm_{D_u}(t)}$: sum of relative term frequencies of term t in all three outlier sets.

Ensemble Heuristics Construction. Ensemble learning is a known approach used in machine learning for combining predictions of multiple models into a final prediction. It is well evidenced [27] that the resulting ensemble model is more accurate than any of the individual models used to build it as long as the models are similarly accurate, are better than random, and their errors are uncorrelated. There is a wide variety of known and well tested ensemble techniques, such as bagging, boosting, majority voting, random forest, naive Bayes, etc. [28]. However, these approaches are usually used for the problem of classification while the core problem presented in this work is ranking. Nevertheless, with the rise of the areas like information retrieval and search engines' web page rankings, ensemble ranking is also gaining attention in the ranking community [29].

One possible—and probably the most typical—approach to designing an ensemble heuristic from a set of base heuristics consists of two steps. In the first step, the task is to select member heuristics for the ensemble heuristic using standard data mining approaches like feature selection. In the second step, equation discovery is used to obtain an optimal combination of member heuristics. The advantage of such approach is that the ensemble creation does not require manual intervention. Therefore, we performed several experiments with this approach; however, the results of an ensemble were even more overfitted to the training domain. Consequently, we decided to manually—based on experience and experimentation—select appropriate base heuristics and construct an ensemble heuristic. As the presentation of numerous experiments, which support our design decisions, is beyond the scope of this chapter, we describe only the final solution, along with some reasoning about choosing the heuristics.

The ensemble heuristic for bridging term discovery, which we constructed based on the experiments, is constructed from two parts: the ensemble voting score and the ensemble position score, which are summed together to give the final ensemble score for every term in the corpus vocabulary. Each term score represents the term's potential for joining the two disjointed domains.

The ensemble voting score (s_t^{vote}) of a given term t is an integer, which denotes how many base heuristics voted for the term. Each selected base heuristic h_i gives one vote ($s_{t_j,h_i}^{vote} = 1$) to each term, which is in the first third in its ranked list of terms and zero votes to all the other terms ($s_{t_j,h_i}^{vote} = 0$). The voting threshold one third ($\frac{1}{3}$) was set empirically grounded on the evaluation of the ensemble heuristic on the migraine-magnesium domain and is based on the number of terms that appear in both domains (not one third of all the terms). Formally, the ensemble voting score of term t_j that is at position p_j in the ranked list of n terms is computed as a sum of individual heuristics' voting scores:

$$s_{t_j}^{vote} = \sum_{i=1}^{k} s_{t_j,h_i}^{vote} = \sum_{i=1}^{k} \begin{cases} 1, & p_j < n/3 \\ 0, & \text{otherwise} \end{cases} \tag{1}$$

Therefore, each term can get a score $s_{t_j}^{vote} \in \{0, 1, 2, ..., k\}$, where k is the number of base heuristics used in the ensemble. The ensemble position score (s_t^{pos}) is calculated as an average of position scores of individual base heuristics. For each heuristic h_i, the term's position score $s^{pos}_{t_j,h_i}$ is calculated as $\frac{n-p_j}{n}$, which results in position scores being in the interval $[0,1)$. For an ensemble of k heuristics, the ensemble position score is computed as an average of individual heuristics' position scores:

$$s^{pos}_{t_j} = \frac{1}{k} \sum_{i=1}^{k} s^{pos}_{t_j,h_i} = \frac{1}{k} \sum_{i=1}^{k} \frac{n-p_j}{n} \tag{2}$$

The final ensemble score is computed as:

$$s_t = s^{vote}_t + s^{pos}_t \tag{3}$$

Using the proposed construction we make sure that the integer part of the ensemble score always presents the ensemble vote score, while the ensemble score's fractional part always presents the ensemble position score. An ensemble position score is strictly lower than 1, therefore a term with a lower ensemble voting score can never have a higher final ensemble score than a term with a higher ensemble voting score. Consequently, every final ensemble score falls into interval $[0, k+1)$, where k is the number of base heuristics used in the ensemble.

The described method for ensemble score calculation is illustrated in Tables 1–5. In Table 1 the base heuristics scores are shown for each term. Table 2 presents terms ranked according to the base heuristics scores. From this table, the voting and position scores are calculated for every term based on its position, as shown in Table 3. For example, all terms at position 2, i.e. t1, t6, and t6, get voting score 1 and position score 4/6. Table 4 shows the exact equation how these base heuristics voting and position scores are combined for each term. Table 5 displays the list of terms ranked by the calculated ensemble scores.

Table 1. Base heuristic scores

Term	h_1	h_2	h_3
t1	0.93	0.46	0.33
t2	0.26	0.15	0.10
t3	0.51	0.22	0.79
t4	0.45	0.84	0.73
t5	0.41	0.15	0.11
t6	0.99	0.64	0.74

Table 2. Terms ranked by base heuristics

Pos.	h_1	h_2	h_3
1	t_6	t_4	t_3
2	t_1	t_6	t_6
3	t_3	t_1	t_4
4	t_4	t_3	t_1
5	t_5	t_2	t_5
6	t_2	t_5	t_2

Table 3. Voting and position scores based on positions in the ranked lists

Pos.	$s^{vote}_{t_j,h_i}$	$s^{pos}_{t_j,h_i}$
1	1	$(6-1)/6 = 5/6$
2	1	$(6-2)/6 = 4/6$
3	0	$(6-3)/6 = 3/6$
4	0	$(6-4)/6 = 2/6$
5	0	$(6-5)/6 = 1/6$
6	0	$(6-6)/6 = 0/6$

Note that at the first sight, our method of constructing the ensemble score looks rather intricate. An obvious way to construct an ensemble score of a term could be simply to sum together individual base heuristics scores; however, the calculation of the ensemble score by our method is well justified by extensive experimental results on the migraine-magnesium dataset described in Sect. 6. The final set of elementary heuristics included in the ensemble is the following:

Table 4. Calculation of ensemble heuristic score

$$\left(s^{vote}_{t_j,h_1} + s^{vote}_{t_j,h_2} + s^{vote}_{t_j,h_3} \right) + \left(s^{pos}_{t_j,h_1} + s^{pos}_{t_j,h_2} + s^{pos}_{t_j,h_3} \right)/k = s^{vote}_{t_j} + s^{pos}_{t_j} = s_{t_j}$$

$s_{t_1} = ($	1	$+$	0	$+$	0	$) + ($	4/6	$+$	3/6	$+$	2/6	$)/3 =$	1	$+$ 9/18	$= 1.50$
$s_{t_2} = ($	0	$+$	0	$+$	0	$) + ($	0/6	$+$	1/6	$+$	0/6	$)/3 =$	0	$+$ 1/18	$= 0.06$
$s_{t_3} = ($	0	$+$	0	$+$	1	$) + ($	3/6	$+$	2/6	$+$	5/6	$)/3 =$	1	$+$ 10/18	$= 1.56$
$s_{t_4} = ($	0	$+$	1	$+$	0	$) + ($	2/6	$+$	5/6	$+$	3/6	$)/3 =$	1	$+$ 10/18	$= 1.56$
$s_{t_5} = ($	0	$+$	0	$+$	0	$) + ($	1/6	$+$	0/6	$+$	1/6	$)/3 =$	0	$+$ 2/18	$= 0.11$
$s_{t_6} = ($	1	$+$	1	$+$	1	$) + ($	5/6	$+$	4/6	$+$	4/6	$)/3 =$	3	$+$ 13/18	$= 3.72$

Table 5. Ranked list of terms produced by the ensemble

t6 (3.72), [t2, t3] (1.56), t1 (1.50), t5 (0.11), t2 (0.06)

- outFreqRelRF
- outFreqRelSVM
- outFreqRelCS

- outFreqSum
- tfidfDomnSum
- freqRatio

Detailed justification is presented in [30].

5.3   Workflows Implementing Individual Steps of the Methodology

The workflow for cross-domain literature mining, presented in Sect. 4.2, is publicly available for sharing and reuse within the TextFlows platform. The workflow integrates the computation of heuristics, described in Sect. 5.2, and is connected to the term exploration interface of the online system CrossBee, which supports the user in advanced document exploration by facilitating document analysis and visualization.

Document Acquisition Workflow (Step 1). The first step of the workflow from Fig. 4 is composed of several components described below. The components are responsible for the following tasks:

1.1. load literature A into annotated document corpus data structure
1.1.1. load raw text data from a file (this component could be replaced by loading documents from the web or by acquiring them using web services), where each line contains a document with exactly three tab-separated entries: (a) document identifier, (b) domain acronym, and (c) the document text,
1.1.2. build the annotated document corpus from the raw data, i.e. parse the loaded raw text data into a collection of documents and assign a domain label (e.g., literature A, docsA, migraine) to the documents to enable their identification after merging with literature B,
1.2. load literature B into the annotated document corpus data structure (individual components are aligned with the components 1.1),

1.3. merge the two literatures into a single annotated document corpus structure,

1.4. optional check of document acquisition by visual inspection of the created corpus.

The document acquisition workflow is shown in Fig. 5. The output is the annotated document corpus consisting of the acquired documents labeled with domain labels.

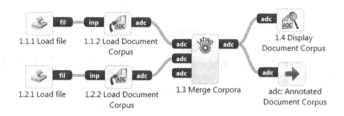

Fig. 5. Document acquisition workflow.

Text Preprocessing Workflow (Step 2). The document acquisition step is followed by the text preprocessing step, which is itself a workflow implemented as shown in Fig. 6. The main components here are tokenization, stopwords labeling and token stemming or lemmatization. The output of this step is structurally equal to the input; however every document in the annotated document corpus now contains additional information about tokens, stopwords and lemmas.

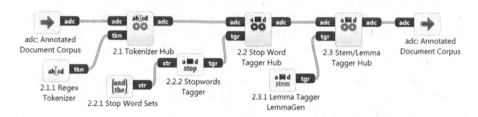

Fig. 6. Document preprocessing workflow.

The individual components perform the following tasks:

2.1 split documents to tokens (the basic units for further text processing),

2.1.1. create tokenizer object (simple tokenizer based on regular expressions),

2.2. tag stopword tokens by using a stopword tagger (component 2.2.2),

2.2.1. load standard English stopwords,

2.2.2. define the stopword tagger using the standard English stopwords only (the detected stopwords are used in candidate B-term extraction step),

2.3. lemmatize tokens by applying the LemmaGen lemmatizer[11] [31],
2.3.1. create an instance of LemmaGen lemmatizer.

Heuristics Specification Workflow (Step 3). While the heuristics specification step is the core part of our methodology, this step only specifies which heuristics are selected and how these heuristics should be combined into the ensemble heuristic. The actual calculation is performed later in the heuristic term score calculation step.

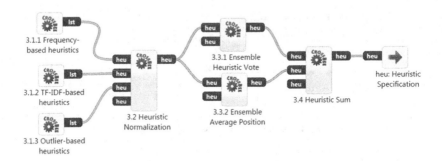

Fig. 7. Heuristic specification.

Heuristic specification displayed in Fig. 7 is the outcome of our research about the base term heuristics and their combination into the ensemble heuristic presented in Sect. 5.2. Which heuristics to use and how to combine them is based on the experiments on the real data that we performed as a part of the research presented in this chapter—these experiments are presented in more detail in [30]. The findings resulted in the setting shown in Fig. 7, which is a good choice when applied on new data. Nevertheless, the setting and the choice of the base heuristics is fully customizable and can be freely configured to better suit the needs of new applications.

The output of this procedure is a specification of a complex ensemble heuristic, which computes the term bisociation scores. The components in the heuristic specification perform the following tasks:

3.1. define base heuristics (see Sect. 5.2 for details about the base heuristics selection),
3.1.1. define TF-IDF based heuristic *tfidfDomnSum*,
3.1.2. define term frequency based heuristic *freqRatio*,
3.1.3. define outlier based heuristics *outFreqRelRF*, *outFreqRelSVM*, *outFreqRelCS*, *outFreqRelSum*
3.2. for every inputted heuristic defines a new heuristic that normalizes the scores to the range [0,1) and outputs a list of new heuristic specifications,

---

[11] LemmaGen is an open source lemmatizer with 15 prebuilted european lexicons. Its source code and documentation is publicly available at http://lemmatise.ijs.si/.

3.3. combine the six heuristics into a single ensemble heuristic
3.3.1. define an ensemble voting heuristic that includes votes of the six heuristics (ensemble voting score, see Eq. 1),
3.3.2. define a calculated heuristic that calculates normalized sum of position scores of the six heuristics (ensemble position score, see Eq. 2),
3.4. define the final ensemble heuristic by summing the ensemble voting heuristics, which results in the number of terms heuristics' votes in the range from 0 to 6 (integer value), and the calculated normalized sum of heuristics scores in the range from 0 to less than 1 (final ensemble score, see Eq. 3).

Candidate B-term Extraction Workflow (Step 4). Another core step of the workflow is candidate B-term extraction, shown in Fig. 8. Although it contains only one component, it has a very important and complex goal of transforming the inputted annotated document corpus into the BoW model in order to represent documents in the form of feature vectors of term occurrences in the documents (for the purpose of visualization of documents and the need of highlighting and emphasizing of specific terms). Another task of this step is to capture the exact parsing procedure, which is needed in order to perform various computations which are performed in the advanced heuristic term scores calculation step. The outputted *BowModelContructor* object also contains the vocabulary of all terms.

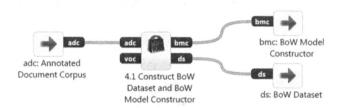

Fig. 8. Candidate B-term extraction.

Heuristic Term Score Calculation Workflow (Step 5). Figure 9 shows a structurally simple methodological step of heuristic term score calculation that contains only one component. The inputs to the procedure are the annotated document corpus, the *BoWModelContructor* and the heuristics specification. Based on the information present in the *BoWModelContructor*, the algorithm calculates various frequency and TF-IDF document features vectors, which are used to calculate the specified heuristics scores for all the terms. The calculation results in the same heuristic structure as defined in the heuristic specification step, however the ensemble heuristic at the top level, as well as all elementary heuristics, now contain their calculated scores of the terms. The scores of the top-level heuristic are intended to represent terms' bisociation scores and are typically used as a basis for the final term ranking.

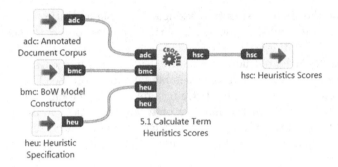

Fig. 9. Heuristic term score calculation.

B-Term Visualization and Exploration Workflow (Step 6). This step of the methodology implements a workflow shown in Fig. 10. It enables visualization and exploration of the ranked list of B-terms. There are four inputs to this step. The first and the most important are the ensemble heuristic scores of the extracted candidate B-terms. Inputs *Annotated Document Corpus* and *BoW Dataset* are used by the online application for cross-context bisociation exploration CrossBee, which needs the exact information about term extraction from documents to be able to align the terms back with the original documents in order to visualize them; while the *BoW Model Constructor* provides the constructed vocabulary. The goals of the created components are the following:

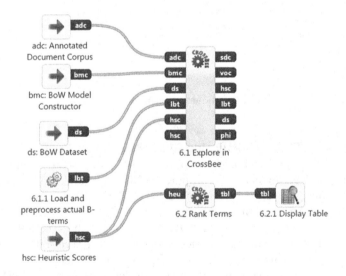

Fig. 10. B-term visualization and exploration.

6.1. explore the final results in a web application CrossBee, which was designed specifically for the purpose of bisociativity exploration (expressed either through terms or through documents),

6.1.1. optional expert specified B-terms may be provided to CrossBee in order to emphasize them in the text and to deliver a feedback about the bisociative quality of the provided ranking. If available, these terms are loaded and preprocessed using the same preprocessing techniques as described in the document preprocessing step,

6.2. rank the terms

6.2.1. display the ranked terms in the form of a table along with their respective scores.

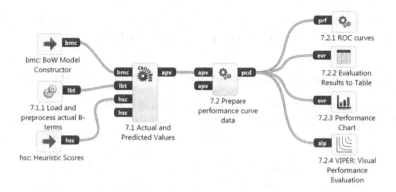

Fig. 11. Methodology evaluation.

Methodology Evaluation Workflow (Step 7). The last step of the proposed methodology is the methodology evaluation step, implemented as a workflow shown in Fig. 11. There are three inputs to the process: the heuristic scores of one or more evaluated heuristics (which presents the result of all the preceding methodological steps), the *BowModelContructor* (which contains the corpus vocabulary) and additional information about the actual B-terms (required in order to assess any kind of quality measures). Note that, in order not to overflow the overall methodology workflow of Fig. 4 with additional information, the list of actual bridging terms was not shown as an additional step of the methodology. Instead, it is implemented as a separate subprocess in the methodology evaluation workflow, which is responsible for loading and preprocessing the actual B-terms.

The components of the methodology evaluation workflow perform the following tasks:

7.1. prepare pairs of actual and predicted values, which are used to calculate different information retrieval measures in step 7.2,

7.1.1. if available, load the actual (expert identified) B-terms, which present the gold standard terms used to evaluate the quality of the methodology and preprocess them using same techniques as in document preprocessing step,

7.2. calculate different measures, such as precision, recall, and the F_1-measure, ROC curves and the AUC (Area Under Curve) values,

7.2.1. display ROC curves graphically,

7.2.2. compare information retrieval measures in the form of a table,

7.2.3. compare information retrieval measures in the form of a bar chart,

7.2.4. display and compare the F_1-scores in the advanced VIPER performance evaluation chart [32] component.

The methodology evaluation functionality presented in this section is not part of the actual workflow for cross-domain knowledge discovery; however, it is indispensable when developing a new approach. Description of this step concludes the section presenting the key parts of the methodology.

5.4 Methodology Empowerment with Controlled Vocabulary

This section describes a new ingredient of the methodology: the use of a controlled vocabulary for improving B-term detection and ranking. The motivation for using predefined controlled vocabularies is to reduce the heuristic search space which, consequently, reduces the running times of B-term discovery algorithms. Controlled vocabularies ensure consistency and resolve ambiguity inherent in normal human languages where the same concept can be given different names. In this way, they improve the quality and organization of retrieved knowledge, given that they consist of predefined, authorized terms that have been pre-selected by the designers of the vocabulary that are experts in the subject area. Controlled vocabularies solve problems of homographs and synonyms by a bijection between concepts and authorized terms.

MeSH (Medical Subject Headings) is a controlled vocabulary used for indexing articles for PubMed, designed by The National Library of Medicine (NLM). Figure 12 shows a top-level example of the MeSH structure and hierarchy. The 2015 version of MeSH contains a total of 27,455 subject headings, also known as descriptors. Each descriptor is assigned a unique tree number (shown in square brackets in Fig. 12) that facilitates search and filtering. Most of the descriptors are accompanied by a short description or definition, links to related descriptors, and a list of synonyms or very similar terms (known as entry terms). Because of these synonym lists MeSH can also be viewed as a thesaurus.

We have implemented a vocabulary construction tool called *MeSH filter* as an interactive widget in the TextFlows platform. This implementation uses synonym lists from the MeSH 2015 database, available online[12]. The interface to the developed interaction widget is designed to enable the selection of descriptors of interest from the hierarchy of descriptors. Its final output is a text file

---

[12] http://www.nlm.nih.gov/mesh/filelist.html.

```
Nervous System Diseases [C10]
   Central Nervous System Diseases [C10.228]
      Brain Diseases [C10.228.140]
         Headache Disorders [C10.228.140.546]
            Headache Disorders, Primary [C10.228.140.546.399]
               Migraine Disorders [C10.228.140.546.399.750]
                  Alice in Wonderland Syndrome [C10.228.140.546.399.750.124]
                  Migraine with Aura [C10.228.140.546.399.750.250]
                  Migraine without Aura [C10.228.140.546.399.750.450]
                  Ophthalmoplegic Migraine [C10.228.140.546.399.750.725]
               Tension-Type Headache [C10.228.140.546.399.875]
               Trigeminal Autonomic Cephalalgias [C10.228.140.546.399.937]
```

Fig. 12. Example of MeSH structure and hierarchy.

containing all the terms that belong to the user selected descriptors from the MeSH hierarchy.

This section describes how we have upgraded the proposed methodology with the ability to use a predefined controlled vocabulary for reducing the B-term search space. This not only increases efficiency of the heuristic calculation algorithms, but also tends to improve the relevance of top ranked B-terms due to reduced ambiguities in human languages. The upgraded methodology is shown in Fig. 13. Compared to the initial methodology shown in Fig. 4, the new workflow[13] includes two new steps: vocabulary acquisition and vocabulary preprocessing.

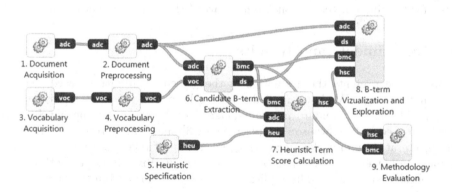

Fig. 13. Methodological steps of the cross-domain literature mining process.

In order to ensure the proper matching between terms from the vocabulary and document corpus, the vocabulary file must be preprocessed using the preprocessing techniques, described in Sect. 5.3, which were also used for preprocessing the document corpus in Step 2. After vocabulary preprocessing in

---

[13] This workflow is publicly available at http://textflows.org/workflow/497/.

Step 4, the produced vocabulary file is used in Step 5 to filter out terms from the document corpus that do not appear in the vocabulary. A procedural explanation of the new steps of the upgraded workflow of Fig. 13 is presented.

Vocabulary Acquisition (Step 3)

- *One term per line*: Every single line in the text file represents one separate term. Only terms which appear in this file are later used in the heuristic calculation steps of the methodology.
- *Synonym format*: Additionally, term synonyms are listed after the term, separated by commas.

$$\text{term}_1 \rightarrow \text{synonym}_{1a}, \text{synonym}_{1b}\dots$$

Every synonym in the document corpus is then substituted with the term, which appears at the first position in the corresponding line.

Vocabulary Preprocessing (Step 4). This step is responsible for applying the same standard text preprocessing to the predefined vocabulary that is used also to preprocess the document corpus. Similarly, the main components here are tokenization, stopwords labeling and token stemming or lemmatization.

Candidate B-Term Extraction (Step 6). After completing the preprocessing steps, the resulting whitelist output is used in Candidate B-term Extraction step for filtering out terms that are not part of the controlled vocabulary.

6   Experiments and Results

This section presents the evaluation of the presented literature based discovery methodology. We have applied different base and ensemble heuristics on two problems: the standard migraine-magnesium literature mining benchmark problem used in the Swanson's experiments [13], and a more recent example of using literature mining for uncovering the nature of relations that might contribute to better understanding of autism, originated in [19,33]. In both cases, our methodology successfully replicated the results known from the literature.

6.1   Experimental Setting

The evaluation was performed based on two datasets (or two domain pairs, since each dataset consists of two domains)—the migraine-magnesium dataset [13] and the autism-calcineurin [33] dataset—which can be viewed as a training and test dataset, respectively. The training dataset is the dataset we employed when developing the methodology, i.e. for creating a set of base heuristics as well as for creating the ensemble heuristic. The results of the evaluation on the training dataset are important, but need to be interpreted carefully due to a danger of overfitting the dataset, as described in [30]. The test dataset is used for the evaluation of the methodology in a real-life setting. The well-researched migraine-magnesium domain pair [13] was used as a training set. In the literature-based discovery process Swanson managed to find more than 60 pairs of articles connecting the migraine domain with the magnesium deficiency via 43 bridging concepts (B-terms), which are listed in Table 6.[14] In testing the developed methodology we aimed at rediscovering the 43 B-terms by ranking them as high as possible in the ranked list of potential B-terms that include Swanson's B-terms and terms that are not in the Swanson's B-term list.

Table 6. B-terms for the migraine-magnesium dataset identified in [13].

1 5 ht	16 convulsive	31 prostaglandin
2 5 hydroxytryptamine	17 coronary spasm	32 prostaglandin e1
3 5 hydroxytryptamine receptor	18 cortical spread depression	33 prostaglandin synthesis
4 anti aggregation	19 diltiazem	34 reactivity
5 anti inflammatory	20 epilepsy	35 seizure
6 anticonvulsant	21 epileptic	36 serotonin
7 antimigraine	22 epileptiform	37 spasm
8 arterial spasm	23 hypoxia	38 spread
9 brain serotonin	24 indomethacin	39 spread depression
10 calcium antagonist	25 inflammatory	40 stress
11 calcium blocker	26 nifedipine	41 substance p
12 calcium channel	27 paroxysmal	42 vasospasm
13 calcium channel blocker	28 platelet aggregation	43 verapamil
14 cerebral vasospasm	29 platelet function	
15 convulsion	30 prostacyclin	

Table 7. B-terms for the autism-calcineurin dataset identified in [33].

1 synaptic	6 bcl 2	11 22q11 2
2 synaptic plasticity	7 type 1 diabetes	12 maternal hypothyroxinemia
3 calmodulin	8 ulcerative colitis	13 bombesin
4 radiation	9 asbestos	
5 working memory	10 deletion syndrome	

For the test dataset we used the autism-calcineurin domain pair [33]. Like Swanson, Petrič et al. also provide B-terms, 13 in total (listed in Table 7), whose importance in connecting autism to calcineurin (a protein phosphatase) is discussed and confirmed by the domain expert. In view of searching for B-terms, this dataset has a relatively different dimensionality compared to the migraine-magnesium dataset. On the one hand it has only about one fourth of the B-terms defined, while on the other hand, it contains more than 40 times

---

[14] Note that Swanson did not state that this was an exclusive list, hence there may exist other important bridging terms which he did not list.

Table 8. Comparison of some statistical properties of the two datasets used in the experiments.

		migraine-magnesium	autism-calcineurin
Retrieval	Source	PubMed	PubMed
	Query terms	"migraine"-"magnesium"	"autism"-"calcineurin"
	Additional conditions	Year < 1988	/
	Part of paper used	Title	Abstract
Document Statistics	Number	8,058 (2,415–5,633)	15,243 (9,365–5,878)
	Doc. with B-term	394 (4.89%)	1,672 (10.97%)
	Avg. words per doc	11	180
Term statistic	Avg. term per doc.	7	173
	Distinct terms	13,525	322,252
	B-term candidates	1,847	78,805
	Defined B-terms	43	13

as many potential B-term candidates. Therefore, the ratio between the actual B-terms and the candidate terms is substantially lower—approximately by factor 160, i.e. the chance to find a B-term among the candidate terms if picking it at random is 160 times lower in the autism-calcineurin dataset then in the magnesium-migraine dataset. Consequently, finding the actual B-terms in the autism-calcineurin dataset is much more difficult compared to the migraine-magnesium dataset.

Both datasets, retrieved from the PubMed database using the keyword query, are formed of titles or abstracts of scientific papers returned by the query. However, we used an additional filtering condition for selecting the migraine-magnesium dataset. For fair comparison we had to select only the articles published before the year 1988 as this was the year when Swanson published his research about this dataset and consequently making an explicit connection between the migraine and magnesium domains.

Table 8 states some properties for comparing the two datasets used in the evaluation. One of the major differences between the datasets is the length of an average document since only the titles were used in the migraine-magnesium dataset, while the full abstracts were used in the autism-calcineurin case. Consequently, also the number of distinct terms and B-term candidates is much larger in the case of the autism-calcineurin dataset. Nevertheless, the preprocessing of both datasets was the same. We can inspect higher numbers in the migraine-magnesium dataset which points to the problem of harder classification of documents in this dataset, which is also partly due to shorter texts.

6.2   Evaluation Procedure

The key aspect of the evaluation is the assessment of how well the proposed ensemble heuristic performs when ranking the terms. Two evaluation measures were used in the evaluation of the developed methodology: the standard Area under the Receiver Operating Characteristic analysis and the amount of B-terms found among the first 5,10, 20, 100, 500 and 2,000 terms in the heuristics' ranked list of terms.

First, we compared the heuristics using the Area under the Receiver Operating Characteristic (AUROC) analysis [34]. The Receiver Operating Characteristic (ROC) space is defined by two axes, where the horizontal axis scales from zero to the number of non-B-terms, and the vertical axis from zero to the number of B-terms. An individual Receiver Operating Characteristic (ROC) curve, representing a single heuristic, is constructed in the following way:

- Sort all the terms by their descending heuristic score.
- For every term of the term list do the following: if a term is a B-term, then draw one vertical line segment (up) in the ROC space, else draw one horizontal line segment (right) on the ROC space.
- If a heuristic outputs the same score for many terms, we cannot sort them uniquely. In such case, we draw a line from the current point p to the point $p+(nb, b)$, where nb is the number of non-B-terms and b is the number of terms that are B-terms among the terms with the same bisociation score. In this way we may produce slanted lines, if such an equal scoring term set contains both B-terms and non-B-terms.

AUROC is defined as the percentage of the area under ROC curve, i.e. the area under the curve divided by the area of the whole ROC space.[15] Besides AUROC we also list the interval of AUROC which tells how much each heuristic varies among the best and the worst sorting of a possibly existing equal scoring term set. This occurs due to the fact that some heuristics do not produce unambiguous ranking of all the terms. Several heuristics assign the same score to a set of terms—including both the actual B-terms as well as non B-terms—which results in the fact that unique sorting is not possible.[16] In the case of equal scoring term sets, the inner sorting is random (which indeed produces different performance estimates), however the constructed ROC curve corresponds to the average ROC curve over all possible such random inner sortings.

From the expert's point of view, the ROC curves and AUROC statistics are not the most crucial information about the quality of a given heuristic. While in general it still holds that a higher AUROC reflects a better heuristic, we are more interested in the ranking from the perspective of the domain expert (the end-user of the our system) who is usually more interested in questions like:

---

[15] If a heuristic is perfect (it detects all the B-terms and ranks them at the top of the ordered list), we get a curve that goes first just up and then just right with an AUROC of 100%. The worst possible heuristic sorts all the terms randomly regardless of being a B-term or not and achieves AUROC of 50%. This random heuristic is represented by the diagonal in the ROC space.

[16] In such cases, the AUROC calculation can either maximize the AUROC by sorting all the B-terms in front of all the other terms inside equal scoring sets or minimize it by putting the B-terms at the back. The AUROC calculation can also achieve many AUROC values in between these two extremes by using different (e.g., random) sortings of equal scoring sets. Preferable are the heuristics with a smaller interval which implies that they produce smaller and fewer equal scoring sets.

(a) how many B-terms are likely to be found among the first n terms in a ranked list (where n is a selected number of terms the expert is willing to inspect, e.g., 5, 20 or 100), or (b) how much one can trust a heuristic if a new dataset is explored. Therefore, we also performed an evaluation using an alternative user oriented approach, which evaluates the ranking results adapted to the user's needs. This evaluation estimates how many B-terms can be found among the first 5, 10, 20, 100, 500 and 2,000 terms on the ranked list of terms produced by a heuristic.

6.3   Results on the Migraine-Magnesium Dataset

Table 9 shows the comparison of ranking performance for the ensemble and all the base heuristics on the migraine-magnesium dataset. The heuristics are ordered by their AUROC. The second and third column in the table represent heuristics' average AUROC score[17] and its AUROC interval, respectively. When looking at the ensemble heuristic scores in Table 9, we notice that it achieves higher

Table 9. Comparison of base and ensemble heuristics capacity to rank the B-terms at the very beginning of the term list for the migraine-magnesium dataset.

Heuristic name	AUROC		Number of B-terms among top n ranked terms								
	Average	Interval	5	10	20	50	100	200	500	1,000	2,000
outFreqRelSvm	58.78%	1.26%	0.12	0.24	0.48	1	1.63	5.88	14.44	29	43
outFreqRelSum	58.19%	0.65%	0	0.28	0.83	1.82	3.68	6	15	27	43
freqDomnRatioMin	57.34%	4.71%	0.14	0.28	0.57	1.42	2.83	5.66	14	28	43
outFreqRelRf	56.85%	1.50%	0.24	0.48	0.95	2	4.15	6.94	14	29	43
outFreqSum	55.41%	4.06%	0	0	0	0	0	2.44	15.06	27.16	43
outFreqRf	55.20%	11.07%	0	0	0	0	0.4	5.15	14.86	26.34	43
outFreqSvm	55.19%	9.38%	0	0	0	0	0.35	3	14.14	26.12	43
outFreqRelCs	54.29%	1.50%	0	0	1	1	2.69	5.07	11	27	43
freqDomnProdRel	53.23%	3.08%	0	0	0	0	0	6	14	27	43
outFreqCs	52.34%	10.51%	0	0	0	0	0	1.43	15.62	24.67	43
tfidfDomnSum	52.11%	2.69%	0	0	0	0	1	2	11	26.14	43
tfidfAvg	51.31%	3.63%	0	0	1	1.79	3.11	5.75	11.84	20.9	43
freqDomnProd	51.20%	3.36%	0	0	0	0	1	3	13.17	27.16	43
tfidfDomnProd	51.18%	2.69%	0	0	0	0	1	3	13.5	27	43
freqRatio	50.51%	39.26%	0	0	1	1	4	5	11.65	23.09	43
appearInAllDomains	50.00%	50.00%	0.11	0.23	0.46	1.15	2.3	4.6	11.49	22.98	43
tfidfSum	49.65%	3.63%	0	0	0	0	0	1	9	25.36	43
freqTerm	49.60%	3.78%	0	0	0	0	0	1	8.91	25.49	43
freqDoc	49.55%	3.82%	0	0	0	0	0	1	8.03	24.79	43
ensemble	59.05%	0.26%	1	1	1	5	6	9	18.57	28	43

---

[17] In contrast to the results reported in [4,5], the AUROC scores presented in this chapter take into account only the terms which appear in both domains. This results in lower AUROC scores, which are thus not directly comparable between the studies. The reason for this approach is in the definition of a bridging term, where the term is required to appear in both domain, as it cannot form a connection otherwise.

AUROC value and lower AUROC interval compared to all the other heuristics. As mentioned in Sect. 5.2, the ensemble was constructed using also two not so well performing heuristics (tfidfDomnSum and freqRatio) in order to avoid overfitting on the training domain. This could have had a negative effect to the ensemble performance, however, the ensemble performance was not seriously affected which gives evidence of right decisions made when designing the ensemble.

As mentioned, such AUROC evaluation does not necessarily aligns well with the methodology evaluation from a user's perspective. Therefore, the right side of Table 9 shows the results of an alternative user oriented evaluation approach, which shows how many B-terms were found among the first 5, 10, 20, 50, 100, 200, 500, 1,000 and 2,000 terms on the ranked list of terms produced by a heuristic. The ensemble heuristic, described in Sect. 5.2, performing ensemble voting of six elementary heuristics, resulted in very favorable results on the training migraine-magnesium domain (as seen in Table 9), where one B-term among the first 5 terms, one B-term (no additional B-terms) among the first 20 terms, 6 B-terms (5 additional) among the first 100 terms, 22 B-terms (16 additional) among first 500 terms and all the 43 B-terms (21 additional) among the first 2,000 terms. Thus, e.g., if the expert limits himself to inspect only the first 100 terms, he will find 6 B-terms in the ensemble ranked term list. These results confirm that the ensemble is the best performing heuristics also from the user's perspective. Even though a strict comparison depends on the threshold of how many terms an expert is willing to inspect, the ensemble is always among the best.

6.4 Results of Using a Controlled Vocabulary on the Migraine-Magnesium Dataset

In this section we demonstrate that by using a predefined controlled vocabulary we can increase the heuristics' capabilities to rank the B-terms at the beginning of the term list. We have repeated the experiments on the migraine-magnesium domain, described in Sect. 6.3, except that we now used a predefined vocabulary constructed from MeSH using the "MeSH filter" widget. As we were particularly interested in the bridging terms between migraine—a disease—and magnesium— a chemical element—as well as the circumstances and processes observed between them, we only selected categories [C] *Diseases*, [D] *Chemicals and drugs* and [G] *Phenomena and Processes*. In the experiment we used the workflow shown in Fig. 13. The generated vocabulary was used in the candidate B-term extraction step as a whitelist filter.

The results of the methodology using a controlled vocabulary on the migraine-magnesium domain are presented in Table 11. The comparison of the heuristics' capabilities to rank the B-terms at the beginning of the term list in the migraine-magnesium domain from Tables 9 and 11 shows an advantage of using the controlled vocabulary. By inspecting the number of B-terms found in the ranked first n terms, we notice that using the controlled vocabulary in the migraine-magnesium domain resulted in a much higher concentration of Swanson's B-terms among the best ranked terms.

Table 10. B-terms for the migraine-magnesium dataset identified in [13]. The 17 terms which are crossed out were not part of the used controlled vocabulary, therefore heuristics were unable to identify them as B-term candidates.

1 5 ht	16 convulsive	31 prostaglandin
2 5 hydroxytryptamine	17 coronary spasm	32 prostaglandin e1
3 5 hydroxytryptamine receptor	18 cortical spread depression	33 prostaglandin synthesis
4 anti aggregation	19 diltiazem	34 reactivity
5 anti inflammatory	20 epilepsy	35 seizure
6 anticonvulsant	21 epileptic	36 serotonin
7 antimigraine	22 epileptiform	37 spasm
8 arterial spasm	23 hypoxia	38 spread
9 brain serotonin	24 indomethacin	39 spread depression
10 calcium antagonist	25 inflammatory	40 stress
11 calcium blocker	26 nifedipine	41 substance p
12 calcium channel	27 paroxysmal	42 vasospasm
13 calcium channel blocker	28 platelet aggregation	43 verapamil
14 cerebral vasospasm	29 platelet function	
15 convulsion	30 prostacyclin	

As explained in Sect. 5.4 a predefined controlled vocabulary can greatly reduce the B-term search space. As a side effect, we were unable to: (a) perform AUROC evaluation comparison due to different number of terms in the vocabulary—As a result, Table 11 provides only evaluation which lists the number of B-terms found in the ranked first n terms, (b) detect all B-terms, identified by Swanson (the crossed out B-terms in Table 10 were not part of the used controlled vocabulary); this could be solved using larger controlled vocabularies, though we must be careful not to overfit the vocabulary to the expected results.

On the other hand, results show that using a predefined controlled vocabulary not only increases the efficiency of the heuristic calculation algorithms, but also tends to improve the relevance of top ranked B-terms. Consequently, the described approach enables the user to perform the exploration task more effectively, potentially leading to new discoveries.

6.5 Results on the Autism-Calcineurin Dataset

In this section we show how our methodology performs on a new independent test dataset—the autism-calcineurin domain—which was not used in the development of the methodology. As discussed, the dimensionality of the autism-calcineurin dataset is considerably different and less favorable compared to the migraine-magnesium dataset.

Table 12 shows that the performance of individual base heuristics significantly changes compared to the migraine magnesium dataset (Table 9), however, the ensemble heuristic is still among the best and exposes small uncertainty. This gives us the final argument for the quality of the ensemble heuristic since it outperforms all the other heuristics (except for the *freqRatio* base heuristic) when comparing the AUROC scores, as well as the numbers of B-terms found in the

Table 11. Comparison of base and ensemble heuristics capacity to rank the B-terms at the very beginning of the term list for the migraine-magnesium dataset using a controlled vocabulary.

Heuristic Name	Number of B-terms among top n ranked terms								
	5	10	20	50	100	200	500	1,000	2,000
freqDomnRatioMin	0.59	1.18	2.37	5.92	13.25	20	26	26	26
outFreqSum	0	1	2.75	5	15.53	17.06	26	26	26
freqDomnProdRel	0	1	2	5.67	9	20	26	26	26
outFreqRf	1	1	2	6.28	12.16	17.5	26	26	26
outFreqSvm	1	1	2.5	5.16	11.74	16.79	26	26	26
outFreqCs	0	0	2.45	5.6	10.22	17.06	26	26	26
tfidfDomnSum	0	1	1	4	10	19	26	26	26
freqDomnProd	0	1	1	4	9	19	26	26	26
tfidfDomnProd	0	1	1	4	9	19	26	26	26
outFreqRelRf	0.67	1.33	2	5	7	14.75	26	26	26
freqDoc	0	0	1	2.5	7.82	17.1	26	26	26
tfidfSum	0	0	1	2.25	7.5	17.35	26	26	26
freqTerm	0	0	1	2.25	7.56	17.43	26	26	26
appearInAllDomains	0.39	0.78	1.56	3.9	7.81	15.62	26	26	26
outFreqRelSum	0.42	0.83	1.29	4	9	15	26	26	26
tfidfAvg	0	1.42	2.47	5.63	7	13	26	26	26
outFreqRelSvm	0.45	0.91	1.82	3.25	10	15	26	26	26
outFreqRelCs	0.31	0.63	1	5	7.06	14	26	26	26
freqRatio	0	1	1	2	5.96	14.56	26	26	26
ensemble	1	3	4	9	13	19	26	26	26

most interesting ranked list lengths (up to 20, 100, 500 terms). The ensemble finds one B-term among 10 ranked terms, 2 among 200 and 3 among 500 ranked terms out of the total of 78,805 candidate terms that the heuristics have to rank. The evidence of the quality of the ensemble can be understood if we compare it to a baseline, i.e. the *appearInAllDomn* heuristic which denotes the performance achievable without developing the methodology presented in this work. The baseline heuristic discovers in average only approximately 0.33 B-terms before position 2,000 in the ranked list while the ensemble discovers 6; not to mention the shorter term lists where the ensemble has even a better ratio compared to the baseline heuristic.

6.6 Results of Using a Controlled Vocabulary on the Autism-Calcineurin Dataset

In this section we replicated the experiments, described in Sect. 6.4, using a predefined controlled vocabulary on the autism-calcineurin dataset. Similarly,

Table 12. Comparison of base and ensemble heuristics capacity to rank the B-terms at the very beginning of the term list for the autism-calcineurin dataset.

Heuristic Name	AUROC		Number of B-terms among top n ranked terms										
	Average	Interval	5	10	20	50	100	200	500	1,000	2,000	5,000	all
freqRatio	95.10%	0.16%	1	1	1	1	1	1	1	3	5	8.99	13
tfidfSum	88.78%	0.05%	0	0	0	0	1	1	1	2	4	5	13
tfidfDomnProd	88.61%	0.05%	0	0	0	0	0	0	1	1	4	6	13
tfidfDomnSum	88.33%	0.02%	0	0	0	0	1	1	2	2	4	5	13
freqTerm	87.80%	0.80%	0	0	0	0	1	1	1	2	3	5	13
freqDomnProd	87.69%	0.73%	0	0	0	0	0	0	0	1	2	6	13
freqDomnProdRel	85.77%	0.69%	0	0	0	0	0	0	0	1	1	6	13
outFreqRf	85.05%	7.91%	0	0	0	0	0	1	1	1.34	4.37	7.4	13
outFreqSum	84.33%	5.80%	0	0	0	0	0	1	1	3	4	8.4	13
outFreqCs	80.50%	10.05%	0	0	0	0	0	1	1	1	4	7.17	13
freqDoc	79.01%	2.53%	0	0	0	0	0	1	1	2	2	5	13
outFreqSvm	75.15%	17.55%	0	0	0	0	1	1	1.46	4	4.67	5.44	13
tfidfAvg	73.56%	0.05%	1	1	1	1	1	1	1	1	3	6	13
outFreqRelRf	72.44%	0.03%	0	0	0	0	1	1	1	1	1	2	13
outFreqRelSum	67.24%	0.03%	0	0	0	0	0	1	1	2	2	2	13
outFreqRelCs	64.40%	0.19%	0	0	0	0	0	0	0	0	0	1.49	13
outFreqRelSvm	58.39%	0.17%	0	0	0	0	0	0	0	0	1.25	2	13
appearInAllDomains	50.00%	50.00%	0	0	0	0.01	0.02	0.03	0.08	0.17	0.33	0.83	13
freqDomnRatioMin	24.93%	1.12%	0	0	0	0	0	0	0	0	0	0	13
ensemble	90.10%	0.00%	0	1	1	1	1	2	3	4	6	8	13

Table 13. B-terms for the autism-calcineurin dataset identified by [33]. The four terms which are crossed out were not part of the used controlled vocabulary, therefore heuristics were unable to identify them as B-term candidates.

1 synaptic	6 bcl 2	11 22q11 2
2 synaptic plasticity	7 type 1 diabetes	12 maternal hypothyroxinemia
3 calmodulin	8 ulcerative colitis	13 bombesin
4 radiation	9 asbestos	
5 working memory	10 deletion syndrome	

we wanted to increase the heuristics' capabilities (in the workflow illustrated in Fig. 13) to rank the B-terms at the beginning of the term list. We used the same predefined vocabulary as with the migraine-magnesium domain, which was constructed from MeSH using the following categories: [C] *Diseases*, [D] *Chemicals and drugs* and [G] *Phenomena and Processes* were used for building the controlled vocabulary (Table 13).

Inspecting the heuristics' capabilities to rank the B-terms at the beginning of the term list in the autism-calcineurin domain (Tables 12 and 14) shows the advantage of using a controlled vocabulary. The increase in the number of B-terms found in the ranked first n terms when using the controlled vocabulary is even more significant than in the migraine-magnesium domain. The ensemble

Table 14. Comparison of base and ensemble heuristics capacity to rank the B-terms at the very beginning of the term list for the autism-calcineurin dataset using a controlled vocabulary.

Heuristic Name	Number of B-terms among top n ranked terms									
	5	10	20	50	100	200	500	1,000	2,000	5,000
outFreqSvm	0	0	0	0.5	2	4	4.8	7	8.92	9
outFreqSum	0	0	0	0	0	4	5.56	7	8	9
tfidfDomnProd	0	0	0	0	0	3	4	7	9	9
freqDomnProd	0	0	0	0	1	3	4	7	9	9
freqRatio	1	1	1	1	2	3	3.6	6.01	9	9
freqDomnProdRel	0	0	0	0	0	1	4	7	9	9
outFreqCs	0	0	0	0	0	2	6.59	7	7.82	9
tfidfSum	0	1	1	1	1	2	3	7	9	9
tfidfDomnSum	0	1	1	1	1	2	3	7	9	9
freqTerm	0	1	1	1	1	2	3	6.21	9	9
freqDoc	0	1	1	1	1	2	3	6	8	9
outFreqRf	0	0	0	0	0	1	2.65	5.59	6.99	9
outFreqRelSvm	0	0	1	1	1	1	2	3	9	9
tfidfAvg	1	1	1	1	1	2	2	4	7	9
outFreqRelCs	0	0	0	0	0	0	2	3	7	9
outFreqRelSum	0	0	0	0	0	1	1	3	7	9
appearInAllDomains	0.01	0.03	0.06	0.14	0.28	0.55	1.38	2.76	5.52	9
outFreqRelRf	0	0	0	0	0	0	0	2	6	9
freqDomnRatioMin	0	0	0	0	0	0	1	2	6	9
ensemble	1	1	1	2	2	2	4	6	8	9

heuristic finds the first B-term among the top 5 ranked terms (before only among top 10) and the second B-term among the top 50 ranked terms (before only among 200). These results confirm the findings that controlled vocabularies can increase the heuristics' capacities to rank the B-terms at the beginning of the term list and, thus, provide a more efficient exploration task to the end-user of the platform.

7   Conclusions and Future Outlook

This chapter presents the TextFlows platform together with its cross-context literature mining facility, which in combination with the term exploration engine CrossBee supports the expert in advanced document exploration, aimed at facilitating document retrieval, analysis and visualization. The combination of the two systems forms a creativity support tool, helping experts to uncover not yet discovered relations between seemingly unrelated domains from large textual databases. As estimating which terms have a high bisociative potential is a challenging research question, we proposed a complex methodology which was developed as a pipeline of natural language processing an literature based discovery components in the TextFlows platform. The visual programming user interface of TextFlows not only enables the user to tailor the methodology steps to his own needs but also allows experiment repeatability and methodology reuse by other users and developers.

This chapter contributes also the evaluation of a number of specially designed heuristic functions that provide a bisociation score quality estimate for each term. These base heuristics can be—based on the type of term features they exploit—divided into the following sets: frequency based, TF-IDF based, similarity based, and outlier based. Another contribution is the development of the improved ensemble-based heuristic, which employs a set of base heuristics to ensure robustness and stable performance across the datasets. We evaluated the ensemble based methodology on two domains, migraine-magnesium and autism-calcineurin, showing that the proposed methodology substantially reduces the end-user's burden in terms of the length of the term list that needs to be inspected to find some B-terms. Furthermore, it was shown that by using a predefined vocabulary we can increase the heuristics' capacities to rank the B-terms at the beginning of the term list. Indeed, by applying this approach in the migraine-magnesium and autism-calcineurin domains we got a higher concentration of B-terms among the best ranked terms. Consequently, the user is presented with a simpler exploration task, potentially leading to new discoveries.

In future work we will introduce additional user interface options for data visualization and exploration as well as advance the term ranking methodology by adding new sophisticated heuristics which will take into account also the semantic aspects of the data. Besides, we will apply the system to new domain pairs to exhibit its generality, investigate the need and possibilities of dealing with domain specific background knowledge, and assist researchers in different disciplines in their explorations which may lead to new scientific discoveries.

This research perfectly demonstrated the importance of the HCI-KDD [35] approach of combining the best of two worlds for getting insight into complex data, which is particularly important for health informatics research, where the human expertise (e.g. a doctor-in-the-loop) is of great help in solving hard problems, which cannot be solved by automatic machine learning algorithms otherwise [36]. There is much research in this area necessary in the future.

Acknowledgements. This work was supported by the Slovenian Research Agency and the FP7 European Commission FET projects MUSE (grant no. 296703) and ConCreTe (grant no. 611733).

References

1. Koestler, A.: The Act of Creation, vol. 13 (1964)
2. Agrawal, R., Mannila, H., Srikant, R., Toivonen, H., Verkamo, A.I., et al.: Fast discovery of association rules. Adv. Knowl. Discov. Data Min. **12**(1), 307–328 (1996)

3. Dubitzky, W., Kötter, T., Schmidt, O., Berthold, M.R.: Towards creative information exploration based on koestler's concept of bisociation. In: Berthold, M.R. (ed.) Bisociative Knowledge Discovery. LNCS (LNAI), vol. 7250, pp. 11–32. Springer, Heidelberg (2012). doi:10.1007/978-3-642-31830-6_2

4. Juršič, M., Cestnik, B., Urbančič, T., Lavrač, N.: Bisociative literature mining by ensemble heuristics. In: Berthold, M.R. (ed.) Bisociative Knowledge Discovery. LNCS (LNAI), vol. 7250, pp. 338–358. Springer, Heidelberg (2012). doi:10.1007/978-3-642-31830-6_24

5. Juršič, M., Cestnik, B., Urbančič, T., Lavrač, N.: Cross-domain literature mining: finding bridging concepts with CrossBee. In: Proceedings of the 3rd International Conference on Computational Creativity, pp. 33–40 (2012)

6. Berthold, M.R. (ed.): Bisociative Knowledge Discovery. LNCS (LNAI), vol. 7250. Springer, Heidelberg (2012)

7. Swanson, D.R.: Medical literature as a potential source of new knowledge. Bull. Med. Libr. Assoc. **78**(1), 29 (1990)

8. Smalheiser, N., Swanson, D., et al.: Using ARROWSMITH: a computer-assisted approach to formulating and assessing scientific hypotheses. Comput. Methods Programs Biomed. **57**(3), 149–154 (1998)

9. Hristovski, D., Peterlin, B., Mitchell, J.A., Humphrey, S.M.: Using literature-based discovery to identify disease candidate genes. Int. J. Med. Inf. **74**(2), 289–298 (2005)

10. Yetisgen-Yildiz, M., Pratt, W.: Using statistical and knowledge-based approaches for literature-based discovery. J. Biomed. Inform. **39**(6), 600–611 (2006)

11. Holzinger, A., Yildirim, P., Geier, M., Simonic, K.M.: Quality-based knowledge discovery from medical text on the web. In: Pasi, G., Bordogna, G., Jain, L.C. (eds.) Qual. Issues in the Management of Web Information. ISRL, vol. 50, pp. 145–158. Springer, Heidelberg (2013)

12. Kastrin, A., Rindflesch, T.C., Hristovski, D.: Link prediction on the semantic MEDLINE network. In: Džeroski, S., Panov, P., Kocev, D., Todorovski, L. (eds.) DS 2014. LNCS (LNAI), vol. 8777, pp. 135–143. Springer, Heidelberg (2014). doi:10.1007/978-3-319-11812-3_12

13. Swanson, D.R.: Migraine and magnesium: eleven neglected connections. Perspect. Biol. Med. **78**(1), 526–557 (1988)

14. Lindsay, R.K., Gordon, M.D.: Literature-based discovery by lexical statistics. J. Am. Soc. Inform. Sci. Technol. **1**, 574–587 (1999)

15. Srinivasan, P.: Text mining: generating hypotheses from medline. J. Am. Soc. Inform. Sci. Technol. **55**(5), 396–413 (2004)

16. Weeber, M., Klein, H., de Jong-va den Berg, L.T.W.: Using concepts in literature-based discovery: simulating swanson's raynaud-fish oil and migraine-magnesium discoveries. J. Am. Soc. Inform. Sci. Technol. **52**(7), 548–557 (2001)

17. Petrič, I., Cestnik, B., Lavrač, N., Urbančič, T.: Outlier detection in cross-context link discovery for creative literature mining. Comput. J. **55**(1), 47–61 (2012)

18. Sluban, B., Juršič, M., Cestnik, B., Lavrač, N.: Exploring the power of outliers for cross-domain literature mining. In: Berthold, M.R. (ed.) Bisociative Knowledge Discovery. LNCS (LNAI), vol. 7250, pp. 325–337. Springer, Heidelberg (2012). doi:10.1007/978-3-642-31830-6_23

19. Urbančič, T., Petrič, I., Cestnik, B., Macedoni-Lukšič, M.: Literature mining: towards better understanding of Autism. In: Bellazzi, R., Abu-Hanna, A., Hunter, J. (eds.) AIME 2007. LNCS (LNAI), vol. 4594, pp. 217–226. Springer, Heidelberg (2007). doi:10.1007/978-3-540-73599-1_29

20. Aggarwal, C.: Outlier Analysis. Springer, Heidelberg (2013)
21. Kranjc, J., Podpečan, V., Lavrač, N.: ClowdFlows: a cloud based scientific work-flow platform. In: Flach, P.A., Bie, T., Cristianini, N. (eds.) ECML PKDD 2012. LNCS (LNAI), vol. 7524, pp. 816–819. Springer, Heidelberg (2012). doi:10.1007/978-3-642-33486-3_54
22. Grčar, M.: Mining text-enriched heterogeneous information networks. Ph.D. thesis, Jožef Stefan International Postgraduate School (2015) (To appear)
23. Bird, S.: Nltk: the natural language toolkit. In: Proceedings of the COLING/ACL on Interactive Presentation Sessions, pp. 69–72. Association for Computational Linguistics (2006)
24. Pedregosa, F., Varoquaux, G., Gramfort, A., Michel, V., Thirion, B., Grisel, O., Blondel, M., Prettenhofer, P., Weiss, R., Dubourg, V., et al.: Scikit-learn: machine learning in python. J. Mach. Learn. Res. **12**, 2825–2830 (2011)
25. Feldman, R., Sanger, J.: The Text Mining Handbook: Advanced Approaches in Analyzing Unstructured Data. Cambridge University Press, New York (2007)
26. Salton, G., Buckley, C.: Term-weighting approaches in automatic text retrieval. Inf. Process. Manage. **24**(5), 513–523 (1988)
27. Dietterich, T.G.: Ensemble methods in machine learning. In: Kittler, J., Roli, F. (eds.) MCS 2000. LNCS, vol. 1857, pp. 1–15. Springer, Heidelberg (2000). doi:10.1007/3-540-45014-9_1
28. Rokach, L.: Pattern classification using ensemble methods. World Scientific (2009)
29. Hoi, S.C., Jin, R.: Semi-supervised ensemble ranking. In: AAAI, pp. 634–639 (2008)
30. Juršič, M.: Text mining for cross-domain knowledge discovery. Ph.D. thesis, Jožef Stefan International Postgraduate School (2015)
31. Juršič, M., Mozetič, I., Erjavec, T., Lavrač, N.: Lemmagen: multilingual lemmatisation with induced ripple-down rules. J. Univ. Comput. Sci. **16**(9), 1190–1214 (2010)
32. Sluban, B., Gamberger, D., Lavrač, N.: Ensemble-based noise detection: noise ranking and visual performance evaluation. Data Mining Knowl. Discov. **28**, 265–303 (2013)
33. Petrič, I., Urbančič, T., Cestnik, B., Macedoni-Lukšič, M.: Literature mining method rajolink for uncovering relations between biomedical concepts. J. Biomed. Inform. **42**(2), 219–227 (2009)
34. Provost, F.J., Fawcett, T., Kohavi, R.: The case against accuracy estimation for comparing induction algorithms. In: ICML, vol. 98, pp. 445–453 (1998)
35. Holzinger, A.: Human-computer interaction and knowledge discovery (HCI-KDD): what is the benefit of bringing those two fields to work together? In: Cuzzocrea, A., Kittl, C., Simos, D.E., Weippl, E., Xu, L. (eds.) CD-ARES 2013. LNCS, vol. 8127, pp. 319–328. Springer, Heidelberg (2013). doi:10.1007/978-3-642-40511-2_22
36. Holzinger, A.: Interactive machine learning for health informatics: when do we need the human-in-the-loop? Springer Brain Inform. (BRIN) **3**, 1–13 (2016)

Visualisation of Integrated Patient-Centric Data as Pathways: Enhancing Electronic Medical Records in Clinical Practice

Joao H. Bettencourt-Silva[1]([✉]), Gurdeep S. Mannu[2], and Beatriz de la Iglesia[3]

[1] Department of Medicine, Clinical Informatics, University of Cambridge,
Cambridge CB2 0QQ, UK
jhb56@medschl.cam.ac.uk
[2] Nuffield Department of Population Health, University of Oxford,
Oxford OX3 7LF, UK
gurdeep.mannu@gtc.ox.ac.uk
[3] School of Computing Sciences, University of East Anglia, Norwich NR4 7TJ, UK
b.iglesia@uea.ac.uk

Abstract. Routinely collected data in hospital Electronic Medical Records (EMR) is rich and abundant but often not linked or analysed for purposes other than direct patient care. We have created a methodology to integrate patient-centric data from different EMR systems into clinical pathways that represent the history of all patient interactions with the hospital during the course of a disease and beyond. In this paper, the literature in the area of data visualisation in healthcare is reviewed and a method for visualising the journeys that patients take through care is discussed. Examples of the hidden knowledge that could be discovered using this approach are explored and the main application areas of visualisation tools are identified. This paper also highlights the challenges of collecting and analysing such data and making the visualisations extensively used in the medical domain.

This paper starts by presenting the state-of-the-art in visualisation of clinical and other health related data. Then, it describes an example clinical problem and discusses the visualisation tools and techniques created for the utilisation of these data by clinicians and researchers. Finally, we look at the open problems in this area of research and discuss future challenges.

Keywords: Visualisation · Big data · Clinical pathways · Data mining · Knowledge discovery · Data quality · Decision making · Medical informatics

1 Introduction

Hospitals routinely collect data related to the interaction of patients with different departments and medical specialties. Traditionally this information was recorded in paper notes yet more recently there has been an increasing shift

© Springer International Publishing AG 2016
A. Holzinger (Ed.): ML for Health Informatics, LNAI 9605, pp. 99–124, 2016.
DOI: 10.1007/978-3-319-50478-0_5

towards the adoption of electronic medical records, as the statistics from the Electronic Medical Record Adoption Model (EMRAM) demonstrate (http://himss.eu/emram), yet in many cases, researchers may still need to collate information manually [1] and methodologies to facilitate this process are relatively unexplored [2]. Clinical data is typically complex and may pertain to diagnoses, admissions and discharges, prescriptions, treatments, biomarkers and blood tests, outcomes and other clinical findings. As a result, patients leave footprints on many hospital systems, but such prints are not often connected to provide a pathway indicative of their journey through care, nor are they presented at the aggregated level. In the context of important diseases such as cancer or stroke, the journey of patients from diagnosis to outcome would provide a unique perspective that could aid clinicians to better understand disease processes and provide valuable information on optimal treatment. Hence, an initial challenge is to gather data from multiple EMR systems and construct meaningful data structures that can encompass all of the relevant information pertaining to a given patient and a given disease over time. We have named such data structures *clinical pathways* and have provided a methodology to build them [2,3]. Note that some researchers refer to clinical pathways as the standardised and normalised therapy pattern recommended for a particular disease [4]. Other researchers have focused on mining common pathways that show typical disease progression based on hierarchical clustering and Markov chains [5]. Our pathways relate to the journey followed by the patient through care and they may align with the recommended guidelines for a particular disease but may also deviate from it.

Visualisations of pathways, at the individual or aggregate level, when well presented and of high quality, could help clinicians to interact with such data and give them a view of patients and disease progression that was otherwise hidden away in databases. This would enable them to utilise the power of the big data in their environment, a very topical subject which currently holds much promise. For example, Shneiderman et al. [6] state that "while clinical trials remain the work horse of clinical research there is now a shift toward the use of existing clinical data for discovery research, leading researchers to analyse large warehouses of patient histories". The visualisation of this big data is a critical topic and the specific subject of this paper.

In the context of medical data mining, clinical pathways, as we define them, require consistent pre-processing techniques, innovative data mining methods and powerful and interactive visualisation techniques. They also present the challenges of data privacy which has to always be maintained when dealing with patients' data. We discuss some of these challenges and present some solutions in this paper, particularly focusing on the visualisation aspects.

This paper is organized as follows: to ensure a common understanding we provide a short glossary in Sect. 2; we examine work on visualisation of medical data that is relevant in the context of the problem we present in Sect. 3; we then provide some background information about clinical pathways, their construction, their visualisation and the challenges of such an approach in Sect. 4.

We then discuss the processes of visualization of aggregated pathways in Sect. 5 and their areas of application in Sect. 6. Finally, we discuss problems in the field and conclude with prospects for the future.

2 Glossary and Key Terms

Electronic Medical Record (EMR): can be characterised as "the complete set of information that resides in electronic form and is related to the past, present and future health status or health care provided to a subject of care" [7].

Medical Informatics: is the interdisciplinary study of the design, development, adoption and application of IT-based innovations in healthcare services delivery, management and planning [8]. Medical informatics is also called health care informatics, health informatics, nursing informatics, clinical informatics, or biomedical informatics.

Data Mining: is an analytic process designed to explore large amounts of data in search of consistent patterns and/or systematic relationships between variables, and then to validate the findings by applying the detected patterns to new subsets of data [9].

Medical Patterns: these are frequently appearing sequences of treatments, diagnoses, etc., that are associated with unusually positive or negative outcomes [10].

Visual Analytics: denotes the science of analytical reasoning facilitated by visual interactive interfaces [11].

Data Quality: includes (physical) quality parameters such as: Accuracy, Completeness, Update status, Relevance, Consistency, Reliability and Accessibility [12].

Clinical Pathway: in the context of this paper it is defined as an ordered set of patient-centric events and information relevant to a particular clinical condition [3]. It can be considered as a suitable data structure for routine data extracted from EMRs that records the actual journey of the patient for a given condition. Others have defined it as "a map of the process involved in managing a common clinical condition or situation" [13]. Hence in the second definition the clinical pathway may embody the *ideal* or recommended pathway and enumerate regular medical behaviours that are expected to occur in patient care journeys and may, therefore, serve as a checkpoint for the performance of the actual pathway.

Temporal abstraction: this refers to the task of creating interval-based concepts or abstractions from time-stamped raw data. In the context of electronic clinical data, data summaries of time-oriented data can help for example when physicians are scanning a long patient record for meaningful trends [14].

Clinical guidelines: are systematically developed statements designed to help practitioners and patients decide on appropriate healthcare for specific clinical conditions and/or circumstances [15]. They may articulate a desired clinical pathway.

3   State-of-the-Art

One of the main characteristics of clinical data is its temporal nature. EMRs are composed of longitudinal event sequences which can sometimes be a concurrent set of treatments for various conditions undertaken by a patient over time. Another important characteristic is the complexity of the data, which can include many different data types, support many levels of granularity and is associated with extensive domain knowledge that may be required for context. Additionally, the type of analysis we want to support may require techniques that take into account individual patients, or aggregate at the cohort level. As we are focusing on visualisation, we need to generate visual user interfaces that can represent such complexity efficiently and effectively without overwhelming the user. We need to provide query engines and mining methods that can deal with the temporal and complex nature of the data with efficient interactions. We also need to ensure that the systems produced are evaluated effectively, which is difficult when evaluation requires the involvement of busy medical practitioners. In this section, we review how researchers have tackled some of these problems so far.

As a starting point, reviews and surveys on the subject of visualisation of EMR data provide a good introduction to this topic. Turkay et al. [16] give a recent introduction to the visualisation of large biomedical heterogeneous data sets and point out the need for mechanisms to improve the interpretability and usability of interactive visual analyses. They also stress the challenge of integrating data from additional sources, such as the "microscopic" world (systems biology), the "omics" world or the "macroscopic" (public health informatics) world, as we move towards precision medicine.

Rind et al. [17] provide a survey comparing a number of state-of-the-art visualisation research systems for EMR, and separately give examples of visualisations produced by commercial systems. They also give a summary of other reviews of this subject. Roque et al. [18] also give comparisons of the key information visualisation systems for clinical data. Similarly, West et al. [19] provide a systematic survey of works between 1996 and 2013. Their article is part of a special issue dedicated to visual analytics to support the analysis of complex clinical data [20]. Lesselroth and Pieczkiewicz [21] discuss a number of strategies for visualising EMRs. More generically, methods for visualising time oriented data have also been surveyed [22].

Time oriented clinical data has been considered to be important by a number of researchers. Early work on visualisation of personal histories [23] produced a system called Lifelines that used graphical time scales to produce a timeline of a single patient's temporal events. Medical conditions could be displayed as horizontal lines, while icons indicated discrete events, such as physician consultations. Line colour and thickness were used to illustrate relationships or the significance of events. Application of Lifelines to medical records was further explored in [24]. Lifelines is the basis for many other systems that visualise time oriented clinical data. The evolution of Lifelines produced a system called Lifelines2 [25] that displays multiple patient histories aligned on sentinel events to enable medical researchers to spot precursor, co-occurring, and after-effect events.

Further work by the same team resulted in LifeFlow [26], which presents a prototype for the visualisation of event sequences involving millions of patients. LifeFlow was one of the first systems to provide an overview and enable the answering of questions such as "what are the most common transfer patterns between services within the hospital". Hence Lifeflow attempts to summarise all possible sequences, together with the temporal spacing of events within the sequences. It provides one visual abstraction that represents multiple timelines so it addresses the problem of aggregation. In terms of the interaction capability, which has become a key issue in visualising clinical information, LifeFlow [26] provides zooming, sorting, filtering and enables further exploration of events by hoovering the cursor over parts of the visualisation. It also enables the user to select non-temporal attributes as the basis for aggregation. This enables comparison between different groups.

Shahar et al. [14] also worked with temporal clinical data. In particular they discuss the extraction of temporal abstractions from electronic data. Such temporal abstractions combine a domain knowledge-base with interval-based concepts. A quoted example is the abstraction of Bone Marrow toxicity from raw individual hematological data. The domain knowledge in this case would establish the context such as following Bone Marrow Transplantation using a particular therapy protocol. A simpler abstraction may be fever from multiple measures of raised temperature over time. Temporal abstractions can support intelligent decision-support systems or be used for the monitoring of clinical guidelines. However, Shahar et al. argue that temporal abstractions can only be truly useful in a clinical setting if they are accompanied by interactive visualisation and exploration capabilities which can also take into account medical domain knowledge. For this, they developed a system called KNAVE-II, a development of a previous system [27]. The work does not provide, however, capabilities for aggregation of patients according to some dynamic criteria. In further work [28], the authors provided such capability under a system called VISITORS.

The issue of introducing context when evaluating patterns in a clinical setting is also important in other scenarios. For example, Duke et al. [29] present a system for incorporating knowledge such as a patient's relevant co-morbidities and risk factors when evaluating drug-drug interactions to improve the specificity of alerts.

Analysis based on comparison of cohorts is also prevalent. Huang et al. [30] describe a system for exploratory data analysis through a visual interactive environment to show disease-disease associations over time. The system simplifies visual complexity by aggregating records over time, clustering patients and filtering association between cohorts. The main visualisation methods used to study disease trajectories over time are Sankey diagrams [31].

Wong et al. [32] proposed INVISQUE, an interactive visualisation to support both medical diagnosis and information analysis and discussed the key issues that need to be addressed when designing interactive visualisation systems for such purposes. CareVis [33] is another system, specifically designed to provide visualisation of medical treatment plans and patient data, including contextual information on treatment steps. It utilises a language called Asbru, designed to represent clinical guidelines and protocols in eXtensible Markup Language (XML). Challenges of the data include hierarchical decomposition, flexible execution order, non-uniform element types and state characteristics of conditions. CareVis utilises multiple integrated views [34] to represent logical and temporal aspects of the treatment data. The views can be coupled with colour, brushing and navigation propagation, hence elements in one view can be linked to the same elements in the other views allowing for interaction with the visualisation.

Another recent work using Asbru, following from CareVis, and specifically designed to analyse compliance with clinical guidelines is presented by Bodesinsky et al. [35]. The authors use visualisation to integrate information about executed treatments with Computer Interpretable Guidelines. Combining views from observation, treatment and guidelines is becoming increasingly important in the clinical setting.

Very recent work on visualisation of temporal queries, which enables clinicians to extract cohorts of patients given temporal constraints is presented by Krause et al. [36]. Retrospective cohort extraction in the traditional way involves a long and complex process and requires involvement from doctors and SQL query specialists. SQL queries do not cater well for temporal constraints and query engines may not optimise well such queries, making the process difficult and inefficient. A system called *COQUITO* is proposed as a visual interface for building COhort QUeries with an ITerative Overview for specifying temporal constraints on databases. The query mechanism is implemented by a visual query user interface and provides real-time feedback about result sets. It also claims to be backed by a Temporal Query Server optimized to support complex temporal queries on large databases. Another system for constructing visual temporal queries is DecisionFlow [37]. DecisionFlow enables interactive queries on high-dimensional datasets (i.e. with thousands of event types).

Given the amount of complex data that needs to be visualised in the context of medical systems, one common problem is the dense display that can result and the difficulty this represents for the user. For example, Kamsu-Foguen et al. [38] discuss the need for intelligent monitoring systems that can help users with the massive information influx. This may require the capturing of domain knowledge to form a physiological/process model as part of the expert interface. It may also require the use of machine learning to improve interaction of machines and humans (e.g. reducing data input by inducing entries based on previous interactions). The software proposed can integrate visual and analytical methods to filter, display, label and highlight relevant medical information from patient-time oriented data. At the same time, it can learn from interactions between medical staff and the system in a particular context, such as modification of a prescription. It could then be used for instance to capture domain expert knowledge in respect to medical guideline compliance.

An issue that is also now receiving attention is the efficiency of visual analytic algorithms as dataset grows. According to Stolper et al. [39] "in the context of medical data, it is common to find datasets with tens of thousand of distinct type of medical events, thousands or even millions of patients and multiple years of medical data per patient." There are typically delays in the workflow of analysts launching queries, inspecting results, refining queries and adjusting parameters and relaunching queries. In this scenario, Stolper et al. propose the use of progressive visual analytics that enable analysts to explore meaningful partial results of an algorithm as they become available and interact with the algorithm to prioritise subspaces of interest. The interface also enables the user to adjust parameters as algorithms are running, re-start the running but also store results obtained until that point so that the user can resume previous run if required.

There are parallels between information visualisation and data mining [40]. Visual Data Mining can integrate the human in the data exploration process and can be seen as a hypothesis generation process based on visualisations [41]. Data Mining analysis is also being applied to clinical data in conjunction with visualisation techniques in order to extract knowledge, for example by identifying outliers and deviations in health care data [42]. For clinical pathways, pathway mining is also prominent and often associated with process mining using clinical workflow logs to discover medical behaviour and patterns [4]. Perer and Wang [10] have integrated frequent pattern mining and visualisation so that the resulting algorithms can handle multiple-levels of detail, temporal context, concurrency and outcome analysis and visualise the resulting frequent event sequences from EMR. This has resulted in a prototype system, Care Pathway Explorer [43], which can correlate medical events such as diagnosis and treatments with patient outcome. The system has a user-centric visual interface which can represent the most frequent patterns mined as bubbles, with the size corresponding to number of times a particular event occurs. It also uses Flow Visualisation to see how the bubbles connect to each other.

Measuring the quality of the data to be used in an important issue, as routinely collected data can be of variable quality. It would be very useful for any system that works with EMR to provide some quality measurements that can be used for the purposes of including or excluding records for further queries and clinical studies. For example, Tate et al. [44] elude to work in this area as part of their attempt to construct a system that enables querying of large primary care databases to select GP practices for clinical trials based on suitability of patient base and measures of data quality.

Another important topic is the visualisation of biological and "omics" data [16]. In systems biology, Jeanquartier et al. [45] carried out a large survey of databases that enable the visual analysis of protein networks. Systems such as the NAViGaTOR 3 extend the basic concept of network visualisation to visual data mining and allow the creation of integrated networks by combining metabolic pathways, protein-protein interactions, and drug-target data [41]. Other techniques, such as multilevel glyphs, have been proposed as a multi-dimensional way to visualise and analyse large biomedical datasets [46] and there is still a high demand for specialized and highly integrative visual analytic approaches in the biomedical domain [40], particularly as we move towards personalised medicine.

The evaluation of information visualisation tools is one of the open challenges in this area. Often carried out by controlled experiments and the production of usability reports, this are however described by Shneiderman and Plaisant [47] as helpful but falling short of expectations. They describe a new paradigm for evaluation in the form of Multi-dimentional In-depth Long-term Case studies (MILCs) that may begin with careful steps to gain entry, permission and participation of subjects and be followed by intense discussions which provide key data for evaluations. As MILCs provide multiple methods, given multiple perspectives on tool usage, they are presented as providing a compelling case for validity and generality. However, they would require substantial investment in longitudinal ethnographic studies of large groups which may not be forthcoming.

In the context of evaluation, Pickering et al. [48] recently proposed a step-wedge cluster randomised trial. This was to test the impact of their system, AWARE (Ambient Warning and Response Evaluation), on information management and workflow on a live clinical intensive care unit setting. Such trials are not commonly conducted, but can give real measures of efficiency of data utilisation and may be a good method of evaluation. They outcome was connected with time spent in data gathering with and without the system and measures were gathered by direct observation and survey.

4   Visualisation of Patient-Centric Pathways

The development of patient-centric pathways and related visualisation tools was first conceptualised as a way to plot and study biomarker trends over time for individual patients with a specific condition. This was carried out in a case study on prostate cancer, where the Prostate Specific Antigen (PSA) was the biomarker test used. The PSA is typically used to measure activity of the cells in the prostate, both benign or malignant, and guidelines for the management and screening or prostate cancer suggest that the PSA test can be read at certain time points to help understand disease progression. As a result, a typical patient will have several PSA readings during their journey through care and in their pathways.

4.1   Pathways

A pathway is comprised of activities each containing the patient identifier, the event code from a pre-defined dictionary of codes, the time when the activity occurred (in days, zeroed at diagnosis date) and the value pertaining to that specific activity. For example, activity A_4 at time 105 (days after diagnosis) describing the surgical removal of the prostate (event code S) for patient id 8 would be described as $A_4 = (8, 105, S,$ "M61.1". In this example, the value pertaining to surgical activity code S is the procedure code for the type of surgical operation. We used the OPCS 4.5 Classification of Interventions and Procedures coding and, in this case, code M61.1 refers to a total excision of prostate and its capsule. The activity in this example would, in turn, be part of a pathway, illustrated in Table 1. The pathway data model is defined in more detail in [3].

4.2   Development of a Graph Plotting System

A first support system was developed to plot the biomarker trends based on the pathways data model [3]. This allowed the computation of charts showing the complete PSA trend for each patient in the dataset. The resulting charts were then divided by treatment type and this provided interesting results and posed additional clinical questions. Analysis of the charts, working together with the clinical team, was critical to determine further system requirements and future developments, including a novel graphical representation of pathways data, described later. The data model can be revisited and data elements can be added or removed, making this approach reproducible in other clinical domains and extensible to different levels of granularity.

The inspection of PSA trend plots made clear that these should contain additional information in order to explain, for example, why the biomarker values dropped from abnormal to normal levels at particular points in time. For example, the most significant drops in PSA should be associated with a particular radical treatment. This led to the development of a more sophisticated visualisation system, capable of interpreting the pathways and transforming them into meaningful yet concise graphical representations. The purpose of such visualizations is to summarise complex clinical information over large periods of time into a single graph.

A graph generating system was developed together with the pathways engine, and comprised an architecture similar to that of the Model-view-controller [49] (MVC). In this implementation, the architecture, specific for building graphical representations of pathways, encompasses the following elements with specific purposes:

- the Data Model, responsible for maintaining the definitions and rules for the interpretation of the pathways data using an extended dictionary that contains information on how events are drawn;
- the Plot Engine, a controller that communicates user or system requests and is responsible for the interaction between the model, the view and the system;
- the Graphical User Interface (containing the view), that receives instructions based on the model and generates a graphical representation of a pathway. This dynamic interface can also allow users to interact with the graphs by communicating information back to the engine.

Figure 1 depicts the architecture of the system. Information available from a Data Store is transformed according to definitions set out by the Data Model and it is then fed to the Plot Engine. In turn, the engine utilises rules on how to draw the graph that is ultimately sent to the Graphical User Interface.

4.3   Graphical Representation

Figure 2 shows the layout of a graph, or pathway plot, and the areas of the graph where information is displayed. The y-axis represents the biomarker values (in

Table 1. Annotated example of a pathway for patient id 8 with 7 activities and 4 distinct data elements (code P - PSA test, D - Diagnosis, G - Histological Gleason Grade and S - Surgery).

Pathway	Activity	Time	Code	Value	Description
$P = \langle$ $A_1 = (8, -51, P, 13.6),$ $A_2 = (8, 0, D, 2),$ $A_3 = (8, 1, G, \text{"}4+3\text{"}),$ $A_4 = (8, 105, S, \text{"M61.1"}),$ $A_5 = (8, 106, G, \text{"}3+4\text{"}),$ $A_6 = (8, 183, P, 0.05),$ $A_7 = (8, 456, P, 0.05)$ $\rangle$	A_1	-51	P	13.6	This patient's first activity was a PSA test (values in ng/ml). In this case the reading was abnormal (>4 ng/ml) 51 days before diagnosis
	A_2	0	D	2	Diagnosis event, value shows tumour staging. In this case stage 2 indicates the tumour is confined to the prostate capsule. At this point, a biopsy was undertaken (poorly recorded in our EMR systems at the time)
	A_3	1	G	$4+3$	The result of the histological assessment of the Gleason grade, that is, the degree of cell differentiation, in this case a Gleason sum of 7
	A_4	105	S	M61.1	The patient then underwent surgery, with an OPCS procedure code of M61.1 indicating total excision of prostate and its capsule
	A_5	106	G	$3+4$	The revised Gleason grade with a more complete sample taken from the surgical operation was still a Gleason sum of 7 but now predominantly showing more of type 3 than type 4
	A_6	183	P	0.05	Post-treatment PSA test was carried out showing a value less than 0.1, denoting effective treatment in reducing the amount of PSA produced in this patient
	A_7	456	P	0.05	Follow-up PSA test reaffirming that the treatment was successful around a year after the treatment was performed

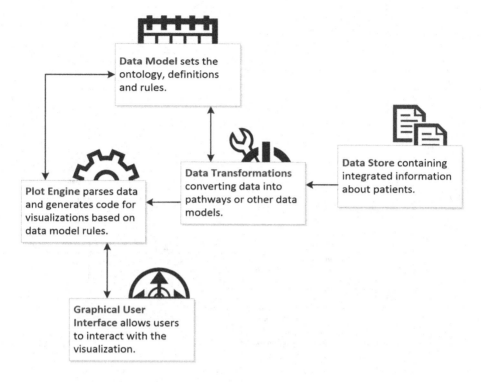

Fig. 1. Architecture of the graph generating system.

this case, PSA) and the x-axis represents time, in days, zeroed at diagnosis date. The biomarker readings are plotted in the center and events (such as treatments or death) are marked with a vertical line (*Line*).

Treatments and other events can be colour-coded and, above the plot, the corresponding pathway code (e.g. S for Surgery) is shown in the *Line headings* area. The *footer area* displays additional information pertaining to events (such as Gleason grades, i.e. the level of cell differentiation seen in the biopsy, or patient age at diagnosis) and the *right column area* on the right of the plot displays additional information on the patient that is not time-dependent, such as deprivation score, additional diagnoses or alerts.

The graph generating system includes additional interaction capabilities and analysis tools. Rather than relying on static graphical representations of the pathways, the MVC architecture embedded within the system, produces real-time plots of the pathways, as they are read from the database. Dynamic interactions were also introduced enabling users to zoom in, re-scale and navigate the pathway plot. This is particularly important as the scales of the plots may render some drawn objects too close to each other. A mechanism for graphical conflict resolution (i.e. avoiding overlapping elements) was also introduced. Examples of pathway plots produced by this system are given in Sect. 6.

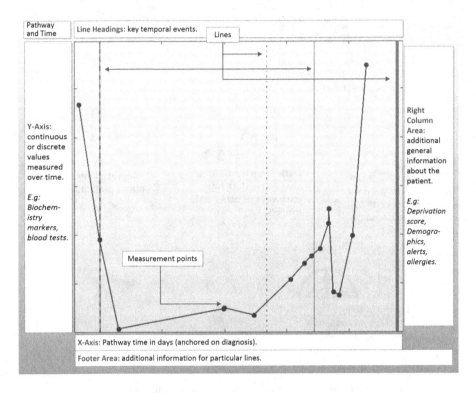

Fig. 2. The schematic layout of a pathway plot.

5   Visualization of Aggregated Pathways

We now explore how to aggregate pathways in a visualisation. The pathways data model enables the production of succinct sequences of activity codes. Truncating the sequence strings (i.e. collapsing sequentially repeating elements into one) enables the aggregation of pathways with similar sequential activities. We developed a web-based software, called ExploraTree, to produce and display an interactive tree of the full cohort of prostate cancer patients based on the available data elements. The technologies used include HTML, CSS, JSON, JavaScript and the InfoVis toolkit. The pathways engine was used to produce the correct data format for a tree representation using JSON and the JavaScript InfoVis toolkit.

In order to accurately aggregate patients with similar sequences of activities, new data elements were introduced in the data dictionary. In the core data dictionary, a patient's death was encoded by only one data element (code Z). In the new encoding, patients who died of prostate cancer were kept with code Z while those who died of other causes were identified with code Y and those who survived, with code X. This ensures that all patients have a terminal element indicating whether they are alive at the end of their follow-up period. Because in this cohort not all patients are followed-up the same amount of time, all terminal elements (X,Y,Z) were given additional child nodes that represent the amount of time the patients were followed-up in years (1 to 5 and '+' for over 5 years). The aggregated pathways tree is illustrated in Fig. 3.

Figure 3 shows the cohort tree and highlighted sequence $\langle P, D, H, P, X \rangle$, that is, patients who started their pathway with one or more PSA tests (code P, n = 1596), followed by a diagnosis of cancer (code D, n = 1502), hormone therapy as first treatment (code H, n = 747), other PSA test(s) (n = 557) and finally were last seen alive in this cohort (code X). 90% of patients with the highlighted pathway (n = 266) were followed-up 3 or more years and one patient was followed-up less than one year.

This aggregation also allows comparing patients that followed similar pathways but who died of prostate cancer ($\langle P, D, H, P, Z \rangle$). In the case of patients with a sequence prefix $\langle P, D, H, P \rangle$, 9% (n = 48) died of prostate cancer (code Z), 13% died of other causes (code Y), 48% survived, and the remaining patients continued with other activities (H - Hormone Therapy, W - Active Surveillance, R - Radiotherapy, S - Surgery).

Visualising the cohort in this manner is important as it enables the selection of subsets of data for specific clinical studies as well as an inspection of the sequential routes that patients take through care. The sequence highlighted in Fig. 3 corresponds to the most common route (with most support on each node sequentially).

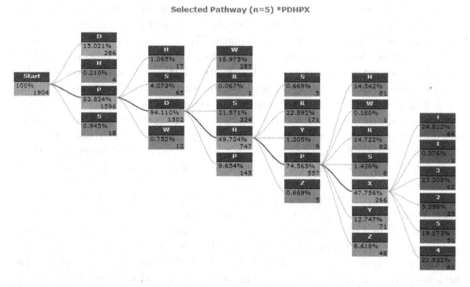

Fig. 3. CaP VIS ExploraTree software displaying a selected pathway (patients with the same sequential activities). The selected pathway nodes are highlighted and terminal nodes are marked as red for patients that died and green for patients that were last seen alive in this cohort. (Color figure online)

It is possible to add more meaning to the visualisation and the pathways by introducing additional data elements and remodeling the data dictionary. For example, instead of using a single code for diagnosis it is possible to have a breakdown of the tumour staging or Gleason grade at diagnosis so as to group similar sequences with this information instead. However, due to the small size of this cohort, increasing granularity in the pathways dictionary would result in fewer patients in each node. For this reason no additional changes were made to the pathways dictionary used for the ExploraTree, but our approach is flexible enough to allow such modifications.

6   Application Areas

This section lists four broad areas where visualisation tools have been applied and are expected to be most useful. Pathway plots illustrating relevant examples are given for each of the areas.

6.1   Decision Support and EMR Enhancement

Recommendations for further research in clinical decision support and expert systems [50] suggest that software that integrates complex data and generates graphical representations is needed to support the analysis and understanding of the data. Visualisations could also be used to enhance EMR systems as these do not typically provide visually meaningful summaries of patient-centric data.

The pathways software was developed so that additional clinical information, such as histopathology text reports, descriptive statistics, and graphical representation could all be available in one place. This created an environment that enables evidence based medicine, supports decision making. Clinicians are able to retrieve similar cases by searching the desired pathway sequences and visually inspect them, thereby gaining insights to support their decisions. In addition, other information derived from domain knowledge such as PSA kinetics (how fast PSA readings are doubling in time and rate of increase, both predictive of outcome) can be shown in the developed system before or after diagnosis and treatment. The flexible pathways data model has also enabled other aspects to be incorporated. For example, rules can be applied to measure adherence to guidelines.

Figure 4 shows four pathway plots for the same patient, a 69 year old diagnosed with tumour stage 3 prostate cancer and a Gleason sum of 9. Plot A shows the original plot where the PSA is seen to have dropped after the patient underwent hormone therapy (code H). The thick red line at the end of the pathway denotes when the patient died. When producing this pathway's plots, the dictionary was extended so that the treatments retrieved from the local cancer registry (and additional source of validation data) appear with a suffix "1" in the vertical lines' headings (code H1). In this case, regarding the date when the patient first commenced hormone therapy, a time discrepancy of 51 days was seen between the two data sources, where the hospital recorded the later date.

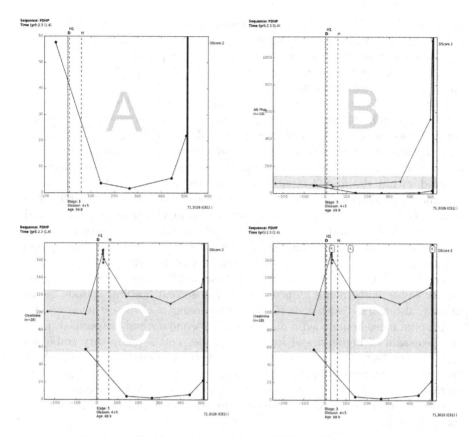

Fig. 4. Four pathway plots of the same patient (175) with sequence $\langle P, D, H, P \rangle$. Plot A shows the original plot with the PSA trend alone. Plot B shows the same information as plot A with additional Alkaline Phosphatase readings and their normal range (shaded area). Plot C shows Creatinine readings and Plot D shows the same information and hospital events (code K). (Color figure online)

Hence this serves to inform on data quality issues (further discussed in the next section). The discrepancy in dates in this case did not introduce uncertainty as the effect of the treatment is seen in the subsequent PSA readings.

The pathway plot in Fig. 4 then shows a PSA relapse in the last two readings. Shortly after the last PSA reading, the patient died of a pulmonary embolism (ICD I26) and prostate cancer (ICD C61) as a secondary condition leading to death. Shortly before death the patient was diagnosed with a secondary and unspecified malignant neoplasm of inguinal and lower limb nodes (ICD C77.4). This was revealed by the additional data collected on hospital episodes and is presented in the visualisation.

Figure 4 Plot B shows an additional element of the pathway, a blood test, Alkaline Phosphatase (ALP) and its normal range in the shaded area. When a patient's advanced cancer metastasises to the bones, ALP can be increased due to active bone formation. Indeed studies have shown that prostate cancer patients with a serum ALP reading of more than twice the normal upper limit had a significantly lower survival rate than their respective counterparts [51]. This is observed in this pathway, although, an increased ALP could be due to other reasons such as an obstructed bile duct or liver disease.

Lastly, plots C and D supplement the pathway with another blood test, Creatinine. Creatinine has been reportedly associated with more advanced disease and decreased survival [52]. However, any condition that impairs the function of the kidneys is likely to raise the creatinine levels in the blood and act as a confounding factor. In plot C, a flare in the values of Creatinine readings was observed within the first 3 months. By introducing additional data elements from the hospital episode statistics in plot D, a hospital episode (marked with pathway code K) was found with an associated primary diagnosis of acute kidney failure. Additional detail on episodes is obtainable by interacting with the visualisation. Although a kidney stone was not coded in this (or any) episode for this patient, a catheterisation of the bladder was performed during the same hospital visit, and an inspection of the patient notes confirmed a kidney stone was the cause of the acute kidney failure. The second hospital episode in this pathway, also marked with code K, was for the removal of the catheter, and the last hospital episode included a diagnosis of a secondary and unspecified malignant neoplasm of inguinal and lower limb nodes and a pulmonary embolism, caused by the first. This level of information that can be added to the pathway would also allow, for example in other cases, to evaluate renal impairment and prostate cancer. Indeed, in this respect, it has been reported that renal impairment in men undergoing prostatectomy represents substantial and unrecognised morbidity [53].

The introduction of additional detail helped to explain the Creatinine flare for this patient and provided interesting insights that would otherwise not be easily explored. The pathway plots provided sufficient information for the interpretation of the pathway yet highlighted potential issues with the quality of the data. Indeed discrepancies in treatment dates across data sources may introduce additional challenges. As such, it is important to be able to differentiate between pathways that have sufficient information and provide an accurate representation of the patient's history and those that do not. The evaluation of the completeness and utility of the generated pathways for investigating biomarker trends is explored in more detail in the next section.

6.2 Data Quality

Methods for the evaluation of data quality dimensions are lacking [54] and visualisation tools can play an important role in quality assurance. Since the development of the pathways framework, one of the first and foremost concerns pertained to the quality of the data being visualised. For the first time since EMR systems were introduced in our hospital, it was possible to visualise integrated data and observe inconsistencies in the ways in which information had been recorded over time. By expanding the data dictionary to include additional information from an external data source, the regional Cancer Registry, it was possible to identify incongruent data across sources.

Figure 5 shows a pathway plot of a patient with Gleason grade 7 prostate cancer who underwent a radical prostatectomy. Information from the Cancer Registry was obtained to validate treatment data and this is included with code S1. In this case, the dates and details of the procedure are in agreement and this patient could easily pass for having a complete record. When plotting the pathway, however, a visual inspection highlighted a significant drop in the PSA values for which there is no clear justification based on the information available. It is unlikely that the PSA values dropped below the 4 ng/ml normal threshold without an intervention. This means that either the treatment date is incorrect in both sources or there is missing information as the patient is likely to have received treatment from another provider while the blood tests continued to be performed by the same laboratory. In this case the plausibility and concordance data quality dimensions were assessed with this visualisation.

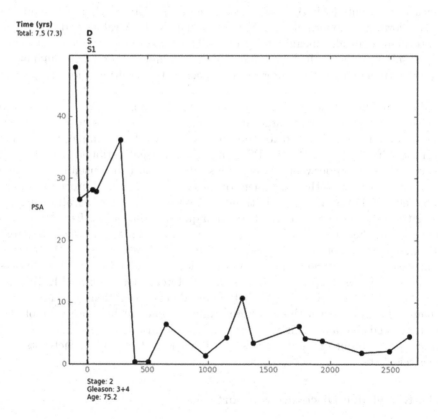

Fig. 5. A Pathway plot for a patient diagnosed with Gleason grade 7 prostate cancer who underwent a radical prostatectomy (code S).

Other data quality examples include mismatch of treatment dates (as seen earlier in Fig. 4) and missing or implausible information. Based on the pathways framework, rules can be devised to inspect individual pathways and determine how complete they might be. For example, in previous work [3] rules pertaining to the availability, positioning and substantiation of the drops in PSA were proposed to determine which pathways would be eligible for further clinical research.

6.3   Cohort Selection, Analysis and Research

Two of the preliminary interests in developing graphical representations of pathways were to compare the shapes of the biomarker curves and also to be able to aggregate patients with similar features. Having pathways expressed as sequences of activity codes has helped to develop the ExploraTree tool, seen in Fig. 3. Depending on how the data points and outcomes are modelled, the trees produced will have varying degrees of granularity and clinical interest. In the example shown earlier, ExploraTree is aggregating patients with similar data points appearing sequentially in time. However, codes for PSA tests (P) could be further broken down into abnormal (say, A) and normal (N) PSA values and this would create more clinically meaningful groups. The ExploraTree software can then help to select relevant cohorts for research, to determine if there are enough members in a particular group of interest and to facilitate recruitment for prospective studies.

Pathway plots allow more detailed and complex information to be presented in a single graphical representation. This enables researchers to observe several data points together and to study new outcomes. For example, Fig. 6 plots Haemoglobin in addition to the PSA and shows normal perioperative bleeding when the patient underwent surgery. This information is not usually examined together yet it enables the assessment of the effect that surgical procedures have on patients and also, the length of time it takes for them to recover after surgery. The latter is an interesting current research question that arose from the visual inspection of the pathways. It is also possible to determine and study different outcomes such as hormone escaped, development of metastases or biochemical recurrence after treatment. Research on services and adherence to guidelines is also possible using the pathway framework [3]. Integration of clinical EMR data with "omics" data is also a topic that should deserve attention in future developments. Pathways with this additional information can be more valuable for precision medicine and their visualisations should also help take knowledge of clinical practice out of the hospitals and bring it to biologists, geneticists and other scientists.

6.4   Knowledge Discovery Support

Visualisation tools are often overlooked when working on knowledge discovery problems in healthcare. One of the most common barriers in machine learning in healthcare is that the models and results produced are not intelligible and work in this area is becoming more topical [55]. Decision trees continue to be the gold standard of intelligible models and more work is needed to create visualisation tools that describe complex models.

Data and process mining techniques are often suggested for the analysis of workflows and pathways, however, most of these techniques have been found unsuitable when applied to heterogeneous routine clinical data. The evaluation of the quality of event logs in process mining relies on trustworthiness (recorded events actually happened), completeness and well defined semantics [56]. These can be achieved by selecting pathways with required data points using the pathways framework. The visualisation system allows for the close inspection and contextualisation of pathways, illustrating particular paths with similar features. It has been reported that a combination of visual analytics with automated process mining techniques would make possible the extraction of more novel insights from event data [56] and further work in this area is needed.

The pathways framework through its graphical representations could also be an interesting way of representing a model, whereby an ideal pathway would be presented and then compared to actual pathways and deviation could be

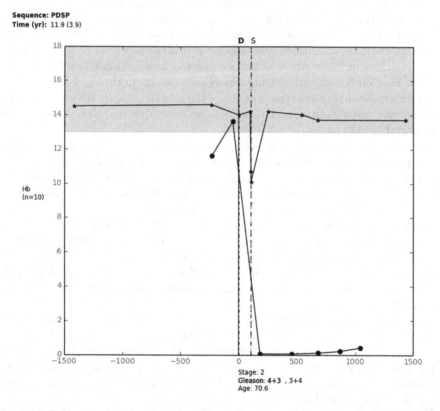

Fig. 6. A Pathway plot showing the effect of a prostatectomy in the Haemoglobin and PSA readings. The green shaded area depicts the normal range for Haemoglobin. (Color figure online)

measured, although further work in this area is required. Additional analysis of the shape of the curves represented (for example, clustering of biomarker trends) is also possible using this framework and some work has already been done in this area using fusion methods [57].

7 Open Problems

Some of the main problems relating to the improvement of health and healthcare with interactive visualisation methods are reviewed by Shneiderman et al. [6], Aigner et al. [58], Caban and Gotz [20], and West et al. [19]. Some of these challenges arise because healthcare must become more "predictive, preemptive, personalised and participative" [6]. Although the efforts described in Sect. 3 and our own efforts are directed to some of this challenges, most systems described to not provide completely satisfactory responses. The open problems summarised from the papers above and from the work presented here include:

- An enduring problem in visualising clinical data is the scale and complexity of the data. Data is not only vast in terms of the number of records but it also includes several different data types (e.g. numeric, categorical, text, images), semantic structures inherent of time data such as cycles and re-occurrences and intertwining conditions and treatment processes. Visual techniques must analyse data in the context of this complexity and summarise it in order to assist busy clinicians with getting timely information in the right format. This requires tools that enable the user to see the overall perspective with powerful yet simple visualisations and then look for anomalies and drill for details of predictable risks early.
- The systems must be capable of scaling up to cohort analysis. Visualising one patient's trajectory can enable monitoring of treatment process for that particular patient. However, it is often necessary to scale the analysis to a cohort of patients as clinicians can then compare responses of diverse patients and assess effectiveness of therapy in the larger scale.
- Context and domain knowledge is very important in clinical decision making so systems must be able to efficiently represent domain knowledge and reason with it to make temporal abstractions, to look at conditions in the context of many clinical parameters such as co-morbidities, medication and history. It may also be desirable to compare cohorts across clinicians, time periods and geographical locations.
- It is increasingly necessary to provide systems that can facilitate multi-disciplinary decision making. Such teams may involve nurses, social workers, physicians and patients. Hence the presentation of knowledge, flexible querying and analysis should accommodate the demands of multiple users with different perspectives and needs. Visualisation tools should play an important role in delivering and interacting with patient data.
- It is often necessary to understand similarity in the context of heterogeneous data but this is not a well developed area of research. Data mining tasks such as classification, clustering, association rules and deviation detection need

to be developed to work with heterogeneous temporal data and to produce intelligible results and meaningful visualisations.

- Data that is routinely collected is plagued by missing values, erroneous values and inaccuracies. Systems that analyse such data must be well equipped to deal with uncertainty. However, uncertainty is a well known open problem in computing. Issues of data quality take their own dimension in a time oriented scenario and can require specific treatment [59]. It is necessary to pre-process the data to uncover data quality issues and exclude dubious data from further analysis. It is also important to quantify data quality dimensions by producing standard measures that can be presented (visually) alongside the data. In addition, presentation of uncertainty in a meaningful way, for example in the context of risk, is still an open research area.
- Currently, according to Kopanitsa et al. [60], there is a gap in transforming knowledge from domain model to interface model. Hence there is a need to turn hard-coded user interfaces into generic methods by a process of standardisation. Standardisation exists for data storage and exchange and they provide a good basis for further efforts. This may also make data more accessible to patients, which may be an important consideration for personalised and participative medicine.
- The design of better interfaces was highlighted as a challenge early on [61] and continues to be an open issue. In particular application of cognitive engineering methods [62] may be beneficial for informing design and for uncovering information needs in clinical systems. There is a requirement for analysing and understanding the process of visual interaction, for example by using logs. Interaction with the visualisation tools is key and must cater for different types of users with different priorities as already discussed.

8   Conclusion and Future Outlook

A picture can arguably be worth a thousand words and in the case of the pathways, a pathway plot is worth, on average, 188 activities using our prostate cancer cohort. For immediate decision-making by clinicians at the point of care, information should be brief and easily interpreted [63] and visualisation tools, if well designed, have a great potential to become part of clinical practice by summarising complex activities in one graphical representation. However, optimal visualisation of clinical data is complex and several open problems remain.

In this paper, clinical pathways were used to demonstrate the potential of visualising routinely collected data using a case study on prostate cancer. The underlying data model enables the summarisation and extension of pathways as well as the aggregation of similar sequences. It is also possible to capture and plot pathways with concurrent elements and to develop algorithms to further explore the data and investigate quality issues. Furthermore, the pathways framework has facilitated interpretation, communication and debate between experts. More work is now needed to assess similar tools in other settings and domains. In this paper, four key areas that hold promise in the future of visualisation in healthcare were identified: decision support and EMR enhancement;

data quality; cohort selection, analysis and research; and knowledge discovery. Further work in each of these areas will bring clinical practice closer to the best available evidence and improve the quality and utility of the *big data* that is available in EMR systems.

References

1. Mannu, G.S., Kyu, M.M., Bettencourt-Silva, J.H., Loke, Y.K., Clark, A.B., Metcalf, A.K., Potter, J.F., Myint, P.K.: Age but not abcd2 score predicts any level of carotid stenosis in either symptomatic or asymptomatic side in transient ischaemic attack. Int. J. Clin. Prac. **69**(9), 948–956 (2015)
2. Bettencourt-Silva, J., De La Iglesia, B., Donell, S., Rayward-Smith, V.: On creating a patient-centric database from multiple hospital information systems. Methods Inf. Med. **51**(3), 210–220 (2012)
3. Bettencourt-Silva, J.H., Clark, J., Cooper, C.S., Mills, R., Rayward-Smith, V.J., de la Iglesia, B.: Building data-driven pathways from routinely collected hospital data: a case study on prostate cancer. JMIR Med. Inform. **3**(3), e26 (2015)
4. Huang, Z., Lu, X., Duan, H.: On mining clinical pathway patterns from medical behaviors. Artif. Intell. Med. **56**(1), 35–50 (2012)
5. Zhang, Y., Padman, R., Patel, N.: Paving the cowpath: learning and visualizing clinical pathways from electronic health record data. J. Biomed. Inform. **58**, 186–197 (2015)
6. Shneiderman, B., Plaisant, C., Hesse, B.W.: Improving healthcare with interactive visualization. Computer **46**(5), 58–66 (2013)
7. Potamias, G.: State of the art on systems for data analysis, information retrieval and decision support. INFOBIOMED project (Deliverable D1) (2006)
8. HiMSS: Healthcare information and management systems society (HiMSS). http://www.himss.org/clinical-informatics/medical-informatics. Accessed 30 Dec 2015
9. Dell Ltd: data mining techniques. http://documents.software.dell.com/statistics/textbook/data-mining-techniques. Accessed 30 Dec 2015
10. Perer, A., Wang, F.: Frequence: interactive mining and visualization of temporal frequent event sequences. In: Proceedings of the 19th International Conference on Intelligent User Interfaces, IUI 2014, pp. 153–162. ACM, New York (2014)
11. Thomas, J.J., Cook, K.A.: Illuminating the path: the research and development agenda for visual analytics. National Visualization and Analytics Ctr (2005)
12. Batini, C., Scannapieco, M.: Data Quality: Concepts, Methodologies and Techniques. Springer, Heidelberg (2006)
13. Hunter, B., Segrott, J.: Re-mapping client journeys and professional identities: a review of the literature on clinical pathways. Int. J. Nurs. Stud. **45**(4), 608–625 (2008)
14. Shahar, Y., Goren-Bar, D., Boaz, D., Tahan, G.: Distributed, intelligent, interactive visualization and exploration of time-oriented clinical data and their abstractions. Artif. Intell. Med. **38**(2), 115–135 (2006)
15. Field, M.J., Lohr, K.N. (eds.): Guidelines for Clinical Practice. Institute of Medicine, National Academy Press, Washington, D.C. (1992). An optional note
16. Turkay, C., Jeanquartier, F., Holzinger, A., Hauser, H.: On computationally-enhanced visual analysis of heterogeneous data and its application in biomedical informatics. In: Holzinger, A., Jurisica, I. (eds.) Knowledge Discovery and Data Mining. LNCS, vol. 8401, pp. 117–140. Springer, Heidelberg (2014)

17. Rind, A., Wang, T.D., Aigner, W., Miksch, S., Wongsuphasawat, K., Plaisant, C., Shneiderman, B.: Interactive information visualization to explore and query electronic health records. Found. Trends Hum. Comput. Interact. **5**(3), 207–298 (2011)
18. Roque, F.S., Slaughter, L., Tkatšenko, A.: A comparison of several key information visualization systems for secondary use of electronic health record content. In: Proceedings of the NAACL HLT 2010 Second Louhi Workshop on Text and Data Mining of Health Documents, Louhi 2010, Stroudsburg, PA, USA, pp. 76–83. Association for Computational Linguistics (2010)
19. West, V.L., Borland, D., Hammond, W.E.: Innovative information visualization of electronic health record data: a systematic review. J. Am. Med. Inform. Assoc. **22**(2), 330–339 (2014)
20. Caban, J.J., Gotz, D.: Visual analytics in healthcare – opportunities and research challenges. J. Am. Med. Inform. Assoc. **22**(2), 260–262 (2015)
21. Lesselroth, B.J., Pieczkiewicz, D.S.: Data visualization strategies for the electronic health record. In: Berhardt, L.V. (ed.) Advances in Medicine and Biology, vol. 16, pp. 107–140. Nova Science Publisher Inc. (2012)
22. Aigner, W., Miksch, S., Schuman, H., Tominski, C.: Visualization of Time-Oriented Data. HCI, 1st edn. Springer, London (2011)
23. Plaisant, C., Milash, B., Rose, A., Widoff, S., Shneiderman, B.: Lifelines: visualizing personal histories. In: Proceedings of the SIGCHI Conference on Human Factors in Computing Systems, CHI 1996, pp. 221–227. ACM, New York (1996)
24. Plaisant, C., Mushlin, R., Snyder, A., Li, J., Heller, D., Shneiderman, B.: Lifelines: using visualization to enhance navigation and analysis of patient records. In: Proceedings of the AMIA Symposium, pp. 76–80 (1998)
25. Wang, T.D., Plaisant, C., Quinn, A.J., Stanchak, R., Murphy, S., Shneiderman, B.: Aligning temporal data by sentinel events: discovering patterns in electronic health records. In: Proceedings of the SIGCHI Conference on Human Factors in Computing Systems, CHI 2008, pp. 457–466. ACM, New York (2008)
26. Wongsuphasawat, K., Guerra Gómez, J.A., Plaisant, C., Wang, T.D., Taieb-Maimon, M., Shneiderman, B.: Lifeflow: visualizing an overview of event sequences. In: Proceedings of the SIGCHI Conference on Human Factors in Computing Systems, CHI 2011, pp. 1747–1756. ACM, New York (2011)
27. Shahar, Y., Cheng, C.: Intelligent visualization and exploration of time-oriented clinical data. In: Proceedings of the 32nd Annual Hawaii International Conference on Systems Sciences, 1999, HICSS-32, vol. Track4, 12 pages, January 1999
28. Klimov, D., Shahar, Y., Taieb-Maimon, M.: Intelligent visualization and exploration of time-oriented data of multiple patients. Artif. Intell. Med. **49**(1), 11–31 (2010)
29. Duke, J.D., Bolchini, D.: A successful model and visual design for creating context-aware drug-drug interaction alerts. In: AMIA Annual Symposium Proceedings 2011, pp. 339–348 (2011)
30. Huang, C.W., Lu, R., Iqbal, U., Lin, S.H., Nguyen, P.A.A., Yang, H.C., Wang, C.F., Li, J., Ma, K.L., Li, Y.C.J., Jian, W.S.: A richly interactive exploratory data analysis and visualization tool using electronic medical records. BMC Med. Inform. Decis. Making **15**(1), 1–14 (2015)
31. Riehmann, P., Hanfler, M., Froehlich, B.: Interactive sankey diagrams. In: IEEE Symposium on Information Visualization, INFOVIS 2005, pp. 233–240, October 2005

32. Wong, B.L.W., Xu, K., Holzinger, A.: Interactive visualization for information analysis in medical diagnosis. In: Holzinger, A., Simonic, K.-M. (eds.) USAB 2011. LNCS, vol. 7058, pp. 109–120. Springer, Heidelberg (2011). doi:10.1007/978-3-642-25364-5_11

33. Aigner, W., Miksch, S.: Carevis: integrated visualization of computerized protocols and temporal patient data. Artif. Intell. Med. **37**(3), 203–218 (2006). Knowledge-Based Data Analysis in Medicine

34. Aigner, W., Miksch, S.: Supporting protocol-based care in medicine via multiple coordinated views. In: Second International Conference on Coordinated and Multiple Views in Exploratory Visualization, Proceedings, pp. 118–129, July 2004

35. Bodesinsky, P., Federico, P., Miksch, S.: Visual analysis of compliance with clinical guidelines. In: Proceedings of the 13th International Conference on Knowledge Management and Knowledge Technologies, i-Know 2013, pp. 12: 1–12: 8. ACM, New York (2013)

36. Krause, J., Perer, A., Stavropoulos, H.: Supporting iterative cohort construction with visual temporal queries. IEEE Trans. Vis. Comput. Graph. **22**(1), 91–100 (2016)

37. Gotz, D., Stavropoulos, H.: Decisionflow: visual analytics for high-dimensional temporal event sequence data. IEEE Trans. Vis. Comput. Graph. **20**(12), 1783–1792 (2014)

38. Kamsu-Foguem, B., Tchuent-Foguem, G., Allart, L., Zennir, Y., Vilhelm, C., Mehdaoui, H., Zitouni, D., Hubert, H., Lemdani, M., Ravaux, P.: User-centered visual analysis using a hybrid reasoning architecture for intensive care units. Decis. Support Syst. **54**(1), 496–509 (2012)

39. Stolper, C., Perer, A., Gotz, D.: Progressive visual analytics: User-driven visual exploration of in-progress analytics. IEEE Trans. Vis. Comput. Graph. **20**(12), 1653–1662 (2014)

40. Sturm, W., Schreck, T., Holzinger, A., Ullrich, T.: Discovering medical knowledge using visual analytics. In: Buhler, K., Linsen, L., John, N.W. (eds.) Eurographics Workshop on Visual Computing for Biology and Medicine. The Eurographics Association (2015)

41. Otasek, D., Pastrello, C., Holzinger, A., Jurisica, I.: Visual data mining: effective exploration of the biological universe. In: Holzinger, A., Jurisica, I. (eds.) Knowledge Discovery and Data Mining. LNCS, vol. 8401, pp. 19–33. Springer, Heidelberg (2014)

42. Lavrac, N., Bohanec, M., Pur, A., Cestnik, B., Debeljak, M., Kobler, A.: Data mining and visualization for decision support and modeling of public health-care resources. J. Biomed. Inform. **40**(4), 438–447 (2007). Public Health Informatics

43. Perer, A., Wang, F., Hu, J.: Mining and exploring care pathways from electronic medical records with visual analytics. J. Biomed. Inform. **56**, 369–378 (2015)

44. Tate, A., Beloff, N., Al-Radwan, B., Wickson, J., Puri, S., Williams, T., van Staa, T., Bleach, A.: Exploiting the potential of large databases of electronic health records for research using rapid search algorithms and an intuitive query interface. J. Am. Med. Inform. Assoc. **21**(2), 292–298 (2014)

45. Jeanquartier, F., Jean-Quartier, C., Holzinger, A.: Integrated web visualizations for protein-protein interaction databases. BMC Bioinform. **16**(1), 1–16 (2015)

46. Müller, H., Reihs, R., Zatloukal, K., Holzinger, A.: Analysis of biomedical data with multilevel glyphs. BMC Bioinform. **15**(6), 1–12 (2014)

47. Shneiderman, B., Plaisant, C.: Strategies for evaluating information visualization tools: multi-dimensional in-depth long-term case studies. In: Proceedings of the 2006 AVI Workshop on BEyond Time and Errors: Novel Evaluation Methods for Information Visualization, BELIV 2006, pp. 1–7. ACM, New York (2006)
48. Pickering, B.W., Dong, Y., Ahmed, A., Giri, J., Kilickaya, O., Gupta, A., Gajic, O., Herasevich, V.: The implementation of clinician designed, human-centered electronic medical record viewer in the intensive care unit: a pilot step-wedge cluster randomized trial. Int. J. Med. Inform. **84**(5), 299–307 (2015)
49. Buschmann, F., Henney, K., Schimdt, D.: Pattern-Oriented Software Architecture: On Patterns and Pattern Language, vol. 5. Wiley, New York (2007)
50. Berner, E.S.: Clinical Decision Support Systems: Theory and Practice, 2nd edn. Springer, New York (2010)
51. Nakashima, J., Ozu, C., Nishiyama, T., Oya, M., Ohigashi, T., Asakura, H., Tachibana, M., Murai, M.: Prognostic value of alkaline phosphatase flare in patients with metastatic prostate cancer treated with endocrine therapy. Urology **56**(5), 843–847 (2000)
52. Weinstein, S.J., Mackrain, K., Stolzenberg-Solomon, R.Z., Selhub, J., Virtamo, J., Albanes, D.: Serum creatinine and prostate cancer risk in a prospective study. Cancer Epidemiol. Biomark. Prev. **18**(10), 2643–2649 (2009)
53. Hill, A.M., Philpott, N., Kay, J., Smith, J., Fellows, G., Sacks, S.: Prevalence and outcome of renal impairment at prostatectomy. Br. J. Urol. **71**(4), 464–468 (1993)
54. Weiskopf, N.G., Weng, C.: Methods and dimensions of electronic health record data quality assessment: enabling reuse for clinical research. J. Am. Med. Inform. Assoc. **20**(1), 144–151 (2013)
55. Caruana, R., Lou, Y., Gehrke, J., Koch, P., Sturm, M., Elhadad, N.: Intelligible models for healthcare: predicting pneumonia risk and hospital 30-day readmission. In: Proceedings of the 21th ACM SIGKDD International Conference on Knowledge Discovery and Data Mining, KDD 2015, pp. 1721–1730. ACM, New York (2015)
56. Van Der Aalst, W., Adriansyah, A., de Medeiros, A.K.A., Arcieri, F., Baier, T., Blickle, T., Bose, J.C., van den Brand, P., Brandtjen, R., Buijs, J., et al.: Process mining manifesto. In: Daniel, F., Barkaoui, K., Dustdar, S. (eds.) Business Process Management Workshops. LNBIP, vol. 99, pp. 169–194. Springer, Heidelberg (2012)
57. Mojahed, A., Bettencourt-Silva, J.H., Wang, W., Iglesia, B.: Applying clustering analysis to heterogeneous data using similarity matrix fusion (smf). In: Perner, P. (ed.) MLDM 2015. LNCS, vol. 9166, pp. 251–265. Springer, Heidelberg (2015). doi:10.1007/978-3-319-21024-7_17
58. Aigner, W., Federico, P., Gschwandtner, T., Miksch, S., Rind, A.: Challenges of time-oriented data in visual analytics for healthcare. In: Caban, J.J., Gotz, D. (eds.) IEEE VisWeek Workshop on Visual Analytics in Healthcare, p. 4. IEEE (2012)
59. Gschwandtner, T., Gärtner, J., Aigner, W., Miksch, S.: A taxonomy of dirty time-oriented data. In: Quirchmayr, G., Basl, J., You, I., Xu, L., Weippl, E. (eds.) CD-ARES 2012. LNCS, vol. 7465, pp. 58–72. Springer, Heidelberg (2012). doi:10.1007/978-3-642-32498-7_5
60. Kopanitsa, G., Hildebrand, C., Stausberg, J., Englmeier, K., et al.: Visualization of medical data based on ehr standards. Methods Inf. Med. **52**(1), 43–50 (2013)
61. Tang, P.C., Patel, V.L.: Major issues in user interface design for health professional workstations: summary and recommendations. Int. J. Bio-Med. Comput. **34**(14), 139–148 (1994). The Health Care Professional Workstation

62. Thyvalikakath, T.P., Dziabiak, M.P., Johnson, R., Torres-Urquidy, M.H., Acharya, A., Yabes, J., Schleyer, T.K.: Advancing cognitive engineering methods to support user interface design for electronic health records. Int. J. Med. Inform. **83**(4), 292–302 (2014)

63. Kay, J.D.: Communicating with clinicians. Ann. Clin. Biochem. **38**, 103 (2001)

Deep Learning Trends for Focal Brain Pathology Segmentation in MRI

Mohammad Havaei[1(✉)], Nicolas Guizard[2], Hugo Larochelle[1,4],
and Pierre-Marc Jodoin[1,3]

[1] Université de Sherbrooke, Sherbrooke, Canada
seyed.mohammad.havaei@usherbrooke.ca
[2] Imagia Inc., Montreal, Canada
[3] Imeka Inc., Sherbrooke, Canada
[4] Twitter Inc., Cambridge, USA

Abstract. Segmentation of focal (localized) brain pathologies such as brain tumors and brain lesions caused by multiple sclerosis and ischemic strokes are necessary for medical diagnosis, surgical planning and disease development as well as other applications such as tractography. Over the years, attempts have been made to automate this process for both clinical and research reasons. In this regard, machine learning methods have long been a focus of attention. Over the past two years, the medical imaging field has seen a rise in the use of a particular branch of machine learning commonly known as deep learning. In the non-medical computer vision world, deep learning based methods have obtained state-of-the-art results on many datasets. Recent studies in computer aided diagnostics have shown deep learning methods (and especially convolutional neural networks - CNN) to yield promising results. In this chapter, we provide a survey of CNN methods applied to medical imaging with a focus on brain pathology segmentation. In particular, we discuss their characteristic peculiarities and their specific configuration and adjustments that are best suited to segment medical images. We also underline the intrinsic differences deep learning methods have with other machine learning methods.

Keywords: Brain tumor segmentation · Brain lesion segmentation · Deep learning · Convolutional Neural Network

1 Introduction

Focal pathology detection of the central nerveous system (CNS), such as lesion, tumor and hemorrhage is primordial to accurately diagnose, treat and for future prognosis. The location of this focal pathology in the CNS determines the related symptoms but clinical examination might to be sufficient to clear identify the underlying pathology. Ultrasound, computer tomography and conventional MRI acquisition protocols are standard image modalities used clinically. The qualitative MRI modalities T1 weighted (T1), T2 weighted (T2), Proton

© Springer International Publishing AG 2016
A. Holzinger (Ed.): ML for Health Informatics, LNAI 9605, pp. 125–148, 2016.
DOI: 10.1007/978-3-319-50478-0_6

density weighted (PDW), T2-weighted FLAIR (FLAIR) and contrast-enhanced T1 (T1C), diffusion weighted MRI and functional MRI are sensitive to the inflammatory and demyelinating changes directly associated with the underlying pathology. As such, MRI is often used to detect, monitor, identify and quantify the progression of diseases.

For instance, in multiple sclerosis (MS), T2 lesions are mainly visible in white matter (WM) but can be found also in gray matter (GM). MS lesions are more frequently located in the peri-ventricular or sub-cortical region of the brain. They vary in size, location and volume but are usually elongated along small vessels. These lesions are highly heterogeneous and include different underlying processes: focal breakdown of the BBB, inflammation, destruction of the myelin sheath (demyelination), astrocytic gliosis, partial preservation of axons and remyelination. Similarly, in Alzheimer's disease (AD), white matter hyperintensity (WMH) which are presumed to be from vascular origin, are also visible on FLAIR images and are believe to be a biomarker of the disease. Similar to vascular hemorrhages, ischemic arterial or venous strokes can be detected with MRI. MRI is also used for brain tumor segmentation which is necessary for monitoring the tumor growth or shrinkage, for tumor volume measurement and also for surgical planning or radiotherapy planning. For glioblastoma segmentation different MRI modalities highlight different tumor sub-regions. For example T1 is the most commonly used modality for structural analysis and distinguishing healthy tissues. In T1C the borders of the glioblastoma are enhanced. This modality is most useful for distinguishing the active part of the glioblastoma from the necrotic parts. In T2, the edema region appears bright. Using FLAIR we can distinguish between the edema and CSF. This is possible because CSF appears dark in FLAIR.

The sub-regions of a glioblastoma are as follows:

- *Necrosis*–The dead part of the tumor.
- *Edema*–Swelling caused by the tumor. As the tumor grows, it can block the cerebrospinal fluid from going out of the brain. New blood vessels growing in and near the tumor can also lead to swelling.
- *Active-enhanced*–Refers to the part of the tumor which is enhanced in T1C modality.
- *Non-enhanced*–Refers to the part of the tumor which is not enhanced in T1C modality.

There are many challenges associated with the segmentation of a brain pathology. The main challenges come from the data acquisition procedure itself (MRI in our case) as well as from the very nature of the pathology. Those challenges can be summarized as follows:

- Certainly *the* most glaring issue with MR images comes from the non-standard intensity range obtained from different scanners. Either because of the various magnet strength (typically 1.5, 3 or 7 Tesla) or because of different acquisition protocol, the intensity values of a brain MRI is often very different from one hospital to another, even for the same patient.

- There is no reliable shape or intensity priors for brain tumors/lesions. Brain pathology can appear anywhere in the brain, they can have any shape (often with fuzzy borders) and come with a wide range of intensities. Furthermore, the intensity range of such pathology may overlap with that of healthy tissue making computer aided diagnosis (CAD) complicated.
- MR images come with a non negligible amount of white Rician noise introduced during the acquisition procedure.
- Homogeneous tissues (typically the gray and the white matter) often suffer from spacial intensity variations along each dimension. This is caused by a so-called *bias field* effect. The MRI bias is a smooth low-frequency signal that affect the image intensities. This problem calls for a bias field correction preprocessing step which typically increase intensity values at the periphery of the brain.
- MR images may have non-isotopic resolution leading to low resolution images, typically along the coronal and the saggital views.
- The presence of a large tumor or lesion in the brain may warp the overall structure of the brain, thus making some procedures impossible to perform. For example, large tumors may affect the overall symmetry of the brain thus making left-right features impossible to compute. Also, brains with a large tumors can hardly be registered onto a healthy brain template.

Methods relying on machine learning also have their own challenges when processing brain images. To count a few:

- Supervised methods require a lot of labeled data in order to generalize well to unseen examples. As opposed to non-medical computer vision applications, acquiring medical data is time consuming, often expensive and requires the non-trivial approval of an ethical committee as well as the collaboration of non-research affiliated staff. Furthermore, the accurate ground truth labeling of 3d MR images is time consuming and expensive as it has to be done by an highly trained personnel (typically a neurologist). As such, publicly-available medical datasets are rare and often made of a limited number of images. One consequence of not having enough labeled data is that the models trained on it are prone to overfitting and perform poorly on new images.
- In supervised learning, we typically estimate maximum likelihoods and thus assumes that the examples are identically distributed. Unfortunately, the intensity variation from one MRI machine to another often violates that assumption. Large variations in the data distribution can be leveraged by having a sufficiently large training dataset, which is almost never the case with medical images.
- Classic machine learning methods rely on computing high dimensional feature vectors which make them computationally inefficient both memory-wise and processing-wise.
- Generally in brain tumor/lesion segmentation, ground truth is heavily unbalanced since regions of interest are very small compared to the whole brain. This is very unfortunate for many machine learning methods such as neural networks whose assumption is that classes have similar size.

– Because of the variability of the data, there is no standard pre-processing
procedure.

Most brain lesion segmentation methods use hand-designed features [22,59].
These methods implement a classical machine learning pipeline according to
which features are first extracted and then given to a classifier whose training
procedure does not affect the nature of those features.

An alternative would be to *learn* such a hierarchy of increasingly complicated
features (i.e. low, mid and high level features). Deep neural networks (DNNs)
have been shown to be successful in learning task-specific feature hierarchies [10].
Importantly, a key advantage of DNNs is that they allow to learn MRI brain-
pathology-specific features that combine information from across different MRI
modalities. Also, convolutions are very efficient and can make predictions very
fast. We investigate several choices for training Convolutional Neural Networks
(CNNs) for this problem and report on their advantages, disadvantages and
performance. Although CNNs first appeared over two decades ago [51], they
have recently become a mainstay for the computer vision community due to their
record-shattering performance in the ImageNet Large-Scale Visual Recognition
Challenge [48]. While CNNs have also been successfully applied to segmentation
problems [4,34,54], most of the previous work has focused on non-medical tasks
and many involve architectures that are not well suited to medical imagery or
brain tumor segmentation in particular.

Over the past two years, we have seen an increasing use of deep learning in
health care and more specifically in medical imaging segmentation. This increase
can be seen in recent Brain Tumor Segmentation challenges (BRATS) which is
held in conjunction with Medical Image Computing and Computer Assisted
Intervention (MICCAI). While in 2012 and 2013 none of the competing methods used DNNs, in 2014, 2 of the 15 methods and in 2015, 7 of the 13 methods
taking part in the challenge were using DNNs. In this work we explore a number of approaches based on deep neural network architectures applied to brain
pathology segmentation.

2   Glossary

Cerebral Spinal Fluid (CSF): a clear, colorless liquid located in the middle
of the brain.

Central Nervous System (CNS): part of the nervous system consisting of
the brain and the spinal cord.

Diffusion Weighted Image (DWI): MR imaging technique measuring the
diffusion of water molecules within tissue voxels. DWI is often used to visualize
hyperintensities.

Deep Neural Network (DNN): an artificial intelligence system modeled on
human brain where through a hierarchy of layers, the model learns low to high
features of the input.

Convolutional Neural Network (CNN): type of DNN adopted for imagery input. Number of parameters in a CNN is significantly less than that of a DNN due to a parameter sharing architecture made feasible by convolutional operations.

FLAIR image: an MRI pulse sequence that suppresses fluid (mainly cerebrospinal fluid (CSF)) while enhancing edema.

Gray Matter (GM): large region located on the surface of the brain consisting mainly of nerve cell bodies and branching dendrites.

High-grade glioma: malignant brain tumors of types 3 and 4.

Low-grade glioma: slow growing brain tumors of types 1 and 2.

Multiple Sclerosis (MS): disease of the central nervous system attacking the myelin, the insulating sheath surrounding the nerves.

Overfitting: in machine learning the *overfitting* phenomenon occurs when the model is too complex relative to the number of observations. Overfitting reduces the ability of the model to generalize to unseen examples.

Proton Density Weighted (PDW) image: MR image sequence used to measure the density of protons; an intermediate sequence sharing some features of both T1 and T2. In current practices, PDW is mostly replaced by FLAIR.

T1-weighted image: one of the basic MRI pulse sequences showing the difference in the T1 relaxation times of tissues [25].

T1 Contrast-enhanced image: a T1 sequence acquired after a gadolinium injection. Gadolinium changes signal intensities by shortening the T1 time in its surroundings. Blood vessels and pathologies with high vascularity appear bright on T1 weighted post gadolinium images.

T2-weighted image: one of the basic MRI pulse sequences. The sequence highlight differences in the T2 relaxation time of tissues [26].

White matter hyperintensity: changes in the cerebral white matter in aged individuals or patients suffering from a brain pathology [64].

3 Datasets

In this section, we describe some of the most widely-used public datasets for brain tumor/lesion segmentation.

BRATS benchmark. The Multimodal BRain Tumor image Segmentation (BRATS) is a challenge held annually in conjunction with MICCAI conference since 2012. The BRATS 2012 training data consist of 10 low- and 20 high-grade glioma MR images whose voxels have been manually segmented with three labels (*healthy*, *edema* and *core*). The challenge data consisted of 11 high- and 5 low-grade glioma subjects no ground truth is provided for this dataset. Using only two basic tumor classes is insufficient due to the fact that the *core* label contains structures which vary in different modalities. For this reason, the BRATS 2013 dataset contains the same training data but was manually labeled into 5 classes; *healthy, necrosis, edema non-enhanced* and *enhanced tumor*. There are also two test sets available for BRATS 2013 which do not come with ground truth; the *leaderboard* dataset which contains the BRATS 2012 challenge dataset plus 10 high-grade glioma patients and the BRATS 2013 challenge dataset which contains 10 high-grade glioma patients. The above mentioned datasets are available for download through the challenge website [2].

For BRATS 2015, the size of the dataset was increased extensively[1]. BRATS 2015 contains 220 brains with high-grade and 54 brains with low grade gliomas for training and 53 brains with mixed high and low grade gliomas for testing. Similar to BRATS'13, each brain from the training data comes with a 5 class segmentation ground truth. BRATS'15 also contains the training data of BRATS'13. The ground truth for the rest of the training brains is generated by a voted average of segmented results of the top performing methods in BRATS'13 and BRATS'12. Although some of these automatically generated ground truths have been refined manually by a user, some authors have decided to remove from their training data brains for which they believe the ground truth was not accurate enough [36,46,79]. This dataset can be downloaded through the challenge website [2].

All BRATS datasets, share four MRI modalities namely; T1, T1C, T2, FLAIR. Image modalities for each subject were co-registered to T1C. Also, all images were skull stripped.

Quantitative evaluation of the model's performance on the test set is achieved by uploading the segmentation results to the online BRATS evaluation system [2]. The online system provides the quantitative results as follows: The tumor structures are grouped in 3 different tumor regions. This is mainly due to practical clinical applications. As described by Menze et al. (2014) [59], tumor regions are defined as:

1. The *complete* tumor region (including all four tumor structures).
2. The *core* tumor region (including all tumor structures exept "edema").
3. The *enhancing* tumor region (including the "enhanced tumor" structure).

Depending on the year the challenge was held, different evaluation metrics have been considered. For each tumor region, they consider *Dice, Sensitivity, Specificity, Kappa* as well as the *Hausdorff* distance. The online evaluation system also provides a ranking for every method submitted for evaluation. This includes methods from the 2013 BRATS challenge published in [59] as well as anonymized unpublished methods for which no reference is available.

ISLES benchmark. Ischemic Stroke Lesion Segmentation (ISLES) challenge started in 2015 and is held in conjunction with the Brain Lesion workshop as

---

[1] Note that the BRATS organizers released a dataset in 2014 but quickly removed it from the web. This version of the dataset is no longer available.

part of MICCAI. ISLES has two categories with individual datasets; sub-acute ischemic stroke lesion segmentation (SISS) and acute stroke outcome/penumbra estimation (SPES) datasets [1].

SISS contains 28 brains with four modalities namely: FLAIR, DWI, T2 TSE (Turbo Spin Echo), and T1 TFE (Turbo Field Echo). The challenge dataset consists of 36 subjects. The evaluation measures used for the ranking were the Dice coefficients, the average symmetric surface distance, and the Hausdorff distance.

SPES dataset contains 30 brains with 7 modalities namely: CBF (Cerebral blood flow), CBV (cerebral blood volume), DWI, T1c, T2, Tmax and TTP (time to peak). The challenge dataset contains 20 subjects. Both datasets provide pixel-accurate level ground truth of the abnormal areas (2 class segmentation). The metrics used to gauge performances are the Dice score, the Hausdorff distance, the recall and precision as well as the average symmetric surface distance (ASSD).

MSGC benchmark. The MSGC dataset which was introduced at MICCAI 2008 [76] provides 20 training MR cases with manual ground truth MS lesion segmentation and 23 testing cases from the Boston Childrens Hospital (CHB) and the University of North Carolina (UNC. For each subject T1, T2 and FLAIR are provided which are co-registered. While lesions masks for the 23 testing cases are not available for download, an automated system is available to evaluate the output of a given segmentation algorithm. The MSGC benchmark provides different metric results normalized between 0 and 100, where 100 is a perfect score and 90 is the typical score of an independent rater [76]. The different metrics (volume difference "VolD", surface distance "SurfD", true positive rate "TPR" and false positive rate "FPR") are measured by comparing the automatic segmentation to the manual segmentation of two experts at CHB and UNC.

4   State-of-the-Art

In this section, we present a brief overview of some methods used to segment brain lesions and brain tumors from MR images.

4.1   Pre Deep Learning Era

These methods can be grouped in two major categories: *semi-automatic* and *automatic* methods. Semi-automatic (or interactive) methods are those relying on user intervention. Many of these methods rely on active deformable models (*e.g.* snakes) where the user initializes the tumor contour [42,84]. Other semi-automatic methods use classification (and yet machine learning) methods whose raw input data is given through regions of interest drawn inside and outside the tumor [8,37,38,44,86]. Semi-automatic methods are appealing in medial imaging applications since the datasets are generally very small [29,40]. Automatic methods on the other hand are those for which no user interaction is made. These methods can be generally divided in two groups; The first group of methods are based on *anomaly* detection where the model estimates intensity similarities between the subject being segmented and an atlas. By doing so, brain regions which deviate from healthy tissue are detected. These techniques have shown good results in structural segmentation when using non-linear registration. When combined with non-local approaches they have proven effective segmentation diffuse and sparse pathologies such as MS [32] as well as more complex multi-label gliomas [45,63,66]. Anomaly detection is not limited to brain tumor/lesion detection but is a key core of health informatics [41].

The second group of methods are *machine learning methods* where a discriminative model is trained using *pre-defined* features of the input modalities. After integrating different intensity and texture features, these methods decide to which class each voxel belongs to. Random forests have been particularly popular. Reza et al. [67] used a mixture of intensity and texture features to train a random forest for voxelwise classification. One problem with this approach is that the model should be trained in a high-dimensional feature space. For example, Festa et al. [24] used a feature space of 300 dimensions and the trained random forest comprised of 50 trees. To train more descriptive classifiers, some methods have taken the approach of adding classes to the ground truth [9,87]. Tustison et al. [78] does this by using Gaussian Mixture Models (GMMs) to get voxelwise tissue probabilities for WM, GM, CSF, edema, non-enhancing tumor, enhancing tumor, necrosis. The GMM is initialized with prior cluster centers learnt from the training data. The voxelwise probabilities are used as input features to a random forest. The intuition behind increasing the number of classes is that the distribution of the healthy class is likely to have different modes for WM, GM and the CSF and so the classifier would be more confidant if it tries to classify them as separate classes. Markov random field (MRF) as well as conditional random field (CRF) are some times used to regularize the predictions [35,52,58,78]. Usually the pairwise weights in these models are either fixed [35] or determined by the input data. They work best in case of weak classifiers such as k-nearest neighbor (kNN) or decision trees and become less beneficial when using stronger classifiers such as convolutional neural networks [70].

Deformable models can also be used as post-processing where the automatic method is used to initialize the counter as opposed to user interaction in semi-automatic methods [39,45,63,66].

4.2   Deep Learning Based Methods

As mentioned before, classical machine learning methods in both automatic and semi-automatic approaches use pre-defined (or hand-crafted) features which might or might not be useful in the training objective. As opposed to that, deep learning methods *learn* features specific to the task at hand. Moreover, these features are learnt in a hierarchy of increasing feature complexity which results in more robust features.

Recently, deep neural networks have proven to be very promising for medical image segmentations. In the past two years, we have seen an increase in use of neural networks applied to brain tumor and lesion segmentations. Notable mentions are the MICCAI's brain tumor segmentation challenge (BRATS) in 2014 and 2015 and the ISLES challenge in 2015 where the top performing methods were taking use of convolutional neural networks [22,23].

In spite of the fact that CNNs were originally developed for image classification, it is possible to use them in a segmentation framework. A simple approach is to train the model in a *patch-wise* fashion as in [15], where for every training (or testing) pixel i, a patch $\mathbf{x}_i$ of size $n \times n$ around i is extracted. Given an image S, the goal is to identify class label y_i given $\mathbf{x}_i$ for all $i \in S$.

Although MRI segmentation is a 3d problem, most methods take a 2D approach by processing the MRI slice by slice. For these methods, training is mostly done patch wise on the axial slices. Zikic et al. [88] use a 3 layer model with 2 convolutional layers and one dense layer. The input size of the model is chosen 19×19, however, since the inputs have been down sampled by a factor of 2, the effective receptive field size is 38×38. *Max pooling* with stride of 3 is used at the first convolutional layer. During test time, down sampled patches of 19×19 are presented to the model in sliding window fashion to cover the entire MRI volume.

The model by Havaei et al. [35] consists of two pathways; a *local pathway* which concentrates on the pixel neighborhood information and a *global pathway* which captures more the global context of the slice. Their local path consists on 2 convolutional layers with kernel sizes of 7×7 and 5×5 respectively while the global path consists of one convolutional layer with 11×11 kernel size. In their architecture, they used *Maxout* [30] as activation function for intermediate layers. Training patch size was 33×33, however during test time, the model was able to process a complete slice making the overall prediction time drop to a couple of seconds. This is achieved by implementing a convolutional equivalent of the dense layers. To preserve pixel density of the label map, they used stride of 1 for max pooling and convolutions.[2] This architecture is shown in Fig. 1.

Havaei et al. [35] also introduced a cascaded method where the class probabilities from a base model are concatenated with input image modalities to train a secondary model similar in architecture than the base model. In their experiments, this approach refined the probability maps produced by the base model and brought them among the top 4 teams in BRATS 2015 [36].

Pereira et al. [61] also adopted a patch wise training with input size experimented with CNNs with small kernel size (i.e. 3×3) as suggested by [74]. This allowed them to have deeper architecture while maintaining the same receptive field as shallow networks with bigger kernels. They trained separate models for

---

[2] Using stride of n means that every n pixel will be mapped to 1 pixel in the label map (assuming the model has one layer). This causes the model to loose pixel level accuracy if full image prediction is to be used at test time. One way to deal with this issue is presented by Pinheiro et al. [62]. Alternatively we can use stride of 1 every where in the model.

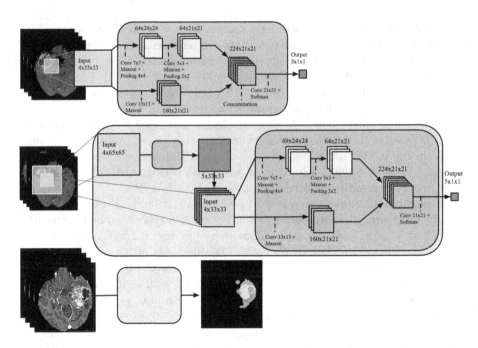

Fig. 1. The proposed architecture by Havaei et al. [35]. First row: TwoPathCNN. The input patch goes through two convolutional networks each comprising of a local and a global path. The feature maps in the local and global paths are shown in yellow and orange respectively. Second row: InputCascadeCNN. The class probabilities generated by TwoPathCNN are concatenated to the input of a second CNN model. Third row: Full image prediction using InputCascadeCNN.

HG and LG tumors. For the HG, their architecture consists of 8 convolutional layers and 3 dense layers while the LG model was a bit shallower containing 4 convolutional layers and 3 dense layers. They used max pooling with stride of 2 and dropout was used only on the dense layers. Leaky rectified linear units (LRLU) [55] was used for activation function. This method achieved good results in BRATS 2015 challenge, ranking them among the top 4 winners. The authors also found *data augmentation* by rotation to be useful. That said, the method comes with a major inconvenience which is for the user to manually decide the type of the tumor (LG or HG) to process.

Dvorak et al. [20] applied the idea of *local structure prediction* [19] for brain tumor segmentation where a dictionary of label patches is constructed by clustering the label patches into n groups. The model is trained to assign an input patch to one of the n groups. The goal is to force the model to take into account labels of the neighboring pixels in addition to the center pixel.

The methods discussed above treat every MRI modality as a channel in CNN the same way color channels are treated in CNN in other computer vision applications. Rao et al. [65] treat these modalities as inputs to separate convolutional

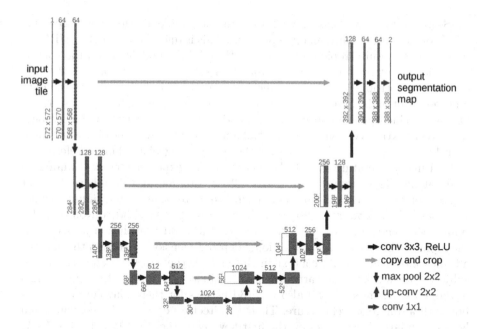

Fig. 2. U-Net: The proposed architecture by Ronneberger et al. [68].

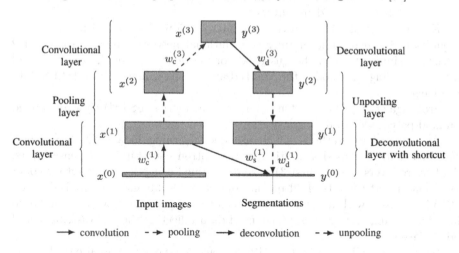

Fig. 3. CEN-s: The proposed architecture by Brosch et al. [11].

streams. In this way, they train 4 separate CNN models each on a different modality. After training, these models are used as feature extractors where features from all 4 models are concatenated to train a random forest classifier. The CNNs share the same architecture of 2 convolutional layers of kernel size 5×5 followed by 2 dense layers. Every CNN takes as input 3 patches of size 32×32 extracted from 3 dimensions (i.e. axial, sagittal, coronal) around the center pixel.

Segmentation problems in MRI are often 3d problems. However, employing CNNs on 3d data remains an open problem. This is due to the fact that MRI volumes are often anisotropic (especially for the FLAIR modality) and the volume resolution is not consistent across subjects. A solution is to pre-process the subjects to be isotropic [32,59]. However, these methods only interpolate the data and the result ends up being severely blurry when the data is highly anisotropic. One way to incorporate information from 3d surroundings is to train on orthogonal patches extracted from axial, sagittal and coronal views. The objective would then be to predict the class label for the intersecting pixel. This is referred to as 2.5d in the literature [65,73]. Havaei et al. [35] experimented by training on 2.5d patches. They argued since BRATS 2013 train and test data have different voxel resolutions, the model did not generalize better than only training on axial view patches. Vaidya et al. [81] and Urban et al. [79] used 3d convolutions for brain lesion and brain tumor segmentation. Using 3d convolution implies that the input to the model has an additional depth dimension. Although this has the advantage of using the 3d context in the MRI, if the gap between slices across subjects varies a lot, the learnt features would not be robust. In a similar line of thoughts, Klein et al. [47] also used 3d kernels for their convolutional layers but with a different architecture. Their architecture consists of 4 convolutional layers with large kernel sizes on the first few layers (i.e. $12 \times 12 \times 12$, $7 \times 7 \times 7$, $5 \times 5 \times 5$, $3 \times 3 \times 3$) with input patch size of $41 \times 41 \times 41$. The convolutional layers are followed by 2 dense layers.

Kamnitsas et al. [43] used a combination [35,61,79] applied to lesion segmentation. In their 11 layer fully convolutional network which consisted of 2 pathways similar to [35], they used 3d convolutions with small kernel sizes of $3 \times 3 \times 3$. Using this model, they ranked among the winners of the ISLES 2015 challenge.

Stollenga et al. [75] used a long short term memories (LSTM) network applied on 2.5d patches for brain segmentation.

As opposed to methods which use deep learning in a CNN framework, Vaidhya et al. [80] used a multi-layer perceptron consisting of 4 dense layers. All feature layers (i.e. the first 3) were pre-trained using denoising auto-encoder as in [83]. Input consists of 3d patches of size $9 \times 9 \times 9$ and training is done on BRATS dataset with a balanced number of class patches. However, similar to [35], fine tuning was done on unbalanced data reflecting the real distribution of label classes.

Inspired by [57], Brosch et al. [12] presented the convolutional encoder networks (CEN) for MS lesion segmentation. The model consists of 2 parts; the encoder part to extract features and up sampling part for pixel level classification[3]. The convolutional encoding part of the model consists of 2 3d convolutional layers in *valid mode*[4] with kernel size $9 \times 9 \times 9$ on both layers followed by an RLU activation function. The up sampling part of the model consists of convolutions

---

[3] In the literature this way of up sampling is some times wrongly referred to as *deconvolution*.

[4] Valid mode is when kernel and input have complete overlap.

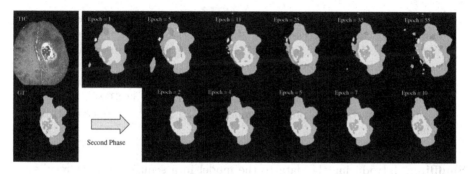

Fig. 4. Effect of second phase training proposed by [35]. The figure shows how the second phase regularizes the predictions and removes false positives.

in *full mode*[5] which results in up sampling the model. Balancing label classes is done by introducing weights per class in the loss function. They improved on this method in [11] by introducing CEN-s, where they combine feature maps from the first hidden layer to the last hidden layer. As shown in Figs. 2 and 3, this model is very similar to the U-Net by Ronneberger et al. [68] with the difference that the U-Net uses interpolation for up sampling as opposed to CEN-s where convolutions are used and transformation weights are learnt during training. Also U-Net is deeper with 11 layers while CEN-s contains only 4 layers. Weights of the model are initialized by RBM unsupervised training. Combining feature maps from shallow layers to higher layers (also referred to as *skip* or *shortcut* connections) are popular in semantic segmentation [33,54].

5   Open Problems

5.1   Preparing the Dataset

Preparing the dataset in a proper way can play a key role in learning. In this chapter we discuss important aspects of dataset preparation for medical imaging.

Pre-processing. As mentioned before, the grayscale distribution of MR images is dependant on the acquisition protocol and the hardware. This makes learning difficult since we expect to have the same data distribution from one subject to another. Therefore, pre-processing to bring all subjects to similar distributions is an important step. Also, it is desirable that all input modalities to the model have the same range so one modality does not have prior advantage over others in deciding the output of the model. Among the many pre-processing approaches reported in the literature, the followings are the most popular:

– Applying the N4/N3 bias field correction [20,31,32,35,49,78,88]. Kleesiek et al. [46] and Urban et al. [79] did not apply bias field correction, instead they

---

[5] Full mode is when minimum overlap is a sufficient condition for applying convolution.

performed intensity normalization with mean CSF value which they claim to be more robust and effective.

- Truncating the 1% or 0.1% quantiles of the histogram to remove outliers from all modalities have also proven to be very effective [35, 78, 80].
- Histogram normalization which is mostly done by matching histogram of every modality to their corresponding template histogram [6, 32, 61, 80].
- Zero mean unit variance on every modality [20, 35] or the selected training patches [61].

Shuffling. Introducing the data to the model in a sequential order results in biasing the gradients and can lead to poor convergence. By sequential order, we mean training first on data extracted from a subject, then training on data extracted from another subject, and so on until the end of the training set. Generally it is a good idea to shuffle the data randomly prior to training. Depending on the dataset, MRI subjects can be are very different in terms of noise and even intensity distribution. Therefore, it is important to shuffle the entire dataset so the model would not overfit to the current training subject and forget it is previous findings. It is desirable that the distribution from which we introduce training examples to the model doesn't change significantly (i.e. the training examples lie on the same manifold). An advantage of patch-wise training over full image training is that in patch-wise training every mini batch contains patches from different slices of different subjects while in full image training, there is no shuffling at pixel level.

Balancing the Dataset. Imbalanced dataset is when class labels are not approximately equally represented. Unfortunately, brain imaging data are rarely balanced due to the small size of the lesion compared to the rest of the brain. For example, the volume of a stroke is rarely more than 1% of the entire brain and a tumor (even large glioblastomas) never occupy more than 4% of the brain. Training a deep network with imbalanced data often lead to very low true positive rates since the system gets to be biased towards the one class that is over represented.

Ideally, we would want to learnt features invariant to the class distribution. This can be done by balancing classes. One approach is to re-sample from the training set so we get an equal number of samples for every class. Another approach is to weight the loss for training examples based on their frequency of appearance in the training data [12, 68]. Sampling from the training set can be done randomly [69–71], or follow an importance sampling criterion to help the model learn things we care about (for example border between classes). For Havaei et al.'s [35] patch-wise training method, the importance sampling is done by computing the class entropy for every pixel in the ground truth and giving training priority to patches with higher entropy. In other words, patches with higher entropy, contain more classes and so would be good candidates to learn the border regions from.

Training on balanced dataset makes the model believe all classes are equiprobable and thus may cause some false positives. In order to compensate for this, one should account for the imbalanced nature of the data in a second training phase during which only the classification layer is trained, the other feature layers being fixed. This allows to regularize the model and remove some false positives. The effect of the second phase training is presented in Fig. 4. Ronneberger et al. [68] took a different approach which is best suited for full image training. In their approach, they compute the distance of every pixel to class borders and, based on that, a weight is assigned to every pixel. A weight map is created for every training image and is used in the loss function to weight every sample differently.

Pereira et al. [61] balance classes mainly by data augmentation. In their case, data augmentation can be a transformation applied on a patch or simply increase the size of the dataset by using patches from similar datasets. For example using patches from brains with high-grade glioma when training a low-grade glioma model.

5.2 Global Information

Adding context information has always been a subject of interest in medical image analysis [3,17,18]. Since anatomical regions in closeup view can appear similar and borders may be diffused in some parts due to lack of contrast or other artifacts, additional context is needed to localize a region of interest.

In CNN, it is possible to encode more contextual information by increasing the portion of the input image each neuron sees (directly or indirectly). Although it is possible to increase the receptive filed of a neuron on the input image through series of convolutional and pooling layers of stride 1, using strides greater than one is computationally more efficient and results in more robust features. By doing so, the model looses precision of spatial information which is needed for segmentation purposes. To take advantage of both worlds, some authors [11,68] learn a global understanding of the input by down sampling the information to smaller size feature maps which are later up sampled and combined with feature maps of lower layer that preserve the spacial information.

Havaei et al. [35] took a different approach where they add a second global convolutional pathway in parallel to a local convolutional pathway. The output feature maps of these two pathways are concatenated before going through the classification layer. This two-pathway approach allows to learn simultaneously global and local contextual features.

5.3 Structured Prediction

Although CNNs provide powerful tools for segmentation, they do not model spatial dependencies. To address this issue, many methods have been proposed to take the information of the neighboring pixels in the label image into account. These methods can be divided into two main categories. The first category are methods which consider the information of the neighboring labels in an *implicit* way while providing no specific pairwise term in the loss function. An example of such approach is provided by Havaei et al. [35] which refine predictions made by the first CNN model by providing the posterior probabilities over classes as extra input to a second CNN model. Roth et al. [70] also use a cascaded architecture to concatenate the probabilities of their first convolutional model with features extracted from multiple scales in a *zoom out* fashion [60]. The second category of methods are ones that *explicitly* define a pairwise term in the loss function which is usually referred to as Conditional Random Field (CRF) in the literature. Although it is possible to train the CNN and CRF end to end, usually for simplicity, the CRF is trained or applied as post processing secondary model to smooth the predicted labels. The weights for the pairwise terms in the CRF can be fixed [37], determined by the input image [37] or learned from the training data [70]. In their work Roth et al. [70] trained an additional convent model between pairs of neighboring pixels.

Post-processing methods based on *connected components* have also proved to be effective to remove small false positive blobs [35,61,80]. In [70], the authors also try 3d isotropic Gaussian smoothing to propagate 2D predictions to 3d and according to them, Gaussian smoothing was more beneficial than using CRF.

5.4   Training on Small or Incomplete Datasets

Deep neural networks generalize better on new data if a large training set is available. This is due to the large number of parameters present in these models. However, constructing a medical imaging dataset is an expensive and tedious task which causes datasets to be small and models trained on these datasets prone to overfitting. Even the largest datasets in this field do not exceed a few hundred subjects. This is much lower than datasets like ImageNet which contains millions of images.

Another problem arises from incomplete datasets. Medical imaging datasets are often multi-modal with images obtained from acquisitions of MRI (T1, T2, proton density, DWI, etc.) [59], or an anatomical MRI image (T1 or T2) coupled with another modality such as SPECT or PET scans [53]. However, not all modalities are available for every subject. How to effectively use the incomplete data rather than simply discarding them is an open question. Another scenario is how to generalize on subjects with missing modalities. In this section we review several effective approaches to train on small and/or incomplete datasets

Data Augmentation. Increasing the size of the dataset by data augmentation is commonly employed in machine learning to enrich a dataset and reduce over-fitting [48]. Flipping the image, applying small rotations, warping the image are common practices for this purpose [16,48,68]. Roth et al. [70] and Ronneberger et al. [68] use non-rigid deformation transformations to increase the size of their dataset and report it to be a key element for their models. The type of data augmentation technique depends on the anatomy of the data and the model being used. For example, Pereira et al. [61] only tested with rotation for data augmentation because the label of the patch is determined by the center pixel. They used angles multiple of 90° and managed to increase the size of the dataset 4 times. They found data augmentation to be very effective in their experiments.

Transfer Learning. Deep learning has made significant breakthroughs in computer vision tasks due to training on very large datasets such as ImageNet. ImageNet contains more than 1.2 million training examples on over 1000 classes. To improve generalization on smaller dataset, it is common to first train a *base* model on a large dataset such as ImageNet and then re-purpose the learnt features to a second *target* model to be *fine tuned* on an application-specific dataset which is often much smaller in size. Yosinski et al. [85] show that the transferability of the features depends on how general those features are and the transferability gap increases as the distance between the tasks increase and features become less general such as the higher level features. But still, transferring weights from a generic pre-trained model to a more specific one is better than initializing weights randomly.

Transfer learning can take 3 forms. The first one is to generate features from the base model and then train a classifier such as SVM or logistic regression with those generated features [5,7,28]. Bar et al. [7] use an ImageNet pre-trained base model to extract features. These features are concatenated with other hand-crafted features before being introduced to an SVM classifier. Van et al. [28] used *overfeat* pre-trained weights to generate features for lung tumor detection. To facilitate with the RGB channels, 3 2D channels are extracted from axial, saggital and coronal views. SVM is used as classifier.

Although this way of transfer learning has proved to be somewhat successful, the degree of it is usefulness depends on how much the source and target datasets are similar. When that is not the case, a transferring method is to fine-tune the features on the target dataset [13,14,27,56]. Gao et al. [27] uses this fine-tuning scheme to detect lung disease in CT images. To accommodate for the RGB channels of the base model which has been pre-trained on ImageNet, three attenuation scales with respect to lung abnormality patterns are captured by rescaling the original 1-channel CT image. Carneiro et al. [13] uses this method to reach state-of-the-art results on the InBreast dataset. Shin et al. [73] reported experimental results in 3 scenarios for Lymph node detection. (1) No transfer learning (2) transfer the weights from another model and only training the classification layer (i.e. weights from other layers are frozen), (3) transfer the weights from another model and fine tune all layers. According to their experiments, the best performance was achieved in the 3rd scenario where the weights of the model are initialized from previously trained model and then all layers are fine tuned on the Lymph node dataset while freezing the weights of the first model achieved least performance. This is expected since the two datasets are very different and the features learnt by model trained on ImageNet are not general enough to be used as on a medical imaging dataset. Tajbakhsh et al. [77] conducted a similar study on transferring pre-trained weights of *AlexNet* on ImageNet to 4 medical imaging datasets. Based on their findings, initializing the weights to a pre-trained model and fine-tuning all layers should be preferred to training from scratch regardless of the size of the dataset. However, if the target dataset is smaller we should be expecting a better gain in performance compared to when the target dataset is sufficiently large. They also observed that transfer learning increases the convergence speed on the target model. Also, since the natural scene image datasets such as ImageNet are very different to medical imaging datasets, we are better off fine-tuning all the layers of the model as opposed to fine tuning only the last few layers. Van et al. [28] cam to a similar conclusion.

A third approach to transfer learning is to initialize the model to weights which have been pre-trained separately in an unsupervised way using models such as *Autoencoders* or *RBMs* [50]. This allows the weights of the main model to be initialized in a better *basin of attraction* [21]. In their lung segmentation problem where they had access to a large un-annotated dataset and a smaller annotated dataset, Schlegl (2014) [72] use convolutional restricted boltzmann machine to pre-train a CNN model in an unsupervised fashion. A shallow model is used as it helps the unsupervised model to learn more general features and less domain specific features.

Missing Modalities. Different modalities in MRI need to be acquired separately and it often happens that different subjects are missing some modalities. The most common practice is to prepare the dataset using modalities which exist in most subjects. This leads to either discarding some subjects from the dataset or discarding some modalities which are not present in all subjects. Another approach is to impute the missing modalities by zero or the mean value of the missing modality. Li et al. [53] used a 3 dimensional CNN architecture to predict a PET modality given a set of MRI modalities. Van et al. [82] proposed to synthesize one missing modality by sampling from the hidden layer representations of a Restricted Boltzmann Machine (RBM). They perform their experiments on BRATS 2013 using patch wise training approach. For every training patch, they train the RBM with every modality to learn the joint probability distribution of the four modalities. At test time, when only one of the modalities is missing they can estimate the missing modality by sampling from the hidden representation vector.

6   Future Outlook

Although deep learning methods have proven to have potential in medical image analysis applications, their performance depends highly on the quality of pre-processing and/or post processing. These methods tend to perform poorly when input data do not follow a common distribution which is often the case. Learning robust representations which are invariant the noise introduced by the acquisition is needed. Unsupervised learning or weakly supervised learning might hold the key to this problem. Also methods based on domain adaptation might help us learn representations which better explain the anatomy of the brain and can better generalize across datasets.

References

1. Isles challenge 2015: Ischemic stroke lesion segmentation. http://www.isles-challenge.org/ISLES2015/. Accessed 11 June 2016
2. Virtual skeleton database. http://www.virtualskeleton.ch/. Accessed 11 June 2016
3. Ali, H., Elmogy, M., El-Daydamony, E., Atwan, A.: Multi-resolution mri brain image segmentation based on morphological pyramid and fuzzy c-mean clustering. Arab. J. Sci. Eng. **40**(11), 3173–3185 (2015)
4. Alvarez, J.M., Gevers, T., LeCun, Y., Lopez, A.M.: Road scene segmentation from a single image. In: Fitzgibbon, A., Lazebnik, S., Perona, P., Sato, Y., Schmid, C. (eds.) ECCV 2012. LNCS, vol. 7578, pp. 376–389. Springer, Heidelberg (2012). doi:10.1007/978-3-642-33786-4_28
5. Arevalo, J., Gonzalez, F.A., Ramos-Pollan, R., Oliveira, J.L., Guevara Lopez, M.A.: Convolutional neural networks for mammography mass lesion classification. In: 37th Annual International Conference of the IEEE Engineering in Medicine and Biology Society (EMBC), pp. 797–800. IEEE (2015)
6. Bakas, S., Zeng, K., Sotiras, A., Rathore, S., Akbari, H., Gaonkar, B., Rozycki, M., Pati, S., Davazikos, C.: Segmentation of gliomas in multimodal magnetic resonance imaging volumes based on a hybrid generative-discriminative framework. In: Proceeding of the Multimodal Brain Tumor Image Segmentation Challenge, pp. 5–12 (2015)
7. Bar, Y., Diamant, I., Wolf, L., Greenspan, H.: Deep learning with non-medical training used for chest pathology identification. In: SPIE Medical Imaging, p. 94140V. International Society for Optics and Photonics (2015)
8. Bauer, S., et al.: A survey of MRI-based medical image analysis for brain tumor studies. Phy. Med. Biol. **58**(13), 97–129 (2013)
9. Bauer, S., Wiest, R., Reyes, M.: segmentation of brain tumor images based on integrated hierarchical classification and regularization. In: proceeding of BRATS-MICCAI (2012)
10. Bengio, Y., Courville, A., Vincent, P.: Representation learning: a review and new perspectives. IEEE Trans. Pattern Anal. Mach. Intell. **35**(8), 1798–1828 (2013)
11. Brosch, T., Tang, L., Yoo, Y., Li, D., Traboulsee, A., Tam, R.: Deep 3D convolutional encoder networks with shortcuts for multiscale feature integration applied to multiple sclerosis lesion segmentation. IEEE Trans. Med. Imaging (2016)
12. Brosch, T., Yoo, Y., Tang, L.Y.W., Li, D.K.B., Traboulsee, A., Tam, R.: Deep convolutional encoder networks for multiple sclerosis lesion segmentation. In: Navab, N., Hornegger, J., Wells, W.M., Frangi, A.F. (eds.) MICCAI 2015. LNCS, vol. 9351, pp. 3–11. Springer, Heidelberg (2015). doi:10.1007/978-3-319-24574-4_1
13. Carneiro, G., Nascimento, J., Bradley, A.P.: Unregistered multiview Mammogram analysis with pre-trained deep learning models. In: Navab, N., Hornegger, J., Wells, W.M., Frangi, A.F. (eds.) MICCAI 2015. LNCS, vol. 9351, pp. 652–660. Springer, Heidelberg (2015). doi:10.1007/978-3-319-24574-4_78
14. Chen, H., Ni, D., Qin, J., Li, S., Yang, X., Wang, T., Heng, P.A.: Standard plane localization in fetal ultrasound via domain transferred deep neural networks. IEEE J. Biomed. Health Informatics **19**(5), 1627–1636 (2015)
15. Ciresan, D., Giusti, A., Gambardella, L.M., Schmidhuber, J.: Deep neural networks segment neuronal membranes in electron microscopy images. In: Advances in Neural Information Processing Systems, pp. 2843–2851 (2012)

16. Cireşan, D.C., Giusti, A., Gambardella, L.M., Schmidhuber, J.: Mitosis detection in breast cancer histology images with deep neural networks. In: Mori, K., Sakuma, I., Sato, Y., Barillot, C., Navab, N. (eds.) MICCAI 2013. LNCS, vol. 8150, pp. 411–418. Springer, Heidelberg (2013). doi:10.1007/978-3-642-40763-5_51

17. Corso, J.J., Sharon, E., Dube, S., El-Saden, S., Sinha, U., Yuille, A.: Efficient multilevel brain tumor segmentation with integrated Bayesian model classification. IEEE Trans. Med. Imaging 27(5), 629–640 (2008)

18. Corso, J.J., Sharon, E., Yuille, A.: Multilevel segmentation and integrated Bayesian model classification with an application to brain tumor segmentation. In: Larsen, R., Nielsen, M., Sporring, J. (eds.) MICCAI 2006. LNCS, vol. 4191, pp. 790–798. Springer, Heidelberg (2006). doi:10.1007/11866763_97

19. Dollár, P., Zitnick, C.: Structured forests for fast edge detection. In: Proceedings of the IEEE International Conference on Computer Vision, pp. 1841–1848 (2013)

20. Dvorak, P., Menze, B.: Structured prediction with convolutional neural networks for multimodal brain tumor segmentation. In: Proceeding of the Multimodal Brain Tumor Image Segmentation Challenge, pp. 13–24 (2015)

21. Erhan, D., Bengio, Y., Courville, A., Manzagol, P.A., Vincent, P., Bengio, S.: Why does unsupervised pre-training help deep learning? J. Mach. Learn. Res. 11, 625–660 (2010)

22. Farahani, K., Menze, B., Reyes, M.: Brats 2014 Challenge Manuscripts (2014). http://www.braintumorsegmentation.org

23. Farahani, K., Menze, B., Reyes, M.: Brats 2015 Challenge Manuscripts (2015). http://www.braintumorsegmentation.org

24. Festa, J., Pereira, S., Mariz, J., Sousa, N., Silva, C.: Automatic brain tumor segmentation of multi-sequence MR images using random dicision forests. In: Proceeding Workshop on Brain Tumor Segmentation MICCAI (2013)

25. Gai, D., Jones, J., et al.: T1 weighted images (2016). http://radiopaedia.org/articles/t1-weighted-image

26. Gai, D., Jones, J., et al.: T1 weighted images (2016). http://radiopaedia.org/articles/t2-weighted-image

27. Gao, M., Bagci, U., Lu, L., Wu, A., Buty, M., Shin, H.C., Roth, H., Papadakis, G.Z., Depeursinge, A., Summers, R.M., et al.: Holistic classification of ct attenuation patterns for interstitial lung diseases via deep convolutional neural networks

28. van Ginneken, B., Setio, A.A., Jacobs, C., Ciompi, F.: Off-the-shelf convolutional neural network features for pulmonary nodule detection in computed tomography scans. In: IEEE 12th International Symposium on Biomedical Imaging (ISBI), pp. 286–289. IEEE (2015)

29. Girardi, D., Küng, J., Kleiser, R., Sonnberger, M., Csillag, D., Trenkler, J., Holzinger, A.: Interactive knowledge discovery with the doctor-in-the-loop: a practical example of cerebral aneurysms research. Brain Informatics, pp. 1–11 (2016)

30. Goodfellow, I.J., et al.: Maxout networks. In: ICML (2013)

31. Gotz, M., Weber, C., Blocher, J., Stieltjes, B., Meinzer, H.P., Maier-Hein, K.: Extremely randomized trees based brain tumor segmentation. In: proceeding of BRATS Challenge-MICCAI (2014)

32. Guizard, N., Coupé, P., Fonov, V.S., Manjón, J.V., et al.: Rotation-invariant multi-contrast non-local means for ms lesion segmentation (2015)

33. Hariharan, B., Arbeláez, P., Girshick, R., Malik, J.: Hypercolumns for object segmentation and fine-grained localization. In: Proceedings of the IEEE Conference on Computer Vision and Pattern Recognition, pp. 447–456 (2015)

34. Hariharan1, B. et al.: Simultaneous detection and segmentation. arXiv preprint arXiv:1407.1808 (2014)

35. Havaei, M., Davy, A., Warde-Farley, D., Biard, A., Courville, A., Bengio, Y., Pal, C., Jodoin, P.M., Larochelle, H.: Brain tumor segmentation with deep neural networks. Medical Image Analysis (2016). http://www.sciencedirect.com/science/article/pii/S1361841516300330

36. Havaei, M., Dutil, F., Pal, C., Larochelle, H., Jodoin, P.-M.: A convolutional neural network approach to brain tumor segmentation. In: Crimi, A., Menze, B., Maier, O., Reyes, M., Handels, H. (eds.) BrainLes 2015. LNCS, vol. 9556, pp. 195–208. Springer, Heidelberg (2016). doi:10.1007/978-3-319-30858-6_17

37. Havaei, M., Jodoin, P.M., Larochelle, H.: Efficient interactive brain tumor segmentation as within-brain knn classification. In: 2014 22nd International Conference on Pattern Recognition (ICPR), pp. 556–561. IEEE (2014)

38. Havaei, M., Larochelle, H., Poulin, P., Jodoin, P.M.: Within-brain classification for brain tumor segmentation. Int. J. Comput. Assist. Radiol. Surg., 1–12 (2015)

39. Ho, S., Bullitt, E., Gerig, G.: Level-set evolution with region competition: automatic 3-D segmentation of brain tumors. In: Proceeding International Conference Pattern Recognition, vol. 1, pp. 532–535 (2002)

40. Holzinger, A.: Interactive machine learning for health informatics: when do we need the human-in-the-loop? Brain Informatics 3(2), 119–131 (2016)

41. Holzinger, A., Dehmer, M., Jurisica, I.: Knowledge discovery and interactive data mining in bioinformatics-state-of-the-art, future challenges and research directions. BMC Bioinformatics 15(Suppl 6), I1 (2014)

42. Jiang, C., Zhang, X., Huang, W., Meinel, C.: Segmentation and quantification of brain tumor. In: IEEE Symposium on Virtual Environments, Human-Computer Interfaces and Measurement Systems, (VECIMS), pp. 61–66 (2004)

43. Kamnitsas, K., Chen, L., Ledig, C., Rueckert, D., Glocker, B.: Multi-scale 3D convolutional neural networks for lesion segmentation in brain MRI. Ischemic Stroke Lesion Segmentation, p. 13 (2015)

44. Kaus, M., Warfield, S.K., Jolesz, F.A., Kikinis, R.: Adaptive template moderated brain tumor segmentation in MRI. In: Evers, H., Glombitza, G., Meinzer, H.-P., Lehmann, T. (eds.) Bildverarbeitung für die Medizin 1999, pp. 102–106. Springer, Heidelberg (1999)

45. Khotanlou, H., Colliot, O., Bloch, I.: Automatic brain tumor segmentation using symmetry analysis and deformable models. In: International Conference on Advances in Pattern Recognition ICAPR, pp. 198–202 (2007)

46. Kleesiek, J., Biller, A., Urban, G., Kothe, U., Bendszus, M., Hamprecht, F.A.: ilastik for multi-modal brain tumor segmentation. In: proceeding of BRATS-MICCAI (2014)

47. Klein, T., Batmanghelich III., Wells III, W.M.: Distributed deep learning framework for large-scale 3D medical image segmentation 18(WS) (2015)

48. Krizhevsky, A., et al.: ImageNet classification with deep convolutional neural networks. In: NIPS (2012)

49. Kwon, D., Akbari, H., Da, X., Gaonkar, B., Davatzikos, C.: Multimodal brain tumor image segmentation using GLISTR. In: proceeding of BRATS Challenge - MICCAI (2014)

50. Larochelle, H., Erhan, D., Courville, A., Bergstra, J., Bengio, Y.: An empirical evaluation of deep architectures on problems with many factors of variation. In: Proceedings of the 24th International Conference on Machine Learning, pp. 473–480. ACM (2007)

51. LeCun, Y., Bottou, L., Bengio, Y., Haffner, P.: Gradient-based learning applied to document recognition. Proc. IEEE 86(11), 2278–2324 (1998)

52. Lee, C.H., Greiner, R., Schmidt, M.: Support vector random fields for spatial classification. In: European Conference on Principles and Practice of Knowledge Discovery in Databases (PKDD), pp. 121–132 (2005)
53. Li, R., Zhang, W., Suk, H.-I., Wang, L., Li, J., Shen, D., Ji, S.: Deep learning based imaging data completion for improved brain disease diagnosis. In: Golland, P., Hata, N., Barillot, C., Hornegger, J., Howe, R. (eds.) MICCAI 2014. LNCS, vol. 8675, pp. 305–312. Springer, Heidelberg (2014). doi:10.1007/978-3-319-10443-0_39
54. Long, J., Shelhamer, E., Darrell, T.: Fully convolutional networks for semantic segmentation. In: Proceedings of the IEEE Conference on Computer Vision and Pattern Recognition, pp. 3431–3440 (2015)
55. Maas, A.L., Hannun, A.Y., Ng, A.Y.: Rectifier nonlinearities improve neural network acoustic models. In: Proceeding ICML, vol. 30, p. 1 (2013)
56. Margeta, J., Criminisi, A., Cabrera Lozoya, R., Lee, D.C., Ayache, N.: Fine-tuned convolutional neural nets for cardiac MRI acquisition plane recognition. Computer Methods in Biomechanics and Biomedical Engineering: Imaging & Visualization, pp. 1–11 (2015)
57. Masci, J., Meier, U., Cireşan, D., Schmidhuber, J.: Stacked convolutional auto-encoders for hierarchical feature extraction. In: Honkela, T., Duch, W., Girolami, M., Kaski, S. (eds.) ICANN 2011. LNCS, vol. 6791, pp. 52–59. Springer, Heidelberg (2011). doi:10.1007/978-3-642-21735-7_7
58. Meier, R., Bauer, S., Slotboom, J., Wiest, R., Reyes, M.: A hybrid model for multimodal brain tumor segmentation. Multimodal Brain Tumor Segmentation, p. 31 (2013)
59. Menze, B.H., Jakab, A., Bauer, S., Kalpathy-Cramer, J., Farahani, K., Kirby, J., Burren, Y., Porz, N., Slotboom, J., Wiest, R., et al.: The multimodal brain tumor image segmentation benchmark (BRATS). IEEE Trans. Med. Imaging **34**(10), 1993–2024 (2015)
60. Mostajabi, M., Yadollahpour, P., Shakhnarovich, G.: Feedforward semantic segmentation with zoom-out features. In: Proceedings of the IEEE Conference on Computer Vision and Pattern Recognition, pp. 3376–3385 (2015)
61. Pereira, S., Pinto, A., Alves, V., Silva, C.A.: Deep convolutional neural networks for the segmentation of gliomas in multi-sequence MRI. In: Crimi, A., Menze, B., Maier, O., Reyes, M., Handels, H. (eds.) BrainLes 2015. LNCS, vol. 9556, pp. 131–143. Springer, Heidelberg (2016). doi:10.1007/978-3-319-30858-6_12
62. Pinheiro, P., Collobert, R.: Recurrent convolutional neural networks for scene labeling. In: Proceedings of The 31st International Conference on Machine Learning, pp. 82–90 (2014)
63. Prastawa, M., Bullitt, E., Ho, S., Gerig, G.: Robust estimation for brain tumor segmentation. In: Ellis, R.E., Peters, T.M. (eds.) MICCAI 2003. LNCS, vol. 2879, pp. 530–537. Springer, Heidelberg (2003). doi:10.1007/978-3-540-39903-2_65
64. Putaala, J., Kurkinen, M., Tarvos, V., Salonen, O., Kaste, M., Tatlisumak, T.: Silent brain infarcts and leukoaraiosis in young adults with first-ever ischemic stroke. Neurology **72**(21), 1823–1829 (2009)
65. Rao, V., Shari Sarabi, M., Jaiswal, A.: Brain tumor segmentation with deep learning. In: MICCAI BraTS (Brain Tumor Segmentation) Challenge, Proceedings Winning Contribution, pp. 31–35 (2014)
66. Rexilius, J., Hahn, H.K., Klein, J., Lentschig, M.G., Peitgen, H.O.: Medical Imaging, p. 65140V (2007)
67. Reza, S., Iftekharuddin, K.: Multi-class abnormal brain tissue segmentation using texture features. In: proceeding of BRATS Challenge - MICCAI (2013)

68. Ronneberger, O., Fischer, P., Brox, T.: U-Net: convolutional networks for biomedical image segmentation. In: Navab, N., Hornegger, J., Wells, W.M., Frangi, A.F. (eds.) MICCAI 2015. LNCS, vol. 9351, pp. 234–241. Springer, Heidelberg (2015). doi:10.1007/978-3-319-24574-4_28
69. Roth, H.R., Farag, A., Lu, L., Turkbey, E.B., Summers, R.M.: Deep convolutional networks for pancreas segmentation in CT imaging. In: SPIE Medical Imaging, p. 94131G. International Society for Optics and Photonics (2015)
70. Roth, H.R., Lu, L., Farag, A., Shin, H.-C., Liu, J., Turkbey, E.B., Summers, R.M.: DeepOrgan: multi-level deep convolutional networks for automated pancreas segmentation. In: Navab, N., Hornegger, J., Wells, W.M., Frangi, A.F. (eds.) MICCAI 2015. LNCS, vol. 9349, pp. 556–564. Springer, Heidelberg (2015). doi:10.1007/978-3-319-24553-9_68
71. Roth, H.R., Lu, L., Seff, A., Cherry, K.M., Hoffman, J., Wang, S., Liu, J., Turkbey, E., Summers, R.M.: A new 2.5D representation for lymph node detection using random sets of deep convolutional neural network observations. In: Golland, P., Hata, N., Barillot, C., Hornegger, J., Howe, R. (eds.) MICCAI 2014. LNCS, vol. 8673, pp. 520–527. Springer, Heidelberg (2014). doi:10.1007/978-3-319-10404-1_65
72. Schlegl, T., Ofner, J., Langs, G.: Unsupervised pre-training across image domains improves lung tissue classification. In: Menze, B., Langs, G., Montillo, A., Kelm, M., Müller, H., Zhang, S., Cai, W.T., Metaxas, D. (eds.) MCV 2014. LNCS, vol. 8848, pp. 82–93. Springer, Heidelberg (2014). doi:10.1007/978-3-319-13972-2_8
73. Shin, H.C., Roth, H.R., Gao, M., Lu, L., Xu, Z., Nogues, I., Yao, J., Mollura, D., Summers, R.M.: Deep convolutional neural networks for computer-aided detection: CNN architectures, dataset characteristics and transfer learning (2016)
74. Simonyan, K., Zisserman, A.: Very deep convolutional networks for large-scale image recognition. arXiv preprint arXiv:1409.1556 (2014)
75. Stollenga, M.F., Byeon, W., Liwicki, M., Schmidhuber, J.: Parallel multi-dimensional lstm, with application to fast biomedical volumetric image segmentation. In: Advances in Neural Information Processing Systems, pp. 2980–2988 (2015)
76. Styner, M., Lee, J., Chin, B., Chin, M., Commowick, O., Tran, H., Markovic-Plese, S., et al.: 3D segmentation in the clinic: a grand challenge ii: MS lesion segmentation. MIDAS **2008**, 1–6 (2008)
77. Tajbakhsh, N., Shin, J., Gurudu, S., Hurst, R., Kendall, C., Gotway, M., Liang, J.: Convolutional neural networks for medical image analysis: Fine tuning or full training? (2016)
78. Tustison, N.J., et al.: Optimal symmetric multimodal templates and concatenated random forests for supervised brain tumor segmentation with ANTsR. Neuroinformatics **13**(2), 209–225 (2015)
79. Urban, G., Bendszus, M., Hamprecht, F., Kleesiek, J.: Multi-modal brain tumor segmentation using deep convolutional neural networks. In: MICCAI BraTS (Brain Tumor Segmentation) Challenge, Proceedings Winning Contribution, pp. 31–35 (2014)
80. Vaidhya, K., Thirunavukkarasu, S., Alex, V., Krishnamurthi, G.: Multi-modal brain tumor segmentation using stacked denoising autoencoders. In: Crimi, A., Menze, B., Maier, O., Reyes, M., Handels, H. (eds.) BrainLes 2015. LNCS, vol. 9556, pp. 181–194. Springer, Heidelberg (2016). doi:10.1007/978-3-319-30858-6_16
81. Vaidya, S., Chunduru, A., Muthuganapathy, R., Krishnamurthi, G.: Longitudinal multiple sclerosis lesion segmentation using 3D convolutional neural networks

82. Tulder, G., Bruijne, M.: Why does synthesized data improve multi-sequence classification? In: Navab, N., Hornegger, J., Wells, W.M., Frangi, A.F. (eds.) MICCAI 2015. LNCS, vol. 9349, pp. 531–538. Springer, Heidelberg (2015). doi:10.1007/978-3-319-24553-9_65

83. Vincent, P., Larochelle, H., Lajoie, I., Bengio, Y., Manzagol, P.A.: Stacked denoising autoencoders: learning useful representations in a deep network with a local denoising criterion. J. Mach. Learn. Res. **11**, 3371–3408 (2010)

84. Wang, T., Cheng, I., Basu, A.: Fluid vector flow and applications in brain tumor segmentation. IEEE Trans. Biomed. Eng. **56**(3), 781–789 (2009)

85. Yosinski, J., Clune, J., Bengio, Y., Lipson, H.: How transferable are features in deep neural networks? In: Advances in Neural Information Processing Systems, pp. 3320–3328 (2014)

86. Zhang, J., Ma, K.K., Er, M.H., Chong, V., et al.: Tumor segmentation from magnetic resonance imaging by learning via one-class support vector machine. In: International Workshop on Advanced Image Technology (IWAIT 2004), pp. 207–211 (2004)

87. Zhao, L., Wu, W., Corso, J.J.: Brain tumor segmentation based on gmm and active contour method with a model-aware edge map. In: BRATS MICCAI, pp. 19–23 (2012)

88. Zikic, D., Ioannou, Y., Brown, M., Criminisi, A.: Segmentation of brain tumor tissues with convolutional neural networks. In: Proceedings MICCAI-BRATS pp. 36–39 (2014)

Differentiation Between Normal and Epileptic EEG Using K-Nearest-Neighbors Technique

Jefferson Tales Oliva$^{(\boxtimes)}$ and João Luís Garcia Rosa

Bioinspired Computing Laboratory, Institute of Mathematics and Computer Science,
University of São Paulo, São Carlos, São Paulo 13566–590, Brazil
jeffersonoliva@usp.br, joaoluis@icmc.usp.br

Abstract. Epilepsy is one of the most common neurological disorder. This disorder can be diagnosed by non-invasive examinations, such as electroencephalography, whose records are called electroencephalograms (EEG). The EEG can be stored in medical databases for reusing in future. In these data, one can apply data mining process supported by machine learning techniques in order to find patterns that can be used for building predictive models. This paper presents an application of the cross-correlation technique and the kNN algorithm for classification in a set with 200 EEG segments in order to differentiate normal and epileptic (abnormal) signals. The results were evaluated using 10-fold cross-validation and contingency table methods. With the evaluation using cross validation, it was not found statistically significant difference for classification using kNN. The contingency table results found that the kNN with $k = 1$ and $k = 7$ performed better for classifying abnormal and normal EEG, respectively. Also, the kNN with $k = 1$ and $k = 7$ were more likely to correctly classify normal and abnormal EEG, respectively.

1 Introduction

According to the World Health Organization (WHO)[1], one in four people will have a mental or neurological disorder. Currently, these disorders reaches approximately 700 million people in the world. Epilepsy is the fourth most common neurological disorder and affects approximately 50 millions people in the world [26,29].

Epilepsy can be diagnosed by electroencephalography, whose records are called electroencephalograms (EEG), which is a non-invasive examination resulting from monitoring of the variation of electrical activity over time generated by neuron populations [4,10]. The EEG signals are stored in databases in order to maintain and to complement the clinical history of patients and be reused by experts to auxiliary in decision making processes for diseases diagnosis [21].

However, with the increasing storage of information in medical databases, their manual analysis becomes an infeasible task. Also, the EEG can contain patterns which are difficult to be identified by naked eye. Thus, methods and

---

[1] http://www.who.int.

© Springer International Publishing AG 2016
A. Holzinger (Ed.): ML for Health Informatics, LNAI 9605, pp. 149–160, 2016.
DOI: 10.1007/978-3-319-50478-0_7

tools must be developed to assist in the analysis and management of such examinations [13].

In this sense, data mining (DM) process supported by machine learning (ML) methods can be applied in different fields to support data analysis and management. This process in conjunction with ML techniques, have motivated several researchers to build descriptive and predictive models [28]. To do so, the data must be in a proper format, e.g., attribute-value table. For EEG signals representation, several features can be extracted from these data [14].

The aim of this study is to classify EEG segments into normal or abnormal (epileptic) class using the ML technique called k-nearest-neighbors (kNN).

This paper is organized as follows: Sect. 2 presents a glossary and key terms related to this work; Sect. 3 reports the EEG database used in this work, the technique applied to extract features in EEG segments and the methods used to build and evaluate the classification performance; Sect. 4 describes the results and discussion in terms of the classification effectiveness obtained with the application of the approach proposed in the database; Sect. 5 presents the final considerations; and Sect. 6 reports proposals for future work.

2   Glossary and Key Terms

Epilepsy is a neurological disorder occasioned by epileptic seizures [19].

Epileptic seizures are signals and/or symptoms due the electrical activity disturbances of the brain [8].

International 10–20 system is a recognized method used in order to distribute electrodes in the scalp for capturing EEG signals. These electrodes are divided into particular locations, considering a distance around between 10 and 20% of the head circumference [10].

Peak value is the maximum value of a time series (TS).

Root mean square is the equivalent voltage of the EEG and it is obtained by multiplying the peak value by a quarter of a sine wave ($sin(45°)$ or 0.707) [16].

Centroid, also called first moment of area, is the geometric center of a wave [6].

Equivalent width is the wave width from the peak value of a wave [6].

Mean square abscissa is the spreading of wave amplitude on the centroid [6].

3   Materials and Methods

3.1   EEG Dataset

The data used in the experiments of this study compose a public EEG database available from [2]. The EEG signals of this database were sampled by a 128-channel amplifier system using an average common reference. These EEG were sampled considering a rate of 173.61 Hz applying 12-bit analog-to-digital conversion and filtered using band-pass at 0.53–40 Hz (12 dB/oct.). The international 10–20 system electrode placement was used for sampling.

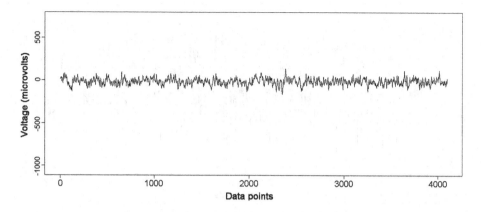

Fig. 1. Normal EEG segment sample.

In this EEG database there are 100 single channel EEG segments with 23.6 s duration sampled, from different subjects. Also, these segments were distributed into five sets and they were selected and removed artifacts, such as eyes movements and muscle activities. Following, the recording conditions of each set are described:

- **A:** Healthy volunteers recordings with eyes open;
- **B:** Healthy volunteers recordings with eyes closed;
- **C:** Recordings of the hippocampal formation of the opposite hemisphere of the brain from patients with epilepsy;
- **D:** Epileptogenic zone recordings from patients with epilepsy;
- **E:** Seizure activity recordings, which were selected from all recording sites showing ictal activity from patients with epilepsy.

Figures 1 and 2 show a normal (health) EEG and an abnormal (epileptic) EEG samples, respectively.

Two sets were used in this work, such as set A (normal) and E (abnormal), according to previous works [3,15]. This way a total of 200 EEG segments were used.

3.2 Feature Extraction

In this work, the cross-correlation (CC) [3] method was applied to extract features in EEG segments in order to represent them in a format suitable for building classifiers. Feature extraction is an essential task for data representation, influencing the performance for building models [15].

CC is a mathematical operation that measures the level of similarity between two signals [22,23] and can be calculated using Eq. 1, where x and y are the signals, n is the signal length and m is the time shift parameter denoted by $m = \{-n + 1, ..., 3, 2, 1, 0, 1, 2, 3, ..., n - 1\}$.

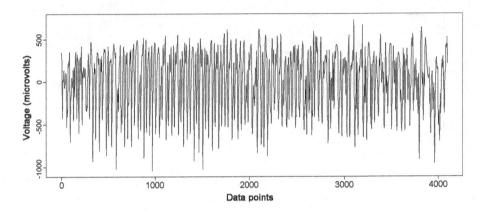

Fig. 2. Epiletic EEG segment sample.

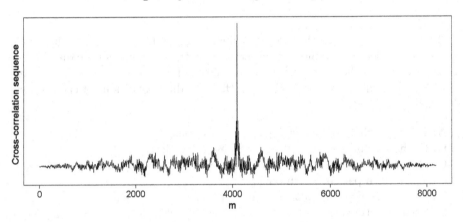

Fig. 3. Cross-correlogram of two healthy EEG segments.

$$CC(x, y, m) = \begin{cases} \sum_{i=0}^{n-m-1} x_{i+m} * y_i & m \geq 0 \\ CC(y, x, -m) & m < 0 \end{cases} \quad (1)$$

So, the CC method generates a cross-correlogram (CCo) with length $2*n-1$, where the *j-th* CCo value is the CC obtained using the time shift $m = j - n$.

Figures 3, 4, and 5 show the CCo of two healthy EEG segments, the CCo of an epileptic and healthy EEG segments, and the CCo of two epileptic EEG segments, respectively.

From CCo, the following features can be extracted [3]:

– **Peak value (PV):**

$$PV = max(CCo) \quad (2)$$

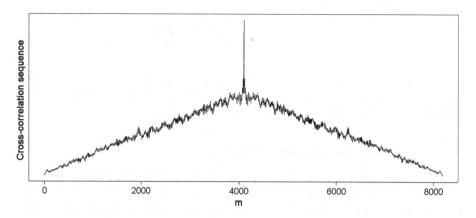

Fig. 4. Cross-correlogram of an epileptic and healthy EEG segments.

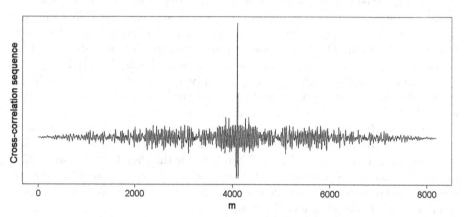

Fig. 5. Cross-correlogram of two epileptic EEG segments.

- **Root mean squared (RMS):**

$$RMS = 0.707 * PV \tag{3}$$

- **Centroid (Ce):**

$$Ce = \frac{\sum_{i=-n}^{n} i * CCo(i)}{\sum_{i=-n}^{n} CCo(i)} \tag{4}$$

- **Equivalent width (EW):**

$$EW = \frac{\sum_{i=-n}^{n} CCo(i)}{PV} \tag{5}$$

- **Mean square abscissa (MSA):**

$$MSA = \frac{\sum_{i=-n}^{n} i^2 * CCo(i)}{\sum_{i=-n}^{n} CCo(i)} \tag{6}$$

For feature extraction based on CCo, initially, an EEG segment is selected as reference, decreasing by 1 the number of instances. Following, this reference EEG is used for building CCo with all other EEG segments [15].

3.3   Building of Classification Models

After feature extraction, the k-nearest-neighbors (kNN) method was used for classification of EEG segments into two classes (normal or abnormal). This method classifies each new example through measuring its similarity with examples previously labeled (training set) by domain experts. For this operation, distance measures can be used to measure similarity among examples, $e.g.$, the Euclidean distance. Also, it is important to emphasize that the kNN technique does not build a classifier (predictive model), $i.e.$, the training set is the classification model itself. The kNN classifies a new example by majority vote of its neighborhood, $i.e.$, the most predominant class in its k-neighbors [1,28].

For binary classifiers, which are applied in two classes classification problem, the k value chosen usually is an odd number in order to avoid ties [12]. In this work, the kNN was applied for $k = 1, 3, 5, 7$, and 9.

The kNN advantages include: easy implementation, fast training, and generalization easy to understand, important characteristic for extracting knowledge in data outside computational area. Therefore, for the classification using kNN, its performance varies according to the value k, $e.g.$, a small value is sensible to noise and a large value, although reducing the noise effect in the classification allows its neighborhood to include examples belonging to another class, $i.e.$, the boundaries between classes can be less distinct [7].

3.4   Model Evaluation

The performance of predictive models are evaluated according to their hits in predicting the class of new examples. The evaluation can be performed by means of cross-validation (CV) method. This method divides the data examples into k equal-sized samples (k folds), which the k-th sample consists of the test set and the k-1 remaining samples compose the training set. Thus, each example of the test set is classified by the kNN using the training set. Afterwards, in the k results of the folds, statistical measures can be calculated, such as average error and standard deviation (SD), to evaluate the classification performance [20]. In addition, statistical tests can be performed to compare the performance of the models in order to verify the existence of the statistically significant difference between them, considering a specific significance level.

Also, the classifiers can be evaluated by means of contingency table (CT) method, which a table type in matrix format used to measure the relationship among nominal variables regarding the class, $i.e.$, the CT verifies whether the variables belong or do not belong to the same class. For example, the CT variables could represent the problem of classifying EEG into normal or abnormal (epileptic) class. Particularly, the following attributes can be calculated from CT [9]:

- **Negative predictive value (NPV):** calculates the percentage of instances without abnormalities in relation to the total of examples that were classified into normal class;
- **Positive predictive value (PPV):** measures the percentage of instances with abnormalities in relation to the total examples that were classified into abnormal class;
- **Specificity:** computes the percentage of instances that were not classified into abnormal class in relation to the total number of examples classified as normal;
- **Sensitivity:** estimates the percentage of instances that were classified into abnormal class related to the total number of examples classified as abnormal.

In this sense, the Java[2] language and the software development platform named NetBeans[3] were used to build a tool for the feature extraction based on CCo. The WEKA tool [18] was used for performing and evaluating the classifiers using the kNN algorithm, which classifies examples of the test set by calculating its similarity with the training set [1]. The software GraphPad Instat© was used to perform statistical analysis.

4   Results and Discussion

The features based on CCo were used and evaluated in previous works. In [15], CCo and other features with ML methods such as Support Vector Machines, Binary Decision Tree and Naive Bayes were used for classification of healthy and epileptic EEG. In [5], CCo with artificial neural network (ANN) was used for heart beat categorization. In [23], CCo with ANN and kNN was used for classification of real high frequency of power transformer windings. In [17], CCo based on logistic regression algorithm was used for classification of motor imagery tasks for brain-computer interface. Also, CCo with ML techniques were used in other related works [11,24,25,27].

In this work, CCo features were extracted from a set of 200 EEG segments. This set is divided into two sets: 100 normal EEG segments (set A) and 100 abnormal EEG (set E). Posteriorly, the first abnormal (epileptic) EEG of a set was selected as reference to build CCo for each remaining EEG. The CCo building method used in this work was implemented in Java using NetBeans.

Subsequently, features based on CCo were extracted, which were used for application of ML techniques to classify EEG segments using kNN algorithm with $k = 1, 3, 5, 7,$ and 9 by WEKA tool.

---

[2] http://www.oracle.com/technetwork/java/index.html.
[3] https://netbeans.org/.

Table 1. Results of applying the CV method to evaluate the classification using kNN.

k value	Average error (%)	Standard Deviation (%)
1	7.22	5.07
3	6.67	5.59
5	7.22	6.67
7	5.00	2.50
9	8.89	6.01

Afterwards, the kNN performance was evaluated for each k value, based on predictive accuracy. This evaluation was performed using the CV and the CT methods, which were performed by WEKA.

The CV method was performed with data divided into ten partitions (10 folds). After, in these partitions, the average error and the SD measures were calculated. Table 1 shows the evaluation results obtained by CV.

Based on this table, it was found that the classification using algorithm kNN with $k = 7$ presents smaller average error and SD than the classification using this algorithm with $k = 1, 3, 5$, and 9. To complement this evaluation, a statistical test was performed for paired data aiming verify the occurrence of a statistically significant difference. The appropriate test type was selected by using the p-value normality test in the error values generated by 10-fold CV for each model. This test found that the classification using kNN with $k = 5$ and 7 were not approved, evidencing that the test to be applied should not be parametric. Thus, the Friedman test [9], considering the significance level of 5%, was applied, resulting in the p-value of 0.4172, considered not significant. Accordingly, it was not possible to observe statistically significant difference for accuracy of the KNN classification with $k = 1, 3, 5, 7$, and 9.

Also, the CT was used to evaluate the classification using kNN. Table 2 shows the correspondent results.

According to this table, the kNN with $k = 7$ was the approach that get better performance for classifying normal EEG, corresponding to 99 signals correctly classified. The kNN with $k = 1$ get better performance for classifying abnormal EEG corresponding to 90 signals correctly classified.

For complement the evaluation using CT, Table 3 presents four precision measures for each built CT.

Based on the Table 3, the kNN with $k = 1$ obtained the highest values for the parameters NPV and sensitivity, which were measured as 91.18% and 90.91%, respectively, finding that this approach was more accurate to correctly classify normal EEG segments and was more likely to rightly categorize abnormal EEG than other approaches used in this work. The kNN with $k = 7$ obtained the highest values for the parameters PPV and specificity, which were measured as 98.88% and 99.00%, respectively, finding that this approach was more accurate to correctly classify abnormal EEG segments and was more likely to rightly categorize normal EEG.

Table 2. CT for the classifier built by the kNN algorithm.

k value	Classification	Normal	Abnormal	Total
1	Normal	93	7	100
	Abnormal	9	90	99
	Total	102	97	199
3	Normal	96	4	100
	Abnormal	10	89	99
	Total	106	93	199
5	Normal	97	3	100
	Abnormal	13	86	99
	Total	110	89	199
7	Normal	99	1	100
	Abnormal	11	88	99
	Total	110	89	199
9	Normal	96	4	100
	Abnormal	14	85	99
	Total	110	89	199

Table 3. Measures calculated using the built CT.

k value	NPV (%)	PPV (%)	Specitivity (%)	Sensitivity (%)
1	91.18	92.78	93.00	90.91
3	90.57	95.70	96.00	89.90
5	88.18	96.63	97.00	86.87
7	90.00	98.88	99.00	88.89
9	87.27	95.51	96.00	85.86

5   Conclusion

In this work, an approach for extracting features based on CCo in EEG segments and for classification these signals using ML techniques was presented. The CCo method was implemented in Java language. The feature extraction was applied in a set with 200 EEG segments. This set consists of 100 normal EEG and 100 abnormal (epileptic) segments. For building CCo, an abnormal EEG segment was selected as reference.

Posteriorly, the kNN algorithm with $k = 1$, 3, 5, 7, and 9, aided by the WEKA tool, was applied for classification of the EEG segments into normal or abnormal class. Afterwards, the results were evaluated according to their hits in predicting the class of the examples.

For performance evaluation of the models, the CV and CT methods by means of WEKA were used. In the evaluation using CV method, the kNN with $k = 7$

reaches lower average error and SD than others k values used in the algorithm. To complement the CV results, the Friedman test was applied in order to verify the existence of the statistically significant difference. The application of this test did not find statistic difference among kNN classification for all k value used in this work.

The performance evaluation of the models using CT found that the kNN with $k = 1$ obtained better performance for classifying abnormal EEG and it was more likely to rightly categorize normal EEG. The kNN with $k = 7$ obtained better performance for classifying normal EEG and it was more likely to rightly categorize abnormal EEG.

6   Future Research

For future works, we include the following activities: performing feature extraction by CCo using other EEG databases, studying and implementing other feature extraction methods to expand the EEG representation; applying the CCo for studying of real EEG related to epilepsy and other diseases diagnosed using this examination, building predictive models using others ML techniques and more classes, and using CCo method in EEG processing for automatic generation of medical reports.

Thereby, with these studies, we expect a greater capacity for prediction of epileptic seizure and other neurological illness, the building of more accurate and representative classifiers, a greater support in the diagnosis of brain diseases, the development of a technique to select EEG segment reference for application of the CC method, the implementation of a tool for filling in medical textual reports automatically, and the support in the decision making processes by medical professionals.

Acknowledgment. J.T. Oliva would like to thank the Brazilian funding agency Coordenação de Aperfeiçoamento de Pessoal de Nível Superior (CAPES) for financial support. J.L.G. Rosa is grateful to the Brazilian agency FAPESP (process 2016/02555-8) for the financial support.

References

1. Alpaydin, E.: Introduction to Machine Learning. MIT press, Cambridge (2014)
2. Andrzejak, R.G., Lehnertz, K., Mormann, F., Rieke, C., David, P., Elger, C.E.: Indications of nonlinear deterministic and finite-dimensional structures in time series of brain electrical activity: Dependence on recording region and brain state. Phy. Rev. E **64**(6), 061907 (2001)
3. Chandaka, S., Chatterjee, A., Munshi, S.: Cross-correlation aided support vector machine classifier for classification of EEG signals. Expert Syst. Appl. **36**(2), 1329–1336 (2009)
4. Chaovalitwongse, W.A., Prokopyev, O.A., Pardalos, P.M.: Electroencephalogram (EEG) time series classification: applications in epilepsy. Ann. Oper. Res. **148**(1), 227–250 (2006)

5. Dutta, S., Chatterjee, A., Munshi, S.: Identification of ECG beats from cross-spectrum information aided learning vector quantization. Measurement **44**(10), 2020–2027 (2011)
6. Easton Jr., R.L.: Fourier Methods in Imaging. Wiley, Danvers (2010)
7. Everitt, B.S., Landau, S., Leese, M., Stahl, D.: Miscellaneous clustering methods. In: Cluster Analysis, pp. 215–255. Wiley, Chichester (2011)
8. Fisher, R.S., Boas, W.E., Blume, W., Elger, C., Genton, P., Lee, P., Engel, J.: Epileptic seizures and epilepsy: definitions proposed by the international league against epilepsy (ILAE) and the international bureau for epilepsy (IBE). Epilepsia **46**(4), 470–472 (2005)
9. Fredman, D., Pisani, R., Ourvers, R.: Statistics. Norton, New York (1988)
10. Freeman, W.J., Quian Quiroga, R.: Imaging Brain Function With EEG: Advanced Temporal and Spatial Analysis of Electroencephalographic Signals. Springer, New York (2013)
11. Gajic, D., Djurovic, Z., Gligorijevic, J., Di Gennaro, S., Savic-Gajic, I.: Detection of epileptiform activity in eeg signals based on time-frequency and non-linear analysis. Frontiers Comput. Neurosci. **9**(38), 1–16 (2015)
12. Hall, P., Park, B.U., Samworth, R.J.: Choice of neighbor order in nearest-neighbor classification. Ann. Stat. **36**(5), 2135–2152 (2008)
13. Han, J.: Data Mining: Concepts and Techniques. Morgan Kaufmann Publishers, San Francisco (2006)
14. Holzinger, A., Scherer, R., Seeber, M., Wagner, J., Müller-Putz, G.: Computational sensemaking on examples of knowledge discovery from neuroscience data: towards enhancing stroke rehabilitation. In: Böhm, C., Khuri, S., Lhotská, L., Renda, M.E. (eds.) ITBAM 2012. LNCS, vol. 7451, pp. 166–168. Springer, Heidelberg (2012). doi:10.1007/978-3-642-32395-9_13
15. Iscan, Z., Dokur, Z., Demiralp, T.: Classification of electroencephalogram signals with combined time and frequency features. Expert Syst. Appl. **38**(8), 10499–10505 (2011)
16. Learnabout Electronics: Measuring the sine wave (2015). http://www.learnabout-electronics.org/ac_theory/ac_waves02.php
17. Li, Y., Wen, P.P.: Modified CC-LR algorithm with three diverse feature sets for motor imagery tasks classification in EEG based brain-computer interface. Comput. Methods Programs Biomed. **113**(3), 767–780 (2014)
18. Machine Learning Group The Universisty of Waikato: Weka 3: data mining software in java (2015). http://www.cs.waikato.ac.nz/ml/weka/
19. Magiorkinis, E., Sidiropoulou, K., Diamantis, A.: Hallmarks in the history of epilepsy: epilepsy in antiquity. Epilepsy Behav. **17**(1), 103–108 (2010)
20. McLachlan, G., Do, K., Ambroise, C.: Analyzing Microarray Gene Expression Data. Wiley, Danvers (2005)
21. Oliva, J.T.: Automating the process of mapping medical reports to estructured database. Master thesis, State University of West Paraná, Foz do Iguaçu, Brazil (2014)
22. Proakis, J.G., Manolakis, D.K.: Digital Signal Processing: Principles, Algorithms, and Application. Prentice Hall, Saddle River (2006)
23. Rahmatian, M., Vahidi, B., Ghanizadeh, A.J., Gharehpetian, G.B., Alehosseini, H.A.: Insulation failure detection in transformer winding using cross-correlation technique with ann and k-NN regression method during impulse test. Int. J. Electr. Power Energy Syst. **53**, 209–218 (2013)

24. Rathipriya, N., Deepajothi, S., Rajendran, T.: Classification of motor imagery ECOG signals using support vector machine for brain computer interface. In: Proceedings of the 15th International Conference Advanced Computing, pp. 63–66, Chennai, India (2013)
25. Ruiz Blondet, M.V., Khalifian, N., Kurtz, K.J., Laszlo, S., Jin, Z.: Brainwaves as authentication method: proving feasibility under two different approaches. In: Proceedings of the 40th Northeast Bioengineering Conference, pp. 1–2, Boston, USA (2014)
26. Shafer, P.O., Sirven, J.I.: Epilepsy statistics (2014). http://www.epilepsy.com/learn/epilepsy-statistics
27. Li, S.Y., Wen, P.: Identification of motor imagery tasks through CC-LR algorithm in brain computer interface. Int. J. Bioinform. Res. Appl. **9**(2), 156–172 (2013)
28. Witten, I., Frank, E., Hall, M.A.: Machine Learning: Practical Machine Learning Tools and Techniques. Morgan Kaufmann, San Francisco (2011)
29. World Health Organization: Epilepsy (2015). http://apps.who.int/gb/ebwha/pdf_files/EB132/B132_8-en.pdf

Survey on Feature Extraction
and Applications of Biosignals

Akara Supratak, Chao Wu, Hao Dong, Kai Sun, and Yike Guo[✉]

William Penney Laboratory, Data Science Institute, Imperial College London,
South Kensington Campus, London SW7 2AZ, UK
{as12212,chao.wu,hao.dong11,kai.sun09,y.guo}@ic.ac.uk

Abstract. Biosignals have become an important indicator not only for medical diagnosis and subsequent therapy, but also passive health monitoring. Extracting meaningful features from biosignals can help people understand the human functional state, so that upcoming harmful symptoms or diseases can be alleviated or avoided. There are two main approaches commonly used to derive useful features from biosignals, which are hand-engineering and deep learning. The majority of the research in this field focuses on hand-engineering features, which require domain-specific experts to design algorithms to extract meaningful features. In the last years, several studies have employed deep learning to automatically learn features from raw biosignals to make feature extraction algorithms less dependent on humans. These studies have also demonstrated promising results in a variety of biosignal applications. In this survey, we review different types of biosignals and the main approaches to extract features from the signal in the context of biomedical applications. We also discuss challenges and limitations of the existing approaches, and possible future research.

Keywords: Feature extraction · Deep learning · Biosignals · Analytical systems

1 Introduction

Biosignals have become an important indicator for medical diagnosis, subsequent therapy and passive health monitoring. They contain information about physiological phenomena which reflect human health and wellbeing [1]. They have been widely used to a variety of applications such as epileptic seizure prediction, sleep stage scoring, affective computing and arrhythmia detection. Recent advances in wearable technology have paved a way to remotely and continuously monitor, record and analyze individuals health status such as number of steps, heart rates, brain signals [2], and glucose level [3]. Tools for analyzing biosignals are vital to understand physiological status of each individual, so that appropriate treatments can be provided in a timely manner. One of the most important research area in biosignals is to develop algorithms to extract features from biosignals

© Springer International Publishing AG 2016
A. Holzinger (Ed.): ML for Health Informatics, LNAI 9605, pp. 161–182, 2016.
DOI: 10.1007/978-3-319-50478-0_8

that can efficiently and compactly represent information relevant to particular problems. There are two main approaches to derive representative features from biosignals: *hand-engineering* and *deep learning*. Hand-engineering feature utilizes ingenuity and expert knowledge to implement algorithms to derive representative features from data. Deep learning, on the other hand, is an approach that utilizes multiple layers of linear and/or non-linear functions to learn useful features from data. In this survey we review feature extraction algorithms developed to transform biosignals into more meaningful features, and the applications to which they have been applied. This survey is useful for those who have basic or advanced knowledge in machine learning, and would like to learn more about different types of biosignals and the algorithms to extract meaningful features from them in order to build analytical tools. The paper is organized as follows: different types of biosignals and the common analytical pipeline will be discussed in Sect. 3. Two main approaches of feature extraction algorithms are explained in Sect. 4. Section 5 demonstrates how these algorithms are applied to different biosignal applications. Challenges and limitations of the existing feature extraction algorithms are discussed in Sect. 6. Finally, possible future research avenues are provided in Sect. 7.

2   Glossary and Key Terms

Biosignals: any signals that can be continually measured/monitored in living organisms.

Hand-engineering Feature: an approach that utilizes ingenuity and expert knowledge to implement algorithms to derive representative features from input data.

Deep Learning: a branch of machine learning that utilizes multi-layer of linear and/or non-linear processing units to learn multi-level of representations that facilitate the subsequent machine learning [4].

Epileptic Seizure: a brief episode of a sign and/or symptom due to abnormal excessive or synchronous neural activity in the brain [5].

Affective Computing: study and development of systems and devices that can assign computers the human-like capabilities of observation, interpretation and generation of affect features [6].

Arrhythmia: a group of conditions in which the heart rhythm or heart rate is irregular.

3   Biosignals

Biosignals refer to any signals that can be continually measured and monitored from living organisms. They can be categorized into two groups: *bioelectrical* and *non-bioelectrical*. In this section, we will discuss examples of bioelectrical and non-bioelectrical signals. Then we will describe the common pipeline of analytical systems for these signals.

3.1 Electrical Biosignals

Bioelectrical signals reflect electrical activity, provoked by electrically active tissue such as nerves and muscles as the result of the changes in the electric currents generated by the sum of electrical potential differences across the tissues. The most commonly used signals include electroencephalogram, electrocardiogram, electromyogram, electrooculogram and electrodermal activity. Table 1 summarizes these signals and examples of their biomedical applications.

Electroencephalogram (EEG) measures and records the electrical activity in the brain. The EEG signals are collected by electrodes which are small, flat metal discs attached on the scalp in certain positions identified by the recordist. The signals reflect voltage fluctuations resulting from ionic current within the neurons in the brain. The amplitudes of EEG signals recorded by electrodes are in the range of microvolts; the main frequencies of interest up to approximately 30 Hz. Based on frequency, EEG waveforms can be broken down into 4 rhythms: β wave (>13 Hz), α wave (8–13 Hz), θ wave (4–8 Hz) and δ wave (<4 Hz). One of the major applications of EEG is diagnosing epilepsy, a condition that causes repeated seizures which can be observed by abnormal patterns in EEG recording (details in Sect. 5). EEG can also be used to investigate other conditions that may affect brain function such as sleep disorders, dementia and brain injuries.

Electrocardiogram (ECG) is a type of biosignals that records the electrical activities of the heart. Electrical changes on the skin that arise from the heart muscle depolarising during each heartbeat are detected by electrodes attached to the body surface. A single beat of an ECG signal consists of three main components: the P wave, QRS complex and the T wave. Variations of these components are associated with different heart characteristics and conditions. Features such as relative positions, magnitudes and shapes of the waves, as well as other derived features such as PR interval, PR segment, QT interval and ST segment, are commonly used by cardiologists while making a diagnosis or investigation. ECG has been used to provide valuable insights into the prevention, diagnosis and treatment of cardiac diseases such as arrhythmia.

Electromyogram (EMG) records the electrical activity produced by muscles. It detects the electrical signals generated by muscle cells when these cells are electrically or neurologically activated. There are two kinds of EMG: surface EMG (sEMG), which measures muscle activity from the surface above the muscle on the skin; and intramuscular EMG, which normally uses electrodes (e.g., needle electrodes) inserted through the skin into a muscle to record electrical signals. EMG can be used to identify neuromuscular diseases including muscular dystrophy, inflammatory myopathy, myasthenia gravis, and others. It can be also used to study biofeedback, functional anatomy of muscles, firing characteristics of motor units and excitability of motor neurons [7].

Electrooculogram (EOG) is used to measure the electrical potential difference between the front (positive pole formed by cornea) and back (negative

Table 1. Different types of bioelectrical signals and application examples.

Biosignal	Tissue/Organ	Applications
Electroencephalogram (EEG)	Brain	Seizures detection, sleep analysis
Electrocardiogram (ECG)	Heart	Arrhythmia detection
Electromyogram (EMG)	Muscles	Neuromuscular disease detection
Electrooculogram (EOG)	Eye	Ophthalmological diagnosis, eye tracking
Electrodermal activity (EDA)	Skin	Stress monitoring, lie detector

pole formed by retina) of the eye. The signals are detected by electrodes placed around the eyes, normally in a range of 5–6 millivolts. EOG is important in the diagnosis of eye diseases such as vitelliform macular dystrophy. Since EOG can detect eye movement and blinks, it is also commonly used in human–computer interaction research.

Electrodermal Activity (EDA) refers to the autonomic changes in the electrical properties of the skin. The skin conductance, which can be non-invasively measured by applying a low constant voltage, is one of the most widely studied electrodermal components [8]. EDA indicates the changes in autonomic sympathetic arousal that are integrated with emotional and cognitive states [9], therefore becomes a common measure of autonomic nervous system activity. EDA has been used in beiofeedback therapy devices for stress monitoring and polygraph devices for lie detecting.

3.2 Non-electrical Biosignals

Biosignals can also be non-electrical, including acoustic signals (e.g., phonocardiogram, respiration), mechanical signals (e.g., mechanomyogram), magnetic signals (e.g., magnetocardiogram), optic signals (e.g., photoplethysmogram) and chemical signals (e.g., partial pressures of oxygen). Measurements such as heart rate and blood pressure, multi-dimensional signals such as video, events such as eye blinking and mouse clicking, can also be considered as non-electrical biosignals and they have been applied to several areas such as affective computing (details will be discussed in Sect. 5.3).

3.3 Common Pipeline of Biosignal Analytical Systems

The common pipeline of analytical systems for biosignals consists of four stages: pre-processing, feature extraction, feature selection (or dimension reduction), and model construction. Firstly, biosignals are pre-processed to ensure that only quality signals can pass to the next stages. This can include removing irrelevant artifacts from signals, correcting inaccurate signals, normalizing signals into a desired range of values, and using a filter to exclude unwanted components. Secondly, features that are meaningful to a certain problem are extracted or derived from the pre-processed signals. The algorithms to extract these features are typically hand-engineered by human experts who know which features are useful for particular problems. Recently, there have been an increasing number of research employing *deep learning* to automate the hand-engineering process. Deep learning, which consists of multiple layers of linear and/or non-linear processing units, is capable of deriving meaningful representations (or features) from high-dimensional input data. Thirdly, it is helpful in some problems to select a subset of extracted features before using machine learning to construct models (i.e., the forth stage). This is because it can speed up the model construction, and can improve the generalization of the constructed models to prevent overfitting. Finally, machine learning algorithms are employed to train and construct models that understand relationships between input (i.e., extracted features) and their desired output (i.e., labels), and generalize observed data to new situations. Depending on the domain for which these models are trained, they are then employed to predict harmful symptoms or classifying diseases.

4 Feature Extraction

4.1 Hand-Engineering Feature

Hand-engineering feature is an approach that utilizes ingenuity and expert knowledge of human being to implement algorithms to derive representative features from data. Generally people tend to employ this approach to build models for a variety of biosignals applications such as classifying diseases and predicting harmful symptoms. This is because it can reduce the amount of data used to build models for such as classifying diseases and predicting harmful symptoms, and the values of extracted features can be easily interpreted as the algorithm details steps to transform from data into features.

Fourier and Wavelet Transforms is a typical tool to extract frequency domain features from time series data. A Fourier transform (DFT) converts a signal into its counterpart in frequency domain, and Fast Fourier transform (FFT) rapidly computes such transformations by factorizing the DFT matrix into a product of sparse factors, including frequency data [10], including magnitude, amplitude, phase, power density, and other computation results. The power density estimation can be made by three different methods: mean squared amplitude (MSA), sum squared amplitude (SSA) and time-integral squared amplitude (TISA). These results could be used as features for prediction or classification (e.g. in EEG [11]).

Another popular time-frequency-transformation for feature extraction comes from wavelet transform. Wavelet transform is designed to address the problem of nonstationary signals. It involves representing a time function in terms of simple, fixed building blocks, termed wavelets. A wavelet series is a representation of a square-integrable (real- or complex-valued) function by a certain orthonormal series generated by a wavelet. They could be treated as features for biosignals such as EEG [12–14]. The WT can be categorized into continuous and discrete.

However, calculating wavelet coefficients for every possible scale can represent a considerable effort and result in a vast amount of data. Therefore, discrete wavelet transform (DWT) is often used.

Principal Component Analysis (PCA) is a statistical procedure that uses an orthogonal transformation to convert a set of observations of possibly correlated variables into a set of values of linearly uncorrelated variables called principal components. The number of principal components is less than or equal to the number of original variables. This transformation is defined in such a way that the first principal component has the largest possible variance (that is, accounts for as much of the variability in the data as possible), and each succeeding component in turn has the highest variance possible under the constraint that it is orthogonal to the preceding components. The resulting vectors are an uncorrelated orthogonal basis set. The principal components are orthogonal because they are the eigenvectors of the covariance matrix, which is symmetric. PCA is sensitive to the relative scaling of the original variables.

4.2   Deep Learning Approach

Deep learning is a branch of machine learning that utilizes multi-layer of linear and/or non-linear processing units to learn multi-level of representations that facilitate the subsequent machine learning [4]. There are many types of deep learning designed to model different types of data. In this section we will describe only three examples of the most commonly used deep learning algorithms in biosignal applications: stacked autoencoder, convolutional neural network and recurrent neural network.

Stacked Autoencoder (SAE) is a neural network consisting of multiple layers of autoencoders in which the outputs of each layer is fed to the input of the next layer [15]. An autoencoder is a neural network consisting of only one hidden layer. It is an unsupervised learning algorithm capable of extracting good feature representations from a plenty of unlabeled data. By setting the target value of the autoencoder to be equal to the input, the autoencoder tries to learn a feature representation that can be used to reconstruct the input. Stacking these autoencoders, therefore, enables the network to learn useful feature representations from EEG data, as the subsequent layers can utilize the features learned from the previous layers to produce even more useful features.

Convolutional Neural Network (CNN) is a neural network consisting of convolutional and pooling layers [16]. Each convolutional layer contains a set of neurons that connect to only a local region or a patch of the input (e.g., a time window in biosignals) in order to detect different patterns. Each neuron contain a number of trainable parameters, or a filter, which are used to convolve each patch location to assess the similarity to the pattern encoded on the parameters. The output generated from all patch locations assemble what is called a feature map. Each pooling layer aggregates consecutive values of the feature maps (such as maximum and mean) resulting from the previous convolutional layer. By properly alternating convolutional and pooling layers, the network can be trained to learn time-invariant local feature detectors from high-dimensional input such as images and biosignals.

Recurrent Neural Network (RNN) is a neural network for handling sequential data. This network maintains what is called a memory (or a hidden state) to learn temporal dependencies between input and output sequences. Depending on the arrangement of the network, it is able to map one input to sequences of output (e.g., image captioning takes an image and outputs a sentence of words), sequences of input to one output (e.g. sentiment analysis where a given sentence is classified as expressing positive or negative sentiment), or input sequences to output sequences (e.g., epileptic seizure prediction where each signal window is classified as preictal or non-preictal). There are many types of RNNs in which update and maintain memory in different ways such as Elman RNN [17], Discrete-time Recurrent Multilayer Perceptrons [18] and Long Short-Term Memory (LSTM) [19].

5   Biosignal Applications

5.1   Epileptic Seizure Detection and Prediction

Almost 60 million people around the world suffer from epilepsy [20]. It is a neurological disorder associated with transient, recurrent and unpredictable epileptic seizures, which are periods of abnormal neural activity in the brain [5]. These seizures can be diagnosed and detected by long-term monitoring of electroencephalograms (EEGs). Thus a system capable of automatically detecting epileptic seizures in real-time can help neurologists to properly provide treatments for patients.

In seizure detection problem, a number of algorithms have been proposed to extract features from EEGs that can be used to differentiate between *ictal* and *non-ictal* states. Fourier transforms have been used to extract features from windowed EEG data such as power spectral density [21,22] and spectral structures that were organized to maintain spatial and temporal information [23]. Later wavelet transform has become more popular compared to the Fourier transforms. Some researchers compared seizure detection performance between these two transforms, and the results showed that the wavelet transforms were better [24,25]. Wavelet transform have been employed to decompose EEG data into frequency bands in order to derive discriminative features such as relative average amplitude, relative scaled energy, relative power, relative derivative and coefficient of variation of amplitude [26,27]; correlation dimension (CD) and largest Lyapunov exponents (LLE) [28–31]; combined seizure index (CSI) [32]; energy, entropy, mean, minimum, maximum and standard deviation [33,34].

Although a system capable of rapidly and accurately detect epileptic seizures is necessary, a more advanced system capable of predict seizures' onsets prior to their presentation would provide even greater benefits. For instance, it might be able to prevent impending seizures through certain therapies, and, therefore, be able to avoid accidents and limit injury [35].

Similar to the detection problem, the seizure prediction is a binary classification problem between *preictal* and *non-preictal* states. Depending on the starting time of seizure symptoms, the preictal state can be a period of several seconds up to several hours before the seizure, and this preictal period varies across differernt patients [36–40].

A majority of existing seizure prediction research concentrates on deriving features from EEG signals. These features can be group into two categories: univariate and multivariate features. The univariate features are extracted from each EEG electrode signal independently such as Lyapunov exponent [41], spectral power [42], wavelet energy and entropy [43], spike rate [44], and repeating EEG patterns [45]. The multivariate features, on the other hand, are derived from pairs or multiple EEG signals in order to represent the relationships (e.g., correlation and synchronizations) among these signals such as phase synchronization [46], and relative spectral power [40]. Several studies have shown that multivariate features demonstrated more promising performance than univariate features [47–49].

Apart from EEG signals, features extracted from ECG signals have also been investigated. Heart rate analysis conducted on ECG signal has been considered as a primary predictor. Ictal tachycardia has been found in some patients of tonic-clonic epilepsy [50], temporal and frontal lobe epilepsies [51,52]. Moreover, tachycardia has also been observed to precede the seizure in some patients with temporal lobe epilepsy [53,54], which has the potential to be used for seizure prediction. Among them, good results have been demonstrated on newborns as the signs of their seizures are more subtle [55,56]. However, for elders, due to complex changes in the ECG occur in physiological and pathological conditions, the ECG-based detection/prediction process is more complicated.

Instead of relying solely on one particular types of biosignals, several studies have introduced approaches that utilizes features extracted from both EEG and ECG signals to improve accuracy and reduce false alarms for seizure detection and prediction. In seizure prediction, Teixeira *et al.* [57] introduced a software package for supporting studies in epileptic seizure prediction including, which includes feature extraction algorithms for EEG and ECG, and data visualization tools. Valderrama *et al.* [58] extracted a large number of time-frequency domain features from EEG and ECG for seizure prediction as they believed that these high-dimensional features could help reduce false alarms. Phomsiricharoenphant *et al.* [59] showed a preliminary results from testing on three events of seizures that the instantaneous frequency of the first mode of Empirical Mode Decomposition (EMD) of EEG was significant dropped down simultaneously with R-R internal variation (inverse of heart beat rate) around 130 s before seizure. Piper *et al.* [60] investigated the synchronization level between heart rate variability and EEG activity during preictal state finding that the synchronization is more significant in the group of right hemispheric temporal lobe epilepsy. Also Greene *et al.* [61] demonstrated the potential of EEG and ECG to complement each other for providing more accurate seizure detection.

There have been several attempts to apply deep learning to implement seizure detection/prediction algorithms that are less dependent on humans. In seizure detection, Guler *et al.* [62] applied Elman RNNs to classify three types of EEG: healthy, seizure free epileptogenic zone, and epileptic seizure segments. The Elman RNNs employing Lyapunov exponents were trained with LevenbergMarquardt algorithm on EEG. The results demonstrated that the proposed RNNs can be useful in discriminating EEG. Supratak *et al.* [63] investigated the possibility of applying SAEs to learn features from raw EEG data. The SAEs was trained with a two-step training including: the greedy layer-wise pretraining [64], and the global fine-tuning to differentiate between ictal and nonictal states. The preliminary results showed that SAEs have potentials to extract features from raw EEG data for seizure detection. In seizure prediction, Petrosian *et al.* [65] made the first attempt to use discrete-time recurrent multilayer perceptrons, one type of RNNs, to predict the onset of epileptic seizures both on scalp and intracranial EEGs. They trained RNNs with raw EEG and its wavelet-decomposed subbands, in contrast to hand-crafted features from EEG, using decoupled extended Kalman filter (DEKF) algorithm. The results showed that it is quite feasible that a preictal period of several minutes preceding seizure existed. Mirowski *et al.* [66] employed CNNs to learn relevant subsets of features. They first extracted four kinds of EEG synchronization features: maximum cross-correlation, nonlinear interdependence, dynamical entrainment and phase synchronization. These features were aggregated to form high-dimensional features, called patterns, which were then used to train CNNs to discriminate preictal from interictal patterns. The results demonstrated that CNNs trained with spatio-temporal patterns of EEG synchronization provided the best seizure prediction performance.

5.2 Sleep Stage Scoring

Sleep is an important biological phenomenon. People spend approximately one-third of their life sleeping. The quality of sleep has a significant impact on people's health. Sleep apnea, insomnia and narcolepsy are common diseases, and about 33% of the world population suffers from insomnia [67]. Thus being able to monitor how well people sleep is essential for both medical research and practice, and could improve the quality of people's life.

EEG signals have been used for monitoring the quantity of sleep and scoring sleep stages. There are two standards for manual sleep stage scoring from EEG [68,69], and American Academy of Sleep Medicine (AASM) is the most commonly used one [69]. AASM classifies sleep into five stages: wake stage (W), rapid eye movement stage (R), and three stages of non-rapid eye movement (N1, N2 and N3).

Features extracted from sleep EEG can be divided into *time-domain* and *frequency-domain*. The reading eye movement, rapid eye movement, slow eye movement, eye blinks and major body movement, k complex, vertex shape waves, sawtooth waves, transient muscle activity from EEG can be considered as time precision features [70–72], which mainly consists of statistical measures of the time series. The frequency features, such as alpha rhythm, low amplitude mixed frequency activity, sleep spindle, slow wave activity, low chin EMG tone, can be extracted by using Morlet wavelets and Fourier transform [73–75]. Apart from these time-domain and frequency-domain features, several studies have proposed other features that can also be used to differentiate sleep stages such as multi-scale entropy [76], spectral entropy [75] and renyi's entropy [73], power-power correlation and autocorrelation [74].

Apart from EEG signal, features extracted from ECG signals have also been investigated [77,78]. For example, the inter-beat interval contains features of heart rate variability (HRV), low frequency (LF, 0.04–0.15 Hz) and high frequency (HF, 0.15–0.4 Hz) of HRV are associated with stage R, N1, N2 and N3. Some nonlinear measures, such as detrended fluctuation analysis (DFA) [79] and fractal component [80], can also be used to classify sleep stages.

Recently, people start to apply deep learning to extract features instead of hand-crafted features [74,81]. This is partly attributed to the tendency of using home-care single channel EEG [82] for sleep stage scoring [73,76,83], which captures less information compared with multi-channel EEG device. Also, sleep stages are scored according to consistent features, but some of the features are not consistent. For instance, about 10% of people did not have alpha activity during walk stage, and another 10% of people had less alpha activity compared with the others (80%) [69]. This introduces what is called variant problem. Deep learning might therefore be a better option to model data with complex structures and variant problem [84].

Deep belief nets (DBNs) [81] was applied to sleep data in order to eliminate the use of hand-crafted features, and it gave a better accuracy compared to fine-turn hand-craft features. Orestis et al. [74] also employed stacked spare autoencoders to reduce the number of features. The results showed a promising performance.

5.3 Affective Computing

Emotion detection and modelling is the core of affective computing [85–87]. Various methods have been proposed to extract features from sensor signals as computational predictors of affect. These features are then used to classify the emotion states in emotion space (e.g. affective dimensions of valence and arousal [88,89], which suggests that emotion is fundamentally organized by these two parameters).

Temporal (and mostly physiological) signals such as skin conductance, heart rate, blood pressure, respiration, pupillary dilation, EEG, speech, and muscle action potentials can provide information regarding the intensity and quality of an individuals internal affect experience. Simple statistical features can be extracted from the average or standard deviation on the time or frequency domains of the raw or normalized signals [90,91]. There are also more complex extractors, e.g. extractors with Legendre and Krawtchouk polynomials [92] and approximate entropy [93,94] using the parameters of linear, quadratic and exponential regression models fitted to a heart rate signal. Some works detected the emotion from speech [91,95], with acoustic features (prosody features, e.g. pitch variables) [96] or speaking rate [97].

Another type of signals comes from events such as user clicking a mouse button, blinking of eyes, etc. Lesh *et al.* [98] proposed a method called "frequent sequence mining", which finds frequent patterns across different discrete modalities, namely gameplay events and discrete physiological events. The count of each pattern was then used as an input feature to an affect detector. The effects of affect on motor-behavior [99] extracted from log-files of mouse and keyboard actions can be used to analyze correlations with affective state. Some other works utilized the mouse clicking and movement as features [100,101].

Multi-dimensional signals [102] such as video were also used for extracting features, through facial expression recognition and gesture recognition [103], where a series of relevant points of the face or body are first detected (e.g., right mouth corner and right elbow) and tracked along frames, then the tracked points are aggregated into discrete or continuous features, such as action units [104] and body contraction index [105]. For gestures recognition, apparentness methods [106] extract apparent features of hand gestures from 2-D images, which 3-D modeling methods [107] extract features by tracking in real 3D environment. Compared to 3-D methods, the apparentness methods are less complicated, and easier to be used in real-time computation, however more efforts should be done to adapt the method into high noise background and the real application. Adopting mixed modeling methods and describing the features of static hand gesture with multiple features (such as local profile features and overall image matrix features) can achieve higher and more robust tracking results [108]. Kapur *et al.* [109] utilized full body skeletal movements captured using video-based sensor, which included 14 markers, each represented as a point in 3D space ($v = [x, y, z]$, where x, y, z are the Cartesian coordinates of the markers position. For each point the velocity (first derivative of position) dv/dt and acceleration (second derivative) d^2v/dt^2 were calculated). During the data collection for gestures recognition, auxiliary equipments such as electromagnetic inductors [110] and optical reflection signs [111] are typically used. For facial expression recognition, parameterized structure of the chief parts of humans face [112], facial action coding system [104], and some other methods [113–115] were used for feature extraction. There were also some multimodal systems, using variety of microphones, video cameras as well as other sensors to enlighten the machine with richer signals from the human [116–118].

Methods of dimensionality reduction on these features include PCA, sequential forward [119], sequential floating forward [120], sequential backwards [121], N-best individuals & perceptron [122], and genetic feature selection [123].

Some recent works tried to achieve automatic feature extraction with deep networks. Stuhlsatz *et al.* [124] used deep networks for discriminative feature extraction from arbitrary distributed raw data, with Generalized Discriminant Analysis [125]. For each considered emotion recognition task, acoustic feature vectors of 6552 dimensions were extracted using the openEAR toolkit as 39 functionals of 56 acoustic Low-Level Descriptors (LLDs) including first and second order delta regression coefficients. In deep network methodologies, information relevant for prediction can be extracted more effectively using dimensionality reduction methods directly on the raw physiological signals than on a set of designer-selected extracted features [126]. Another good property of deep networks is that it can handle both discrete and continuous signals; a lossless transformation can convert a discrete signal into a binary continuous signal, which can potentially be fed into a deep network. Neural networks and Deep networks, including CNN, can also be used for object recognition in images and thus be utilized for feature extraction in multi-dimensional signals. Some existing works include [127–129].

5.4   Arrhythmia Detection

Arrhythmia detection is one of the major biomedical applications of ECG [130]. Arrhythmia is a group of conditions in which the heart rhythm or heart rate is irregular. There are various types of arrhythmias, including supraventricular tachycardia, atrial fibrillation, ventricular tachycardia, ventricular fibrillation, heart block and sick sinus syndrome, each type is considered to be associated with a patten. Irregular heartbeats produce different morphology or wave frequency compared with normal heartbeats, and such alterations can be identified by ECG signals. Different approaches have been proposed for extracting meaningful features from ECG signals and constructing models for arrhythmia detection. Li *et al.* [131] introduced an algorithm based on WT to detect QRS complex of ECG signals. Bachler *et al.* [132] developed an algorithm suitable for online real time and offline ECG analysis. In this approach, a set of wavelet coefficients were extracted from the ECG signal using WT, and used to distinguish ECG waves from noise, artefacts and baseline drift. WT-based approaches were proved to be powerful for ECG feature extraction [131,133,134] and subsequently, a number of methods that combine feature extraction using WT and classification using machine learning algorithms such as SVM [135,136] and probabilistic neural network (PNN) [137] have been proposed in different studies for rhythm classification and arrhythmia detection. Feature extraction methods such as Linear discriminant analysis (LDA) [138], PCA [139], and independent component analysis (ICA) [140] are also been applied to ECG signals to extract features from various waveform properties. Recently, deep learning approaches have been applied to automated learn and identify features from ECG signals for arrhythmia detection. For example, Kiranyaz *et al.* proposed a patient-specific ECG classification and monitoring system based on adaptive 1D convolutional neural networks (CNNs) [141]. In another study, Yang *et al.* used a SAE to extract feature vector from normalised ECG data, and then used a softmax regression model as a classifier to differentiate premature ventricular contraction (PVC) beats and non-PVC beats [142]. Restricted Boltzmann machine was used by Yan *et al.* to learn features from ECG data and build a deep belief network for ECG classification [143].

6   Open Problems

Most of the hand-engineering algorithms are designed specifically to extract useful features from biosignals for particular applications. Even though these algorithms have demonstrated promising results in a number of applications, designing algorithms to extract features that generalize past experience well to new situation is, however, still an active research problem. This might be due to the fact that most of these approaches rely on assumptions or past experiences observed from a limited set of data. Also most of these algorithms always extract the same set of features which may not be optimal, as for each patient the features that can best represent the characteristics of the underlying problem may be different. Therefore, these hand-engineering algorithms might not perform well when applied to new patients. Recent studies have started to apply deep learning to learn representative features from biosignals. They believe that deep learning might be able to learn more meaningful features that are not covered by hand-engineered features [126]. Although these deep learning approaches are able to achieve relatively good performance compared to the hand-engineering ones, the process to training deep learning algorithms is, however, computational expensive. This makes it difficult to frequently incorporate new data into the trained model. Moreover, in the domain of biosignals, it is also difficult to interpret and understand the features learned by deep learning, which is different from other domains such as computer vision.

7   Future Research

Very important is to implement algorithms that integrate knowledge from more than one types of biosignals to enhance the performance of analytical systems. Recent advances in wearable technology have paved a way to remotely and continuously monitor and record multiple types of biosignals from millions of people around the world. Even though the quality of the signals might not be as good as the ones recorded from hospitals or research labs, this allows us to have access to continuous data that might capture interesting information that could be analyzed to improve the quality of the treatments in a variety of the diseases and generate alarms when abnormal patterns are detected. Another future research area could be to develop algorithms that combine features from both hand-engineering and deep learning approaches. As deep learning is a data-driven approach, it might be able to learn features that are complement to the hand-crafted ones, so that the performance of analytical systems are improved. By investigating features learned by deep learning, we may have a better understanding of the characteristics of many diseases. One problem with this approach is that such automatic approaches need many training sets, in health informatics we are often confronted with a small number of data sets or rare events, where automatic algorithms suffer of insufficient training samples, here interactive machine learning with a "doctor-in-the-loop" [145] may be of help.

References

1. Kaniusas, E.: Biomedical Signals and Sensors I. Biological and Medical Physics, Biomedical Engineering. Springer, Heidelberg (2012)
2. Looney, D., Kidmose, P., Park, C., Ungstrup, M., Rank, M., Rosenkranz, K., Mandic, D.: The in-the-ear recording concept: user-centered and wearable brain monitoring. IEEE Pulse **3**(6), 32–42 (2012)
3. Yao, H., Marcheselli, C., Afanasiev, A., Lahdesmaki, I., Parviz, B.A.: A soft hydrogel contact lens with an encapsulated sensor for tear glucose monitoring. In: Proceedings of the IEEE International Conference on Micro Electro Mechanical Systems (MEMS), pp. 769–772, February 2012
4. Bengio, Y., Courville, A., Vincent, P.: Representation learning: a review and new perspectives. IEEE Trans. Pattern Anal. Mach. Intell. **35**(8), 1798–1828 (2012)
5. Fisher, R.S., Van Emde Boas, W., Blume, W., Elger, C., Genton, P., Lee, P., Engel, J.: Epileptic seizures and epilepsy: definitions proposed by the International League Against Epilepsy (ILAE) and the International Bureau for Epilepsy (IBE). Epilepsia **46**(4), 470–472 (2005)
6. Tao, J., Tan, T.: Affective computing: a review. In: Tao, J., Tan, T., Picard, R.W. (eds.) ACII 2005. LNCS, vol. 3784, pp. 981–995. Springer, Heidelberg (2005). doi:10.1007/11573548_125
7. Türker, K.S.: Electromyography: some methodological problems and issues. Phy. Ther. **73**(10), 698–710 (1993)
8. Braithwaite, J.J., Watson, D.G., Jones, R., Rowe, M.: A guide for analysing electrodermal activity (EDA) & skin conductance responses (SCRS) for psychological experiments. Psychophysiology **49**, 1017–1034
9. Critchley, H.D.: Book review: electrodermal responses: what happens in the brain. Neuroscientist **8**(2), 132–142 (2002)
10. Ahmed, N., Natarajan, T., Rao, K.R.: Discrete cosine transfom. IEEE Trans. Comput. **1**, 90–93 (1974)
11. Polat, K., Güneş, S.: Classification of epileptiform eeg using a hybrid system based on decision tree classifier and fast fourier transform. Appl. Math. Comput. **187**(2), 1017–1026 (2007)
12. Subasi, A.: EEG signal classification using wavelet feature extraction and a mixture of expert model. Expert Syst. Appl. **32**(4), 1084–1093 (2007)
13. Jahankhani, P., Kodogiannis, V., Revett, K.: EEG signal classification using wavelet feature extraction and neural networks. In: IEEE John Vincent Atanasoff 2006 International Symposium on Modern Computing, JVA 2006, pp. 120–124. IEEE (2006)
14. Subasi, A.: Application of adaptive neuro-fuzzy inference system for epileptic seizure detection using wavelet feature extraction. Comput. Biol. Med. **37**(2), 227–244 (2007)
15. Bengio, Y.: Learning Deep Architectures for AI, vol. 2 (2009)
16. LeCun, Y., Bengio, Y.: Convolutional networks for images, speech, and time series. In: The Handbook of Brain Theory and Neural Networks (November 1997), vol. 3361, pp. 255–258 (1995)
17. Elman, J.L.: Finding structure in time. Cogn. Sci. **14**(2), 179–211 (1990)
18. Hush, D., Horne, B.G.: Progress in Supervised Neural Networks: What's New Since Lip (1993)
19. Hochreiter, S., Schmidhuber, J.: Long short-term memory. Neural Comput. **9**(8), 1735–1780 (1997)

20. Witte, H., Iasemidis, L., Litt, B.: Special issue on epileptic seizure prediction. IEEE Trans. Biomed. Eng. **50**(5), 537–539 (2003)
21. Polat, K., Gunes, S.: Classification of epileptiform EEG using a hybrid system based on decision tree classifier and fast Fourier transform. Appl. Math. Comput. **187**(2), 1017–1026 (2007)
22. Tzallas, A.T., Tsipouras, M.G., Fotiadis, D.I.: Epileptic seizure detection in EEGs using time-frequency analysis. IEEE Trans. Inform. Technol. Biomed. **13**(5), 703–710 (2009)
23. Shoeb, A., Guttag, J.: Application of machine learning to epileptic seizure detection. In: Proceedings of the 27th International Conference on Machine Learning (ICML-2010), pp. 975–982 (2010)
24. Kiymik, M.K., Güler, I., Dizibüyük, A., Akin, M.: Comparison of STFT and wavelet transform methods in determining epileptic seizure activity in EEG signals for real-time application. Comput. Biol. Med. **35**(7), 603–616 (2005)
25. Logesparan, L., Casson, A.J., Imtiaz, S.A., Rodriguez-Villegas, E.: Discriminating between best performing features for seizure detection and data selection. In: Proceedings of the Annual International Conference of the IEEE Engineering in Medicine and Biology Society, EMBS, pp. 1692–1695 (2013)
26. Saab, M.E., Gotman, J.: A system to detect the onset of epileptic seizures in scalp EEG. Clin. Neurophysiol. **116**(2), 427–442 (2005)
27. Kuhlmann, L., Burkitt, A.N., Cook, M.J., Fuller, K., Grayden, D.B., Seiderer, L., Mareels, I.M.Y.: Seizure detection using seizure probability estimation: comparison of features used to detect seizures. Ann. Biomed. Eng. **37**(10), 2129–2145 (2009)
28. Adeli, H., Ghosh-Dastidar, S., Dadmehr, N.: A wavelet-chaos methodology for analysis of EEGs and EEG subbands to detect seizure and epilepsy. IEEE Trans. Biomed. Eng. **54**(2), 205–211 (2007)
29. Ghosh-Dastidar, S., Adeli, H., Dadmehr, N.: Mixed-band wavelet-chaos-neural network methodology for epilepsy and epileptic seizure detection. IEEE Trans. Biomed. Eng. **54**(9), 1545–1551 (2007)
30. Ghosh-Dastidar, S., Adeli, H., Dadmehr, N.: Principal component analysis-enhanced cosine radial basis function neural network for robust epilepsy and seizure detection. IEEE Trans. Biomed. Eng. **55**(2), 512–518 (2008)
31. Ghosh-Dastidar, S., Adeli, H.: A new supervised learning algorithm for multiple spiking neural networks with application in epilepsy and seizure detection. Neural Networks **22**(10), 1419–1431 (2009)
32. Zandi, A.S., Javidan, M., Dumont, G.A., Tafreshi, R.: Automated real-time epileptic seizure detection in scalp EEG recordings using an algorithm based on wavelet packet transform. IEEE Trans. Biomed. Eng. **57**(7), 1639–1651 (2010)
33. Gandhi, T., Panigrahi, B.K., Bhatia, M., Anand, S.: Expert model for detection of epileptic activity in EEG signature. Expert Syst. Appl. **37**(4), 3513–3520 (2010)
34. Ahammad, N., Fathima, T., Joseph, P.: Detection of epileptic seizure event and onset using EEG. BioMed Research International 2014, p. 7 (2014)
35. Ramgopal, S., Thome-Souza, S., Jackson, M., Kadish, N.E., Fernández, S.I., Klehm, J., Bosl, W., Reinsberger, C., Schachter, S., Loddenkemper, T.: Seizure detection, seizure prediction, and closed-loop warning systems in epilepsy. Epilepsy Behav. **37**, 291–307 (2014)
36. Litt, B., Esteller, R., Echauz, J., D'Alessandro, M., Shor, R., Henry, T., Pennell, P., Epstein, C., Bakay, R., Dichter, M., Vachtsevanos, G.: Epileptic seizures may begin clinical study hours in advance of clinical onset: a report of five patients. Neuron **30**(1), 1–14 (2001)

37. Le Van Quyen, M., Martinerie, J., Navarro, V., Boon, P., D'Havé, M., Adam, C., Renault, B., Varela, F., Baulac, M.: Anticipation of epileptic seizures from standard EEG recordings. Lancet **357**(9251), 183–188 (2001)

38. Le Van Quyen, M., Navarro, V., Martinerie, J., Baulac, M., Varela, F.J.: Toward a neurodynamical understanding of ictogenesis. Epilepsia **44**(Suppl 1), 30–43 (2003)

39. Litt, B., Lehnertz, K.: Seizure prediction and the preseizure period. Current Opinion Neurol. **15**(2), 173–177 (2002)

40. Bandarabadi, M., Teixeira, C.A., Rasekhi, J., Dourado, A.: Epileptic seizure prediction using relative spectral power features. Clin. Neurophysiol. **126**(2), 237–248 (2015)

41. Sackellares, J.C., Shiau, D.S., Principe, J.C., Yang, M.C.K., Dance, L.K., Suharitdamrong, W., Chaovalitwongse, W.A., Pardalos, P.M., Iasemidis, L.D.: Predictability analysis for an automated seizure prediction algorithm. J. Clin. Neurophysiol. **23**(6), 509–520 (2006). Official publication of the American Electroencephalographic Society

42. Park, Y., Luo, L., Parhi, K.K., Netoff, T.: Seizure prediction with spectral power of EEG using cost-sensitive support vector machines. Epilepsia **52**(10), 1761–1770 (2011)

43. Gadhoumi, K., Lina, J.M., Gotman, J.: Seizure prediction in patients with mesial temporal lobe epilepsy using EEG measures of state similarity. Clin. Neurophysiol. **124**(9), 1745–1754 (2013)

44. Li, S., Zhou, W., Yuan, Q., Liu, Y.: Seizure prediction using spike rate of intracranial EEG. IEEE Trans. Neural Syst. Rehabil. Eng. **21**(6), 880–886 (2013)

45. Eftekhar, A., Juffali, W., El-Imad, J., Constandinou, T.G., Toumazou, C.: Ngram-derived pattern recognition for the detection and prediction of epileptic seizures. PLoS ONE **9**(6), e96235 (2014)

46. Zheng, Y., Wang, G., Li, K., Bao, G., Wang, J.: Epileptic seizure prediction using phase synchronization based on bivariate empirical mode decomposition. Clin. Neurophysiol. **125**(6), 1104–1111 (2014). Official journal of the International Federation of Clinical Neurophysiology

47. Lehnertz, K., Litt, B.: The first international collaborative workshop on seizure prediction: summary and data description. Clin. Neurophysiol. **116**(3), 493–505 (2005)

48. Mormann, F., Kreuz, T., Rieke, C., Andrzejak, R.G., Kraskov, A., David, P., Elger, C.E., Lehnertz, K.: On the predictability of epileptic seizures. Clin. Neurophysiol. **116**(3), 569–587 (2005)

49. Mormann, F., Andrzejak, R.G., Elger, C.E., Lehnertz, K.: Seizure prediction: the long and winding road. Brain **130**(2), 314–333 (2007)

50. Oppenheimer, S.M., Gelb, A., Girvin, J.P., Hachinski, V.C.: Cardiovascular effects of human insular cortex stimulation. Neurology **42**(9), 1727–1732 (1992)

51. Leutmezer, F., Schernthaner, C., Lurger, S., Potzelberger, K., Baumgartner, C.: Electrocardiographic changes at the onset of epileptic seizures. Epilepsia **44**(3), 348–354 (2003)

52. Opherk, C., Coromilas, J., Hirsch, L.J.: Heart rate and EKG changes in 102 seizures: analysis of influencing factors. Epilepsy Res. **52**(2), 117–127 (2002)

53. Di Gennaro, G., Quarato, P.P., Sebastiano, F., Esposito, V., Onorati, P., Grammaldo, L.G., Meldolesi, G.N., Mascia, A., Falco, C., Scoppetta, C., Eusebi, F., Manfredi, M., Cantore, G.: Ictal heart rate increase precedes EEG discharge in drug-resistant mesial temporal lobe seizures. Clin. Neurophysiol. **115**(5), 1169–1177 (2004)

54. Weil, S., Arnold, S., Eisensehr, I., Noachtar, S.: Heart rate increase in otherwise subclinical seizures is different in temporal versus extratemporal seizure onset: Support for temporal lobe autonomic influence. Epileptic Disorders **7**(3), 199–204 (2005)

55. Clancy, R.R., Legido, A., Lewis, D.: Occult neonatal seizures. Epilepsia **29**(3), 256–261 (1988)

56. Murray, D.M., Boylan, G.B., Ali, I., Ryan, C.A., Murphy, B.P., Connolly, S.: Defining the gap between electrographic seizure burden, clinical expression and staff recognition of neonatal seizures. Arch. Disease Childhood **93**(3), F187–F191 (2008). Fetal And Neonatal Edition

57. Teixeira, C.A., Direito, B., Feldwisch-Drentrup, H., Valderrama, M., Costa, R.P., Alvarado-Rojas, C., Nikolopoulos, S., Le Van Quyen, M., Timmer, J., Schelter, B., Dourado, A.: EPILAB: a software package for studies on the prediction of epileptic seizures. J. Neurosci. Methods **200**(2), 257–271 (2011)

58. Valderrama, M., Alvarado, C., Nikolopoulos, S., Martinerie, J., Adam, C., Navarro, V., Le Van Quyen, M.: Identifying an increased risk of epileptic seizures using a multi-feature EEG-ECG classification. Biomed. Signal Process. Control **7**(3), 237–244 (2012)

59. Phomsiricharoenphant, W., Ongwattanakul, S., Wongsawat, Y.: The preliminary study of EEG and ECG for epileptic seizure prediction based on Hilbert Huang Transform. In: BMEiCON 2014–7th Biomedical Engineering International Conference, pp. 1–4. IEEE (2015)

60. Piper, D., Schiecke, K., Leistritz, L., Pester, B., Benninger, F., Feucht, M., Ungureanu, M., Strungaru, R., Witte, H.: Synchronization analysis between heart rate variability and EEG activity before, during, and after epileptic seizure. Biomed. Eng./Biomedizinische Technik **59**(4), 343–355 (2014)

61. Greene, B.R., Boylan, G.B., Reilly, R.B., de Chazal, P., Connolly, S.: Combination of EEG and ECG for improved automatic neonatal seizure detection. Clin. Neurophysiol. **118**(6), 1348–1359 (2007)

62. Güler, N.F., Übeyli, E.D., Güler, I.: Recurrent neural networks employing Lyapunov exponents for EEG signals classification. Expert Syst. Appl. **29**(3), 506–514 (2005)

63. Supratak, A., Li, L., Guo, Y.: Feature extraction with stacked autoencoders for epileptic seizure detection. In: Annual International Conference of the IEEE Engineering in Medicine and Biology Society, pp. 4184–4187 (2014)

64. Bengio, Y., Lamblin, P., Popovici, D., Larochelle, H.: Greedy layer-wise training of deep networks. Adv. Neural Inform. Process. Syst. **19**(1), 153 (2007)

65. Petrosian, A., Prokhorov, D., Homan, R., Dasheiff, R., Wunsch, D.: Recurrent neural network based prediction of epileptic seizures in intra- and extracranial EEG. Neurocomputing **30**(1–4), 201–218 (2000)

66. Mirowski, P., Madhavan, D., LeCun, Y., Kuzniecky, R.: Classification of patterns of EEG synchronization for seizure prediction. Clin. Neurophysiol. **120**(11), 1927–1940 (2009)

67. Ohayon, M.M.: Epidemiology of insomnia: what we know and what we still need to learn. Sleep Med. Rev. **6**(2), 97–111 (2002)

68. Rechtschaffen, A., Kales, A.: A manual of standardized terminology, techniques and scoring system for sleep stages of human subjects, public health service, U.S. government printing office, Washington, DC (1968)

69. Schulz, H.: The AASM manual for the scoring of sleep and associated events (2007)

70. Yetton, B.D., Niknazar, M., Duggan, K.A., McDevitt, E.A., Whitehurst, L.N., Sattari, N., Mednick, S.C.: Automatic detection of Rapid Eye Movements (REMs): a machine learning approach. J. Neurosci. Methods **259**, 72–82 (2015)

71. Cona, F., Pizza, F., Provini, F., Magosso, E.: An improved algorithm for the automatic detection and characterization of slow eye movements. Med. Eng. Phy. **36**(7), 954–961 (2014)

72. Marshall, H., Robertson, B., Marshall, B., Carno, M.A.: Polysomnography for the Sleep Technologist: Instrumentation, Monitoring, and Related Procedures. Elsevier Health Sciences (2013)

73. Fraiwan, L., Lweesy, K., Khasawneh, N., Wenz, H., Dickhaus, H.: Automated sleep stage identification system based on time-frequency analysis of a single EEG channel and random forest classifier. Comput. Methods Programs Biomed. **108**(1), 10–19 (2012)

74. Tsinalis, O., Matthews, P.M., Guo, Y.: Automatic sleep stage scoring using time-frequency analysis and stacked sparse autoencoders. Ann. Biomed. Eng. (2015)

75. Lajnef, T., Chaibi, S., Ruby, P., Aguera, P.E., Eichenlaub, J.B., Samet, M., Kachouri, A., Jerbi, K.: Learning machines and sleeping brains: Automatic sleep stage classification using decision-tree multi-class support vector machines. J. Neurosci. Methods, pp. 1–12 (2014)

76. Liang, S.F., Kuo, C.E., Hu, Y.H., Pan, Y.H., Wang, Y.H.: Automatic stage scoring of single-channel sleep EEG by using multiscale entropy and autoregressive models. IEEE Trans. Instrum. Meas. **61**(6), 1649–1657 (2012)

77. Adnane, M., Jiang, Z., Yan, Z.: Sleep-wake stages classification and sleep efficiency estimation using single-lead electrocardiogram. Expert Syst. Appl. **39**(1), 1401–1413 (2012)

78. Xiao, M., Yan, H., Song, J., Yang, Y., Yang, X.: Sleep stages classification based on heart rate variability and random forest. Biomed. Signal Process. Control **8**(6), 624–633 (2013)

79. Penzel, T., Kantelhardt, J.W., Lo, C.C., Voigt, K., Vogelmeier, C.: Dynamics of heart rate and sleep stages in normals and patients with sleep apnea. Neuropsychopharmacology **28**(Suppl 1), S48–S53 (2003). Official publication of the American College of Neuropsychopharmacology

80. Togo, F., Yamamoto, Y.: Decreased fractal component of human heart rate variability during non-REM sleep. Am. J. Physiol. Heart Circulatory Physiol. **280**, H17–H21 (2001)

81. Längkvist, M., Karlsson, L., Loutfi, A.: Sleep stage classification using unsupervised feature learning. Adv. Artif. Neural Syst. **2012**, 1–9 (2012)

82. Chi, Y.M., Jung, T.P., Cauwenberghs, G.: Dry-contact and non-contact biopotential. IEEE Rev. Biomed. Eng. **3**, 106–119 (2010)

83. Berthomier, C., Drouot, X., Herman-Stoïca, M., Berthomier, P., Prado, J., Bokar-Thire, D., Benoit, O., Mattout, J., D'Ortho, M.P.: Automatic analysis of single-channel sleep EEG: validation in healthy individuals. Sleep **30**(11), 1587–1595 (2007)

84. Glorot, X., Bordes, A., Bengio, Y.: Deep sparse rectifier neural networks. Aistats **15**, 315–323 (2011)

85. Picard, R.W., Picard, R.: Affective Computing. MIT press, Cambridge (1997)

86. Picard, R.W.: Affective computing: challenges. Int. J. Hum Comput Stud. **59**(1), 55–64 (2003)

87. Stickel, C., Ebner, M., Steinbach-Nordmann, S., Searle, G., Holzinger, A.: Emotion detection: application of the valence arousal space for rapid biological usability testing to enhance universal access. In: Stephanidis, C. (ed.) UAHCI 2009. LNCS, vol. 5614, pp. 615–624. Springer, Heidelberg (2009). doi:10.1007/978-3-642-02707-9_70

88. Gomez, P., Danuser, B.: Affective and physiological responses to environmental noises and music. Int. J. Psychophysiol. **53**(2), 91–103 (2004)

89. Lang, P.J., Greenwald, M.K., Bradley, M.M., Hamm, A.O.: Looking at pictures: affective, facial, visceral, and behavioral reactions. Psychophysiology **30**, 261 (1993)

90. Picard, R.W., Vyzas, E., Healey, J.: Toward machine emotional intelligence: analysis of affective physiological state. IEEE Trans. Pattern Anal. Mach. Intell. **23**(10), 1175–1191 (2001)

91. Ververidis, D., Kotropoulos, C.: Automatic speech classification to five emotional states based on gender information. In: 12th European Signal Processing Conference, pp. 341–344. IEEE (2004)

92. Giakoumis, D., Tzovaras, D., Moustakas, K., Hassapis, G.: Automatic recognition of boredom in video games using novel biosignal moment-based features. IEEE Trans. Affective Comput. **2**(3), 119–133 (2011)

93. Yannakakis, G.N., Hallam, J.: Entertainment modeling through physiology in physical play. Int. J. Hum Comput Stud. **66**(10), 741–755 (2008)

94. Holzinger, A., Stocker, C., Bruschi, M., Auinger, A., Silva, H., Gamboa, H., Fred, A.: On applying approximate entropy to ECG signals for knowledge discovery on the example of big sensor data. In: Huang, R., Ghorbani, A.A., Pasi, G., Yamaguchi, T., Yen, N.Y., Jin, B. (eds.) AMT 2012. LNCS, vol. 7669, pp. 646–657. Springer, Heidelberg (2012). doi:10.1007/978-3-642-35236-2_64

95. Sang-TaeLee, B., ChungyongLee, D.H.: Speaker dependent emotion recognition using speech signals. In: The Proceedings of the 6th International Conference on Spoken Language Processing (2000)

96. Scherer, K.R.: Vocal affect expression: a review and a model for future research. Psychol. Bull. **99**(2), 143 (1986)

97. Petrushin, V.A.: Emotion recognition in speech signal: experimental study, development, and application. Studies **3**, 4 (2000)

98. Lesh, N., Zaki, M.J., Ogihara, M.: Mining features for sequence classification. In: Proceedings of the fifth ACM SIGKDD International Conference on Knowledge Discovery and Data Mining, pp. 342–346. ACM (1999)

99. Zimmermann, P., Guttormsen, S., Danuser, B., Gomez, P.: Affective computinga rationale for measuring mood with mouse and keyboard. Int. J. Occup. Safety Ergonomics **9**(4), 539–551 (2003)

100. Mueller, F., Lockerd, A.: Cheese: tracking mouse movement activity on websites, a tool for user modeling. In: CHI 2001 Extended Abstracts on Human Factors in Computing Systems, pp. 279–280. ACM (2001)

101. Scheirer, J., Fernandez, R., Klein, J., Picard, R.W.: Frustrating the user on purpose: a step toward building an affective computer. Interact. Comput. **14**(2), 93–118 (2002)

102. Cowie, R., Douglas-Cowie, E., Tsapatsoulis, N., Votsis, G., Kollias, S., Fellenz, W., Taylor, J.G.: Emotion recognition in human-computer interaction. IEEE Sig. Process. Mag. **18**(1), 32–80 (2001)

103. Caridakis, G., Asteriadis, S., Karpouzis, K., Kollias, S.: Detecting human behavior emotional cues in natural interaction. In: 17th International Conference on Digital Signal Processing (DSP), pp. 1–6. IEEE (2011)

104. Ekman, P., Friesen, W.V.: Facial Action Coding System (1977)
105. Kleinsmith, A., Bianchi-Berthouze, N.: Affective body expression perception and recognition: a survey. IEEE Trans. Affective Comput. **4**(1), 15–33 (2013)
106. Pavlovic, V., Sharma, R., Huang, T.S., et al.: Visual interpretation of hand gestures for human-computer interaction: a review. IEEE Trans. Pattern Anal. Mach. Intell. **19**(7), 677–695 (1997)
107. Aggarwal, J.K., Cai, Q.: Human motion analysis: a review. Comput. Vis. Image Underst. **73**(3), 428–440 (1999)
108. Gavrila, D.M.: The visual analysis of human movement: a survey. Comput. Vis. Image Underst. **73**(1), 82–98 (1999)
109. Kapur, A., Kapur, A., Virji-Babul, N., Tzanetakis, G., Driessen, P.F.: Gesture-based affective computing on motion capture data. In: Tao, J., Tan, T., Picard, R.W. (eds.) ACII 2005. LNCS, vol. 3784, pp. 1–7. Springer, Heidelberg (2005). doi:10.1007/11573548_1
110. O'Brien, J.F.: Bodenheimer Jr., R.E., Brostow, G.J., Hodgins, J.K.: Automatic joint parameter estimation from magnetic motion capture data (1999)
111. Azarbayejani, A., Wren, C., Pentland, A.: Real-time 3-D tracking of the human body. In: IMAGE'COM, Bordeaux, France (1996)
112. Etcoff, N.L., Magee, J.J.: Categorical perception of facial expressions. Cognition **44**(3), 227–240 (1992)
113. Black, M.J., Yacoob, Y.: Recognizing facial expressions in image sequences using local parameterized models of image motion. Int. J. Comput. Vision **25**(1), 23–48 (1997)
114. Essa, I., Pentland, A.P., et al.: Coding, analysis, interpretation, and recognition of facial expressions. IEEE Trans. Pattern Anal. Mach. Intell. **19**(7), 757–763 (1997)
115. Schiano, D.J., Ehrlich, S.M., Rahardja, K., Sheridan, K.: Face to interface: facial affect in (hu)man and machine. In: Proceedings of the SIGCHI Conference on Human Factors in Computing Systems, pp. 193–200. ACM (2000)
116. Chen, L.S., Huang, T.S., Miyasato, T., Nakatsu, R.: Multimodal human emotion/expression recognition. In: Proceedings, Third IEEE International Conference on Automatic Face and Gesture Recognition, pp. 366–371. IEEE (1998)
117. De Silva, L.C., Miyasato, T., Nakatsu, R.: Facial emotion recognition using multimodal information. In: Proceedings of 1997 International Conference on Information, Communications and Signal Processing, ICICS 1997, vol. 1, pp. 397–401. IEEE (1997)
118. Yoshitomi, Y., Kim, S.I., Kawano, T., Kilazoe, T.: Effect of sensor fusion for recognition of emotional states using voice, face image and thermal image of face. In: Proceedings, 9th IEEE International Workshop on Robot and Human Interactive Communication, RO-MAN 2000, pp. 178–183. IEEE (2000)
119. Lee, C.M., Narayanan, S.S.: Toward detecting emotions in spoken dialogs. IEEE Trans. Speech Audio Process. **13**(2), 293–303 (2005)
120. Vyzas, E., Picard, R.W.: Affective pattern classification. In: Proceeding AAAI Fall Symposium Series: Emotional and Intelligent: The Tangled Knot of Cognition, pp. 176–182 (1998)
121. Wagner, J., Kim, J., André, E.: From physiological signals to emotions: Implementing and comparing selected methods for feature extraction and classification. In: IEEE International Conference on Multimedia and Expo, ICME 2005, pp. 940–943. IEEE (2005)
122. Yannakakis, G.N., Martínez, H.P., Jhala, A.: Towards affective camera control in games. User Model. User-Adap. Inter. **20**(4), 313–340 (2010)

123. Martínez, H.P., Yannakakis, G.N.: Genetic search feature selection for affective modeling: a case study on reported preferences. In: Proceedings of the 3rd International Workshop on Affective Interaction in Natural Environments, pp. 15–20. ACM(2010)
124. Stuhlsatz, A., Meyer, C., Eyben, F., Zielke, T., Meier, G., Schuller, B.: Deep neural networks for acoustic emotion recognition: raising the benchmarks. In: IEEE International Conference on Acoustics, Speech and Signal Processing (ICASSP), pp. 5688–5691. IEEE (2011)
125. Stuhlsatz, A., Lippel, J., Zielke, T.: Discriminative feature extraction with deep neural networks. In: The 2010 International Joint Conference on Neural Networks (IJCNN), pp. 1–8. IEEE (2010)
126. Martinez, H.P., Bengio, Y., Yannakakis, G.N.: Learning deep physiological models of affect. IEEE Comput. Intell. Mag. 8(2), 20–33 (2013)
127. LeCun, Y., Bengio, Y.: Convolutional networks for images, speech, and time series. In: The Handbook of Brain Theory and Neural Networks, vol. 3361(10) (1995)
128. Matsugu, M., Mori, K., Mitari, Y., Kaneda, Y.: Subject independent facial expression recognition with robust face detection using a convolutional neural network. Neural Networks 16(5), 555–559 (2003)
129. Rifai, S., Bengio, Y., Courville, A., Vincent, P., Mirza, M.: Disentangling factors of variation for facial expression recognition. In: Fitzgibbon, A., Lazebnik, S., Perona, P., Sato, Y., Schmid, C. (eds.) ECCV 2012. LNCS, vol. 7577, pp. 808–822. Springer, Heidelberg (2012). doi:10.1007/978-3-642-33783-3_58
130. Mayer, C., Bachler, M., Holzinger, A., Stein, P., Wassertheurer, S.: The effect of threshold values and weighting factors on the association between entropy measures and mortality after myocardial infarction in the cardiac arrhythmia suppression trial (cast). Entropy 18(4) (2016)
131. Li, C., Zheng, C., Tai, C.: Detection of ECG characteristic points using wavelet transforms. IEEE Trans. Biomed. Eng. 42(1), 21–28 (1995)
132. Bachler, M., Mayer, C., Hametner, B., Wassertheurer, S., Holzinger, A.: Online and offline determination of QT and PR interval and QRS duration in electrocardiography. In: Zu, Q., Hu, B., Elçi, A. (eds.) ICPCA/SWS 2012. LNCS, vol. 7719, pp. 1–15. Springer, Heidelberg (2013). doi:10.1007/978-3-642-37015-1_1
133. Saxena, S., Kumar, V., Hamde, S.: Feature extraction from ECG signals using wavelet transforms for disease diagnostics. Int. J. Syst. Sci. 33(13), 1073–1085 (2002)
134. Saritha, C., Sukanya, V., Murthy, Y.N.: ECG signal analysis using wavelet transforms. Bulg. J. Phys 35(1), 68–77 (2008)
135. Zhao, Q., Zhang, L.: ECG feature extraction and classification using wavelet transform and support vector machines. In: ICNN&B 2005, International Conference on Neural Networks and Brain, vol. 2, pp. 1089–1092. IEEE (2005)
136. Übeyli, E.D.: Ecg beats classification using multiclass support vector machines with error correcting output codes. Digit. Signal Proc. 17(3), 675–684 (2007)
137. Yu, S.N., Chen, Y.H.: Electrocardiogram beat classification based on wavelet transformation and probabilistic neural network. Pattern Recogn. Lett. 28(10), 1142–1150 (2007)
138. Song, M.H., Lee, J., Cho, S.P., Lee, K.J., Yoo, S.K.: Support vector machine based arrhythmia classification using reduced features. Int. J. Control Autom. Syst. 3(4), 571 (2005)
139. Martis, R.J., Chakraborty, C., Ray, A.K.: An integrated ecg feature extraction scheme using pca and wavelet transform. In: 2009 Annual IEEE India Conference (INDICON), pp. 1–4. IEEE (2009)

140. Yu, S.N., Chou, K.T.: Selection of significant independent components for ECG beat classification. Expert Syst. Appl. **36**(2), 2088–2096 (2009)
141. Kiranyaz, S., Ince, T., Gabbouj, M.: Real-Time Patient-Specific ECG Classification by 1D Convolutional Neural Networks (2015)
142. Yang, J., Bai, Y., Li, G., Liu, M., Liu, X.: A novel method of diagnosing premature ventricular contraction based on sparse auto-encoder and softmax regression. Bio-Med. Mater. Eng. **26**(s1), 1549–1558 (2015)
143. Yan, Y., Qin, X., Wu, Y., Zhang, N., Fan, J., Wang, L.: A restricted boltzmann machine based two-lead electrocardiography classification. In: IEEE 12th International Conference on Wearable and Implantable Body Sensor Networks (BSN), pp. 1–9. IEEE (2015)
144. Zeiler, M.D., Fergus, R.: Visualizing and understanding convolutional networks. In: Fleet, D., Pajdla, T., Schiele, B., Tuytelaars, T. (eds.) ECCV 2014. LNCS, vol. 8689, pp. 818–833. Springer, Heidelberg (2014). doi:10.1007/978-3-319-10590-1_53
145. Holzinger, A.: Interactive machine learning for health informatics: when do we need the human-in-the-loop? Brain Inform. **3**, 1–13 (2016)

Argumentation for Knowledge Representation, Conflict Resolution, Defeasible Inference and Its Integration with Machine Learning

Luca Longo[✉]

School of Computing, College of Sciences and Health,
Dublin Institute of Technology
ADAPT:
The Global Centre of Excellence for Digital Content and Media Innovation,
Dublin, Republic of Ireland
luca.longo@dit.ie

Abstract. Modern machine Learning is devoted to the construction of algorithms and computational procedures that can automatically improve with experience and learn from data. Defeasible argumentation has emerged as sub-topic of artificial intelligence aimed at formalising common-sense qualitative reasoning. The former is an inductive approach for inference while the latter is deductive, each one having advantages and limitations. A great challenge for theoretical and applied research in AI is their integration. The first aim of this chapter is to provide readers informally with the basic notions of defeasible and non-monotonic reasoning. It then describes argumentation theory, a paradigm for implementing defeasible reasoning in practice as well as the common multi-layer schema upon which argument-based systems are usually built. The second aim is to describe a selection of argument-based applications in the medical and health-care sectors, informed by the multi-layer schema. A summary of the features that emerge from the applications under review is aimed at showing why defeasible argumentation is attractive for knowledge-representation, conflict resolution and inference under uncertainty. Open problems and challenges in the field of argumentation are subsequently described followed by a future outlook in which three points of integration with machine learning are proposed.

Keywords: Defeasible reasoning · Argumentation · Conflict resolution · Knowledge-representation · Interactive machine learning · Medicine
·

1 Introduction

The fast-growing field of Machine Learning (ML) is devoted to the construction of algorithms and computational procedures that can automatically improve with experience and learn from data. Although ML is increasing in popularity with a plethora of applications in several fields, and it has proved to be useful in the identification and extraction of meaningful patterns of data and rules,

© Springer International Publishing AG 2016
A. Holzinger (Ed.): ML for Health Informatics, LNAI 9605, pp. 183–208, 2016.
DOI: 10.1007/978-3-319-50478-0_9

it is often based upon algorithms that implement quantitative manipulation of training data. These algorithms are frequently used as 'black-boxes' and the inference process that lead to the quantitative output is neglected. In the last two decades, Defeasible Reasoning (DR) has emerged as sub-topic of artificial intelligence (AI) aimed at formalising common-sense qualitative reasoning. This type of reasoning is often performed in contexts characterised by high uncertainty, such as medicine and health care, where available information is usually fragmented, partial, conflicting, noisy and multi-dimensional. Defeasible reasoning can be combined to machine learning inference techniques and a great challenge for theoretical and applied research in AI is their integration. This challenge is highly connected to the notion of interactive Machine Learning (iML) [1,2] being proposed in this book. In particular, as Fig. 1 depicts, on one hand machine learning might support defeasible reasoning by providing it with quantitative evidence for enhancing reasoning processes. On the other hand, defeasible reasoning might contribute to extend and enhance the inferential mechanisms behind machine learning techniques with more qualitative and transparent reasoning and by incorporating intelligence and argumentative capacity. The integration of these two subfields of AI is likely to impact and contribute to design and develop intelligence agents with greater knowledge extraction, predictive power as well as argumentative and reasoning capabilities [3]. Machine learning is a more mature branch of research within artificial intelligence than formal defeasible reasoning. Therefore the main focus of this chapter is on the latter paradigm with emphasis on argumentation theory and argument-based systems, the computational approaches to implement defeasible reasoning in practice. The rest of this document is organised as it follows. Firstly, a glossary describes the core definitions and terms of this desk research. Argumentation theory is subsequently introduced with an emphasis on its role in defeasible reasoning. This is complemented by a detailed description of the multi-layered pattern upon which argument-based systems are usually built. An overview of practical applications of argumentation in clinical domains is then presented followed by a description of the main features and advantages of defeasible reasoning and argumentation theory in decision-making and knowledge representation. Open problems and challenges in applied research are then discussed and a summary concludes this chapter with a future outlook for argumentation and its integration with machine learning.

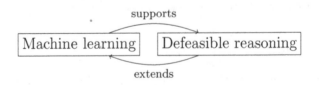

Fig. 1. Interaction of argumentation and machine learning

2 Glossary and Key Terms

Machine learning (ML): subfield of computer science devoted to the design of computational procedures able to learn from and perform prediction of data.

Default knowledge: kn owledge routinely employed by humans in a reasoning process even if the preconditions for its application are only partially known.

Defaults: specific inference rules employed in default knowledge.

Monotonicity: property of a reasoning process in which conclusions are not affected by new pieces of evidence and, as a consequence, the set of available conclusions monotonically increases.

Non-monotonicity: property of a reasoning process in which conclusions can be retracted in the light of new pieces of evidence, and as a consequence, the set of available conclusions can decrease in cardinality.

Defeasible reasoning(DR): a type of reasoning with the non-monotonicity property based upon reasons that are defeasible. This reasoning does not produce a complete and final demonstration of a claim, instead it acknowledges corrigibility and fallibility of a conclusion.

Argumentation theory (AT): a multidisciplinary area of artificial intelligence that provides state-of-the-art computational models of defeasible reasoning.

Argument: piece of evidence considered in a defeasible reasoning process. Typically an argument is built upon a set of assumptions or premises, a method of reasoning and a conclusion.

Undermining attack: a type of conflict in which an argument is attacked on one of its premises by another argument whose conclusion negates that premise.

Rebutting attack: a type of conflict that occurs when an argument negates the conclusions of another argument.

Undercutting attack: a type of conflict that occurs when an argument uses a defeasible inference rule that is attacked by another argument arguing that there is a special case that does not allow the application of the rule itself.

Semantics: a formal criterion to determine which arguments of an argumentation graph can be accepted.

3 State-of-the-Art: Defeasible Argumentation Theory

3.1 Defeasible Reasoning

The capability of deriving defeasible conclusions with partial information is an important aspect of modern medical systems. In order to achieve such a capability, humans routinely resort to the so-called *default knowledge*, a main feature of which is that it can be used in a reasoning process even if the preconditions for its application are only partially known. These preconditions, whose truth is not explicitly verified, are assumed to hold defeasibly, that means in the absence of explicit information to the contrary. In the event that new information becomes available and the falsity of such preconditions can be deduced, then the conclusions derived from the application of the default knowledge have to be retracted. This type of reasoning is known as *defeasible reasoning* [4]. Default knowledge is represented by using *defaults* that are specific inference rules. These are expressions of the form: $p(x) : j_1(x), ..., j_n(x) \longrightarrow c(x)$ where $p(x)$ is the prerequisite of the default, $j(x)$ is the justification and $c(x)$ is the consequent. If $p(x)$ is known and if $j(x)$ consistent with what is known, then $c(x)$ can be defeasibly deduced. In other words, if it is believed that the prerequisite is true, and each of the n conditions (justifications) can be assumed since they are consistent with current beliefs, then this leads to believe the truth of the conclusion. Defeasible reasoning, unlike standard deductive reasoning, is *non-monotonic*. Intuitively this means that adding new premises may lead to removing, rather than adding new conclusions. More specifically, if the conclusion p follows from a set of premises A (denoted as $A \vdash p$), in standard monotonic reasoning it also holds that $A, B \vdash p$ namely t, if and only if any additional set of premises B is added to A, the conclusion p is still valid. This property is called *monotonicity*: conclusions are not affected by new evidence hence the set of conclusions monotonically increases. This is not the case in real life in general and in medicine, health care in particular where reasoning is often non-monotonic: conclusions can be retracted when new evidence is available. Consider the following example [5]:

- *X has undergone breast cancer surgery and subsequently radiotherapy.*
- *Radiotherapy minimises the risk of cancer recurrence*, so possibly
- *X has a low risk of breast cancer recurrence.*

If in addition to the fact that *X has undergone cancer surgery and subsequently radiotherapy*, it is found out that

- *X had a cancer with high degree of lymph node involvement,*

then the conclusion that *X has a low risk of cancer recurrence* has to be retracted, as a special exception has been raised.

Non-monotonic logic relies on the idea that the pieces of knowledge employed in a reasoning activity such as *X has a low risk of cancer recurrence* may admit exceptions and it is impossible to include a full list of exceptions within the reasoning rules [4]. In these cases, the premise of a certain rule is only partially specified and a conclusion can be derived from the premises, assuming that no exception occurs, that means that all the implicit premises of the rule are satisfied. In the case where an exception subsequently arises then the derived conclusion has to be retracted. The basic idea of non-monotonic inferences is that, when more information is obtained, some previously accepted inference may no longer hold. Defeasible reasoning has increasingly gained attention in the medical sector because it supports reasoning over partial, incomplete and dynamic evidence and knowledge, where several exceptions can arise according to various circumstances. Argumentation theory (AT), an important sub-field of artificial intelligence (AI), provides state-of-the-art computational models of defeasible reasoning (DR).

3.2   Argumentation Theory

Argumentation theory (AT), often referred to as argumentation, is a multi-disciplinary research subject ranging from law to philosophy and linguistic, with aspects borrowed from psychology and sociology [6,7]. AT has gained interest in artificial intelligence as it provides the basis for computational models inspired by the way humans reason [8]. These models have extended classical reasoning approaches, based on deductive logic, that were proving increasingly inadequate for problems requiring non-monotonic reasoning and explanatory reasoning not available in standard non-monotonic logics [9]. AT focuses on how pieces of evidence, seen as arguments, can be represented, supported or discarded in a defeasible reasoning process, and it investigates formal approaches to assess the validity of the conclusions inferred [6]. AT has been employed for tasks like practical reasoning, decision support, dialogue and negotiation [6,10–12] as well as for knowledge representation [13,14]. It differs from many traditional mono-lithic non-monotonic logics because it envisages a modular and intuitive process, supporting the explanation of each reasoning step, making the reasoning and inference processes more explanatory.

In a nutshell, argumentation deals with the interactions between possibly conflicting arguments, arising when different parties, participants or artificial agents argue for and against some conclusions or when different pieces of evidence, even conflicting, are available [12]. Arguments can be regarded as 'tentative proofs for propositions' [15] in a logical language whose axioms represent premises in the domain under consideration. In general, the premises are not consistent because they may lead to incompatible conclusions. These conflicts may arise either during the defeasible reasoning activity of a single human/agent or in the context of a dialogue between multiple humans or artificial agents. These modes are referred to as monological and dialogical argumentation, respectively. Accordingly, *monological models* [16] focus on the internal structure of an argument, meaning its components (like premises, rules, conclusions) and their relations. *Dialogical models* focus instead on argument conflicts and their resolution and typically regard arguments as monolithic entities, whose internal structure is abstracted away as far as the conflict resolution process is concerned. Roughly speaking, monological models concern the production and construction of arguments while dialogical models concern management of their conflicts, that means the actual arguing process. A third classification of models, referred to as *rhetorical models*, has also been proposed (Table 1) in which neither the monological nor the dialogical structure is considered [16]. Here, the rhetorical nature of arguments is stressed. More specifically, the audience's perception of arguments and how they can be employed as a means of persuasion is taken into account [17,18].

In the literature of argumentation, models belonging to one category difficultly belong to the other categories. For instance, dialogical models do not address the internal representation of an argument and do not consider their perception by an audience. However, according to [16], in order to design intelligent systems that incorporate powerful argumentative capabilities, the micro-

Table 1. Classification of argumentation models

	Monological	Dialogical	Rhetorical
Structure	Micro	Macro	Persuasive
Foundation	Arguments as tentative proofs	Defeasible reasoning	Audience's perception of arguments
Linkage	Connecting a set of premises to a claim at the level of argument	Connecting a set of arguments in a dialogical structure	Connecting arguments in a persuasive way

structure of an argument, its relation with other arguments as well as the rhetorical structure should be addressed. The internal representation of an argument should clearly relate premises to conclusions, and at an external level, the argument should be considered within the set of the other arguments it interacts with. Eventually, the perception by an audience is important because in real life implementations, arguments are built to achieve predefined objectives, according to the participating agents' believes. The general idea is that argumentation systems formalise non-monotonic reasoning as the internal construction of arguments (micro-structure) as well as their comparisons for and against certain conclusions (macro-structure). The construction of arguments, based on a theory, is monotonic that means an argument remains the same even if the theory is expanded with new information. Non-monotonicity is expressed in terms of interaction between conflicting arguments. This is because the additional information may generate stronger arguments that in turn defeat previous arguments.

Argumentation systems and the notion of an argument are typically constructed upon an *underlying logical* language and around an associated notion of *logical consequence*. As mentioned before, this notion of consequence is monotonic. New information can not invalidate existing arguments as constructed, but can only be responsible for the generation of new counterarguments. Some argument-based applications assume a particular and well-defined logic whereas other leave the underlying logic part of the context of application or even totally undefined. In the case the logic is left unspecified, the system can be instantiated with different alternative logics, thus they are often referred to as frameworks rather then systems. Beside the chosen underlying language, argumentation systems are generally built upon five layers [19] (Fig. 2):

1. definition of the internal structure of arguments
2. definition of conflicts between arguments
3. evaluation of conflicts and definition of valid attacks
4. definition of the dialectical status of arguments
5. accrual of acceptable arguments

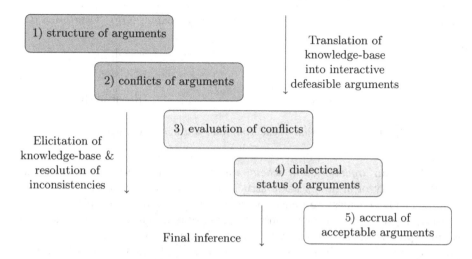

Fig. 2. Five layers upon which argumentation systems are generally built

3.3   Layer 1: Definition of the Internal Structure of Arguments

The internal representation of arguments is addressed by monological models. Often an argument is internally represented with a set of premises $(P_1, P_2, ..., P_n)$, and a conclusion (C) follows from them with the application of some rule $(\rightarrow)$.

$$Argument : P_1, P_2, ..., P_n \rightarrow C$$

Many argumentation systems do not make any distinction between premises. However, arguments actually used in human reasoning may follow a more articulated structure where different premises play different roles, as in the argument model first introduced by Toulmin [20] composed of six parts (Fig. 3).

- *Claim (C)*: an assertion/claim (conclusion) potentially controversial;
- *Data (D)*: statements specifying facts/beliefs previously established related to a situation in which the claim is made;
- *Warrant (W)*: statement that justifies the derivation of conclusion from data;
- *Backing (B)*: a set of information that ensures the trustworthiness of a warrant. It is the grounds underlying the reason. A backing is invoked when the warrant is challenged;
- *Qualifier (Q)*: a statement that expresses the degree of certainty associated with the claim;
- *Rebuttal (R)*: a statement introducing a situation in which the conclusion might be defeated.

Toulmin's model plays a significant role in highlighting the elements that form a natural argument, providing a useful basis for knowledge representation. Another well-known monological paradigm has been proposed by Reed and Walton to model the notion of *arguments as product* [21,22]. It is based upon

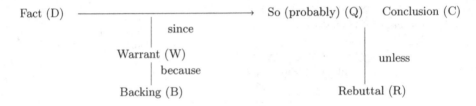

Fig. 3. An illustration of the Toulmin's argument representation

the notion of an *argumentation scheme* and it is useful for identifying and evaluating a variety of argumentation structures in everyday discourse [16]. These argumentation schemes are aimed at capturing common stereotypical patterns of reasoning that are non-monotonic and defeasible in nature [13]. Consider the example presented in [8] in which two parts, A and B, are discussing chemotherapy, and that B is not in favour of it because P thinks that it has a high emotional impact on the person due to the risk of alopecia phenomenon and should be discouraged. B's argument is:

Argument: *Dr. B (expert in psychology) says that chemotherapy affects the emotional state of the patient*

It appears that B's argument is implicitly *an appeal to expert opinion*. In addition, it is evidently an instance of *argument from consequences*. These two schemes can be used by B to build a point of view. B is claiming that negatively affecting the emotional state is a bad consequence of an action. The argument is based upon the assumption that, since the bad outcome is a consequence of chemotherapy, therefore chemotherapy should not be applied. This can be represented by the following argumentation chain:

– *Dr. B., an expert psychologist, says that chemotherapy negatively affects emotional state, because he has knowledge of patients emotions;*
– *chemotherapy negatively affects emotional state;*
– *negatively affecting the emotional state is a bad thing;*
– *anything that leads to bad consequences is a bad practice;*
– *chemotherapy is a bad practice.*

Walton identified 25 different argumentation schemes, each including a set of *critical questions* such as:

'*is the expert E in a position to know about the proposition P?*'

Critical questions provide a sort of checklist about the validity conditions for the application of a specific argument scheme. Intuitively, critical questions make the defeasibility of argument schemes explicit and indicate some canonical ways to build the relevant counterarguments. For further information on monological approaches to argumentation, readers can refer to [16]. The Toulmin's model [20] as well as the Reed and Walton's approach [21,22] do not specify the way different argument structures can be aggregated nor how they can interact or conflict in the dynamics of an argumentation process.

3.4   Layer 2: Definition of the Conflicts Between Arguments

Monological models, aimed at representing the internal structure of arguments are complemented by dialogical models, focused on the relationships between arguments and, in particular, their conflicts. The latter investigates the issue of invalid arguments that appear to be valid (fallacious arguments). *Conflicts*, often referred to attacks or defeats, and sometimes with slightly different meanings, are the key notions in argumentation theory. In the AT literature several kinds of conflicts have been considered. Here the classification proposed in [23] is stressed. This encompasses three classes of conflicts (Figs. 4, 5, and 6):

- *undermining attack*: occurs when an argument is attacked on one of its premises by another whose conclusion negates that premise;
- *rebutting attack* occurs when an argument negates the conclusions of another;
- *undercutting attack* occurs when an argument uses a defeasible inference rule and is attacked by arguing that there is a special case that does not allow the application of the rule itself [24].

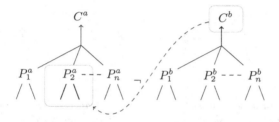

A: *'alcohol consumption is low according to X so X has a low risk of recurrence'*   B: *the alcohol level from a blood test is high so X has a high alcohol consumption*

Fig. 4. Undermining attack: A is undermined by B

3.5   Layer 3: Evaluation of Conflicts and Definition of Valid Attacks

Conflict between arguments, although an important notion, does not embody any approach for the determination of the success of an attack, from one argument to its target. Generally an attack, sometimes referred to as 'defeat', has a form of a binary relation between two arguments. Some authors distinguish a relation in a weak form (attacking another argument and not weaker) or in a strong form (attacking another argument and stronger) [25]. The former is generally referred to as 'defeat' whereas the latter as 'strict defeat' [23]. Defeat relations are determined in various ways, influenced by the domain of application and are usually defeasible. For example, in those domains where observations are important, defeats might depend on the reliability of tests or the expertise of the observers. Evaluating an attack can occur through:

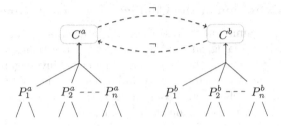

A: ' *radiotherapy minimises risk so X has*   B: '*X is an old patient, the strongest risk*
a low risk of breast cancer recurrence   *for breast cancer is age, so the risk of*
                                                                              recurrence is high'.

Fig. 5. Rebutting attack: A is rebutted by B and viceversa

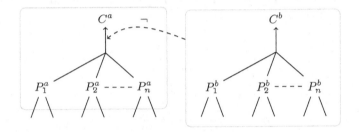

A: '*radiotherapy minimises the risk of*   B: '*paper Z demonstrated that*
recurrence so X has a low risk of breast   *radiotherapy failed several times in*
cancer recurrence'   *curing breast cancer so it is not always*
                                                                            an effective method to reduce recurrence'.

Fig. 6. Undercutting attack: A is undercut by B

– the notion of *preferentiality of arguments* or *strength of arguments*
– the notion of *preferentiality of attacks* or *strength of an attack relation.*

Strength of Arguments. To establish whether an attack can be considered a successful defeat, a trend in AT is devoted to the consideration of the *strength* of arguments. In this respect a key concept is represented by the inequality of the strength of arguments that has to be accounted for in the computation of sets of arguments and counterarguments [26]. Several works have adopted the notion of *preferentiality* among arguments [27]. For example, in [28,29], the authors formalised the role of preferences and if an arguments X undercuts another argument Y, then X is a successful attack (defeat) if Y is not stronger than X. Other approaches adopt preferentiality at a more abstract level. For instance, in the *Preference-based Argumentation Framework (PAF)* proposed by [30], an attack from X to Y is successful only if Y is not preferred to X. [31] proposed a *Value-based argumentation framework (VAF)* in which an attack from X to Y is successful only if the value promoted by X is ranked higher or equal than the valued promoted by Y, in accordance to a given ordering on values. Figure 7 illustrates these various scenarios of preferentiality, given an attack set and the resulting defeat (successful attack) set.

Starting attack set:

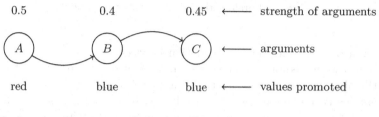

Preference of arguments: $[B > A > C]$ Rank of values: $[red > blue]$

Resulting successful attack set:

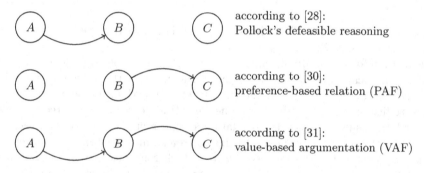

Fig. 7. Implementations of preferentiality between arguments

The information necessary to decide whether an attack between two arguments is successful is often assumed to be pre-specified, and implemented as an ordering of values or a given partial preference. However, according to [27], the information related to preferentiality of arguments might be contradictory, as the preferences may vary depending on the context and on different subjects who can assign different strengths, to different arguments, employing different criteria. This led the author to propose the concept of *meta-level argument*: a simple node in a graph of nodes where preferentiality is abstractly defined, by creating a new attack relation that comes from a preference argument. Meta-level arguments allow no commitment regarding the definition of the preferences of arguments, rendering the reasoning process simpler. To model the preference relation among arguments, the notion of fuzziness has been used in [32] where a *fuzzy preference argumentation framework* (FPAF) has been proposed. Here,

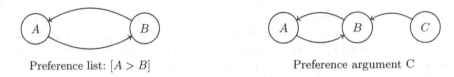

(a) Standard preferentiality   (b) Meta-level argument

Fig. 8. Standard preferentiality and meta-level arguments

a value X attached to a preference relation between two arguments A, B corresponds to the degree of credibility by which A is strictly preferred to B. To clarify the above notions, consider the example of Fig. 8 where two arguments A, B, claiming two different conclusions rebut each other. Suppose the existence of a pre-defined preference list in which argument A is preferred to argument B (part a). According to Modgil [27], this situation can be expressed as in the graph (part b) where another meta-level argument C is added to the reasoning process, undercutting the inference link of argument B.

Strength of Attack Relations. Preferentiality, as reviewed so far, is implemented by assigning to arguments an importance value. This is usually predefined, in form of a full or partial priority list of available arguments, or in form of a numerical value attached to each of them, explicitly provided or implicitly derived from the strength of the rules used within the argument. In turn preferentiality allows to establish whether an attack can be considered successful, thus formalising a proper defeat relation, or considered a weak/false attack, thus being disregarded. As opposite to this approach, another branch of argumentation is devoted to associate weights to attack relations instead to arguments. In [26] the role of adding weights on the attack links between arguments has been investigated, introducing the notion of *inconsistency budget*. This quantifies the amount of inconsistency a designer of an argumentation system is willing to tolerate. With an inconsistency budget α, the designer is open to disregard attacks up to a total weight α. It turns out that, increasing this threshold, more solutions can be achieved progressively as less attack would be disregarded. As a consequence, this gives a preference order over solutions, and the solutions having a lower inconsistency budget are preferred. A similar recent approach that considers the strength of attacks is incorporated in [33] resulting in a *varied-strength attacks argumentation framework* (VSAAF). Here, each attack relation is assigned a type, and the framework is equipped with a partial ordering over the types. Let us consider the example of Fig. 9 where the type of attack from an argument A to B is i and from B to C is j. Intuitively, depending on whether the type j is higher, lower or equally ranked than the type i, different ranges of solutions are possible. Beside this relation of attack, another approach has been proposed [34] by employing the notion of *fuzzy relations* borrowed from Fuzzy

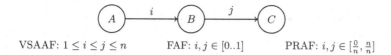

VSAAF: $1 \leq i \leq j \leq n$ FAF: $i, j \in [0..1]$ PRAF: $i, j \in [\frac{0}{n}, \frac{n}{n}]$

Fig. 9. Types of the strength of attack relations

Logic [35,36]. This approach allows the representation of the degree to which an argument attacks another one, creating a *fuzzy argumentation framework* (FAF).

Strength of arguments and defeat relations has been considered also in [37]. Here, probabilities are assigned both to arguments and defeats, introducing the notion of *probability argumentation framework* (PRAF). Probabilities refer to the likelihood of the existence of a specific argument or defeat relation, thus capturing the inherent uncertainties in the argumentation system. The idea is that all possible arguments neither definitely are disregarded nor they definitely exist: they have different chances of existing. In the approach proposed in [38] two fictitious people have to be confronted, endorsing respectively the roles of proponent and opponent of the argument. Situation of conflicts are subsequently analysed employing the paradigm of *game theory* [38].

3.6 Layer 4: Definition of the Dialectical Status of Arguments

Defeat relations, as per layer 3, focus on the relative strength of two individual arguments and do not tell yet what arguments can be seen as justifiable. The final state of each argument depends on the interaction with the others and a definition of their *dialectical status* is needed. Layer 4 of the multi-layer schema of Fig. 2 is aimed at determining the outcome of an argumentation system usually by splitting the set of arguments in two classes, those that support a certain decision/action and those that do not. Sometimes a further class can contain those arguments that leave the dispute in an undecided status. Multiple actions or decisions can be accounted for in a defeasible reasoning process, thus the number of classes can increase. Modern implementations for computing the dialectical status of arguments are usually built upon the theory of Dung [9] which, historically speaking, derives from other more practical and concrete works on argumentation such as [24,39]. Dung's *abstract argumentation frameworks* (AF) allow comparisons of different systems by translating them into his abstract format [39]. The underlying idea is that given a set of abstract arguments (the internal structure is not considered) and a set of defeat relations, a decision to determine which arguments can ultimately be accepted has to be taken. AF is a directed graph in which arguments are presented as nodes and the attacks as arrows (Fig. 10). Solely looking at an argument's defeaters to decide the status of an argument is not enough: it is also important to investigate whether the defeaters are defeated themselves. Generally, an argument B *defeats* A if and only if B is a reason against A.

Given an AF, the issue is to decide which arguments should ultimately be accepted. In Fig. 10, A is attacked by B, and apparently A should not be accepted

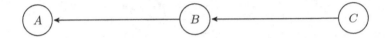

Fig. 10. Argument and reinstatement

since it has a counterargument. However, B is itself attacked by C that, in turn, is not attacked by anything, thus C should be accepted. But if C is accepted, then B is ultimately rejected and does not form a reason against A anymore. Therefore A should be accepted as well. In this scenario it is said that C *reinstates* A and in order to determine which arguments of an AF can be accepted, a formal criterion is necessary. This criterion is known as *acceptability semantics*, and given an AF, it specifies zero or more *extensions* (sets of acceptable arguments) [40]. Using the labelling approach proposed in [41], each argument is either *in*, *out* or *undec* according to two conditions:

1. an argument is labelled *in* if, only if all its defeaters are labelled *out*, and
2. an argument is labelled *out* if, only if it has at least one defeater labelled *in*.

Informally speaking, an argument labelled *in* means it has been accepted, *out* means it has been rejected and *undec* means it can not be neither accepted nor rejected. In the AF of Fig. 10, for argument C it holds that all its defeaters are labelled *out* (trivial as C is not defeated by any argument), thus C has to be labelled *in*. B now has a defeater labelled *in* thus it has to be labelled *out*. For A, it holds that all its defeaters are labelled *out*, so it has to be labelled *in*. As a consequence the resulting status of each argument is: $Lab(A) = in$, $Lab(C) = in$ and $Lab(B) = out$. Thus, A and C can be accepted and argument B has to be rejected. A set of arguments is called *conflict-free* if and only if it does not contain any argument A and B such that A defeats B. A set of arguments $Args$ is said to *defend* an argument C if and only if each defeater of C is defeated by an argument in $Args$. These basic notions drive the proposal of the *complete semantics* aimed at computing *complete extensions* [9]. The idea is that a complete labelling might be viewed as a subjective and reasonable point of view that a designer can consider with respect to which arguments are accepted, rejected or considered undecided. Each point of view can be certainly questioned by someone, but its internal inconsistency cannot be pointed out. The set of complete labellings can be seen as the reasonable positions available to a designer [41].

Complete semantics have an important property: more than one complete extension might exist. However, sometimes it is advantageous to take a skeptical approach, thus a semantics that is guaranteed to generate exactly one extension is the *grounded semantics*. The idea is to select the complete labelling Lab in which the set of *in*-labelled arguments is minimal. The grounded extension coincides with the complete labelling in which *in* is minimised, *out* is minimised and *undec* is maximised and can be the empty set. In Fig. 10, the grounded extension is $\{A, C\}$. However, this skeptical approach might be replaced by a more credulous one, known as *preferred semantics* [9]. The idea is that, instead of maximising *undec* arguments, it maximises *in* arguments (and also *out* arguments). They are based on the notion of *admissibility*. A set of arguments is admissible if and only if it is conflict-free and defends at least itself. The empty set is admissible in every AF as it is conflict-free and trivially defends itself against each of its defeaters (none). For any AF, there exists at least one preferred extension. Every grounded and every preferred extension is a complete extension. In Fig. 10, the admissible sets are $\{C\}$, $\{A, C\}$. $\{B\}$ and $\{A\}$ are not admissible as they do not defend themselves respectively against C and B. Only one preferred extension exists: $\{A, C\}$. Grounded and preferred semantics have been conceived by Dung and firstly described in his topical work [9]. However, other semantics have been proposed such as the ideal semantics [42,43], semi-stable [44], stage [45], non-admissibility based semantics [46] and CF2 semantics [47]. For further readings on argumentation semantics, the reader is referred to [40,48].

3.7 Layer 5: Accrual of Acceptable Arguments

Multiple acceptable extensions of arguments may be computed from the previous layer coinciding with possible consistent points of view that can be considered for describing the knowledge being modelled and thus employed for decision-making and defeasible inference. However, sometimes for practical purposes, as in the medical domain, a single decision must be takes or a single action must be performed. Thus a fifth layer is sometimes added to the argumentative schema aimed at extracting the most credible or consistent point of view for informing such a decision or action. It includes a strategy for computing, for instance, a degree of credibility of each extension that can be used for purposes of comparison. The most credible can be eventually selected and employed to support decision-making. Various strategies have been proposed in the literature for selecting such an extension [49,50]. These include the consideration of the strength of arguments, or a preference list among them defined in layer 3. Alternatively, the extension with higher cardinality can be considered, that is the larger conflict-free set of arguments. In the literature of argumentation and defeasible reasoning, this layer is probably the less developed and further works should be carried out.

4 Application Areas

The previously described five layers (Fig. 2) give an overall idea of the main components that are usually considered in an argumentative process, and are strictly connected. The first layer deals with monological argumentation while the other layers with dialogical argumentation. Some of these layers can be neglected or merged together. For example, when the strength of arguments or attack relations is not considered, layer 3 can be discarded. Also, the strength of arguments and their preferentiality may be considered in the 5th layer and not only in the 3rd layer. The literature of defeasible reasoning and its theoretical works is vast in the logic and artificial intelligence communities. Readers can refer to [16] for a taxonomy of argument-based models and to [51] for a review of defeasible reasoning implementations. In this section, applications of defeasible reasoning and argumentation in medicine and health-care are described. Argumentation was adopted in the context of the *Aspic* project [52]: a general model for argumentation services. The goal was to develop a theoretical framework for inference, decision-making, dialogue and learning that could be used, for example, in the identification of patients treatment options given multiple and conflicting pieces of evidence. An application of this framework includes a multi-agent scenario where three agents collaborate exchanging pros and cons of alternative interventions and diagnoses towards settling on a justifiable treatment for a patient with chest pain [53]. *Aspic* has been also used as method for genetic counselling aimed at providing patients and clinicians with an aid for customising, evaluating, visualising and communicating care plans. Another application concerned a simulation where eight cancer genetic counsellors participated in an experiment in which they had to counsel a woman carrying a risk-increasing gene mutation. Information was visually displayed in an organised-fashion, in the form of structured arguments. These arguments helped counsellors enhancing their discussion with the patient and explaining the options available for mitigating the risk of cancer [54]. In the *Aspic* project, arguments are constructed from a knowledge-base of facts, internally modelled with strict and defeasible inference rules. These rules are composed by a set of premises supporting a claim and an argument can embed different rules organised as a tree. Each argument has a numerical degree of belief attached (1 for strict arguments and a partial degree, less than 1, for defeasible arguments), and this can be computed employing different principles. These include the 'weakest link' principle in which the minimum of the strength of an argument's premises and its links is computed, or the 'last link' principle in which the maximum strength of an argument's links, with no accrual of reasons is considered [55]. Once arguments are defined, the *Aspic* framework allows the explication of a set of attack relations between them, always according to the knowledge-base of facts. Dung's calculus of opposition [9] is employed to compute a dialectical (justification) status of arguments. Eventually, from the claim of the justified arguments, a final inference is drawn, this being usually a decision, a diagnosis or a treatment recommendation.

Argumentation has been used for medical group-decision support [56]. In this context, expert clinicians participated in a group discussion to decide on the best treatment for a given patient or case. A web-prototype to build arguments was presented to a group of oncologists who were asked to discuss on treatment therapies for patients having cancer in the head-to-neck region. Arguments were modelled as natural language propositions constructed upon a particular piece of evidence, acquired from the literature, and linked to a particular treatment choice. Each argument was also accompanied by a value indicating the strength of the underlying evidence. A machinery that extended Dung's calculus of opposition [9] was proposed, followed by a preference-based accrual of arguments [56]. Further research studies adopted the *Aspic* framework in the context of consensus on explanations and it focused on understanding how two clinicians, with a disagreement in relation to an anomalous patient's response to treatment, exchanged arguments in order to arrive at a consensus [57]. Gorogiannis et al. employed argumentation for investigating treatment efficacy and their work was motivated by the fact that, although there was a rapidly-growing dataset of trial results, this dataset was inconsistent, incomplete and required a significant effort to be sensibly aggregated for the inference of a single correct decision [58]. The authors proposed an argument-based framework to analyse the available knowledge and present the different possible results. In this framework, the monological structure of arguments was modelled as a triple $< A, B, C >$ with A the set of evidence from a clinical trail, B an inference rule that linked evidence to a claim C. The claim was a comparison between the outcomes of two generic treatments $t1$ and $t2$ (only two-arm comparisons were treated) that can be either $t1 > t2$ ($t1$ is statistically superior to $t2$), $t2 < t1$ (viceversa) or $t1 \sim t2$ (no statistical difference). Regarding the dialogical structure, arguments (clinical tests) conflicted with each other if they entailed contradicting claims and contradictions were resolved with the Dung's calculus of opposition. This framework was extended in [59] by allowing the expression of preferences among arguments and by employing descriptive logic to further specify their monological structure. In this extension, authors performed a case study on ovarian cancer data showing how the introduction of the dialogical Dung's calculus of opposition could support the selection of relevant/undisputed clinical evidence in a large and fragmented dataset of cases.

Argumentation has been employed for predicting the recurrence of breast cancer in patients who have undergone a surgery [60]. In this circumstance, the knowledge-base of a cancer expert has been translated into arguments with premises supporting either recurrence or non-recurrence of cancer. This monological structure has been subsequently extended adding conflicts among arguments organised dialogically, always according to the expert's knowledge-base. In turn, they were evaluated with the Dung's calculus of opposition. A strategy based on the largest cardinality was implemented for selecting the most credible preferred extension, and thus recommending a justifiable outcome (recurrence or non-recurrence). [61] describes an application of argumentation to the field of organ transplant called *Carrel+*. Human-organ is a decision-making process that often illustrates conflicts among medical experts: what may be sufficient for one doctor to discard an organ may not be for another one. This application allows doctors to express their arguments about the viability of an organ and employs monological argumentation techniques, namely argumentation schemes [20] and critical questions [21] to combine arguments, to identify inconsistencies and to propose a valid solution considering their relative strength as well as the available evidence about the organ and the donor. Other ways to elaborate and construct arguments exist and they differ because of the variability of their monological structure. For instance, [58,59] are different from [61–63]. In the former studies, arguments are built directly from clinical trial results with a uniform structure that makes the approach less domain-dependent and scalable to large-volume data. In the latter works, arguments are hand-crafted and ad-hoc constructs built by relying on domain specific expertise and therefore they have a variable internal structure.

Ultimately, [64] is probably the most complete work applying argumentation to medical decision support. This work is closely adhering to the 5-layer schema previously introduced (Sect. 3). First, the available evidence, collected from experts or literature, is converted into a monological argument structured as an inference rule. Second, a medical expert can set up preference relations by assigning a weight to each arguments (argument A can be preferred to B because, despite having comparable effects, A has fewer side effects than B). Third, meta-arguments can be built about the quality of arguments created in the first stage (an argument based on a non-randomised small sample is weaker than another based on the evidence collected on a large randomised sample). Forth, the dialogical structure is arranged in a Dung style argumentation graph and an argumentation semantics is used for computing their dialectical and acceptability status from which consistent conclusions can be suggested to the decision makers. The study proposes several case studies: diagnosis of glaucoma, treatment of hypertension and treatments of pre-eclampsia.

In summary, Table 2 gives a panoramic of the contributions reviewed so far, classified according to the 5-layer schema introduced in Fig. 2 The aim is at providing the reader with a high-level snapshot describing the current effort devoted towards producing argument-based systems in medicine and health-care.

4.1 Features of Argumentation

Theoretically, argumentation and defeasible reasoning have a set of features that are generally appealing and specifically interesting for clinicians and practitioners in the field of medicine and health-care [7,60].

- *Inconsistency/incompleteness:* argumentation provides a methodology for reasoning on available evidence, even if this evidence is partial and inconsistent as it often happens in medicine and health-care;
- *Expertise/uncertainty:* argumentation captures expertise in an organised fashion, employing the notion of arguments and it can handle vagueness and the uncertainty associated with clinical evidence;
- *Intuitiveness:* argumentation is close to the way humans reason. Vague knowledge bases can be structured as arguments built with familiar linguistic terms, which is extremely appealing for clinicians;
- *Explainability:* argumentation leads to explanatory reasoning thanks to its incremental, modular way of reasoning with available evidence. It provides approaches for computing the justification status of arguments, allowing the final decision of a reasoning process to be better explained;
- *Dataset independency:* argumentation does not require a complete dataset and it may be useful for emerging knowledge, where quantitative evidence has not yet been gathered or is limited;

Table 2. Argument-based systems in medicine and health-care: applications

Ref	Domain	Layer 1	Layer 2	Layer 3	Layer 4	Layer 5
[52,53]	argumentation services, patient treatment options	a tree of premises→claim + degree of belief	abstract attacks	degree of belief	dung	n/a
[54]	genetic consueling, care plans	Toulmin	n/a	n/a	n/a	n/a
[56]	group-decision support	natural language propositions + strength of evidence	abstract attacks	preference list	dung +	preference-based
[57]	consensus, explanations	a tree of premises→claim + degree of belief	abstract attacks	degree of belief	dung	n/a
[60]	cancer prediction	premises→claim	abstract attacks	n/a	dung	extension cardinality
[58]	treatment efficacy	premises→claim	abstract attacks	preference list	dung	n/a
[59]	identification of relevant evidence	descriptive logic	abstract attacks	preference relation-ships	dialectical tree	n/a
[61]	organ transplant confirmation	argument schemes + critical questions	abstract attacks	argument strength	dung	n/a
[62]	breast cancer care	Evidence-based guideline	n/a	n/a	n/a	n/a
[64]	Treatments of diseases	inference rule	argument strength	meta arguments	dung	utility theory

- *Extensibility/updatability:* argumentation is an extensible paradigm that allows a decision to be retracted in the light of new evidence. An argumentation system can be updated with new arguments when they become available;
- *Knowledge-bases comparability:* argumentation allows comparisons of different subjective knowledge-bases. Two clinicians might build their own argumentation frameworks, identify differences in the definition of their beliefs, expertise and intuitions as well as compare their inferential capacity;
- *Consensus building:* argumentation is a useful approach for decision-making and achieving consensus between contradicting perspectives of knowledge.

Although argumentation has a great potential for supporting decision-making, enhancing knowledge representation and performing defeasible inference in the light of fragmented, partial, vague and inconsistent knowledge, it has some limitations [10,11]. The aforementioned features are appealing at the theoretical level, however, there are more practical, open problems for applied research. The following section is aimed at describing these problems and present future challenges for enabling wide-spread application of argumentation at the more practical level. Readers can refer to [11] for a further discussion on the role of argumentation and argumentation-based applications in modern computing.

5   Open Problems and Challenges

Bench-Capon and Dunne discussed limitations of argumentation in artificial intelligence and computer science [10], identifying a set of challenges concerning the widespread deployment of argumentation technology. These challenges are still valid and their resolution requires the union of theoretical work with more practical engineering work. Probably, the most important limitation concerns the adoption of argumentation methods and systems in practical fields, these including medicine and health care. However, other limitations exist:

- lack of engineering solutions for application/automation of argumentation
- lack of a strong link between argumentation and other formalisms for dealing with uncertainty;
- scalability of argument-based applications and their widespread;
- ambiguity of the communication protocols and language that can be used by artificial agents incorporating argumentative capabilities.

Firstly, as it often happens in real-world knowledge-engineering, pieces of knowledge are abundant, so the amount of arguments that can be built upon them. However, engineering and software tools for the monological representation of arguments are limited, despite advances in technology and interfaces. Diagrammatic representations of arguments have been proposed [20,21,65] but their implementation in practice is still narrow. Human reasoning over graphical diagrams is fundamental to enable human experts to translate their knowledge bases and beliefs in a computable form employable for reasoning and inference. User-friendly interfaces are necessary for enabling human operators to link arguments together, for modelling their conflicts and for performing inference through the execution of acceptability semantics for the resolution of these conflicts. These bottlenecks must be addressed to support the deployment and adoption of argument-based applications. Advances in user-interface design and deployment as well as the availability of web-based tools (javascript) are valid candidates for tackling these bottlenecks.

Secondly, in order to facilitate the impact of argument-based applications in the arena of intelligent computer systems, a further challenge is the construction of a stronger link with other formalisms for dealing with uncertainty within the broader field of artificial intelligence. Examples include probability and Bayesian theories, Dempster-Shafer theory and Game Theory [38] for applications requiring the interaction of multiple parties, participants [56] or Fuzzy Sets and Logic [32,34–36] for representation of vague knowledge. Further formalisms concerning the supporting of collaborative work/learning or decision-making [52] include Organisational Theory [66,67] and Decision theory [68].

Thirdly, another important challenge refers to the scalability of applications of argumentation and their widespread. This means that in order to demonstrate the impact of argument-based technologies to knowledge representation and reasoning, several applications have to be deployed and tested in different disciplines such as education, medicine [54,56,57,64], psychology, biology extending traditional fields of application such as artificial intelligence [10], computer science, philosophy, linguistic and human-computer Interaction [69–71]. The scalability challenge also refers to a more technical issue concerning the deployment of engineering systems that can easily scale, such as in [72], and let a great amount of parties, participants or artificial agents to be engaged in a large-scale argumentative process and enabling collective intelligence [73]. Assuming the above challenges can be resolved there is another important challenge referred to the development of the protocols for allowing artificial agents, incorporating argumentative capabilities, to communicate, argue and negotiate with each other in a distributed digital world [11,74]. Recent advances in the field of multi-agent systems might offer valid approaches to tackle this problem.

6   Future Outlook

This chapter has presented an overview of argumentation for knowledge representation, conflict resolution and defeasible reasoning, with an informal description of the multi-layer pattern usually adopted for implementing in practice such reasoning. A literature review of applications of argumentation showed how defeasible reasoning has been employed so far in the medical and health-care sectors. Advantages and features of argumentation have been proposed emphasising the benefits for defeasible inference under uncertainty. Open problems and challenges have been identified, these mainly referring to the practical applicability of argumentation rather than the development of new theoretical formalisms. The lack of user-friendly tools and procedures employable by humans to build arguments, connect them in a dialogical structure and enable defeasible reasoning in practice is the most important challenge for applied research. From a more theoretical perspective, future work should be focused on the integration of argumentation theory and machine learning as two different but complementary methods for enhancing knowledge representation and extraction, reasoning and classification with fragmented, partial and conflicting information [75]. This integration could be tackled through 3 points of interaction (Fig. 11, A, B, C).

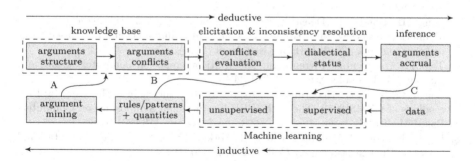

Fig. 11. Integration of machine learning and defeasible argumentation

On one hand, argumentation represents a theory and belief-driven deductive paradigm to reasoning over pieces of evidence, potentially conflicting and fragmented towards a final inference. On the other hand, machine learning, is a data-driven inductive paradigm aimed at exploring data, extracting patterns and building learning models from it so classification can be performed and predictions can be made. Through these models, new arguments can be built and incorporated in existing knowledge-bases thus enhancing reasoning processes (A) [76]. The rules and patterns emerged from unsupervised machine learning techniques and the predictions, probabilistic values available in supervised machine learning classifiers can support the resolution of potential inconsistencies in a defeasible reasoning process, providing it with numerical attributes useful for formalising preferences and deciding between conflicting arguments (B). Eventually, the inference produced by a defeasible reasoning process can provide machine learning with a useful theoretical background for identifying deceptive chains of inference that might lead to erroneous results (C). Hybrid models employing both the paradigms can benefit from the advantages of each approach and tackle their pitfalls and they are expected to perform better in term of representation, clustering of knowledge and in term of prediction and inference.

References

1. Holzinger, A.: Interactive machine learning for health informatics: when do we need the human-in-the-loop? Brain Inform. **3**, 1–13 (2016)
2. Holzinger, A., Plass, M., Holzinger, K., Crişan, G.C., Pintea, C.-M., Palade, V.: Towards interactive Machine Learning (iML): applying ant colony algorithms to solve the traveling salesman problem with the human-in-the-loop approach. In: Buccafurri, F., Holzinger, A., Kieseberg, P., Tjoa, A.M., Weippl, E. (eds.) CD-ARES 2016. LNCS, vol. 9817, pp. 81–95. Springer, Heidelberg (2016). doi:10.1007/978-3-319-45507-5_6
3. Gomez, S.A., Chesnevar, C.I.: Integrating defeasible argumentation with fuzzy art neural network for pattern classification. J. Comp. Sci. Technol. **4**(1), 45–51 (2004)
4. Baroni, P., Guida, G., Mussi, S.: Full nonmonotonicity: a new perspective in defeasible reasoning. In: ESIT 1997, European Symposium on Intelligent Techniques, pp. 58–62 (1997)
5. Longo, L., Dondio, P.: Defeasible reasoning and argument-based medical systems: an informal overview. In: 27th International Symposium on Computer-Based Medical Systems, pp. 376–381. IEEE, New York (2014)
6. Toni, F.: Argumentative agents. In: The Multiconference on Computer Science and Information Technology, pp. 223–229 (2010)
7. Longo, L., Kane, B., Hederman, L.: Argumentation theory in health care. In: Proceedings of CBMS 2012, The 25th IEEE International Symposium on Computer-Based Medical Systems, June 20–22, Rome, Italy, pp. 1–6 (2012)
8. Longo, L.: Formalising Human Mental Workload as a Defeasible Computational Concept. PhD thesis, Trinity College Dublin (2014)
9. Dung, P.M.: On the acceptability of arguments and its fundamental role in non-monotonic reasoning, logic programming and n-person games. Artif. Intell. **77**(2), 321–358 (1995)
10. Bench-Capon, T.J., Dunne, P.E.: Argumentation in artificial intelligence. Artif. Intell. **171**(10–15), 619–641 (2007)

11. Rahwan, I., McBurney, P.: Argumentation technology (guest editors). IEEE Intell. Syst. **22**(6), 21–23 (2007)
12. Matt, P.A., Morgem, M., Toni, F.: Combining statistics and arguments to compute trust. In: International Conference on Autonomous Agents and Multiagent Systems (2010)
13. Dondio, P., Longo, L.: Computing trust as a form of presumptive reasoning. In: 2014 IEEE/WIC/ACM International Joint Conferences on Web Intelligence (WI) and Intelligent Agent Technologies (IAT), vol. I, Warsaw, Poland, August 11–14, pp. 274–281 (2014)
14. Longo, L.: A defeasible reasoning framework for human mental workload representation and assessment. Behav. Inf. Technol. **34**(8), 758–786 (2015)
15. Krause, P., Ambler, S., Elvang-Gransson, M., Fox, J.: A logic of argumentation for reasoning under uncertainty. Comput. Intell. **11**(1), 113–131 (1995)
16. Bentahar, J., Moulin, B., Blanger, M.: A taxonomy of argumentation models used for knowledge representation. Artif. Intell. Rev. **33**(3), 211–259 (2010)
17. Grasso, F.: Towards a framework for rhetorical argumentation. In: Proceedings of the 6th Workshop on the Semantics and Pragmatics of Dialogue, pp. 53–60 (2002)
18. Pasquier, P., Rahwanm, I., Dignum, F., Sonenberg, L.: Argumentation and persuasion in the cognitive coherence theory. In: The 1st International Conference on Computational Models of Argument, pp. 223–234 (2006)
19. Prakken, H., Vreeswijk, G.: Logics for defeasible argumentation. In: Gabbay, D.M., Guenthner, F. (eds.) Handbook of Philosophical Logic, vol. 4, pp. 219–318. Springer, Heidelberg (2002)
20. Toulmin, S.: The use of argument. Cambridge University Press, Cambridge (1958)
21. Walton, D.: Argumentation Schemes for Presumptive Reasoning (Studies in Argumentation Theory). Lawrence Erlbaum Associates, Inc., Hillsdale (1996)
22. Reed, C., Walton, D.: Argumentation schemes in argument-as-process and argument-as-product. In: Proceedings of the Conference Celebrating Informal Logic, vol. 25 (2003)
23. Prakken, H.: An abstract framework for argumentation with structured arguments. Argument and Comput. **1**(2), 93–124 (2011)
24. Pollock, J.L.: Justification and defeat. Artif. Intell. **67**(2), 377–407 (1994)
25. Martínez, D.C., García, A., Simari, G.R.: Strong and weak forms of abstract argument defense. In: Proceedings of the 2008 Conference on Computational Models of Argument: Proceedings of COMMA 2008, pp. 216–227. IOS Press (2008)
26. Dunne, P.E., Hunter, A., McBurney, P., Parsons, S., Wooldridge, M.: Weighted argument systems: basic definitions, algorithms, and complexity results. Artif. Intell. **175**(2), 457–486 (2011)
27. Modgil, S.: Reasoning about preferences in argumentation frameworks. Artif. Intell. **173**(9–10), 901–934 (2009)
28. Pollock, J.L.: Defeasible reasoning. Cognitive Sci. **11**(4), 481–518 (1987)
29. Prakken, H., Sartor, G.: Argument-based extended logic programming with defeasible priorities. J. Appl. Non-Class. Logics **7**, 25–75 (1997)
30. Amgoud, L., Cayrol, C.: A reasoning model based on the production of acceptable arguments. Ann. Math. Artif. Intell. **34**(1–3), 197–215 (2002)
31. Bench-Capon, T.J.: Persuasion in practical argument using value-based argumentation frameworks. J. Logic Comput. **13**(3), 429–448 (2003)
32. Kaci, S., Labreuche, C.: Argumentation framework with fuzzy preference relations. In: 13th International Conference on Information Processing and Management of Uncertainty, pp. 554–563 (2010)

33. Martinez, D.C., Garcia, A.J., Simari, G.R.: An abstract argumentation framework with varied-strength attacks. In: International Conference on Principles of Knowledge Representation and Reasoning, pp. 135–143 (2008)
34. Janssen, J., De Cock, M., Vermeir, D.: Fuzzy argumentation frameworks. In: Information Processing and Management of Uncertainty in Knowledge-based Systems, pp. 513–520, June 2008
35. Zadeh, L.A.: Fuzzy sets. Inf. Control **8**(3), 338–353 (1965)
36. Zadeh, L.A.: Fuzzy Sets, Fuzzy Logic, Fuzzy Systems. World Scientific Press (1966)
37. Li, H., Oren, N., Norman, T.J.: Probabilistic argumentation frameworks. In: Modgil, S., Oren, N., Toni, F. (eds.) TAFA 2011. LNCS (LNAI), vol. 7132, pp. 1–16. Springer, Heidelberg (2012). doi:10.1007/978-3-642-29184-5_1
38. Matt, P.-A., Toni, F.: A game-theoretic measure of argument strength for abstract argumentation. In: Hölldobler, S., Lutz, C., Wansing, H. (eds.) JELIA 2008. LNCS (LNAI), vol. 5293, pp. 285–297. Springer, Heidelberg (2008). doi:10.1007/978-3-540-87803-2_24
39. Vreeswijk, G.: Defeasible dialectics: a controversy-oriented approach towards defeasible argumentation. J. Logic Comput. **3**, 3–27 (1993)
40. Baroni, P., Caminada, M., Giacomin, M.: An introduction to argumentation semantics. Knowl. Eng. Rev. **26**(4), 365–410 (2011)
41. Wu, Y., Caminada, M., Podlaszewski, M.: A labelling based justification status of arguments. Stud. Logic **3**(4), 12–29 (2010). 13th International Workshop on Non-Monotonic Reasoning
42. Dung, P.M., Mancarellab, P., Toni, F.: Computing ideal sceptical argumentation. Artif. Intell. **171**(10–15), 642–674 (2007)
43. Caminada, M.W.A.: A labelling approach for ideal and stage semantics. Argument Comput. **2**(1), 1–21 (2006)
44. Caminada, M.W.A., Carnielli, W.A., Dunne, P.E.: Semi-stable semantics. J. Logic Comput. **22**(5), 1207–1254 (2012)
45. Caminada, M.W.A.: An algorithm for stage semantics. In: Baroni, P., Cerutti, F., Giacomin, M., Simari, G.R. (eds.): Frontiers in Artificial Intelligence and Applications, Proceedings of the 3rd International Conference on Computational Models of Argument (COMMA 2010), vol. 216, pp. 147–158. IOS Press (2010)
46. Jakobovits, H., Vermeir, D.: Robust semantics for argumentation frameworks. Logic. Comput. **9**(2), 215–261 (1999)
47. Baroni, M., Giacomin, M., Guida, G.: Scc-recursiveness: a general schema for argumentation semantics. Artif. Intell. **168**(1–2), 165–2010 (2005)
48. Baroni, P., Giacomin, M.: Semantics of abstract argument systems. In: Simari, G., Rahwan, I. (eds.): Argumentation in Artificial Intelligence, pp. 25–44. Springer, Heidelberg (2009)
49. Konieczny, S., Marquis, P., Vesic, S.: On supported inference and extension selection in abstract argumentation frameworks. In: Destercke, S., Denoeux, T. (eds.) ECSQARU 2015. LNCS (LNAI), vol. 9161, pp. 49–59. Springer, Heidelberg (2015). doi:10.1007/978-3-319-20807-7_5
50. Coste-Marquis, S., Konieczny, S., Marquis, P., Akli Ouali, M.: Selecting extensions in weighted argumentation frameworks. In: Computational Models of Argument, COMMA (2012)
51. Bryant, D., Krause, P.: A review of current defeasible reasoning implementations. Knowl. Eng. Rev. **23**(3), 227–260 (2008)
52. Fox, J., Glasspool, D., Grecu, D., Modgil, S., South, M., Patkar, V.: Argumentation-based inference and decision making-a medical perspective. IEEE Intell. Syst., 21–23 (2007)

53. Fox, J., Black, L., Glasspool, D., Modgil, S., Oettinger, A., Patkar, V., Williams, M.: Towards a general model for argumentation services. In: AAAI Spring Symposium Series (2006)
54. Glasspool, D., Fox, J., Oettinger, A., Smith-Spark, J.: Argumentation in decision support for medical care planning for patients and clinicians. In: AAAI Spring Symposium: Argumentation for Consumers of Healthcare, pp. 58–63 (2006)
55. Pollock, J.L.: Defeasible reasoning with variable degrees of justification. Artif. Intell. **133**, 233–282 (2001)
56. Chang, C.F., Miller, A., Ghose, A.: Mixed-initiative argumentation: group decision support in medicine. In: Kostkova, P. (ed.) eHealth 2009. LNICSSITE, vol. 27, pp. 43–50. Springer, Heidelberg (2010). doi:10.1007/978-3-642-11745-9_8
57. Grando, M.A., Moss, L., Sleeman, D., Kinsella, J.: Argumentation-logic for creating and explaining medical hypotheses. Artif. Intell. Med **58**(1), 1–13 (2013)
58. Gorogiannis, N., Hunter, A., Patkar, V., Williams, M.: Argumentation about treatment efficacy. In: Riaño, D., Teije, A., Miksch, S., Peleg, M. (eds.) KR4HC 2009. LNCS (LNAI), vol. 5943, pp. 169–179. Springer, Heidelberg (2010). doi:10.1007/978-3-642-11808-1_14
59. Williams, M., Hunter, A.: Harnessing ontologies for argument-based decision-making in breast cancer. In: ICTAI (2), pp. 254–261 (2007)
60. Longo, L., Hederman, L.: Argumentation theory for decision support in healthcare: a comparison with machine learning. In: Imamura, K., Usui, S., Shirao, T., Kasamatsu, T., Schwabe, L., Zhong, N. (eds.) BHI 2013. LNCS (LNAI), vol. 8211, pp. 168–180. Springer, Heidelberg (2013). doi:10.1007/978-3-319-02753-1_17
61. Tolchinsky, P., Cortes, U., Modgil, S., Caballero, F., Lopez-Navidad, A.: Increasing human-organ transplant availability: argumentation-based agent deliberation. IEEE Intell. Syst. **21**(6), 30–37 (2006)
62. Patkar, V., Hurt, C., Steele, R., Love, S., Purushotham, A., Williams, M., Thomson, R., Fox, J.: Evidence-based guidelines and decision support services: a discussion and evaluation in triple assessment of suspected breast cancer. Br. J. Cancer **95**(11), 1490–1496 (2006)
63. Fox, J., Das, S.: Safe and Sound: Artificial Intelligence in Hazardous Applications, 1st edn. AAAI Press (2000)
64. Hunter, A., Williams, M.: Argumentation for aggregating clinical evidence. In: ICTAI (1), pp. 361–368 (2010)
65. Prakken, H.: Ai & law, logic and argument schemes. Argumentation (Special Issue on The Toulmin Model Today) **19**, 303–320 (2005)
66. Jones, G.R.: Organizational Theory, Design, and Change: Text and Cases, 6th edn. Pearson Prentice Hall, Upper Saddle River, NJ (2010)
67. Daft, R.L.: Organization Theory and Design, 9th edn. Thomson South-Western, Mason, OH (2007)
68. Rapoport, A.: Decision Theory and Decision Behaviour. Springer (1989)
69. Longo, L., Rusconi, F., Noce, L., Barrett, S.: The importance of human mental workload in web-design. In: 8th International Conference on Web Information Systems and Technologies, pp. 403–409, April 2012
70. Longo, L.: Formalising human mental workload as non-monotonic concept for adaptive and personalised web-design. In: Masthoff, J., Mobasher, B., Desmarais, M.C., Nkambou, R. (eds.) UMAP 2012. LNCS, vol. 7379, pp. 369–373. Springer, Heidelberg (2012). doi:10.1007/978-3-642-31454-4_38

71. Longo, L., Dondio, P.: On the relationship between perception of usability and subjective mental workload of web interfaces. In: IEEE/WIC/ACM International Conference on Web Intelligence and Intelligent Agent Technology, WI-IAT 2015, Singapore, December 6–9, vol. I, pp. 345–352 (2015)

72. Dondio, P., Longo, L.: Trust-based techniques for collective intelligence in social search systems. In: Bessis, N., Xhafa, F. (eds.) Next Generation Data Technologies for CCI, SCI, vol. 352, pp. 113–135. Springer, Heidelberg (2011)

73. Longo, L., Dondio, P., Barrett, S.: Enhancing social search: a computational collective intelligence model of behavioural traits, trust and time. Trans. Comput. Collective Intell. **2**, 46–69 (2010)

74. Luca, L., Stephen, B., Pierpaolo, D.: Information foraging theory as a form of collective intelligence for social search. In: Nguyen, N.T., Kowalczyk, R., Chen, S.-M. (eds.) ICCCI 2009. LNCS (LNAI), vol. 5796, pp. 63–74. Springer, Heidelberg (2009). doi:10.1007/978-3-642-04441-0_5

75. Možina, M., Žabkar, J., Bratko, I.: Argument based machine learning. Artif. Intell. **171**(10–15), 922–937 (2007). Argumentation in Artificial Intelligence

76. Lippi, M., Torroni, P.: Argument mining: a machine learning perspective. In: Black, E., Modgil, S., Oren, N. (eds.) TAFA 2015. LNCS (LNAI), vol. 9524, pp. 163–176. Springer, Heidelberg (2015). doi:10.1007/978-3-319-28460-6_10

Machine Learning and Data Mining Methods for Managing Parkinson's Disease

Dragana Miljkovic[1]([✉]), Darko Aleksovski[1], Vid Podpečan[1], Nada Lavrač[1], Bernd Malle[2], and Andreas Holzinger[2,3]

[1] Knowledge Technologies Department, Jožef Stefan Institute, Ljubljana, Slovenia
dragana.miljkovic@ijs.si

[2] Holzinger Group, Institute for Medical Informatics, Statistics and Documentation, Medical University Graz, Graz, Austria
a.holzinger@hci-kdd.org

[3] Institute of Information Systems and Computer Media, Graz University of Technology, Graz, Austria

Abstract. Parkinson's disease (PD) results primarily from dying of dopaminergic neurons in the Substantia Nigra, a part of the Mesencephalon (midbrain), which is not curable to date. PD medications treat symptoms only, none halt or retard dopaminergic neuron degeneration. Here machine learning methods can be of help since one of the crucial roles in the management and treatment of PD patients is detection and classification of tremors. In the clinical practice, this is one of the most common movement disorders and is typically classified using behavioral or etiological factors. Another important issue is to detect and evaluate PD related gait patterns, gait initiation and freezing of gait, which are typical symptoms of PD. Medical studies have shown that 90% of people with PD suffer from vocal impairment, consequently the analysis of voice data to discriminate healthy people from PD is relevant. This paper provides a quick overview of the state-of-the-art and some directions for future research, motivated by the ongoing PD_manager project.

Keywords: Machine learning · Data mining · Parkinson's disease

1 Introduction

We present the results of a literature-based study of data mining methods used for Parkinson's disease management. The study was motivated by requirements of the EU H2020 project PD_manager[1], which aims to develop an innovative, mobile-health, patient-centric platform for Parkinson's disease management. One part of the data mining module of this platform will include predictive data mining algorithms designed to predict the changes in patients symptoms as well as their severity. The second segment will include descriptive data mining methods, which will analyze and provide deeper insight in the patients condition by discovering new disease patterns.

---

[1] http://www.parkinson-manager.eu/.

© Springer International Publishing AG 2016
A. Holzinger (Ed.): ML for Health Informatics, LNAI 9605, pp. 209–220, 2016.
DOI: 10.1007/978-3-319-50478-0_10

Data mining algorithms search for patterns and/or models in data, which are interesting and valid according to the user-defined criteria of interestingness and validity. Both predictive as well as descriptive data mining methods are lately rapidly used in the healthcare domain. Use of data mining methods brings numerous advantages in healthcare, such as lowering the cost of the available medical solutions, improving the detection of disease causes and proper identification of treatment, drug recommendation and providing support in personalized health [1].

There are several symptoms that are important for diagnosis, management and treatment of Parkinson's disease patients. It appears that one of the crucial roles in managing Parkinson's disease is the detection and classification of tremor. Tremor, which is a primary symptom of the disease, is an involuntary, rhythmical, forwards and backwards movement of a body part and is assessed in some studies with Hidden Markov models, neural networks and different methods for time domain and spectral analysis. Besides tremor, freezing of gait (FoG) is one of the advanced symptoms in Parkinson's disease. Very few computational methods have been developed so far to detect it and they can be grouped into the following categories: analysis of electromyography signals, 3D motion analysis, foot pressure analysis and motion signal analysis using accelerometers and gyroscopes. The problem of gait initiation, the transient state between standing and walking, is studied in terms of differentiation between normal and abnormal gait initiation. In addition to these symptoms, medical studies have shown that over 90% of people with Parkinson's disease suffer from some form of vocal impairment. The analysis of voice can be used for successfully diagnosing Parkinson's disease.

There were several EU projects devoted to different aspects of Parkinson's disease, which is the topic of this research. On the basis of the state-of-art search, this work proposes the design and the functionality of a data mining module that will be implemented within the mobile e-health platform for the purpose of the PD_manager project.

2   Glossary and Key Terms

Parkinson's disease (PD) results primarily from dying of dopaminergic neurons in the Substantia Nigra, a part of the Mesencephalon (midbrain), which is not curable to date. PD medications treat symptoms only, none halt or retard dopaminergic neuron degeneration [2].

ClowdFlows is an open source cloud-based platform for composition, execution, and sharing of interactive machine learning and data mining workflows, which is based on the principles of service-oriented knowledge discovery and features interactive scientific workflows [3].

Hyper heuristics are a way of selecting or configuring algorithms by searching a space of lower level heuristics instead of searching the solution (parameter) space itself.

3   Data Mining

This section overviews the basic concepts and provides a state-of-the-art literature review of data mining methods used in PD diagnosis, prediction, analysis and management.

3.1   Basic Concepts

Data mining algorithms search for patterns and/or models in data that are interesting and valid according to the user-defined criteria of interestingness and validity. There are two main machine learning approaches used in data mining algorithms: supervised learning takes classified examples as input for training the classification/prediction model, while unsupervised learning takes as input unclassified examples [4]. Consequently, data mining methods can be classified into two main categories:

– Predictive data mining methods result in models for prediction and classification. In classification, data are class labeled and the task of a classifier is to determine the class for a new unlabeled example. The most commonly used predictive methods are rule and decision tree learning methods. The classification rule model consists of if-then rules in a format: if Conditions then Class, where Conditions represent conjunctions of attribute values, and rule consequent is a Class label. The decision tree model consists of nodes and arcs. Non-leaf nodes in a decision tree represent a test on a particular attribute, each arc is test output (one or more attribute values in case of nominal attributes, or an interval in case of numeric attributes) and each leaf is a class label.
– Descriptive data mining methods are used for finding individual data patterns, such as associations, clusters, etc. Association rule induction, clustering and subgroup discovery are among the most popular descriptive data mining methods. Association rule learning is an unsupervised learning method where an association rule is given in a form $X \rightarrow Y$, where X and Y are sets of items. The goal of association rule learning is to find interesting relationships among sets of data items. Clustering is another unsupervised learning method where data instances are clustered into groups based on their common characteristics. On the other hand, subgroup discovery is a supervised learning method, aimed at finding descriptions of interesting population subgroups.

Data mining is used extensively in various domains, such as business management, market analytics, insurance policies, healthcare, etc. In the last decade, data mining has made its breakthrough and since then its use in the healthcare domain is rapidly growing. The use of data mining methods brings numerous advantages to healthcare, such as lowering the cost of medical solutions, detection of disease causes and proper identification of treatment methods, developing personalized health profiles, drug recommendation systems, etc. [5]. This literature review specifically focuses on data mining applications for Parkinson's disease, which is the topic of the next section.

3.2   State-of-the-art Review

This section presents a survey of the data mining methods used for diagnosing, predicting, analyzing and managing PD. It is structured according to the particular tasks in PD domain for which data mining algorithms were employed.

Tremor Assessment. One of the crucial roles in the management and treatment of PD patients is the detection and classification of tremors. In clinical practice, this is one of the most common movement disorders and is typically classified using behavioral or etiological factors [6]. During early stages of PD, tremor is mostly present at rest, while at later stages postural action tremor can be observed. The two are hard to distinguish with automated methods using only their base frequencies (3.5–7.5 Hz vs. 4–12 Hz) so the recognition of body posture is also essential. Because clinical tremor assessment is most commonly based on subjective methods such as clinical scales, handwriting and drawing assessment [7,8], there is a great need for objective, computational methods for the detection and quantification of tremors.

Several approaches to computational assessment of tremor have been proposed. Methods such as time domain analysis [9], spectral analysis [10] and nonlinear analysis [10] have addressed the detection and quantification of tremor. Much of the recent work is based on body fixed sensors (BFS) for long-term monitoring of patients [11,12]. Recent work by Rigas et al. [13] on the assessment of tremor activity tries to overcome the limitations of older methods using the following approach. First, six body sensors are used to collect raw data in real time. Then, signal pre-processing is performed to separate lower frequency events (not interesting) and higher frequency events (relevant for tremor assessment). Following data pre-processing, two sets of features are extracted from signal data. The first set of features is used for posture recognition while the second set is used for tremor detection and quantification. The obtained data is used to train two Hidden Markov Models (HMM), one for posture recognition and the other for tremor classification. By using the combined output of both models, tremor can be accurately assessed. The authors report high accuracy on a set of 23 subjects which indicates that the method is efficient for tremor assessment in practice. A less popular, invasive approach to data collection for tremor assessment is using deep brain electrodes implanted in PD patients [14]. Wu et al. have demonstrated the performance of radial basis function neural network in detecting tremor and non-tremor patterns. These patterns allowed them to predict the tremor onset in PD patients.

Gait Analysis. Muniz et al. [15] study the effects of deep brain stimulation (DBS) on ground reaction force (GRF) during gait. They are interested in the ability to discriminate between normal and PD subjects. They report using the Principal Component Analysis (PCA) of the walking trials data to extract PC features from the different GRF components. Then, the aim of the paper is to investigate which classification method is the most successful for the addressed discrimination task. The methods tested are Support Vector Machines (SVM), Probabilistic Neural Networks (PNN) and Logistic Regression (LR). They conclude that the PNN and SVM models show the best performance.

The problem of discriminating between normal and PD gait pattern is analyzed also in a study by Tahir and Manap [16]. Beside the GRF data, the authors use additional spatio-temporal (e.g., stride time, cadence, step length) and kinematic (e.g., hip, knee, ankle angle) data, acquired by using reflective markers on the subjects skin and an infrared camera. The methods they compare are SVMs using linear, radial basis function and polynomial kernels, and Neural Networks (NN). Their results suggest that the kinematic features are not informative for this task, and that the SVM classifier performs better than the NNs.

Freezing of Gait Detection. Besides tremor, freezing of gait (FoG) is one of the advanced symptoms in Parkinson's disease. Three types of FoG are distinguished:

- inability to start walking or continue movement,
- complete absence of movement, and
- shuffling with very short steps [17].

Automated assessment of FoG events is of crucial importance because (a) it becomes more frequent and disabling with the progression of Parkinson's disease and (b) because FoG is a common cause of falls and has a great impact on the quality of life. Clinical assessment of FoG is performed using different scales and questionnaires [18]. Such scales are largely subjective and lack validation against the onset and duration of events. This calls for the development of automated computational methods that are able to detect and assess FoG accurately.

Surprisingly, only few computational methods have been developed so far. The methods can be classified into four categories:

- analysis of electromyography signals [19],
- 3D motion analysis [20],
- foot pressure analysis [21], and
- motion signal analysis using accelerometers and gyroscopes [22–24].

The methods from the last category are specially important because they are based on body sensor data analysis and can therefore be integrated with the detection and assessment of other PD symptoms and movement disorders (e.g., tremor assessment described above). In their recent work, Tipoliti et al. [22] developed a methodology for FoG detection using six wearable accelerometers and two gyroscopes. The method is based on signal processing and feature extraction, followed by classification using four well-known machine learning algorithms. The methodology has four stages: (1) missing data imputation, (2) low pass filtering, (3) extraction of features using a sliding window, (4) classification using one the well-known machine learning algorithms (Naive Bayes, Random forest, Decision tree, Random tree). The evaluation was performed on a set of 16 patients: 5 patients diagnosed with PD and history of FoG events,

6 patients with PD exhibiting other symptoms, and 5 healthy control subjects. The proposed approach is interesting because it can be fully integrated into clinical practice and exhibits high accuracy of 96.11% in classification.

Gait Initiation. The problem of gait initiation, the transient state between standing and walking, was addressed in the study of Muniz et al. [25]. The authors target only the long-term effects of DBS on gait initiation, as the disease progresses. Their hypothesis is that as the disease progresses, the gait initiation worsens. The methods used to test this include PCA of the GRF components, selection of the most informative PCs, and analysis of standard distance[2]. The authors also use logistic regression to identify a threshold over the standard distance data, which would discriminate between normal and abnormal gait initiation. They conclude that the standard distance based on PCA of gait initiation GRF data is increased on long-term.

Vocal Impairment of PD Patients. Medical studies have shown that over 90% of people with PD suffer from some form of vocal impairment [26]. The analysis of voice can be used for successfully diagnosing PD. The study of Das [27] distinguishes the healthy individuals from the ones with PD based on the vocal recordings from 31 people where 23 were with PD. The author has performed a comparative study where performance of several classification algorithms was evaluated (Neural Networks, DMneural, Regression and Decision Tree) and showed that Neural Network achieved the highest accuracy of 92.9%.

The remote tracking of PD patients using acoustic data was done by Eskidere et al. [28] and Chen et al. [29]. The data they use are publicly available [30, 31] deposited in the UCI machine learning repository[3,4].

Eskidere et al. [28] compare standard SVM, Multilayer Perceptron Neural Networks (MLPNN), General Regression Neural Networks (GRNN) and Least Square Support Vector Machines (LS-SVM). The target variables correspond to the Unified Parkinson's Disease Rating Scale (UPDRS), and are the total-UPDRS and motor-UPDRS, which are numeric variables and denote the presence and severity of symptoms. The authors conclude that a logarithmic transformations of extracted vocal features along with Least Square Support Vector Machines (LS-SVM) shows best overall mean-square results.

Chen et al. [29] use data consisting of vocal measurements of 31 people, and are interested in discriminating healthy people from those with PD. The authors use the fuzzy k-nearest neighbour approach (FKNN) and compare its performance to two different SVM variants. In the discussion they also state that a lot of different methods have been tried on this classification task, with different results: decision trees, SVMs, Neural Networks, to name a few. The method asso-

---

[2] Standard distance: a statistic mainly used for spatial GIS data, to measure compactness of a distribution.

[3] https://archive.ics.uci.edu/ml/datasets/Parkinsons+Telemonitoring.

[4] https://archive.ics.uci.edu/ml/datasets/Parkinsons.

ciated with the best classification accuracy is obtained by the fuzzy-based non-linear transformation method in combination with the SVM classifier [32]. Additionally, the authors claim that their 10-times 10-fold cross-validation results suggest that FKNN shows even higher classification accuracy.

Analysis of Combined PD Symptoms. System PERFORM, containing a data mining module with the Predictor and Associator part, represents an effort to combine tracking of several PD symptoms [33]. Based on the initial patients examination and medications taken the Predictor part can predict each PD symptom separately covering 15 different PD symptoms in total. Its prediction accuracy ranges from 57.1% to 77.4% depending on the symptom where the highest accuracy is achieved for tremor detection. The Associator generates association rules from the patients dataset and can discover new insights for the disease.

4   Open Problems Addressed in the PD_manager Project

Data mining methods are used within the PD_manager project for the analysis of various types of data, such as sensor data in the form of time series, lifestyle, therapy, etc. in order to create new, valuable and improved knowledge in the domain of PD. Moreover, the problem of prediction of PD symptoms and their severity are addressed. Both of these tasks have the goal to help decision support systems monitoring patients status, evaluating the current therapy and, when necessary, suggesting a new therapy plan.

Two research phases are carried out within the data mining module. The first one involves raw patients data, therapy, patient profiles and other available data to analyze the patients status where the analysis is done throughout the rule discovery process with association rule mining algorithms. The second phase includes developments of automatic recognition of symptoms based on time series data from patients. This prediction is based on decision trees where we aim to improve the prediction accuracy compared to the existing study [33]. The recognized symptoms, therapy information and other available patients data are the starting point for the rule discovery process in the second phase.

The PD_manager data mining module consists of workflows for data processing and data mining algorithms and is included into the novel web-based data mining platform ClowdFlows[5]. The implementation of this module in the form of workflows provides the benefits of repeatability of such workflows and potential sharing results between different users. The main advantage of using a web-based platform to analyze patients data and predict symptoms is that no installation is required, which also eliminates the problem of building island solutions which may contain data of great interest and value, but do not expose them to the whole research community [3]. Moreover, focusing on isolated implementations

---

[5] http://www.clowdflows.org/.

usually involves much technological effort (as described in [34]) which would be better invested in improving core research.

The platform has a user-friendly graphical user interface which enables its easy utilization by the end users (clinicians). We expect that the proposed PD_manager data mining module, implemented in the ClowdFlows platform, will exhibit several advantages (such as efficient feature selection, and wider selection of applicable data mining and machine learning algorithms) and will enable data analysis in clinical practice.

5   Future Challenges

Building on the initial implementation of the data mining module, one could take several possible research routes to improve the effectiveness of our methods. The use of a centralized, Web based graphical workflow system will prove especially useful in those endeavors, as it bundles not only data, but the experimental results of all experts involved with that platform, which can be useful to experiment with. This follows the concept of an "expert-in-the-loop" to solve problems which would otherwise be computationally hard [35] (for clinical examples refer to: [36–38]). This "glass-box"-approach [39] may be an alternative to the often criticized fully-automatic "black-box"-approach.

5.1   Heterogeneous Data Linkage

As we have seen, the field of Parkinson's disease comprises several sub-problems which are amenable to different machine learning approaches and feature their own, distinctive input data sets. Coming from EEG, EMG, implanted body sensors and force resisting sensors, these data sets have distinct attribute domains, which are—via their time dimension, and probably via many other biological attributes—interlinkable with one another. Usually, studies are only concerned about using a single one of those data sources and applying different methods to it. However, a more holistic approach would be to fuse those data sets along a certain dimension (time, spectral, etc.) in order to achieve a richer representation of the underlying problem. A resulting data-set might take the form of a graph structure, in which individual entities from the originating sets are linked by meaningful connection rules (which will have to be learned in the first place). For example, [40] introduced the concept of authority ranking for heterogeneous networks, where the impact is transferred along edges to simultaneously rank nodes of different types.

5.2   Meta Machine Learning

Meta-learning applies learning algorithms on data collected about machine learning experiments. As one of the first papers regarding this topic, [41] defined the 'Algorithm Selection Problem', which was first recognized as a meta learning problem by the machine learning community in the 1990s. He describes several spaces in which the Algorithm Selection Problem plays out, comprising the problem space, feature space, the pool of suitable algorithms, performance measures (metric space) as well the criteria space defining the weights assigned to performance measures.

In our scenario we are concerned with the selection of workflow components and their parameters based on the tackled problems, their features, available learning algorithms, preprocessing methods, parameters and performance measures. Several approaches and successful applications of this principle exist and we will follow the best practices [42]. The greatest advantage of using Meta ML in combination with a centralized, Web based workflow system lies in the fact that users may profit from their colleagues' meta data by building up a collective Meta ML database: input data plus algorithm parameters plus success metrics.

5.3 Hyper Heuristics

Hyper heuristics are a way of selecting or configuring algorithms by searching a space of lower level heuristics instead of searching the solution (parameter) space itself. Hyper heuristics are different from meta learning in that they work independently of the problem domain and therefore promise to be generally applicable; the challenges lie in producing algorithms that do not need to be optimal, but rather good-enough, soon-enough, cheap-enough [43].

Although the field of Parkinson's disease in itself is not broad enough to be a suitable proving ground for hyper heuristic research, the ClowdFlows platform will provide us with meta-data about experiments in many diverse areas. We fully agree with [44] who concludes that there is still little interaction between research communities, a problem whose solution could lead to the extension of algorithms to both new problem domains and new methodologies through cross-fertilization of ideas. A huge challenge in the future is in privacy aware machine learning [45].

Acknowledgments. The work of the authors was supported by the PD_manager project, funded within the EU Framework Programme for Research and Innovation Horizon 2020, under grant number 643706.

References

1. Holzinger, A.: Trends in interactive knowledge discovery for personalized medicine: cognitive science meets machine learning. IEEE Intell. Inf. Bull. **15**, 6–14 (2014)
2. Dauer, W., Przedborski, S.: Parkinson's disease: mechanisms and models. Neuron **39**, 889–909 (2003)
3. Kranjc, J., Podpečan, V., Lavrač, N.: ClowdFlows: a cloud based scientific workflow platform. In: Flach, P.A., Bie, T., Cristianini, N. (eds.) ECML PKDD 2012. LNCS (LNAI), vol. 7524, pp. 816–819. Springer, Heidelberg (2012). doi:10.1007/978-3-642-33486-3_54

4. Mladenic, D., Lavrač, N., Bohanec, M., Moyle, S. (eds.): Data Mining and Decision Support: Integration and Collaboration. The Springer International Series in Engineering and Computer Science. Springer, Heidelberg (2003)

5. Tomar, D., Agarwal, S.: A survey on data mining approaches for healthcare. Int. J. Bio Sci. Bio Technol. **5**, 241–266 (2013)

6. Findley, L.J.: Classification of tremors. J. Clin. Neurophysiol. **13**, 122–132 (1996)

7. Budzianowska, A., Honczarenko, K.: Assessment of rest tremor in parkinson's disease. Polish J. Neurol. Neurosurg. **42**, 12–21 (2008)

8. Jankovic, J.: Parkinson's disease: clinical features and diagnosis. J. Neurol. Neurosurg. Psychiatry **79**, 368–376 (2008)

9. Timmer, J., Gantert, C., Deuschl, G., Honerkamp, J.: Characteristics of hand tremor time series. Biol. Cybern. **70**, 75–80 (1993)

10. Riviere, C.N., Reich, S.G., Thakor, N.V.: Adaptive fourier modelling for quantification of tremor. J. Neurosci. Methods **74**, 77–87 (1997)

11. Patel, S., Hughes, R., Huggins, N., Standaert, D., Growdon, J., Dy, J., Bonato, P.: Using wearable sensors to predict the severity of symptoms and motor complications in late stage parkinson's disease. In: Conference Proceedings: Annual International Conference of the IEEE Engineering in Medicine and Biology Society, pp. 3686–3689 (2008)

12. Patel, S., Lorincz, K., Hughes, R., Huggins, N., Growdon, J., Standaert, D., Akay, M., Dy, J., Welsh, M., Bonato, P.: Monitoring motor fluctuations in patients with parkinson's disease using wearable sensors. IEEE Trans. Inf. Technol. Biomed. **13**, 864–873 (2009)

13. Rigas, G., Tzallas, A.T., Tsipouras, M.G., Bougia, P., Tripoliti, E., Baga, D., Fotiadis, D.I., Tsouli, S., Konitsiotis, S.: Assessment of tremor activity in the parkinson's disease using a set of wearable sensors. IEEE Trans. Inf. Technol. Biomed. **16**, 478–487 (2012)

14. Wu, D., Warwick, K., Ma, Z., Burgess, J., Pan, S., Aziz, T.: Prediction of parkinson's disease tremor onset using radial basis function neural networks. Expert Syst. Appl. **37**, 2923–2928 (2010)

15. Muniz, A.M., Liu, H., Lyons, K., Pahwa, R., Liu, W., Nobre, F.F., Nadal, J.: Comparison among probabilistic neural network, support vector machine and logistic regression for evaluating the effect of subthalamic stimulation in parkinson disease on ground reaction force during gait. J. Biomech. **43**, 720–726 (2010)

16. Tahir, N.M., Manap, H.H.: Parkinson disease gait classification based on machine learning approach. J. Appl. Sci. **12**, 180–185 (2012)

17. Bloem, B.R., Hausdor, J.M., Visser, J.E., Giladi, N.: Falls and freezing of gait in parkinson's disease: a review of two interconnected, episodic phenomena. Mov. Disorders J. **19**, 871–884 (2004)

18. Giladi, N., Tal, J., Azulay, T., Rascol, O., Brooks, D.J., Melamed, E., Oertel, W., Poewe, W.H., Stocchi, F., Tolosa, E.: Validation of the freezing of gait questionnaire in patients with parkinson's disease. Mov. Disorders J. **24**, 655–661 (2009)

19. Nieuwboer, A., Dom, R., De Weerdt, W., Desloovere, K., Janssens, L., Stijn, V.: Electromyographic profiles of gait prior to onset of freezing episodes in patients with parkinson's disease. Brain **127**, 1650–1660 (2004)

20. Delval, A., Snijders, A.H., Weerdesteyn, V., Duysens, J.E., Defebvre, L., Giladi, N., Bloem, B.R.: Objective detection of subtle freezing of gait episodes in parkinson's disease. Mov. Disorders J. **25**, 1684–1693 (2010)

21. Hausdor, J.M., Schaafsma, J.D., Balash, Y., Bartels, A.L., Gurevich, T., Giladi, N.: Impaired regulation of stride variability in parkinson's disease subjects with freezing of gait. Exp. Brain Res. **149**, 187–194 (2003)

22. Tripoliti, E.E., Tzallas, A.T., Tsipouras, M.G., Rigas, G., Bougia, P., Leontiou, M., Konitsiotis, S., Chondrogiorgi, M., Tsouli, S., Fotiadis, D.I.: Automatic detection of freezing of gait events in patients with parkinson's disease. Comput. Methods Prog. Biomed. **110**, 12–26 (2013)

23. Han, J.H., Lee, W.J., Ahn, T.B., Jeon, B.S., Park, K.S.: Gait analysis for freezing detection in patients with movement disorder using three dimensional acceleration system. In: Conference Proceedings: Annual International Conference of the IEEE Engineering in Medicine and Biology Society, vol. 2, pp. 1863–1865. Medicine and Biology Society (2003)

24. Bächlin, M., Plotnik, M., Roggen, D., Giladi, N., Hausdor, J.M., Tröster, G.: A wearable system to assist walking of parkinson s disease patients. Methods Inf. Med. **49**, 88–95 (2010)

25. Muniz, A.M., Nadal, J., Lyons, K., Pahwa, R., Liu, W.: Long-term evaluation of gait initiation in six parkinson's disease patients with bilateral subthalamic stimulation. Gait Posture **35**, 452–457 (2012)

26. Little, M.A., McSharry, P., Hunter, E.J., Spielman, J., Ramig, L.O.: Suitability of dysphonia measurements for telemonitoring of parkinsons disease. IEEE Trans. Biomed. Eng. **56**, 1015–1022 (2009)

27. Das, R.: A comparison of multiple classification methods for diagnosis of parkinson disease. Expert Syst. Appl. **37**, 1568–1572 (2010)

28. Eskidere, O., Ertaç, F., Hanilçi, C.: A comparison of regression methods for remote tracking of parkinsons disease progression. Expert Syst. Appl. **39**, 5523–5528 (2012)

29. Chen, H.L., Huang, C.C., Yu, X.G., Xu, X., Sun, X., Wang, G., Wang, S.J.: An efficient diagnosis system for detection of parkinsons disease using fuzzy k-nearest neighbor approach. Expert Syst. Appl. **40**, 263–271 (2013)

30. Little, M.A., McSharry, P.E., Roberts, S.J., Costello, D.A.E., Moroz, I.M.: Exploiting nonlinear recurrence and fractal scaling properties for voice disorder detection. BioMed. Eng. OnLine **6**, 23 (2007)

31. Tsanas, A., Little, M., McSharry, P.E., Ramig, L.O.: Accurate telemonitoring of parkinson's disease progression by noninvasive speech tests. IEEE Trans. Biomed. Eng. **57**, 884–893 (2010)

32. Li, D.C., Liu, C.W., Hu, S.C.: A fuzzy-based data transformation for feature extraction to increase classification performance with small medical data sets. Artif. Intell. Med. **52**, 45–52 (2011)

33. Exarchos, T.P., Tzallas, A.T., Baga, D., Chaloglou, D., Fotiadis, D.I., et al.: Using partial decision trees to predict parkinsons symptoms: a new approach for diagnosis and therapy in patients suffering from parkinsons disease. Comput. Biol. Med. **42**, 195204 (2012b)

34. Sculley, D., Holt, G., Golovin, D., Davydov, E., Phillips, T., Ebner, D., Chaudhary, V., Young, M.: Machine learning: the high interest credit card of technical debt. In: SE4ML: Software Engineering for Machine Learning (NIPS 2014 Workshop) (2014)

35. Holzinger, A.: Interactive machine learning for health informatics: when do we need the human-in-the-loop? Brain Inf. (BRIN) **3**, 119–131 (2016)

36. Hund, M., Böhm, D., Sturm, W., Sedlmair, M., Schreck, T., Ullrich, T., Keim, D.A., Majnaric, L., Holzinger, A.: Visual analytics for concept exploration in subspaces of patient groups: making sense of complex datasets with the doctor-in-the-loop. Brain Inf. **3**(4), 233–247 (2016)

37. Girardi, D., Küng, J., Kleiser, R., Sonnberger, M., Csillag, D., Trenkler, J., Holzinger, A.: Interactive knowledge discovery with the doctor-in-the-loop: a practical example of cerebral aneurysms research. Brain Inf. **3**(3), 133–143 (2016)

38. Yimam, S.M., Biemann, C., Majnaric, L., Sabanovic, S., Holzinger, A.: An adaptive annotation approach for biomedical entity and relation recognition. Brain Inf. **3**, 1–12 (2016)

39. Holzinger, A., Plass, M., Holzinger, K., Crişan, G.C., Pintea, C.-M., Palade, V.: Towards interactive machine learning (iML): applying ant colony algorithms to solve the traveling salesman problem with the human-in-the-loop approach. In: Buccafurri, F., Holzinger, A., Kieseberg, P., Tjoa, A.M., Weippl, E. (eds.) CD-ARES 2016. LNCS, vol. 9817, pp. 81–95. Springer, Heidelberg (2016). doi:10.1007/978-3-319-45507-5_6

40. Sun, Y., Han, Y.: Mining Heterogeneous Information Networks: Principles and Methodologies. Synthesis Lectures on Data Mining and Knowledge Discovery. Morgan & Claypool Publishers, San Francisco (2012)

41. Rice, J.R.: The algorithm selection problem. Adv. Comput. **15**, 65–117 (1975)

42. Lemke, C., Budka, M., Gabrys, B.: Metalearning: a survey of trends and technologies. Artif. Intell. Rev. **44**, 117–130 (2015)

43. Burke, E., Kendall, G., Newall, J., Hart, E., Ross, P., Schulenburg, S.: Hyperheuristics: an emerging direction in modern search technology. International Series in Operations Research and Management Science, pp. 457–474 (2003)

44. Burke, E.K., Gendreau, M., Hyde, M., Kendall, G., Ochoa, G., Özcan, E., Qu, R.: Hyper-heuristics: a survey of the state of the art. J. Oper. Res. Soc. **64**, 1695–1724 (2013)

45. Malle, B., Kieseberg, P., Weippl, E., Holzinger, A.: The right to be forgotten: towards machine learning on perturbed knowledge bases. In: Buccafurri, F., Holzinger, A., Kieseberg, P., Tjoa, A.M., Weippl, E. (eds.) CD-ARES 2016. LNCS, vol. 9817, pp. 251–266. Springer, Heidelberg (2016). doi:10.1007/978-3-319-45507-5_17

Challenges of Medical Text and Image Processing: Machine Learning Approaches

Ernestina Menasalvas[✉] and Consuelo Gonzalo-Martin

Center of Biomedical Technology, Universidad Politecnica de Madrid, Madrid, Spain
{consuelo.gonzalo,ernestina.menasalvas}@upm.es

Abstract. The generalized adoption of Electronic Medical Records (EMR) together with the need to give the patient the appropriate treatment at the appropriate moment at the appropriate cost is demanding solutions to analyze the information on the EMR automatically. However most of the information on the EMR is non-structured: texts and images. Extracting knowledge from this data requires methods for structuring this information. Despite the efforts made in Natural Language Processing (NLP) even in the biomedical domain and in image processing, medical big data has still to undertake several challenges. The ungrammatical structure of clinical notes, abbreviations used and evolving terms have to be tackled in any Name Entity Recognition process. Moreover abbreviations, acronyms and terms are very much dependant on the language and the specific service. On the other hand, in the area of medical images, one of the main challenges is the development of new algorithms and methodologies that can help the physician take full advantage of the information contained in all these images. However, the large number of imaging modalities used today for diagnosis hinders the availability of general procedures as machine learning is, once again, a good approach for addressing this challenge. In this chapter, which concentrates on the problem of name entity recognition, we review previous approaches and look at future works. We also review the machine leaning approaches for image segmentation and annotation.

Keywords: Natural language processing · Electronic medical record (EMR) · Medical image processing · Name entity recognition · Image annotation · Image segmentation

1 Introduction

In addition to the enormous use that medical data has in the diagnosis and treatment of individual patients, the great value of these data is provided by the possibility of extracting knowledge from a large number of patient medical records. The wisdom, knowledge and experience of a large number of physicians are hidden in electronic medical records. Complex computer algorithms oriented to supporting clinical diagnostic methods, description of diseases as well as the dimensioning of the chances of success of a particular treatment

© Springer International Publishing AG 2016
A. Holzinger (Ed.): ML for Health Informatics, LNAI 9605, pp. 221–242, 2016.
DOI: 10.1007/978-3-319-50478-0_11

will make it possible to go from clinical judgement to evidence-based medicine. Electronic Medical Records (EMR) (also called Electronic Health Records (EHR)) are one of the main sources of information as they contain the medical history of the patient, diagnoses, medications, treatment plans, immunization dates, allergies, images (radiology, etc., and laboratory and test results. Most of the information contained in the EMR is consequently non-structured (natural text and images). Understanding this information requires methods for structuring this information for example by labelling or annotating text and images respectively. However it is still a daunting task as most of the existing methods for other domains do not perform well on medical images and clinical notes. Once the information is structured, the challenge lies in mining the structured information. Clinical notes are frequently not grammatically correct, they include abbreviations and acronyms that are often not standard and the medical terms contained evolve almost continuously. Name Entity Recognition (NER) is a paramount step in the natural language process in which words or tokens representing a particular entity are found. NER encompasses analyzing terms that refer to treatments, diseases or body parts, amongst others, as well as analysing the relationship between these concepts. The use of dictionaries and ontologies such as SNOMED, LOINC, etc., plays an important role in this task. The previous features of text in EMR increase the complexity of NERs for clinical notes that have to deal with the disambiguation of abbreviations and multilingual issues for example. On the other hand, these peculiarities of clinical text makes NER for biomedical domains less precise in clinical notes. Several approaches have been proposed for the task. We will review these approaches in this chapter, in which machine learning is applied and will highlight the open problems and look at future developments. On the other hand, it should be noted that medical imaging currently constitutes one of the main sources of information used by physicians for diagnosis and therapy. As a consequence, medical imaging technologies have evolved rapidly; and a large number of new imaging modalities and methodologies have emerged. Just to mention some of them: positron-emission tomography (PET)/CT, conebeam/multi-slice CT, 3D ultrasound imaging, tomosynthesis, diffusion-weighted magnetic resonance imaging (MRI), electrical impedance tomography or diffuse optical tomography. The analysis and interpretation of this huge volume of data requires the development of new algorithms and methodologies that help the physician take full advantage of the information contained in all these images. Since the extraction of the information from the images depends on many factors, such as: modality, registration conditions, devices, and many others, it is not possible to have general procedures available to locate and identify objects such as anatomical structures or lesions in medical images. Machine learning currently plays an essential role in the analysis of medical images, and it has been used for image segmentation, image registration, image fusion, image annotation and content-based image retrieval. In this chapter we concentrate on the challenges behind medical image segmentation and annotation. We will review the challenges that have to be tackled when annotating medical images and the existing approaches that have been proposed from the machine learning community. We will also analyse these problems and the future outlook.

Consequently, we believe that computer scientists and data scientists will find this chapter especially interesting in identifying the challenges and problems still to be tackled both in the field of NER in clinical notes and medical image annotation and segmentation. On the other hand, we recommend that healthcare professionals also read the chapter so that they may appreciate the value of the data they generate and then look at the existing approaches to extract this value. In a sense, this chapter tries to bridge the gap between data scientists, who will better understand open problems, and healthcare professionals, who will discover the value behind the data they generate and how they can make use of this value as feedback by producing better quality data that will be easier to analyze automatically. By closing the loop between health care practitioners and data scientists, the solutions demanded for a better health care practice will become a reality.

The rest of the chapter has been organized as follows: The beginning of Sect. 2 contains the list of terms and acronyms that are used to understand the chapter fully. Section 3.2 dissects the problem of analyzing natural medical text. We cover the Natural Language Process and we focus the attention on the NER and on the solutions from machine learning to approach this problem. In Sect. 3.3, first we describe the image analysis challenges and then proceed to analyse the efforts made in machine learning towards image processing. Despite these efforts, there is still a long way to go both in image segmentation and annotation as well as NER and consequently in Sect. 4 we highlight the open problems and we end with the future outlook in Sect. 5.

2   Glossary and Key Terms

Active learning techniques aim to select the most effective samples actively to present to the users for feedback, fully using human effort [1].

Cluster analysis divides data into meaningful or useful groups (clusters).

Deep learning is a new area of machine learning, which deals mainly with the optimization of deep neural networks.

Image Annotation is a technique that assigns a set of linguistic terms to images in order to categorize the images conceptually and provide a means for accessing images from databases effectively [2].

Image Mining can be defined as the set of techniques and processes that allow the extraction of knowledge contained in images stored in large databases.

Image Segmentation refers to the partition of an image into a set of homogeneous regions that cover the whole image and in which the regions do not overlap.

Machine Learning can be defined as a set of methods that can automatically detect patterns in data, and then use these patterns to predict future data, or carry out other types of decision making under conditions of uncertainty (such as planning how to collect more data!) [3].

Natural Language Processing (NLP) refers to the Artificial Intelligent method of communicating with intelligent systems using a natural language such as English.

Named Entity Recognition (NER) is the task of identifying elements in text belonging to predefined categories such as the names of persons, organizations, locations, expressions of times, quantities, monetary values, percentages, etc.

Part-Of-Speech Tagger is a piece of software that reads text in a language and assigns parts of speech to each word (and other tokens), such as noun, verb, adjective, etc. [4].

Support Vector Machines is a discriminative classifier formally defined by a separating hyperplane: given labelled training data (supervised learning), the algorithm outputs an optimal hyperplane which categorizes new examples.

3   State-of-the-art

3.1   Machine Learning for Text

Today, a major part of the patient's clinical observations, including radiology reports, operative notes, and discharge summaries are recorded as narrative text, even laboratory and medication records are sometimes only available as natural text notes [5]. After a patient visit, diagnosis codes are assigned to the medical records by trained coders by reviewing all the documents associated with the visit. This is a very complex task for which computational approaches to the code assignment have been proposed in recent years [6]. For example in [7], logistic regression is used to learn a string similarity measure from a dictionary, useful for softstring matching. In fact, the notes are written in the official language of the country so one issue is that of multilingualism. In this chapter however we will concentrate on the English language and the solutions that have been proposed for this language.

Even though NLP techniques can enable the meaning from a natural language input to be derived automatically, the process is not straightforward due to the inherent ambiguity of the language at different levels: (i) lexicographic: the same word can have several meanings, (ii) structural: it is required to disambiguate the semantic dependence of different phrases that lead to the construction of different syntax trees, (iii) detection of the affected subject: especially in healthcare information in which patient information plays a very important role in detecting the subject of a disease, whether it be denied or hypothetical is paramount to understanding clinical notes.

The problem of being able to extract knowledge from texts and querying the system in natural language and even extracting patterns from clinical notes lies in natural language processing which is far beyond that of information retrieval. In fact, in medical texts, the work is even more challenging as the terminology changes, sentences can contain the negation of facts that are discriminated in order to know the factors of a disease, there are numbers that indicate either lab result texts, doses of treatments, and several acronyms can be ambiguous and have to be expanded depending on the context. Consequently, after the process of tokenizing and syntactically analyzing the text there are two important tasks related to entity recognition, that is to say recognizing whether a certain work (or part of a sentence) corresponds to a certain disease, treatment, gene, drug, etc. and the relationships among the entities discovered.

Over recent decades, a lot of effort has been made to apply NLP technologies to clinical texts. As a result of this effort, several systems were developed such as the Linguistic String Project [8] or the Medical Language Extraction and Encoding System (MedLEE) [9]. Recent efforts including cTAKES [10] and HiTEX [11] have also been introduced into the community. One common feature of clinical NLP systems is that they can extract various types of named entities from clinical texts and link them to concepts in the Unified Medical Language System (UMLS).

In this section, first we describe the different stages of the NLP to concentrate on a specific problem that, as we will see, is paramount in the medical domain: the detection of entities. We will first explore the challenges and then the machine learning approaches that have been proposed to resolve them.

The processing of medical texts normally starts with spelling correction, finding dates, doses, disambiguation of acronyms [12] and the expansion of abbreviations [13]. Then the Natural Language Process is applied which is made up of several steps: (i) sentence detector: sentences are found (ii) tokenization: a token is an instance of a sequence of characters, at this stage the sentence is divided into all possible tokens, (iii) part of speech: based on its use and functions, words (tokens) are categorized into several types or parts of speech (in the English grammar 8 major parts of speech are defined: noun, pronoun, verb, adverb, adjective, conjunction, preposition, and interjection); (iv) shallow parsing also called chunking: the process of analyzing a sentence identifying the constituents (noun groups, verb groups, etc.) and (v) entity recognition: recognizing words or phrases as medical terms that represent the domain concepts and understanding the relationships between the identified concepts. The process of determining an appropriate Part-Of-Speech (PoS) tag for each word in a text is called PoS tagging. Each language has its own structure and rules for the construction of sentences. Therefore, a PoS tagger is a language specific tool. A PoS Tagger is a piece of software that reads text in a particular language and assigns parts of speech to each word. A Java implementation of the log-linear part-of-speech taggers is described in [14].

A tagset is a list of predefined PoS tags. The size of the tagset can differ from several types to hundreds of types. The Penn Treebank [MSM93] corpus for English texts uses 48 tags, of which 12 tags are punctuation and currency symbols. Many machine learning methods have also been applied to the problem of PoS tagging. Methods such as SVM, Maximum Entropy classifier, Perceptron, and Nearest-neighbour have all been tried, and most can achieve an accuracy of more than 95%.

In [15] a PoS tagger that achieves more than 97% accuracy in MEDLINE citations is presented. In fact, two studies are presented in [16] and [17] in which it is shown how training a PoS-tagger on a relatively small set of clinical notes improves the performance of the PoStagger trained on Penn Treebank from 90% to 95% in the first case and from 79% to 94% in the second case. PoS taggers are out of the scope of this chapter. For the interested reader, one can find a list of several PoS taggers in [18], as one of the main challenges behind obtaining a good medical PoS tagger is the availability of an annotated medical corpus, such as PoS taggers trained in medical data, reports better results than those being trained on a general purpose corpus. In [19] a comprehensive review of the state-of-art and open problems in biomedical text mining is presented.

3.2 Name Entity Recognition

Named Entity Recognition (NER), as has been seen, labels sequences of words in a text which are the names of things. Typical examples include person, locations and company names. For the medical domain, the entities to be identified are diseases, genes, drugs, or protein names amongst others. The problem of finding entities requires the extraction of the features of the words that can help to identify them later and which sometimes requires dictionaries, as we shall see.

NER in medicine is crucial to understanding any clinical note, be it a radiological report, a discharge summary or whatever type of clinical text, as it helps to identify terms that make reference to names of diseases, treatments, doses, etc., and make it possible to find associations among them. Biomedical names are very complex; they include acronyms, and morphological, derivational and orthographic variants. These variants of the same term have to be clearly identified in a non-ambiguous way.

In the literature we find references to NER as the task that involves identifying the boundaries of the name in the text while the term Name Entity Classification (NEC) is used for the task of classifying or assigning a semantic class to the entity based on a dictionary or ontology of terms. However, both tasks are often grouped under the name of NER, and this is the term that we will use in this chapter.

Research indicates that even state-of-the-art NER systems developed for one domain do not typically perform well in other domains [20]. In fact, this is one of the challenges to tackle when analysing clinical notes. A great deal of effort has been dedicated to the biomedical domain since 1998, in particular for gene recognition and later in finding out the name of a drug, but as we will see there is a paucity of works in which clinical notes are analyzed.

We will briefly review the efforts of NER in general domains and then we will analyze the efforts in the biomedical field with emphasis on these machine learning approaches.

A classification of NER methods in dictionary and statistical-based methods is in [21]. In statistical based approaches, NER is formalised as a classification task in which an input expression is either classified as an entity or not. As in any supervised problem in the training phase, the parameters of the NER model are learned from the annotated data and then the trained model is used for name entity detection in unseen documents. Supervised learning methods are reported to achieve a performance superior to unsupervised ones (those only based on dictionaries), but previously annotated data are essential for training supervised models [22]. Consequently, the main drawback of supervised systems is the manual effort needed for the creation of labelled training data. Reducing the annotation work for NER can be achieved through a dynamic selection of sentences to be annotated [23] or through active learning [24,25].

A dictionary-based recognizer does not need labelled text as training data. A dictionary is a collection of phrases that describe named entities. The UMLS [26] is a repository of biomedical vocabularies developed by the US National Library of Medicine. The UMLS integrates over 2 million names for some 900 K concepts from more than 60 families of biomedical vocabularies, as well as 12 million relationships among these concepts. Vocabularies integrated in the UMLS Metathesaurus include the NCBI taxonomy, Gene Ontology, the Medical Subject Headings (MeSH), OMIM and the Digital Anatomist Symbolic Knowledge Base. Many NER methods (applied to both the clinical narrative and the biomedical literature texts) use UMLS Meta and tools developed within the UMLS. One of the main drawbacks of a dictionary-based NER is that the quality of the dictionary used can be very much dependant on local terms especially in the case of dealing with clinical notes. In [27] the construction of a resource that provides semantic information on words and phrases to facilitate the processing of medical narrative is presented, concluding that automatic methods can be used to construct a semantic lexicon from existing UMLS sources. The semantic information obtained this way can aid natural language processing programs that analyze medical narrative, provided that lexemes with multiple semantic types are kept to a minimum, however further work is still needed to increase the coverage of the semantic lexicon and to exploit contextual information when selecting semantic senses.

In clinical notes one problem is shared with traditional biomedical systems; local terminology is paramount to mapping concepts. In the biomedical case, as they have been developed independently of each other, they do not have a common structure, nor do they share a common data dictionary or data elements. Consequently, in [28], the authors propose to improve the mapping of the UMLS by using supplementary information based on WordNet, however as shown in the conclusions, synonyms are of almost no use as there are very few of them in WordNet and a relatively low similarity between some definitions has been shown. Despite all these limitations, the method helped to solve mappings that were not solved in UMLS. Consequently, in clinical notes for dictionary-based methods, it would be interesting to have lexicons developed for each service, sector or hospital to improve the efficacy of the NER.

Supervised NER Approaches. Named entity recognition using machine learning models have the main drawback, as has been previously highlighted, that training data (i.e. annotated corpora) have to be available. Methods such as Conditional Random Fields or Support Vector Machines have shown that they can outperform dictionary based NERs in terms of accuracy. However, the dearth of training data (i.e. annotated corpora) makes it difficult for machine learning-based Named Entity Recognizers to be used in building practical information extraction systems.

In [29] one can find a survey covering the results of research into NER from 1991 to 2006. In this paper, the main efforts from the machine learning community are specified. Consequently, the following are reported as supervised methods: Hidden Markov Models (HMM) [30], Decision Trees [31], Maximum Entropy Models (ME) [32], Support Vector Machines (SVM) [33], and Conditional Random Fields (CRF) [34]. In this work, the authors also review the work on semisupervised learning, as obtaining results in some problems that can be compared to those of supervised learning [35].

Finally, in unsupervised methods, they highlight clustering as the most important approach in which, for example, one can try to gather named entities from clustered groups based on the similarity of context. The techniques rely on lexical resources such as WordNet, on lexical patterns and on statistics computed on a large unannotated corpus.

Focusing on the supervised approaches for NER, not specific for the clinical domain the work presented in [34] is the pioneering work in CRF. Lexicon-based features, which are used to build the training set, report 84% for the English language. The main disadvantage of CRFs is the computational cost of training. In [36], one can find a Java implementation of this technique.

The results of the sixteen systems that participated in the CoNLL- 2003 shared task are compared in [37]. They used a wide variety of machine learning techniques (Maximum Entropy Model, Hidden Markov Models, AdaBoost.MH, Conditional Markov Models, Memory-Based Learning, Support Vectors Machines and Conditional Random Fields) as well as system combination. Almost all participants used lexical features as well as part-of-speech tags. Orthographic information, affixes, and chunk information were also incorporated into most systems. The best performance for both languages has been obtained using a combined-learning system that used Maximum Entropy Models, transformation-based learning, Hidden Markov Models as well as robust risk minimization [38]. It is worth mentioning that in this paper, the authors also highlight that in the CoNLL-2002 shared task they found out that the choice of features is at least as important as the choice of the learning approach for a good NER.

The work presented in [38] combines a robust linear classifier, Maximum Entropy, transformation-based learning, and hidden Markov model. The authors report the results using features based on the words with their lemmas, PoS tags, text chunks, prefixes and suffixes, form of the word, gazetteers, proper names, and organizations. When no gazetteer or other additional training resources are used, the combined system attains a 91.6% F-measure performance on the English data. However, when trained on more general data integrating name, location and person gazetteers, the F-measure is reduced by a factor of 15 to

21%. However, these works have not been trained on medical data. Since the late 1990's, there has been a great deal of interest in entity identification in molecular biology, bioinformatics, and natural medical language processing communities. The most common entity of interest in that domain has been names of genes and gene products. There has also been considerable interest in the recognition of chemical entities and drugs in the context of the CHEMDNER competition, with 27 teams participating in this task [39].

Meystre et al. review information extraction from clinical narrative [40]. In this paper it is very interesting to see the difference that the author makes between biomedical data and clinical data. In fact, in this work, biomedical text refers to be the kind of text that appears in books, articles, literature abstracts, posters, and so forth. Clinical texts, on the other hand, are defined as texts written by clinicians in a clinical setting. These texts describe patients, their pathologies, their personal, social, and medical histories, findings made during interviews or procedures, and in general all the information in the patient's records.

In general, clinical notes differ from biomedical texts. Certain features of clinical notes that can make NER trained on biomedical text not work on clinical notes are worth mentioning, such as the number of abbreviations (often ambiguous), acronyms, misspelling errors, numbers with different meanings (doses in treatment, number of lab tests), repetitions due to cutting and pasting from other reports and frequently a lack of grammatical structure. Consequently, we review the efforts we have found in the literature, noting that in these clinical notes, they can be similar to biomedical texts in structure and content, so that in research reports, for example, one could think that existing techniques should behave in a similar way [40].

In particular, a two-phase named entity recognizer for the biomedical domain based on SVMs is described in [41]. The approach consists of two subtasks: a boundary identifier and a semantic classifier of named entities. This separation of the NER task allows the use of the appropriate SVM classifier and the relevant features for each subtask, resulting in a reduction in computational complexity and an improvement in performance. A hierarchical classification method is used for a semantic classification that used 22 semantic classes that are based on the GENIA ontology [42].

As has already been mentioned, reducing the annotation effort for NER can be achieved through the dynamic selection of sentences to be annotated [23] or active learning [25]. These methods could be of value for the annotation of clinical notes because the existing collections of annotated clinical notes are significantly smaller than those in medical literature (most dataset owners report gold standards of around 160 notes [43, 44]. The F-scores achieved for a statistical NER in these collections range from low 70% [44] to 86% [45].

More recent approaches include the work on novel feature exploration presented in [46] for identifying the entities of the text into 5 types: protein, DNA, RNA, cell-line and cell-type. They apply Semi-CRFs that label a segment not as a single word like in other conditional random field model approaches.

The approach is a two-phase method: (i) term boundary detection and semantic labelling. The new feature sets are reused to improve the performance.

Furthermore, in the biomedical field, the works presented in [47] compare Hidden Markov Model and Conditional Random Fields in the biomedical domain and experiments are conducted on the GENETAG [48] and JNLPBA corpora.

An optimization method for two-phase recognition using Conditional Random Fields is proposed in [49]. First, each named entity boundary is detected to distinguish all real entities and then the semantic class of the entity detected is labelled. The model training process is implemented using MapReduce. The approach tries to improve the recognition performance by reducing the training time which is now crucial due to the volume of biological data.

Another field that has been increasing in interest in recent years in the medical domain is that of recognizing the names of drugs. In this sense, a machine learning-based approach to recognize the names of drugs in biomedical texts is presented in [50], in which experimental results achieve an F-score of 92.54% on the test set of DDIExtraction2011. In this approach, a drug name dictionary is first constructed using DrugBank and PubMed. Then a semi-supervised learning method, feature-coupling generalization, is used to filter this dictionary. Finally, the drug name dictionary is combined with a Conditional Random Field (CRF) model to recognize drug names.

RapTAT, a token-order-specific naïve Bayes-based machine learning system that predicts associations between phrases and concepts, is presented in [51]. The performance was assessed using a reference standard generated from 2,860 VA discharge summaries containing 567,520 phrases that had been mapped to 12,056 distinct clinical terms in SNOMED CT. In this work, the authors demonstrate the feasibility of rapidly and accurately mapping phrases into a wide range of medical concepts based on a token-order-specific naïve Bayes model and machine learning.

In the biomedical domain, for example, several annotated corpora such as GENIA [52], PennBioIE [53], and GENETAG [48] have been created and made publicly available, but the named entity categories annotated in these corpora are tailored to their specific needs and not always sufficient or suitable for text mining tasks that other researchers need to carry out.

Drug NER using limited or no manually annotated data is researched in [23]. An algorithm is proposed for combining methods based on annotations and dictionaries. The drug NER recall is improved using suffix patterns that were calculated by genetic programming. Drug NER performances improved by aggregating heterogeneous drug NER methods (Aggregating drug NER methods, based on gold-standard annotations, dictionary knowledge and patterns). The experiments show that combining heterogeneous models can achieve a similar or comparable classification performance with that of our best performing model trained on gold-standard annotations. In particular, the authors have shown that in the pharmacology domain, static knowledge resources such as dictionaries actually contain more information than is immediately apparent, and therefore can be used in other, non-static contexts. It remains to be seen whether a larger annotated collection of clinical notes will prove to be beneficial for statistical NER.

A novel approach in which interactive machine learning with the human-in-the-loop [54] is applied to solving medical problems is presented in [55]. The novelty behind the approach is that contrary to classic machine learning, it does not operate on predefined training or test sets, and human input to improve the system is supplied iteratively. Then during annotation, a machine learning model is built on previous annotations and used to propose labels for subsequent annotations. The iterative and interactive process is shown to improve the learning process.

Following the interactive machine learning approach, in [56] the authors present an innovative approach in which rather than using established ontologies they allow users to annotate and create their own ontologies of concepts which could later be integrated with known ontologies. The experiments conducted in the paper lead to the understanding that users in the process of learning are a very good asset to improve the overall learning process and can help to outperform methods already used in the literature. Moreover, the human can help to solve computational hard problems, an experimental proof for the human-in-the-loop approach can be found in [57].

3.3   Machine Learning for Medical Image Analysis

The use of modern machine learning techniques in medical imaging has suffered a considerable delay compared to other fields such as business intelligence, detection of e-mail spam, or fraud and credit scoring [58]. However, machine learning currently plays an essential role in the area of medical imaging, and it has been used in many applications, such as: image segmentation [59,60], image registration [61], image fusion [62], image annotation [63] and content-based image retrieval [64] amongst others, and for almost any imaging modality. There are a huge number of conferences, workshops and scientific papers on all these issues [65]. A simple search of the terms "machine learning medical image"? in Google Scholar provides 731,000 results and the similar search "machine learning medical imaging" obtains 215,000 results.

Given the difficulty in addressing the overall problem and taking into account space restrictions, this document will focus on the theme of machine learning for medical image mining, in particular in the processes of segmentation and annotation.

Image mining can be defined as the set of techniques and processes that allow the extraction of knowledge contained in images stored in large databases. Even though standard data mining methods can be used to mine structured information contained in images, image mining is more than just an extension of data mining to the image domain. Different and complex processes should be applied to transform images into some form of quantitative data or, in other words, into structured information, as a first step for the further application of data mining algorithms. Two of the main processes involved in this transformation are the segmentation of the images into homogeneous objects and the annotation of the images with semantic concepts.

Machine Learning for Medical Images Segmentation. The goal of a segmentation process is to separate objects of interest from the background. Since the definition of the background depends on the kinds of objects that we are looking for, a priori knowledge on the objects of interest is generally needed in order to obtain an optimal segmentation. Thus, for example, depending on what we are looking for, vital organs such as: lungs, liver, heart; or for pathological tissues inside one of these organs, different segmentations should be done. Since segmentation is the first step in the chain of processes to be analysed and interpret images, the accuracy of the final results depends strongly on the quality of the segmentation.

Several works can be found in the literature that address the use of machine learning in both challenges: organ identifications and pathological tissues. Thus, [66] presented a review on machine learning techniques for the automatic segmentation of liver images. In this review, they describe three main types of technique: based on Neural Networks, based on Support Vector Machines and based on Clustering. They conclude that even though a comparative evaluation of these methods it is not possible, since different dataset and different error measures are used, it seems that hybrid methods that combines different machine learning techniques provide better results than individual techniques.

In order to avoid the problem of the lack of a uniform dataset to carry out machine learning technique validation, the competitions proposed in recent years with the goal of finding the best segmentation algorithm for particular cases should be mentioned. For that, they provide annotated datasets, real cases for which the ground truth information is known, as is the validation protocol. Thus, it is ensured that the results provided by different algorithms are technically comparable. In 2007, the Retinopathy Online Challenge (ROC) was organized by the University of Iowa [1]. Diabetic retinopathy is the second largest cause of blindness in the US and Europe. Even though there are a lot of studies and researchers, they have not been implanted into clinical practice. The objective of the competition was to make the use of these results in clinical practice possible. The set of data used for the competition consisted of 50 training images with the available reference standard and 50 test images from which the reference standard was withheld by the organizers. The main conclusion was that there is room for improvement. One of the most active organizations in this direction is the Medical Image Computing and Computer Assisted Intervention Society (MICCAI[2]).

Many competitions sponsored by the different workshops organized in the framework of the annual conference of this society, have been held. Just some examples will be mentioned here. One of the main challenges addressed in recent years has been the 3D segmentation as a part of the "3D segmentation in the

---

[1] http://webeye.ophth.uiowa.edu/ROC/.

[2] http://www.miccai.org.

clinic: A grand challenge"? workshops, in which different competitions have been held. In 2007, the proposed challenges were: (i) extraction of the liver from CT and (ii) and extraction of the caudate nucleus from brain MRI data [67]. In 2008, the Coronary Artery Tracking competition was organized. Three different challenges were proposed in this competition: (i) automatic tracking; (ii) tracking with minimal user-interaction and (iii) interactive tracking [68]. One of the most significant challenges, from the point of view of its difficulty, is perhaps the *Multimodal Brain Tumour Image Segmentation* (BRATS). The segmentation of the brain tumours is one of the most difficult tasks in medical image analysis. This is due to their unpredictable appearance and shape, as well as their non-normal behaviour in particular image modalities, requiring the use of different image modalities simultaneously. Even though, this problem has been addressed by researchers for more than 20 years [69,70], there is no consensus as regards the best algorithm that have to be used. The results of the BRATS (2012–2013) are published in [71]. These results were obtained for twenty, state-of-the-art tumour segmentation algorithms applied to a set of 65 multi-contrast MR scans of low-and high-grade glioma patients. All these images were manually annotated by up to four raters. The evaluation was performed automatically by an online tool [72]. All the discussed challenges are already open, since different problems have not been solved yet. A summary of them will be detailed and discussed in the Sect. 4.

Machine Learning for Medical Image Annotation. The objective of imaging annotation is to generate words that describe the content of the image. In fact, the annotation consists of a set of words capable of describing the image. Traditionally imaging annotation is carried out manually by humans. However, this process has some disadvantages such as, the time cost and the subjectivity of the operator. Although the same operator delimits and annotates the same image at different times, the annotation will not necessarily be the same. The alternative approach is automatic or semi-automatic annotation done by machine. In the latter approach, humans participate in some way in the annotation, but in the automatic approach, all work is done by the machine. Two main steps are involved in this approach: feature extraction and final annotation, which is done mainly by a classification process.

In the case of medical image annotation, the contributions of the ImageCLEF association should be mentioned. ImageCLEF aims to provide an evaluation forum for the cross–language annotation and retrieval of images. ImageCLEF was launched in 2003 as part of the Cross Language Evaluation Forum (CLEF). Its goal is to provide support for the evaluation of (i) language-independent methods for the automatic annotation of images with concepts, (ii) multimodal information retrieval methods based on the combination of visual and textual features, and (iii) multilingual image retrieval methods. Since 2005, the medical automatic image annotation task exists in ImageCLEF. It can be highlighted that among the 10 most cited papers under the search "medical image annotation" are the overview of the results of these tasks for the years 2005 [73],

2007 [63], 2008 [74] and 2009 [75]. During the different competitions several key aspects of these problems were addressed. Thus, for example, in 2005, the aim was to explore and promote the use of automatic annotation techniques to allow semantic information to be extracted from little-annotated medical images. The complexity of the tasks has been increased in order to evaluate the performance of state-of-the-art methods for the completely automatic annotation of medical images based on visual properties. The evolution of the tasks and the results during the period 2005–2007 is described in [63], the conclusions being that the application of techniques developed in the machine learning and computer vision domain for object recognition in different areas, not necessarily in medical images and based on local image descriptors and discriminative models, provide reasonable predictions. The quality of content-based image retrieval and image classification by means of overall signatures was the task driven by the ImageCLEF 2008 medical association. An innovation in this competition was the introduction of the hierarchy of reference in the IRMA reference code [76]. A scoring scheme was defined to penalise incorrect classification in early code positions over those in later branches of the code hierarchy, and to penalise false category associations in the assignment of a "unknown" code. In total, 12,076 images were used, and 24 runs of 6 groups were submitted. In 2009, a classification scheme using SVM and local descriptors outperformed the other methods was the winner.

Many other papers have been published in the last 10 years regarding automatic medical image annotation by machine learning such as [77–85] amongst others. In [85] a good summary of some of these methods such as: Multilevel, IRMA code ii, Visual Bag of Words (BOW), Neural Network, Surf detector or Hausdorff distance, can be found. From all of them it can be concluded that even though most of them are classified as an automatic method, they required a previous manual annotation. As has already been mentioned, this task is time consuming and depends greatly on the operator. In addition it has not completely solved the semantic "gap" between the description of the image at low level features and its semantic interpretation at a high level. These issues will be discussed in the Sect. 4.

4   Open Problems

In this paper we have reviewed existing works from the machine learning community for the problem of NER in medical notes and for the segmentation and annotation of medical images. The analysis of the literature highlights the problems that remain open despite the efforts to date.

In particular, the following remains as open lines of research:

- **Creation of annotated corpora**. There is a need have an annotated corpora from clinical notes. This is a crucial step in order to be able to evaluate NER algorithms. One important problem to be tackled here is confidentiality as the data from the clinical notes could contain information that has to be made anonymous prior to making the corpus available for researchers.

- **Multilingualism.** Techniques and approaches that have been analysed are mainly for the English language. The performance of NER is very much dependant on language so it remains an open issue how to deal with information, which to the contrary of biomedical literature does not have to be in English.
- **Abbreviations and acronyms.** It remains as an open problem how to deal with the large evolving amount of ambiguous and local terms. This problem is also related to multilingualism as acronyms and abbreviations differ from one language to another, from a medical service to another and even from one physician to another.
- **Scope of the entity.** It is still an open problem how to deal, for example, with expressions containing numbers such as doses of treatments, or lab results.

On the other hand, in the segmentation and annotation of medical imaging from our perspective, there are two main problems that are worth highlighting and the subject of future research:

- **The availability of annotated open data sets.** Independently the problem considered (segmentation, annotation) the use of machine learning requires the availability of labelled images, from which the machine learning can learn. In order to compare the performance of different machine learning methods to solve a particular problem, the existence of correctly annotated open data sets is essential. It has been mentioned that there have been a significant number of competitions to date trying to resolve this situation; however, two aspects remain yet unsolved: (i) The size of the training data sets. In an appreciable number of the papers reviewed in Sect. 3.3 it has been detected that the number of cases used for the training phase are not large enough to generate accurate and general models that perform adequately. (ii) Specificity of the models. The methods developed work only for specific organs, when not for particular pathologies and sometimes, only for a particular age or sex.
- **Bridging the "semantic gap".** Even though the automatic image annotation with low level features (gray level, texture, shape, etc.) has evolved satisfactorily in recent years, this kind of annotation is not enough to interpret the content of the image, or to search for images in the same way as text documents. For this, the annotation of the images with semantic concepts is required. This gap between the low level features and semantic concepts associated to images is known as the "semantic gap". A lot of knowledge of the specific work domain is required to bridge it.

5 Future Outlook

In this paper we have concentrated on analysing two problems that are currently worrying the scientific community: on the one hand, that related to information extraction from clinical notes and in particular the problem of NER and, on the other hand, the problem of image annotation and segmentation.

As regards NER, since 1998, there has been a great deal of interest in entity identification in the molecular biology, bioinformatics, and medical natural language processing communities. The most common entity of interest in this domain is names of genes and gene products. There has also been considerable interest in the recognition of chemical entities and drugs [39]. However, little effort has been dedicated to analyzing NER for clinical notes and despite the similarities one can find between biomedical and clinical note, research has indicated that NER systems developed for one domain do not typically perform well in other domains [20].

We have also analyzed how clinical texts differ from biomedical text, which implies a special challenge to NLP tasks and in particular to NER. The lack of grammatical structure combined with the number of abbreviations, acronyms, and local dialectal shorthand phrases, misspellings and duplications due to cutting and pasting means that the NER trained on biomedical texts not necessarily perform alike. On the other hand, there is another aspect that makes NER in the medical field challenging that is the constant evolution of terms in the health sector (proteins, genes, diseases, drugs, organs, DNA and RNA are almost constantly evolving).

As we have already mentioned most NER systems relay a set of feature functions that represent a machine-readable characteristic of a word. The choice of features for an NER system is the most important aspect of any NER system. Some feature datasets have already been used in the approaches that have been reviewed in similar general domains. However is has been also shown that the performance depends as much on the algorithm used to train as the decision on the feature set. Finally, we have analyzed the problem of the lack of training data (annotated corpora) that makes the task of learning challenging and evaluation difficult to compare with different corpora containing a small number of annotated clinical notes.

From the discussion of the aforementioned open problems regarding medical imaging, it is obvious that a critical challenge for smart medical image mining is automatic-semantic imaging annotation. On the other hand, the need for a lot of expert knowledge to bridge the "semantic gap"? has also been referred to.

A possible approach to manage these issues is to benefit from user interactions and feedback. Active learning techniques aim to select the most effective samples actively to present to the users for feedback, fully utilizing human effort [1]. This strategy first allows the time spent by manual annotation to be reduced in order to generate models for automatic annotation [86] and moreover, it is possible to include mechanisms in the active learning framework to tackle the bridging of the semantic gap [87].

Recently a new area of machine learning, known as deep learning, has emerged. Deep learning mainly deals with the optimization of deep neural networks or, in other words, neural networks with multiple hidden layers. The number of layers that a neural network has determines its depth. Since in the network, each layer learns patterns from the previous layer, the complexity of the patterns captured by the neurons depends on the depth of the layer in which the neurons are located. In this way, the deep learning architectures learn multiple levels of the representation and abstraction of data and, in particular, images. These ideas are not new. However, their implementation has not been possible in the past for different reasons, mainly the problem of training them. Nevertheless, deep neural networks are now possible because of the development of new techniques to train them efficiently, even though the training data are unlabeled, and the computational power and the huge amounts of data are increasing. Nowadays, researchers are aware of the enormous number of possible applications of this new technique in many different areas and for different kinds of data, such as: image classification [88,89], image segmentation [90], among others. However, to our knowledge, they have not been exploited for medical imaging annotation in order to avoid the lack of training data and to bridge the "semantic gap". From our perspective, we consider that this line of research will be a source of solutions for the problems detected in the application of machine learning to Electronic Health Records.

Having said all this and given the rapid adoption of EMR it is necessary to provide healthcare practitioners with solutions for evidence-based medicine. There is an urgent need for data scientists and physicians to cooperate to accelerate the developments.

We can foresee that the machine learning community has an opportunity to provide solutions that will definitely boost the development of evidence-based medicine solutions. In this sense improving NER algorithms with specific methods for the expansion and disambiguation of abbreviations and numerical expressions will be paramount for all languages. There is also an urgent need to have annotated corpora that can be used by all the community to evaluate algorithms. In this sense, the organization of a conference challenge to produce this annotated corpora and solutions for NER will once again accelerate the development of solutions as a consequence of the joint efforts of physicians and data scientists.

In the same way, there is a need to share images and their reports with confidentiality so the barriers to annotating images can be removed. In this field it is once again remarkable that the development of solutions will only come as a hand-in-hand effort of image processing professionals and physicians.

References

1. Huang, T.S., Dagli, C.K., Rajaram, S., Chang, E.Y., Mandel, M., Poliner, G.E., Ellis, D.P., et al.: Active learning for interactive multimedia retrieval. Proc. IEEE **96**(4), 648–667 (2008)
2. Wei, C.H., Chen, S.Y.: Annotation of medical images. In: Intelligent Multimedia Databases and Information Retrieval: Advancing Applications and Technologies, pp. 74–90 (2012)
3. Murphy, K.P.: Machine Learning: A Probabilistic Perspective. John Wiley & Sons Ltd., Chichester (2012)
4. Toutanova, K., Klein, D., C.M., Singer, Y.: Feature-rich part-of-speech tagging with a cyclic dependency network. In: Proceedings of HLT-NAACL (2003)
5. Holzinger, A., Geierhofer, R., Modritscher, F., Tatzl, R.: Semantic information in medical information systems: utilization of text mining techniques to analyze medical diagnoses. J. Univ. Comput. Sci. **14**(22), 3781–3795 (2008)

6. Kavuluru, R., Rios, A., Lu, Y.: An empirical evaluation of supervised learning approaches in assigning diagnosis codes to electronic medical records. Artif. Intell. Med. **65**(2), 155–166 (2015). Intelligent healthcare informatics in big data era

7. Tsuruoka, Y., McNaught, J., Tsujii, J., Ananiadou, S.: Learning string similarity measures for gene/protein name dictionary look-up using logistic regression. Bioinformatics **23**(20), 2768–2774 (2007)

8. http://www.cs.nyu.edu/cs/projects/lsp/. Accessed 5 Dec 2015

9. http://www.medlingmap.org/taxonomy/term/80. Accesed 5 Dec 2015

10. Savova, G.K., Masanz, J.J., Ogren, P.V., Zheng, J., Sohn, S., Kipper-Schuler, K.C., Chute, C.G.: Mayo clinical text analysis and knowledge extraction system (cTAKES): architecture, component evaluation and applications. J. Am. Med. Inf. Assoc. **17**(5), 507–513 (2010)

11. Goryachev, S., Sordo, M., Zeng, Q.T.: A suite of natural language processing tools developed for the I2B2 project, Boston, Massachusetts, Decision Systems Group. Brigham and Women's Hospital, Harvard Medical School (2006)

12. Joshi, M., Pakhomov, S., Pederson, T., Chute, C.: A comparative study of supervised learning as applied to acronym expansion in clinical reports. In: AMIA Annual Symposium Proceedings, pp. 399–403 (2006)

13. Pakhomov, S., Pedersen, T., Chute, C.G.: Abbreviation and acronym disambiguation in clinical discourse. In: AMIA Annual Symposium Proceedings, pp. 589–593 (2005)

14. Toutanova, K., Manning, C.D.: Enriching the knowledge sources used in a maximum entropy part-of-speech tagger. In: Joint SIGDAT Conference on Empirical Methods in Natural Language Processing and Very Large Corpora (EMNLP/VLC-2000), Hong Kong (2000)

15. Smith, L., Rindflesch, T., Wilbur, W.J.: MedPost: a part-of-speech tagger for bio-Medical text. Bioinformatics (Oxford, England) **20**(14), 2320–2321 (2004)

16. Wermter, J., Hahn, U.: Really, is medical sublanguage that different? Experimental counter-evidence from tagging medical and newspaper corpora. In: 11th World Congress on Medical Informatics (MEDINFO) (2004)

17. Pakhomov, S.V., Coden, A., Chute, C.G.: Developing a corpus of clinical notes manually annotated for part-of-speech. Int. J. Med. Inf. **75**(6), 418–429 (2006)

18. http://www-nlp.stanford.edu/links/statnlp.html. Acessed 5 Dec 2015

19. Holzinger, A., Schantl, J., Schroettner, M., Seifert, C., Verspoor, K.: Biomedical text mining: state-of-the-art, open problems and future challenges. In: Holzinger, A., Jurisica, I. (eds.) Interactive Knowledge Discovery and Data Mining in Biomedical Informatics. LNCS, vol. 8401, pp. 271–300. Springer, Heidelberg (2014)

20. Poibeau, T., Kosseim, L.: Proper name extraction from non-journalistic texts. In: Daelemans, W., Sima'an, K., Veenstra, J., Zavrel, J., (eds.) CLIN, vol. 37 of Language and Computers - Studies in Practical Linguistics, Rodopi, pp. 144–157 (2000)

21. Demner-Fushman, D., Chapman, W.W., McDonald, C.J.: What can natural language processing do for clinical decision support? J. Biomed. Inf. **42**(5), 760–772 (2009)

22. Ananiadou, S., Mcnaught, J.: Text Mining for Biology and Biomedicine. Artech House Inc., Norwood (2005)

23. Korkontzelos, I., Piliouras, D., Dowsey, A.W., Ananiadou, S.: Boosting drug named entity recognition using an aggregate classifier. Artif. Intell. Med. **65**(2), 145–153 (2015). Intelligent healthcare informatics in big data era

24. Dagan, I., Engelson, S.P.: Committee-based sampling for training probabilistic classifiers. In: Proceedings of the Twelfth International Conference on Machine Learning, pp. 150–157. Morgan Kaufmann (1995)

25. Tomanek, K., Wermter, J., Hahn, U.: An approach to text corpus construction which cuts annotation costs and maintains reusability of annotated data. In: Proceedings of EMNLP/CoNLL07, pp. 486–495 (2007)
26. Bodenreider, O.: The unified medical language system (UMLS): integrating biomedical terminology. Nucleic Acids Res. **32**, D267–D270 (2004)
27. Johnson, S.B.: A semantic lexicon for medical language processing. J. Am. Med. Inf. Assoc. **6**(3), 205–218 (1999)
28. Mougin, F., Burgun, A., Bodenreider, O.: Using wordnet to improve the mapping of data elements to UMLS for data sources integration. In: AMIA Annual Symposium Proceedings, vol. 2006, p. 574. American Medical Informatics Association (2006)
29. Nadeau, D., Sekine, S.: A survey of named entity recognition and classification. Lingvisticae Investigationes **30**(1), 3–26 (2007)
30. Bikel, D.M., Miller, S., Schwartz, R., Weischedel, R.: Nymble: a high-performance learning name-finder. In: Proceedings of the Fifth Conference on Applied Natural Language Processing, pp. 194–201. Association for Computational Linguistics (1997)
31. Satoshi Sekine, N.: Description of the Japanese NE system used for MET-2. In: Proceedings of MUC-7, Verginia, USA, pp. 1314–1319 (1998)
32. Borthwick, A., Sterling, J., Agichtein, E., Grishman, R.: NYU: description of the MENE named entity system as used in MUC-7. In: Proceedings of the Seventh Message Understanding Conference (MUC-7). Citeseer (1998)
33. Asahara, M., Matsumoto, Y.: Japanese named entity extraction with redundant morphological analysis. In: Proceedings of the 2003 Conference of the North American Chapter of the Association for Computational Linguistics on Human Language Technology, vol. 1, pp. 8–15. Association for Computational Linguistics (2003)
34. McCallum, A., Li, W.: Early results for named entity recognition with conditional random fields, feature induction and web-enhanced lexicons. In: Proceedings of the Seventh Conference on Natural Language Learning at HLT-NAACL 2003 (CONLL 2003), Stroudsburg, PA, USA, vol. 4, pp. 188–191. Association for Computational Linguistics (2003)
35. Nadeau, D., Turney, P.D., Matwin, S.: Unsupervised named-entity recognition: generating gazetteers and resolving ambiguity. In: Lamontagne, L., Marchand, M. (eds.) AI 2006. LNCS (LNAI), vol. 4013, pp. 266–277. Springer, Heidelberg (2006). doi:10.1007/11766247_23
36. http://nlp.stanford.edu/software/CRF-NER.shtml. Accessed 5 Dec 2015
37. Sang, E.F.T.K., De Meulder, F.: Introduction to the CoNLL-2003 shared task: language-independent named entity recognition. In: Proceedings of the Seventh Conference on Natural Language Learning at HLT-NAACL 2003, vol. 4, pp. 142–147. Association for Computational Linguistics (2003)
38. Florian, R., Ittycheriah, A., Jing, H., Zhang, T.: Named entity recognition through classifier combination. In: Proceedings of CoNLL-2003, pp. 168–171 (2003)
39. Krallinger, M., Leitner, F., Rabal, O., Vazquez, M., Oyarzabal, J., Valencia, A.: Overview of the chemical compound and drug name recognition (CHEMDNER) task. In: BioCreative Challenge Evaluation Workshop, vol. 2, p. 2 (2013)
40. Meystre, S., Savova, G., Kipper-Schuler, K., Hurdle, J.: Extracting information from textual documents in the electronic health record: a review of recent research. Yearb. Med. Inf. **35**, 128–144 (2008)
41. Ananiadou, S., Friedman, C., Tsujii, J.: Introduction: named entity recognition in biomedicine. J. Biomed. Inf. **37**(6), 393–395 (2004)

42. Ohta, T., Tateisi, Y., Kim, J.D.: The GENIA corpus: an annotated research abstract corpus in molecular biology domain. In: Proceedings of the Second International Conference on Human Language Technology Research (HLT 2002), San Francisco, CA, USA, pp. 82–86. Morgan Kaufmann Publishers Inc. (2002)

43. Ogren, P.V., Savova, G.K., Chute, C.G.: Constructing evaluation corpora for automated clinical named entity recognition. In: LREC. European Language Resources Association (2008)

44. Roberts, A., Gaizauskas, R.J., Hepple, M., Demetriou, G., Guo, Y., Roberts, I., Setzer, A.: Building a semantically annotated corpus of clinical texts. J. Biomed. Inf. 42(5), 950–966 (2009)

45. Li, D., Kipper-Schuler, K., Savova, G.: Conditional random fields and support vector machines for disorder named entity recognition in clinical texts. In: Proceedings of the HLT Workshop on Current Trends in Biomedical Natural Language Processing, Ohio, USA (2008)

46. Yang, L., Zhou, Y.: Exploring feature sets for two-phase biomedical named entity recognition using semi-CRFs. Knowl. Inf. Syst. 40(2), 439–453 (2014)

47. Wang, X., Yang, C., Guan, R.: A comparative study for biomedical named entity recognition. Int. J. Mach. Learn. Cybern. 1–10 (2015). Springer

48. Tanabe, L., Xie, N., Thom, L.H., Matten, W., Wilbur, W.J.: GENETAG: a tagged corpus for gene/protein named entity recognition. BMC Bioinf. 6(Suppl 1), 1 (2005)

49. Tang, Z., Jiang, L., Yang, L., Li, K., Li, K.: CRFs based parallel biomedical named entity recognition algorithm employing mapreduce framework. Cluster Comput. 18(2), 493–505 (2015)

50. He, L., Yang, Z., Lin, H., Li, Y.: Drug name recognition in biomedical texts: a machine-learning-based method. Drug Disc. Today 19(5), 610–617 (2014)

51. Gobbel, G.T., Reeves, R., Jayaramaraja, S., Giuse, D., Speroff, T., Brown, S.H., Elkin, P.L., Matheny, M.E.: Development and evaluation of RapTAT: a machine learning system for concept mapping of phrases from medical narratives. J. Biomed. Inf. 48, 54–65 (2014)

52. Kim, J.D., Ohta, T., Tateisi, Y., Ichi Tsujii, J.: GENIA corpus - a semantically annotated corpus for bio-textmining. ISMB (Suppl. Bioinf.) 19, 180–182 (2003)

53. Seth, K., Bies, A., Liberman, M., Mandel, M., Mcdonald, R., Palmer, M., Schein, A.: Integrated annotation for biomedical information extraction. In: Proceedings of the BioLINK 2004 (2004)

54. Holzinger, A.: Interactive machine learning for health informatics: when do we need the human-in-the-loop? Brain Inf. 3(2), 119–131 (2016)

55. Yimam, S.M., Biemann, C., Majnaric, L., Šabanović, Š., Holzinger, A.: An adaptive annotation approach for biomedical entity and relation recognition. Brain Inf. 3(3), 1–12 (2016). Springer

56. Girardi, D., Küng, J., Kleiser, R., Sonnberger, M., Csillag, D., Trenkler, J., Holzinger, A.: Interactive knowledge discovery with the doctor-in-the-loop: a practical example of cerebral aneurysms research. Brain Inf. 3(3), 1–11 (2016). Springer

57. Holzinger, A., Plass, M., Holzinger, K., Crişan, G.C., Pintea, C.-M., Palade, V.: Towards interactive machine learning (iML): applying ant colony algorithms to solve the traveling salesman problem with the human-in-the-loop approach. In: Buccafurri, F., Holzinger, A., Kieseberg, P., Tjoa, A.M., Weippl, E. (eds.) CD-ARES 2016. LNCS, vol. 9817, pp. 81–95. Springer, Heidelberg (2016). doi:10.1007/978-3-319-45507-5_6

58. Wernick, M.N., Yang, Y., Brankov, J.G., Yourganov, G., Strother, S.C.: Machine learning in medical imaging. IEEE Signal Process. Mag. 27(4), 25–38 (2010)

59. Powell, S., Magnotta, V.A., Johnson, H., Jammalamadaka, V.K., Pierson, R., Andreasen, N.C.: Registration and machine learning-based automated segmentation of subcortical and cerebellar brain structures. NeuroImage **39**(1), 238–247 (2008)
60. Ling, H., Zhou, S.K., Zheng, Y., Georgescu, B., Sühling, M., Comaniciu, D.: Hierarchical, learning-based automatic liver segmentation. In: CVPR 2008, pp. 1–8 (2008)
61. Glocker, B., Zikic, D., Haynor, D.R.: Robust registration of longitudinal spine CT. Med. Image Comput. Comput. Assist. Interv. **17**, 251–258 (2014)
62. Wang, Z., Ma, Y.: Medical image fusion using m-PCNN. Inf. Fus. **9**(2), 176–185 (2008)
63. Deselaers, T., Deserno, T.M., Müller, H.: Automatic medical image annotation in ImageCLEF 2007: overview, results, and discussion. Pattern Recogn. Lett. **29**(15), 1988–1995 (2008)
64. Müller, H., Michoux, N., Bandon, D., Geissbuhler, A.: A review of content-based image retrieval systems in medical applications—clinical benefits and future directions. Int. J. Med. Inf. **73**(1), 1–23 (2004)
65. Shen, D., Wu, G., Zhang, D., Suzuki, K., Wang, F., Yan, P.: Machine learning in medical imaging. Comput. Med. Imaging Grap. Official J. Comput. Med. Imaging Soc. **41**, 1–2 (2015)
66. Singh, S.: Review on machine learning techniques for automatic segmentation of liver images. Int. J. Adv. Res. Comput. Sci. Softw. Eng. **3**(4), 666–670 (2013)
67. Van Ginneken, B., Heimann, T., Styner, M.: 3D segmentation in the clinic: a grand challenge. In: 3D Segmentation in the Clinic: A Grand Challenge, pp. 7–15 (2007)
68. Metz, C., Schaap, M., van Walsum, T., van der Giessen, A., Weustink, A., Mollet, N., Krestin, G., Niessen, W.: 3D segmentation in the clinic: a grand challenge II-coronary artery tracking. Insight J. **1**(5), 6 (2008)
69. Angelini, E.D., Clatz, O., Mandonnet, E., Konukoglu, E., Capelle, L., Duffau, H.: Glioma dynamics and computational models: a review of segmentation, registration, and in silico growth algorithms and their clinical applications. Curr. Med. Imaging Rev. **3**, 262–276 (2007)
70. Bauer, S., Wiest, R., Nolte, L.P., Reyes, M.: A survey of MRI- based medical image analysis for brain tumor studies. Phys. Med. Biol. **58**, R97–R129 (2013)
71. Menze, B.H., et al.: The multimodal brain tumor image segmentation benchmark (BRATS). IEEE Trans. Med. Imaging **34**(10), 1993–2024 (2015)
72. Shattuck, D.W., Prasad, G., Mirza, M., Narr, K.L., Toga, A.W.: Online resource for validation of brain segmentation methods. Neuroimage **45**(2), 431–439 (2009)
73. Deselaers, T., Müller, H., Clough, P., Ney, H., Lehmann, T.M.: The CLEF 2005 automatic medical image annotation task. Int. J. Comput. Vis. **74**(1), 51–58 (2007)
74. Peters, C., et al. (eds.): CLEF 2008. LNCS, vol. 5706. Springer, Heidelberg (2009)
75. Peters, C., Caputo, B., Gonzalo, J., Jones, G.J.F., Kalpathy-Cramer, J., Müller, H., Tsikrika, T. (eds.): CLEF 2009. LNCS, vol. 6242. Springer, Heidelberg (2010)
76. Lehmann, T.M., Schubert, H., Keysers, D., Kohnen, M., Wein, B.B.: The IRMA code for unique classification of medical images. In: Medical Imaging 2003, pp. 440–451. International Society for Optics and Photonics (2003)
77. Mueen, A., Zainuddin, R., Baba, M.S.: Automatic multilevel medical image annotation and retrieval. J. Digital Imaging **21**(3), 290–295 (2007)
78. Ko, B.C., Lee, J., Nam, J.Y.: Automatic medical image annotation and keyword-based image retrieval using relevance feedback. J. Digital Imaging **25**(4), 454–465 (2011)

79. Wei, C.H., Chen, S.Y.: Annotation of Medical Images (2012)
80. An, K., Prasad, B.G.: Automated image annotation for semantic indexing and retrieval of medical images. Int. J. Comput. Appl. **55**(3), 26–33 (2012)
81. Burdescu, D.D., Mihai, C.G., Stanescu, L., Brezovan, M.: Automatic image annotation and semantic based image retrieval for medical domain. Neurocomputing **109**, 33–48 (2013)
82. Dumitru, D.B., Stanescu, L., Brezovan, M.: Information extraction from medical images: evaluating a novel automatic image annotation system using semantic-based visual information retrieval (2014)
83. Villena Román, J., González Cristóbal, J.C., Goñi Menoyo, J.M., Martínez Fernández, J.L.: Miracles naive approach to medical images annotation (2005)
84. Setia, L., Teynor, A., Halawani, A., Burkhardt, H.: Grayscale medical image annotation using local relational features. Pattern Recognit. Lett. **29**(15), 2039–2045 (2008)
85. Khademi, S.M., Pakize, S.R., Tanoorje, M.A.: A review of methods for the automatic annotation and retrieval of medical images. Int. J. Adv. Res. Comput. Sci. Softw. Eng. **4**(7), 1–5 (2014)
86. Wang, M., Hua, X.S.: Active learning in multimedia annotation and retrieval: a survey. ACM Trans. Intell. Syst. Technol. **2**(2), 10 (2011)
87. Tang, J., Zha, Z.J., Tao, D., Chua, T.S.: Semantic-gap-oriented active learning for multilabel image annotation. IEEE Trans. Image Process. **21**(4), 2354–2360 (2012)
88. Ciresan, D., Meier, U., Schmidhuber, J.: Multi-column deep neural networks for image classification. In: 2012 IEEE Conference on Computer Vision and Pattern Recognition (CVPR), pp. 3642–3649. IEEE (2012)
89. Krizhevsky, A., Sutskever, I., Hinton, G.E.: Imagenet classification with deep convolutional neural networks. In: Advances in Neural Information Processing Systems, pp. 1097–1105 (2012)
90. Ciresan, D., Giusti, A., Gambardella, L.M., Schmidhuber, J.: Deep neural networks segment neuronal membranes in electron microscopy images. In: Advances in Neural Information Processing Systems, pp. 2843–2851 (2012)

Visual Intelligent Decision Support Systems in the Medical Field: Design and Evaluation

Hela Ltifi[1,2(✉)] and Mounir Ben Ayed[1,3]

[1] REsearch Groups on Intelligent Machines,
National School of Engineers (ENIS),
University of Sfax, BP 1173, 3038 Sfax, Tunisia
{hela.ltifi,mounir.benayed}@ieee.org
[2] Faculty of Sciences and Techniques of Sidi Bouzid,
University of Kairouan, Kairouan, Tunisia
[3] Computer Sciences and Communication Department,
Faculty of Sciences of Sfax, Route Sokra Km 3.5, BP 1171, 3000 Sfax, Tunisia

Abstract. The tendency for visual data mining applications in the medical field is increasing, because it is rich with temporal information, furthermore visual data mining is becoming a necessity for intelligent analysis and graphical interpretation. The use of interactive machine learning allows to improve the quality of medical decision-making processes by effectively integrating and visualizing discovered important patterns and/or rules. This chapter provides a survey of visual intelligent decision support systems in the medical field. First, we highlight the benefits of combining potential computational capabilities of data mining with human judgment of visualization techniques for medical decision-making. Second, we introduce the principal challenges of such decision systems, including the design, development and evaluation. In addition, we study how these methods were applied in the medical domain. Finally, we discuss some open questions and future challenges.

Keywords: Decision support systems · Data mining · Visualization · Medical field

1 Introduction

Medical data and knowledge have become increasingly numerous over last years with advances in imaging, development of biological tests and therapeutic procedures [60, 41] Human memory is limited and physicians have to keep in mind all the medical knowledge they need for their daily practice. Therefore, a patient care following good medical practices requires that physicians must be assisted to perform these complex tasks. This is the purpose of medical Decision Support Systems (DSS) that occupy many researchers in bioinformatics for many recent years [60].

Machine learning techniques have been increasingly integrated in medical DSSs to automatically assist decision-makers in their analytical procedures [41]. The efficient use of these techniques supports evidence-based decision-making and assist in realizing the primary objectives of personalized medicine. Medical DSSs must allow decision-makers

© Springer International Publishing AG 2016
A. Holzinger (Ed.): ML for Health Informatics, LNAI 9605, pp. 243–258, 2016.
DOI: 10.1007/978-3-319-50478-0_12

to make more accurate and effective decisions while minimizing medical errors, improving patient care and reducing costs [25]. From these intelligent techniques, we are particularly interested in those of data mining [19, 24]. Data mining extends the possibilities for decision support by discovering patterns and hidden relationships in data therefore enabling an inductive approach to data analysis [38, 83] including methods from machine learning. A main constituent of iDSS is visualization; it enables humans to perceive, use, and communicate abstract data and amplify cognition. Such visual aids provide *interactive machine learning* [28] for making more precise decisions [41]. Over the last years, several medical DSS based on visualization and data mining have been developed. This chapter reviews and summarizes a number of recent studies for modeling and evaluating such kind of systems.

This chapter is organized as follows: we start by providing some background information about the DSS based on visualization and data mining (Sect. 3). In Sect. 4, we focus on a literature review of the modeling approaches. In Sect. 5 we provide some existing utility and usability evaluation methods. In Sect. 6, we discuss the provided review and we propose future challenges. Finally we conclude in Sect. 7.

2   Glossary and Key Terms

Medical Decision Support System (DSS): is an interactive computerized system that helps decision makers using medical data and models in resolving unstructured and semi-structured clinical problems [69].

Machine Learning: represent a computer science field that develops a set of automated, learnable and improvable algorithms, which can be used for predictions [28]. Data mining can include these algorithms for extracting knowledge.

Visual Data Mining: is a combination of interactive visualization and data mining methods allowing users to explore, gain insight and interact with data for drawing conclusions [37].

Software Engineering (SE): is a discipline that incorporates various methods and models to design, develop and maintain software [79].

Human-Computer Interaction (HCI): is a discipline that includes the design and use of computer technology, focusing particularly on the interfaces between users and computers [68].

Cognitive Modeling: is a discipline that deals with simulating human problem solving and mental task processes in a computerized model for the purposes of comprehension and prediction [67].

Multi-Agent System (MAS): is a computerized system that involves various interacting intelligent agents (autonomous entities) to solve complex problems within a distributed environment [86].

Usability Evaluation: it refers to the system ease of use. It can be evaluated with criteria like learnability, efficiency, memorability, less errors and user satisfaction [37].

Utility Evaluation: it concerns the relevance and efficacy evaluation of the developed system [37].

3   Decision Support in the Medical Field: Current Trends

3.1   The Medical Decision-Making

Decision support systems (DSS) are computerized systems that support business and organizational decision making activities. Medical DSS have an increased attention in many domains of healthcare. They integrate different sources of health information and assert intelligent access to relevant medical knowledge by helping in the process of structuring health decisions. DSS can employ machine-learning methods to automatically solve problems by formal techniques. Information can include clinical knowledge and guidance, intelligently filtered and presented at the appropriate time.

Medical databases are characterized by the complexity and diversity of their data. They incorporate large amount of complex data about patients, hospitals' resources, disease diagnosis, electronic patient records and medical devices, etc. This high amount of data is an important resource to be processed and analyzed for knowledge extraction that enables support for decision-making. Data mining presents a set of tools and techniques that can be applied for discovering hidden patterns [19, 24]. These patterns provide healthcare professionals with an additional source of knowledge for making decisions. Thus, we address in particular the data mining based DSS: *intelligent DSS (iDSS)*. In fact, several literature research efforts tried to develop iDSS by exploiting data mining tools, addressing efficient new classes of decision making discipline [83].

3.2   Intelligent Decision Support Systems

Data mining technology has attracted significant interest during the past decades and was applied in many medical domains providing a large number of medical applications [83]. These applications range from medical diagnosis to quality assurance [25]. Data Mining can be defined as the process that starting from apparently unstructured data tries to extract unknown interesting patterns [19]. During this process, machine learning algorithms are used (cf. Fig. 1). While Data Mining applies machine-learning techniques, it can also drive its advancement.

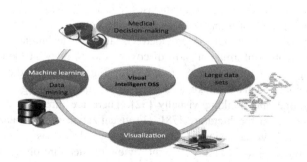

Fig. 1. Involved interdisciplinary fields

Using automated data mining techniques to support pre-established DSS tasks is one implementation of emerging technologies (cf. Fig. 1). An intelligent DSS does not require a priori decision-maker knowledge. It is developed to find new interesting patterns and relationships in a given data set and then applies such discovered knowledge to a new data set [25].

Several examples of medical iDSS in the literature highlight the significant impact of data mining for DSS. Leonard et al. (2002) [47] applied the Bayesian Network to mine biomedical literature for references to genes and proteins and evaluate the relevance of each reference assignment. Walsh et al. (2004) [84] developed a neural network technique to predict the bronchiolitis disposition for children in emergency situations. Gordon et al. (2005) [23] applied logistic regression models to compare hospital profiles based on risk-adjusted mortality of non-cardiac surgery and identification of hospitals with quality problems. Kumar et al. (2009) [43] proposed the integration of different data mining techniques (such as decision tree and association rules) to analyze medical data for decision-making tasks. Kuo et al. (2011) [44] introduced a rule-based iDSS to interpret multiple medical data in health examinations. Ltifi et al. (2012) [50] suggested the application of the Dynamic Bayesian Networks technique for daily calculating Nosocomial Infections probabilities in the Intensive Care Units. Tsolis et al. (2013) [82] introduced a medical iDSS that combines efficient data mining, artificial intelligence and web services to support diagnosis and treatment planning. El-Sappagh et al. (2014) [17] proposed an open distributed medical DSS architecture taking advantage of Electronic Health Record (EHR), data mining techniques, clinical databases and domain expert knowledge bases, to provide decision-making support for healthcare professionals.

iDSS were treated continually in the literature by applying data mining algorithms for decision making tasks. One of the current trends in iDSS is the visualization aiming at exploring and understanding data and discovered knowledge: visual iDSS (viDSS).

3.3   Visual Intelligent Decision Support Systems

Since the human brain can treat a small amount of information, it can recognize a limited number of different visual objects instantly. Consequently, the conversion of numerical data to images is an important visualization process computationally done. For this, information visualization has received increased attention by developing visualization techniques for exploring databases [37, 49, 52, 78].

The emerging results of information visualization community can be an important contribution in iDSS community if provided visualization techniques enables iDSS using the available information to discover more relevant knowledge for decision-making: *visual intelligent DSS* (viDSS) (cf. Fig. 1). This kind of DSS aims at significantly helping decision-makers to treat data and knowledge more rapidly, reducing work time and thinking visually [52]. There are three visual data mining paradigms presented in the literature [78]: (1) visualization of the data, (2) patterns visualization, and (3) visualization of data mining algorithm steps.

In this section, we provide a brief recent review of literature on the viDSS in the medical field. We aim in particular to demonstrate the progressive application of visualization in the medical iDSS. There have been numerous developed systems for visualizing discovered temporal medical patterns to be recognized and exploited by decision makers (PatternFinder [18], OutFlow [87], and EventFlow [58]). Perer et al. (2014) [65] presented a system that integrates data mining and visualization for finding frequent medical patterns to handle different levels of detail, temporal aspect, concurrency, and medical result analysis. Basole et al. (2015) [5] introduced a viDSS that allows decision makers obtaining ideas for care process data, spot trends, visualize patterns and recognize outliers. Ltifi et al. (2015) [52] suggested the integration of temporal visualization techniques in the knowledge discovery stages for the fight against nosocomial infections in Intensive Care Units. Otasek et al. (2014) [64], Müller et al. (2014) [59] and Jeanquartier et al. (2015) [32] underlined the enormous challenge of the visualization of EHR data and Omics data for knowledge discovery, particularly in future and personalized medicine.

As indicated in the literature, the integration of visual data mining in DSS can lead to significantly improve solutions in practical medical applications and enable tackling complex and real-time health care problems. Such improvements highlight the benefits of combining potential computational capabilities of data mining with the human judgment of the visualization techniques for the medical decision-making [28].

4 Design and Development Approaches

viDSS are systems that deal with problems based on automatic analysis (using data mining techniques) combined with visual analytics (using visualization techniques). It becomes difficult to develop such kind of system that fits exactly to the users' (decision-makers) needs. To overcome this difficulty, many research works on the design and development of effective DSS are discussed in literature using: (1) design models, (2) cognitive modeling methods or (3) Multi-agent architectures.

4.1 Design Models

Finding appropriate DSS design and development models is a critical topic, which has kept researchers in the DSS community. Studies on DSS development conducted us to begin by investigating the field of Software Engineering (SE). From this field are derived traditional models, including the waterfall [72], V [54] and Spiral [9] models, and more recent development cycles, including the Y model [3] and the Unified Process (UP) [31]. These models are often oriented towards the technical aspect while non-directed towards the user. Such models most often come with little explanation for users consideration. The design and evaluation of Human-Computer Interaction (HCI) aspects are rarely specific in these models [6]. For this reason, we examine enriched models under the HCI angle. Among them, we can cite the Long and Denley's model [48]; the Star model [26]; the Nabla model [40]; or the U model [1]. These models are difficult to use because they are not sufficiently complete and show insufficiencies relating to the iterative development and the early evaluation.

Furthermore, several approaches specific to DSS are proposed. Examples are: the evolutionary approach [13], the development process [63], the MODESTI model [15] and ADESIAD approach [46]. These approaches present interesting aspects, in particular, the expert consideration, the reusability and the knowledge integration. However, they don't consider the data mining tasks. Consequently, none of these models are adapted to develop such kind of DSS.

For this reason, hybrid models are suggested in literature. Examples are: (1) the Context-Based Approach of [21] that considers the context of the DSS during the development process by combining the benefits-realization approach with the realization feedback process; (2) the U/UP model [6] (cf. Fig. 2) based on two complementary methods: an adapted U model to include the data mining specificities (from the field of the HCI), and the Unified Process (from the field of the SE); and (3) the ExUP [51] that consists of extending the Unified Process activities by integrating the HCI and the data mining aspects.

This brief literature review of the design models is not exhaustive but only provides some of representative models. Currently, it is challenging to develop DSS facing complex, uncertain, visual and real-time environments. So, these design models become insufficient. Design considerations of visualization integration in the data mining phases are suggested in several works such as [52, 28]. In such complex dynamic situations, it seems to be essential to model the cognitive behavior of the decision-maker.

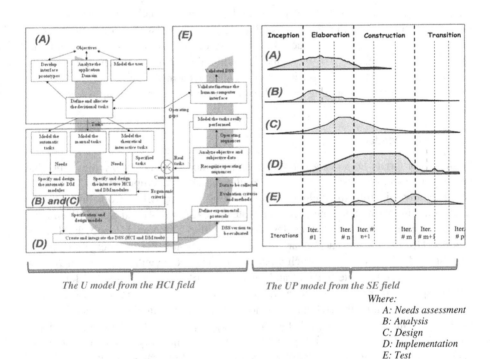

Fig. 2. The U/UP model adapted from [6]

4.2 Cognitive Modeling Approaches

Cognitive modeling of dynamic DSS deals with formulating human problem solving and mental task processes (understanding, intentions, processing and knowledge). It integrates decision-makers as part of the dynamic situation and reacts to the human operator's actions [27]. Several cognitive models are proposed to design and develop DSSs.

Dearden et al. (2000) [14] and Millot (2014) [57] suggested adaptive task allocation to the machine. Jungerman and Fischer (2005) [35] specified a cognitive model to understand the dynamics of cooperative decision-making situations, examining in particular, the acceptance or the reject of an expert advice. Tran (2010) [80], Burnett (2011) [10] and Yu et al. (2013) [88] introduced trust assessment models in open, dynamic, untrusted and uncertain environments.

Simoff et al. (2008) [78] proposed two strategies of evaluating human cognition in visual data mining: (1) the guided cognition to simulate the human cognitive mechanisms to discover the visual forms, interact with them and conduct meaningful interpretations; and (2) the validated cognition to confirm the results of human perception of the visualized forms. Ltifi et al. (2015) [53] introduced a viDSS cognitive model that specifies and applies the cognitive causal links between the data acquisition, understanding the situation, the analysis and the dynamic knowledge integration in the dynamic decision-making process (cf. Fig. 3). Benmohamed et al. (2015) [8] studied the Bloom's cognitive taxonomy for the development of the concentric circles technique to visualize the patterns extracted by a Dynamic Bayesian Networks for the fight against nosocomial infections.

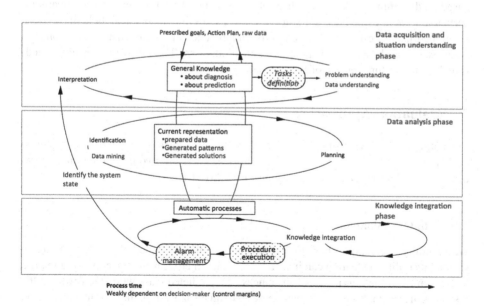

Fig. 3. The viDSS cognitive model adapted from [53]

viDSS cognitive modeling is interesting because it considers the main notions of dynamic situation, cooperative modeling and human cognition supporting in visualization and data mining technologies; Another interesting design domain to investigate is the Multi-Agent Systems.

4.3   Agent-Oriented Modeling Approaches

Intelligent agents are autonomous software or hardware entities that perform a set of tasks on behalf of a user or another program [4]. It applies artificial intelligence techniques such as machine learning, inductive or deductive reasoning.

DSS applied Multi-Agent System (MAS) in order to delegate complex tasks for intelligent agents, which allows: (1) automating the repetitive tasks, (2) extracting and filtering information from complex data and (3) learning and making recommendations to users concerning a particular action course by employing some knowledge of the user's purposes or desires [4]. MAS based DSS have been designed and applied to a great variety of fields for modeling complex reality: e.g. Krzywicki et al. (2014) [42] who studied the applicability of agent-oriented Meta heuristics to DSS and how the MAS can fulfill scalability and performance requirements. Jemal et al. (2015) [33] suggested a MAS-DSS architecture that integrates intelligent agents in the health delivery process of hospital organizations. Ellouzi et al. (2015) [16] proposed a new MAS-based viDSS for the fight against nosocomial infections while Ben Jemmaa et al. (2015) [7] suggested a MAS-based architecture of a Remote Health Care Monitoring system based on the visual data mining.

As presented above, the MAS architecture is used to design and develop DSS even based on data mining and/or visualization. This technology has proven its applicability, particularly in the medical domain. Several viDSS in the medical field have been developed using design models, cognitive approaches or MAS. Their evaluation was addressed to understand their potential and limitations. The following section is dedicated to a literature review of the evaluation approaches.

5   Evaluation Approaches

Evaluation of a viDSS prototype is one of the hottest topics of the field. The objective of this section is *to evaluate in order to improve*. There are two traditional dimensions of evaluation in the HCI field: utility and usability [61, 74, 75].

5.1   Utility Evaluation

viDSS utility evaluation relates to its relevance or efficacy. Since viDSS is a predictive system, its utility evaluation can investigate specific metrics using the confusion matrix. The columns of the matrix list the instances of a predicted class while the rows list the instances of an actual class. This matrix allows detailed analysis of the system's prediction ability by calculating a set of associated performance metrics [70]. These metrics are: sensitivity (true positive rate), specificity (true negative rate), precision (positive predictive value), negative predictive value, false positive rate, false discovery rate, false negative rate, Accuracy and the F1 score (the harmonic mean of precision and sensitivity).

5.2 Usability Evaluation

As viDSSs are interactive systems that include visual interfaces, its usability evaluation must be addressed in particular to the generated visualization. Numerous alternatives to assess visualization tools exist in the literature [30]. We present in Table 1 some selected evaluation approaches discussed in the literature.

Table 1. Usability evaluation methods

Method	Principle
Usability Testing	Includes typical methods imported from Human-Computer Interaction such as observations and questionnaires. It consists in assessing visualizations usability by interpreting and comparing results against a predefined usability specification [26]
Controlled experiments	Controlled experiments [12] have been used in many studies to evaluate visualizations. It consists in applying: (1) independant variables to control the tool's tasks, data, and participant classes and (2) dependent variables to measure accuracy (such as precision, error rates, etc.) and efficiency (calculating time to achieve predefined tasks). Controlled experiments allowed effectiveness comparison of visualisation tools in numerous studies [29, 39])
Heuristic evaluation (analytic evaluation)	Analytical evaluation of the interfaces by experts through heuristics [61]. It examines the effects of visualization techniques usage. Examples of used metrics in the literature are: expressiveness and effectiveness criteria [55], design guidelines [76], visual properties, effectiveness [11], representation and interaction criteria [20], evaluation cognitive models [34] and preattentive processing and perceptual independence [85]
Case Studies in realistic settings	To evaluate the impact of visualization tools on real users' practices, specific case studies have been discussed. Examples of such studies are: the workplace study in Gonzales et al. (2003) [22], the field study in Rieman (1996) [71] and the case study in Shneiderman et al. (2006) [77]
Focus groups	Collecting qualitative data from users using specific interviews. Focus group interviews include (1) open-ended questions aiming at exploring user attitudes and beliefs, and (2) cognitive questions aiming at exploring visualization tools cognitive tasks [56]
Insight based evaluation	An evaluation method based on the characteristics of data insight and allowing identifying and quantifying it in the user tests [73, 62]
Inspection based evaluation	It consists in using critical inspection as a form of evaluating visualization tools [45]. It can be done: (1) by the tools authors themselves, (2) by external experts [81], or also (3) by visual experts such as graphic designers, illustrators and artists [36, 2]

In this chapter, we tried to provide a survey on the design and evaluation methods that can be applied in the context of viDSS. The following section discusses the presented brief review and presents future challenges.

6 Discussion and Open Questions

6.1 On ViDSS Design and Development

The structure of today's DSS environment becomes very complex due to the data mining and visualization technology integration. In this context, DSS development process is not simple and needs an adequate design method able to manage different tools to achieve decision-maker's requirements. In Table 2, we provide some conclusions on the presented design approaches (cf. Sect. 3).

Table 2. Conclusions on the design methods

Approaches	Conclusions
Software Engineering models	- The way of designing viDSS is different from that of a classic information system - viDSS cannot be developed using the classical methods of software engineering
HCI models	- User-centred design models are applicable for interactive systems - These methods are insufficient for DSS because the conditions that decision-makers faces are continually changing and the decision problems are unstructured
Hybrid approaches	- Specific models for DSS (where some of them integrate the data mining tasks) - As far as we know, visualization design is absent in such approaches
Cognitive approaches	Several interesting cognitive models are proposed taking into account: decision-makers behaviour, dynamic situations, data mining and visualization tasks and processes
MAS architexture	Intelligent architecture are suitable for designing complex viDSS in by assigning agents to data mining and visualization tasks

Making adaptations to hybrid approaches, cognitive models and/or MAS architecture are promising for the viDSS design and development. It is a major future challenge that can improve the quality of viDSS tools, especially for the medical decision-makers where decisions are critical and based on temporal data. Another future work lies in the visualization process of temporal medical data and its consideration in the viDSS development cycle.

6.2 On ViDSS Evaluation

We discuss in this section the presented usability evaluation methods (cf. Table 1). Concerning usability testing and controlled experiments, North (2005) [62] supposed that these methods limit the user's thinking and performance, which is inappropriate as the evaluation aims at informing the development of a visualization tool. Analytic evaluation is more difficult to use since it implicates a list of heuristics and cannot identify any unexpected problems [56]. Focus groups and case studies in realistic settings allow uncovering these problems [56]. Unfortunately, they consume time to conduct evaluation and results could not be generalized [66]. Insight and inspection based evaluations are more novel and interesting, but based just on user tasks and data characteristics which is insufficient to judge the visualizations usability for intelligent decision-making tasks. To better measure the usefulness of visualizations in intelligent DSS, we need a new evaluation approach that focuses on the visualizations ability to generate knowledge and allows the intelligent analysis of the evaluation results. In this context, we plan to propose a new evaluation methodology consisting of two main steps: (1) a questionnaire including relevant metrics in relation to the visual analytics tasks of the viDSS, and (2) a fuzzy logic technique to interpret and analyze questionnaire evaluation results. As an improvement of this work, the evaluation can learn in real-time, based on user environmental feedback and past experience. To do so, it is possible to apply an intelligent technique of machine learning such as the neural network method.

7 Conclusion and Future Outlook

Medical decision support systems have employed visualization and data mining techniques to assist physicians in making more accurate decisions within a reasonable time period. Such DSS (named visual intelligent DSS) requires adequate design and evaluation methods. In this chapter, we provided first a brief literature review of the existing viDSS tools in the medical field in order to underline the benefits of combining the potential computational capabilities of the data mining with the human judgment of the visualization techniques for the medical decision-making.

As DSS based on visualization and data mining is a complex system, its design and evaluation must be able to manage these different technologies to achieve decision-maker's requirements. For this reason, we have provided a literature review on the design models (from SE, HCI, DSS, cognitive modeling and MAS fields) and the visualization evaluation methods (to evaluate the viDSS interfaces characterized by their visual aspect). This review allowed us to discuss these models and methods and provide possible future challenges on viDSS design, development and evaluation.

In addition, another major future research area in medical viDSS includes big data. To face such high levels of data volume, characterized by its variety and variability, traditional analytic techniques may easily fall short of storing, analyzing and processing these for decision-making. Key success factors of managing big data and exploiting them for medical decision making include the improvement of data mining algorithms efficiency, the improvement of speed and accuracy of decision-making, the ability to predict and a better understanding of physicians' needs. Turning big data into biomedical field will therefore become one of the major challenges in the viDSS discipline by looking for novel and innovative methodologies, theories, techniques and systems.

Another important future outlook concerns the integration of visual data mining technology in the Remote Healthcare Monitoring Systems (RHMS), which are currently in the front of several bioinformatics research works. These systems aim to monitor elderly and dependent people in their own homes. Data mining integration allows analyzing the real-time data collected from numerous ambient captors for detecting risk situations and generating appropriate decisions to the remote monitoring center. Such analysis can be improved using visualization techniques.

Acknowledgements. The authors would like to acknowledge the financial support for this research by grants from the ARUB program under the jurisdiction of the General Direction of Scientific Research (DGRST) (Tunisia).

References

1. Abed, M., Bernard, J.M., Angué, J.C.: Task analysis and modeling by using SADT and Petri Networks. In: Proceedings Tenth European Annual Conference on Human Decision Making and Manual Control, Liege, Belgium (1991)
2. Acevedo, D., Jackson, C.D., Drury, F., Laidlaw, D.H.: Using visual design experts in critique-based evaluation of 2D vector visualization methods. IEEE Trans. Visual Comput. Graphics **14**(4), 877–884 (2008)
3. André, J.: Moving From Merise to Schlaer and Mellor, 3rd edn. SIG-Publication, New York (1994)
4. Lee, J., Barley, M. (eds.): PRIMA 2003. LNCS (LNAI), vol. 2891. Springer, Heidelberg (2003). doi:10.1007/b94219
5. Basole, R.C., Braunstein, M.L., Kumar, V., Park, H., Kahng, M., Chau, D.H., et al.: Understanding variations in pediatric asthma care processes in the emergency department using visual analytics. J. Am. Med. Inform. Assoc. **22**(2), 318–323 (2015)
6. Ayed, M.B., Ltifi, H., Kolski, C., Alimi, M.A.: A user-centered approach for the design and implementation of KDD-based DSS: a case study in the healthcare domain. Decis. Support Syst. **50**(1), 64–78 (2010)
7. Ben Jemmaa, A., Ltifi, H., Ayed, M.B.: Multi-agent architecture for visual intelligent remote healthcare monitoring system. In: The 15th International Conference on Hybrid Intelligent Systems (HIS 2015) in Seoul, South Korea, pp. 211–221 (2015)
8. Benmohamed, E., Ltifi, H., Ayed, M.B.: Using Bloom's taxonomy to enhance interactive concentric circles representation. In: The 12th ACS/IEEE International Conference on Computer Systems and Applications, Marrakech, Moroco (2015)
9. Boehm, B.: A spiral model of software development and enhancement. Computer **21**, 61–72 (1988)
10. Burnett, C.: Trust assessment and decision-making in dynamic multi-agent systems, Ph.D. Dissertation, Department of Computing Science, University of Aberdeen (2011)
11. Cleveland, W.S.: The Elements of Graphing Data. Hobart Press, Summit (1994)
12. Chen, C., Czerwinski, M.: Empirical evaluation of information visualizations: an introduction. Int. J. Hum.-Comp. Studies **53**, 631–635 (2000)
13. Courbon, J.C., Grageof, J., Tomasi, J.: L'approche évolutive. Informatique et Gestion **21**, 29–34 (1981)
14. Dearden, A., Harrison, M., Wright, P.: Allocation of function: scenarios, context and the economics of effort. Int. J. Hum.-Comp. Studies **52**, 289–318 (2000)

15. Duribreux-Cocquebert, M.: MODESTI: vers une méthodologie interactive de développe-ment de Systèmes à Base de Connaissances, Ph.D. Thesis, University of Valenciennes, France (1995)
16. Ellouzi, H., Ltifi, H., Ayed, M.B.: New Multi-agent architecture of visual intelligent decision support systems: application in the medical field. In: The 12th ACS/IEEE International Conference on Computer Systems and Applications, Morocco (2015)
17. El-Sappagh, S.H., El-Masri, S.: A distributed clinical decision support system architecture. J. King Saud Univ. Comput. Inf. Sci. **26**(1), 69–78 (2014)
18. Fails, J., Karlson, A., Shahamat, L., Shneiderman, B.: A visual interface for multivariate temporal data: finding patterns of events across multiple histories. In: IEEE Symposium on Visual Analytics Science and Technology, pp. 167–174 (2006)
19. Fayyad, U.M., Piatetsky-Shapiro, G., Smyth, P.: Knowledge discovery and data mining: towards a unifying framework. In: Proceedings of the 2nd International Conference on Knowledge Discovery and Data Mining, pp. 82–88. AAAI Press, Portland, August 1996
20. Freitas, C., Luzzardi, P., Cava, R., Pimenta, M., Winckler, A., Nedel, L.: Evaluating usability of information visualization techniques. In: Proceeding Advanced Visual Interfaces (AVI 2002), pp. 373–374 (2002)
21. Gachet, A., Sprague, R.: A context-based approach to the development of decision support systems. Encycl. Decis. Making Decis. Support Technol. **2**, 93–101 (2008)
22. Gonzales, V., Kobsa, A.: A workplace study of the adoption of information visualization systems. In: Proceeding I-KNOW 2003, Third International Conference Knowledge Management, pp. 92–102 (2003)
23. Gordon, H.S., Johnson, M.L., Wray, N.P., et al.: Mortality after noncardiac surgery: prediction from administrative versus clinical data. Med. Care **43**, 159–167 (2005)
24. Han, J., Kamber, M.: Data Mining: Concepts and Techniques, 2nd edn. Morgan Kaufman, Los Altos (2006)
25. Hardin, J.M., Chhieng, D.C.: Data mining and clinical decision support systems. In: Berner, E.S. (ed.) Clinical Decision Support Systems Theory and Practice. Health Informatics, pp. 44–63. Springer, New York (2007)
26. Hartson, H., Hix, D.: Developing User Interfaces: Ensuring Usability through Product and Process. Wiley, New York (1993)
27. Hoc, J.M., Amalberti, R.: Diagnosis: Some theoretical questions raised by applied research. Current Psychol. Cogn. **14**(1), 73–101 (1995)
28. Holzinger, A.: Interactive machine learning for health informatics: when do we need the human-in-the-loop? Brain Informatics, pp 1–13 (2016)
29. Irani, P., Ware, C.: Diagramming information structures using 3D perceptual primitives. ACM Trans. Comput.-Hum. Interact. **10**(1), 1–19 (2003)
30. Isenberg, T., Isenberg, P., Chen, J., Sedlmair, M., Möller, T.: A systematic review on the practice of evaluating visualization. IEEE Trans. Visual Comput. Graph. **19**(12), 2818–2827 (2013)
31. Jacobson, I., Booch, G., Rumbaugh, J.: The Unified Software Development Process. Addison Wesley Longman, Boston (1999)
32. Jeanquartier, F., Jean-Quartier, C., Holzinger, A.: Integrated web visualizations for protein-protein interaction databases. BMC Bioinformatics **16**(1), 195 (2015)
33. Jemal, H., Kechaou, Z., Ayed, M.B., Alimi, A.M.: A multi agent system for hospital organization. Int. J. Mach. Learn. Comput. **5**(1), 51–56 (2015)
34. Juarez, O.: CAEVA: cognitive architecture to evaluate visualization applications. In: Proceeding International Conference Information Visualization (IV 2003), pp. 589–595 (2003)

35. Jungermann, H., Fischer, K.: Using expertise and experience for giving and taking advice. In: Betsch, T., Haberstroh, S. (eds.) The Routines and Decision Making. Lawrence Erlbaum, Mahwah (2005)

36. Keefe, D.F., Karelitz, D.B., Vote, E.L., Laidlaw, D.H.: Artistic collaboration in designing VR visualizations. IEEE Comput. Graph. Appl. 25(2), 18–23 (2005)

37. Keim, D.A.: Information visualization and visual data mining. IEEE Trans. Visual Comput. Graph. 8(1), 1–8 (2002)

38. Khademolqorani, S., Hamadani, A.Z.: An adjusted decision support system through data mining and multiple criteria decision-making. In: Social and Behavioral Sciences, vol. 73, pp. 388–395 (2013)

39. Kobsa, A.: An empirical comparison of three commercial information visualization systems. In: Proceeding IEEE InfoVis, pp. 123–130 (2001)

40. Kolski, C.: A call for answers around the proposition of an HCI-enriched model. ACM SIGSOFT Softw. Eng. Notes 3, 93–96 (1998)

41. Kountchev, R., Iantovics, B. (eds.): Advances in Intelligent Analysis of Medical Data and Decision Support Systems. Studies in Computational Intelligence, vol. 473. Springer, Heidelberg (2013)

42. Krzywicki, D., Faber, L., Byrski, A., Kisiel-Dorohinicki, M.: Computing agents for decision support systems. Future Gener. Comput. Syst. 37, 390–400 (2014)

43. Kumar, A., Gosain, A.: Analysis of health care data using different data mining techniques. in: International Conference on Intelligent Agent & Multi-Agent Systems (IAMA), Chennai, pp. 1–6 (2009)

44. Kuo, K.-L., Fuh, C.-S.: A rule-based clinical decision model to support interpretation of multiple data in health examinations. J. Med. Syst. 35(6), 1359–1373 (2011)

45. Kosara, R.: Visualization criticism – the missing link between information visualization and art. In: Proceeding Information Visualization, pp. 631–636. IEEE Computer Society, Los Alamitos (2007)

46. Lepreux, S.: Approche de Développement centré décideur et à l'aide de patrons de Systèmes Interactifs d'Aide à la Décision, PhD Thesis, Valenciennes, France (2005)

47. Leonard, J.E., Colombe, J.B., Levy, J.L.: Finding relevant references to genes and proteins in Medline using a Bayesian approach. Bioinformatics 18, 1515–1522 (2002)

48. Long, J.B., Denley, I.: Evaluation for practice: tutorial. In: Ergonomics Society Annual Conference (1990)

49. Ltifi, H., Ayed, M.B., Lepreux, S., et al.: Survey of information visualization techniques for exploitation in KDD. In: IEEE AICCSA, Rabat, Morocco, pp. 218–225. IEEE Computer Society, New York (2009)

50. Ltifi, H., Trabelsi, G., Ayed, M.B., Alimi, A.M.: Dynamic decision support system based on Bayesian Networks, application to fight against the Nosocomial Infections. Int. J. Adv. Res. Artif. Intell. (IJARAI) 1(1), 22–29 (2012)

51. Ltifi, H., Kolski, C., Ayed, M.B., et al.: Human-centered design approach for developing dynamic decision support system based on knowledge discovery in databases. J. Decis. Syst. 22(2), 69–96 (2013)

52. Ltifi, H., Mohamed, E.B., Ayed, M.B.: Interactive visual KDD based temporal decision support system. Inform. Visual. 14(1), 1–20 (2015)

53. Ltifi, H., Kolski, C., Ayed, M.B.: Combination of cognitive and HCI modeling for the design of KDD-based DSS used in dynamic situations. Decis. Support Syst. 78, 51–64 (2015)

54. McDermid, J., Ripkin, K.: Life Cycle Support in the ADA Environment. Cambridge University Press, Cambridge (1984)

55. Mackinlay, J.D.: Automating the design of graphical presentations of relational information. ACM Trans. Graphics 5, 110–141 (1986)

56. Mazza, R., Berre, A.: Focus group methodology for evaluating information visualization techniques and tools. In: 11th International Conference on Information Visualization, IV 2007, Zurich, pp. 74–80. IEEE (2007)
57. Millot, P.: Cooperative organization for Enhancing Situation Awareness. In: Millot, P. (ed.) Risk Management in Life Critical Systems, pp. 279–300. ISTE-Wiley, London (2014)
58. Monroe, M., Lan, R., del Olmo, J.M., Shneiderman, B., Plaisant, C., Millstein, J.: The challenges of specifying intervals and absences in temporal queries: a graphical language approach. In: Proceedings of the SIGCHI Conference on Human Factors in Computing Systems, CHI 2013, pp. 2349–2358. ACM, New York (2013)
59. Müller, H., Reihs, R., Zatloukal, K., Holzinger, A.: Analysis of biomedical data with multilevel glyphs. BMC Bioinformatics 15(Suppl 6), S5 (2014)
60. Musen, M.A., Shahar, Y., Shortliffe, E.H.: Clinical Decision-Support Systems, Biomedical Informatics. Part of the series Health Informatics, pp. 698–736 (2006)
61. Nielsen, J.: Usability Engineering. Morgan Kaufmann Publishers Inc., San Francisco (1993)
62. North, C.: Toward measuring visualization insight. IEEE Comput. Graphics Appl. 11(4), 443–456 (2005)
63. Nykanen, P.: Decision support system from a health informatics perspective, Ph.D. Thesis, University of Tampere (2000)
64. Otasek, D., Pastrello, C., Holzinger, A., Jurisica, I.: Visual data mining: effective exploration of the biological universe. In: Holzinger, A., Jurisica, I. (eds.) Interactive Knowledge Discovery and Data Mining in Biomedical Informatics: State-of-the-Art and Future Challenges. LNCS, vol. 8401, pp. 19–34. Springer, Heidelberg (2014)
65. Perer, A., Wang, F.: Frequence: interactive mining and visualization of temporal frequent event sequences. In: Proceedings of the 19th International Conference on Intelligent User Interfaces, IUI 2014, pp. 153–162. ACM, New York (2014)
66. Plaisant, C.: The challenge of information visualization evaluation, In: AVI 2004, Proceeding Advanced visual interfaces, pp. 109–116 (2004)
67. Polk, T., Seifert, C.: Cognitive Modeling. Bradford Books series, A Bradford Book, 1292 pages (2002)
68. Posard, M.: Status processes in human-computer interactions: does gender matter? Comput. Hum. Behav. 37(37), 189–195 (2014)
69. Power, D.: Decision Support Systems: Frequently Asked Questions. iUniverse, Inc., 252 pages (2004)
70. Power, D.: Evaluation: from precision, recall and F-measure to ROC, informedness, markedness & correlation. J. Mach. Learn. Technol. 2(1), 37–63 (2011)
71. Rieman, J.: A field study of exploratory learning strategies. ACM Trans. Comput.-Hum. Interact. 3, 189–218 (1996)
72. Royce, W.: Managing the development of large software systems: concepts and techniques. WESCON, Technical Papers (1970)
73. Saraiya, P., North, C., Duca, K.: An insight-based methodology for evaluating bioinformatics visualizations. IEEE Trans. Visual Comput. Graphics 11(4), 443–456 (2005)
74. Sears, A., Jacko, J.A. (eds.): The Human Computer Interaction Handbook: Fundamentals, Evolving Technologies and Emerging Applications, 2nd edn. Lawrence Erlbaum Associates, Mahwah (2008)
75. Shibl, R., Lawley, M., Debuse, J.: Factors influencing decision support system acceptance. Decis. Support Syst. 54(2), 953–961 (2013)
76. Shneiderman, B.: The eyes have it: a task by data type taxonomy. In: Proceeding IEEE Symposium Visual Languages 1996, pp. 336–343 (1996)

77. Shneiderman, B., Plaisant, C.: Strategies for evaluating information visualization tools: multi-dimensional in-depth long-term case studies. In: Proceeding BELIV, pp. 81–87. ACM, New York (2006)
78. Simoff, S.J., Böhlen, M.H., Mazeika, A. (eds.): Visual Data Mining. LNCS, vol. 4404. Springer, Heidelberg (2008). doi:10.1007/978-3-540-71080-6
79. Sommerville, I.: What is Software Engineering? 8th edn, p. 7. Pearson Education, Harlow (2007). ISBN 0-321-31379-8
80. Tran, T.T.: Protecting buying agents in e-marketplaces by direct experience trust modelling. Knowl. Inf. Syst. 22(1), 65–100 (2010)
81. Tory, M., Moller, T.: Evaluating visualizations: do expert reviews work? IEEE Comput. Graphics Appl. 25(5), 8–11 (2005)
82. Tsolis, D., Paschali, K., Tsakona, A., Ioannou, Z.-M., Likothanasis, S., Tsakalidis, A., Alexandrides, T., Tsamandas, A.: Development of a clinical decision support system using AI, medical data mining and web applications. In: Iliadis, L., Papadopoulos, H., Jayne, C. (eds.) EANN 2013. CCIS, vol. 384, pp. 174–184. Springer, Heidelberg (2013). doi:10.1007/978-3-642-41016-1_19
83. Turban, E., Aronson, J.E., Liang, T.P.: Decision Support Systems and Intelligent Sytems, 7th edn. Prentice Hall, Englewood Cliffs (2004)
84. Walsh, P., Cunningham, P., Rothenberg, S.J., O'Doherty, S., Hoey, H., Healy, R.: An artificial neural network ensemble to predict disposition and length of stay in children presenting with bronchiolitis. Eur. J. Emerg. Med. 11, 259–564 (2004)
85. Ware, C.: Information Visualization: Perception for Design. Morgan Kaufmann, San Francisco (2004)
86. Wooldridge, M.: An Introduction to Multi-Agent Systems, p. 366. Wiley (2002)
87. Wongsuphasawat, K., Gotz, D.: Outflow: visualizing patient flow by symptoms and outcome. IEEE, Providence (2011)
88. Yu, H., Shen, Z., Leung, C., Miao, C., Lesser, V.: A survey of multi-agent trust management systems. IEEE Access 1(1), 35–50 (2013)

A Master Pipeline for Discovery and Validation of Biomarkers

Sebastian J. Teran Hidalgo[1], Michael T. Lawson[2], Daniel J. Luckett[2],
Monica Chaudhari[2], Jingxiang Chen[2], Arkopal Choudhury[2],
Arianna Di Florio[3], Xiaotong Jiang[2],
Crystal T. Nguyen[2], and Michael R. Kosorok[2]([✉])

[1] Department of Biostatistics, Yale University, Hew Haven, CT, USA
`sebastian.teranhidalgo@yale.edu`
[2] Department of Biostatistics, University of North Carolina, Chapel Hill, NC, USA
`jgxchen@email.unc.edu`,
{`mtlawson,luckett,mcunc12,arkopal,xiaotong,ctn92`}`@live.unc.edu`,
`kosorok@bios.unc.edu`
[3] Division of Psychological Medicine and Clinical Neurosciences, Cardiff University, Cardiff, Wales, UK
`diflorioa@cardiff.ac.uk`

Abstract. A major challenge in precision medicine is the development of biomarkers which can effectively guide patient treatment in a manner which benefits both the individual and the population. Much of the difficulty is the poor reproducibility of existing approaches as well as the complexity of the problem. Machine learning tools with rigorous statistical inference properties have great potential to move this area forward. In this chapter, we review existing pipelines for biomarker discovery and validation from a statistical perspective and identify a number of key areas where improvements are needed. We then proceed to outline a framework for developing a master pipeline firmly grounded in statistical principles which can yield better reproducibility, leading to improved biomarker development and increasing success in precision medicine.

Keywords: Biomarker discovery · Reproducibility · Data mining · Machine learning

1 Introduction

Biomarkers occupy a position of fundamental importance in biomedical research and clinical practice. They can be employed for a variety of tasks, such as diagnostic tools or surrogate endpoints for clinical outcomes; Table 1 gives several examples of biomarkers and their uses. In this chapter, we will primarily focus on **prognostic biomarkers**, which provide information on the natural history of a disease and help in estimating a patient's overall outcome or prognosis, and **predictive biomarkers**, which provide information on the likelihood that a patient will respond to a therapeutic intervention and help in identifying the

© Springer International Publishing AG 2016
A. Holzinger (Ed.): ML for Health Informatics, LNAI 9605, pp. 259–288, 2016.
DOI: 10.1007/978-3-319-50478-0_13

Table 1. Examples of biomarkers and their significance in medicine

Biomarker	How it is measured	Relevance
Body mass index (BMI)	Person's weight in kilograms divided by the square of height in meters	Associated with a number of health outcomes, including obesity [6] and death [7]
Periodic variation of R-R intervals (heart rate variability)	Calculated from continuous electrocardiogram record	Indicator of the activity of the autonomic nervous system [8], predictor of survival after heart attack [8,9]
Glycosolated hemoglobin (HbA1c)	Assayed from blood samples	Diagnostic marker for diabetes [10]; an indicator of glycemic control in patients with diabetes [11]
KRAS Somatic mutations	Assayed from tumor samples	Associated with treatment response in colorectal cancer [12]
BRCA1 Germline mutations	Assayed from human buccal cells or blood	Associated with the risk of breast and ovarian cancer [13]

most effective course of treatment. Note that some biomarkers, such as estrogen receptor status in breast cancer, can be both prognostic and predictive [1].

The emergence of "-omics" approaches has enabled new biomarkers to step into the limelight, holding promise for precision medicine, an emerging field that builds individual variability in biological and environmental factors into its approach to treating disease [2]. Parallel advances in high-throughput technologies have generated an unprecedented amount of data ("big data"). The sheer scale and variety of information available, along with its structural and functional heterogeneity and often its inconsistencies, have led to the current paradox: biomarker discovery is more possible than it has ever been before, but it is also more problematic and inefficient. Of the hundreds of thousands of disease-associated markers that have been reported, only a small fraction have been validated and proven clinically useful [3–5].

It has become abundantly clear, given the current difficulties, that research practices in biomarker discovery must be firmly grounded in statistical and biomedical practices. In this chapter, we outline a framework for developing a master pipeline for biomarker discovery and validation that is aimed at increasing the reliability and reproducibility of biomarker discovery experiments.

We will first review various approaches to study design, highlighting those that are relevant to biomarker discovery trials. We will then discuss the challenges of ensuring data quality in the world of "big data" and propose strategies for data collection and curation. We will introduce several statistical analysis techniques, devoting special attention to the role of machine learning techniques. We will emphasize the role of traditional statistical considerations, such as power analysis, in biomarker studies, regardless of the specific analysis technique. We will then mention several approaches to the validation and evaluation of biomarkers. We will conclude by discussing the clinical interpretation of biomarkers and the central role it plays, and by providing some directions for future research.

2 Glossary

Accelerated Failure Time (AFT) Model: specifies the regression model $\lambda(t|Z) = e^{-\beta'Z(t)}\lambda_0\left(e^{-\beta'Z(t)}\right)$ for the hazard function.

Biomarkers or *biological markers*: quantifiable, objectively measured and evaluated indicators of physiological and pathogenic processes, responses to interventions, and environmental exposures.

Biclustering: a clustering method which considers groupings of rows (experimental subjects) and columns (covariates) both together and independently.

Classification: a supervised learning method with a binary, ordinal, or multi-category outcome variable. The focus of classification is placing observations into the correct class based on covariates.

Cluster Analysis: aims to group together individuals who are more similar to each other than the individuals assigned to other clusters. Examples include k-means, hierarchical, and spectral clustering.

Cox Proportional Hazard Model: specifies the semiparametric regression model $\lambda(t|Z) = \lambda_0(t)e^{\beta'Z(t)}$ for the hazard function.

Dimension Reduction: reduces the number of covariates and converts data to a lower dimensional space that is easier to analyze. Examples include principal component analysis (PCA), linear discriminant analysis (LDA), and classical multidimensional scaling (MDS).

False Discovery Rate (FDR): The average proportion of false discoveries (V) among all discoveries R, or rejections of the null hypothesis, in a study, i.e. $FDR = E[V/R]$.

Family-wise Error Rate (FWER): The probability that even one false discovery (V) will be made in a study, i.e. $FWER = \Pr(V \geq 1)$.

G-Estimation: a method for estimating causal effects in structural nested models, while accounting for time-varying confounders and mediators.

Least Absolute Shrinkage and Selection Operator (LASSO): an L_1-penalized regression technique for the linear model $Y = X\beta + \epsilon$. The L_1 penalization causes the estimates of coefficients for unimportant covariates to shrink to exactly zero, thereby performing model selection.

Machine Learning Methods: flexible, nonparametric methods derived from the field of computer science, which arose from the study of pattern recognition in artificial intelligence. Machine learning methods are well-suited for prediction in a variety of complex data scenarios, but many do not have well-studied inferential properties.

Negative predictive value (NPV): the probability that a subject is disease negative given that they test negative.

Nonparametric Methods: assume that the data arise from a complicated process whose set of explanatory parameters is not fixed. Offer flexibility at the expense of interpretability and efficiency.

Non-penalized Methods: estimate parameters by directly maximizing a likelihood function.

Outcome Weighted Learning: a machine learning method suited to identifying predictive biomarkers within a randomized trial or observational study for binary treatments with substantial treatment heterogeneity.

Parametric Methods: assume that the data arise from a known probability distribution that is determined by a small, fixed number of parameters. Offer interpretability and efficiency at the expense of strong assumptions.

Penalized Methods: estimate parameters by maximizing a likelihood function that is modified by a penalty term. Penalized methods are used to regularize parameter estimates, which aids in prediction by reducing overfitting.

Positive predictive value (PPV): the probability that a subject is disease positive given that they test positive.

Power: the probability that a null hypothesis that is actually false will correctly be rejected.

Predictive Biomarker: a biomarker that helps in determining which of several possible treatments will be most beneficial to a patient. Causal in nature.

Prognostic Biomarker: a biomarker that helps in ascertaining or predicting disease status. Not causal in nature.

Q-Learning: a regression-based machine learning method that estimates optimal personalized treatment strategies by directly estimating the Q-functions.

Random Forests: nonparametric machine learning tools that combine decision trees, which provide low bias without strong assumptions, bootstrap aggregation, which reduces the variance of the tree-based estimate, and feature randomization, which reduces the correlation between trees for further variance reduction.

Receiver Operating Characteristic (ROC) Curve: a plot of the sensitivity and specificity of a diagnostic test over all possible cutoff values.

Regression: a supervised learning technique that poses a model for the mean of an outcome variable that depends on the covariates of interest and the inherent variability of the sample.

Reproducibility: the ability of a study's results to be corroborated or confirmed by similar experiments in similar settings.

Semiparametric Methods: assume that the data arise from a process containing a parametric piece and a nonparametric piece. Offer a middle ground between the flexibility of nonparametric methods and the efficiency and interpretability of parametric methods.

Sensitivity: the probability of a positive test given that a subject is disease positive; also called the true positive fraction.

Singular Value Decomposition (SVD): the factorization of a data matrix $X = UDV^T = \sum_{k=1}^{r} s_k u_k v_k^T$, where r is the rank of X, U is a matrix of orthonormal left singular vectors, V is a matrix of orthonormal right singular vectors, D is a diagonal matrix with positive singular values on its diagonal. X can be approximated $X \approx X^{(K)} \equiv \sum_{k=1}^{K} u_k s_k v_k^T$ where $X^{(K)}$ is the closest rank-K approximation of X [14].

Specificity: the probability of a negative test given that a subject is disease negative; one minus specificity is also called the false positive fraction.

Supervised Learning: a class of learning methods that explicitly incorporate an outcome variable. Supervised learning methods can be used to predict future values of the outcome, assess the effect of covariates on the outcome, or both.

Support Vector Machine (SVM): a supervised learning method that classifies data points with a binary outcome based on the optimal separating hyperplane.

Unsupervised Learning: a type of machine learning that uses unlabeled data to conduct statistical inference, where the covariates of interest are known but the outcome variables are not given.

3   Biomarker Discovery and Validation Pipeline

3.1   Study Design

While the role a biomarker plays in a study—prognostic or predictive—is important, trouble can arise if investigators focus too much on the details specific to that role and lose sight of the fundamentals of study design. In *Anna Karenina*, Leo Tolstoy wrote that "Happy families are all alike; every unhappy family is unhappy in its own way." A similar statement can be made about biomarker studies. Successful studies will address similar minimal criteria at each phase of development, while unsuccessful studies can fail to do so in any number of unique and creative ways. Study objectives, outcome measures and their reliability, availability of appropriate analysis methods, and the biomarker's clinical context should all play an essential role in determining the study design.

Studies involving prognostic biomarkers tend to focus on the development and evaluation of clinical assays and screening tests for a disease. Pepe et al. (2001) [15] suggest five phases for prognostic biomarker studies:

1. **Phase 1: Pre-clinical Exploratory Studies** Phase 1 studies identify and prioritize potentially useful biomarkers from a large pool of candidates. A biomarker's utility is based on how significantly its levels differ between disease cases and healthy controls, which are often matched to account for patient heterogeneity.
2. **Phase 2: Clinical Assay Development** Phase 2 studies develop reliable clinical assays based on the biomarkers identified in phase 1. Clinical assays employ non-invasively obtained specimens that are simple to collect.
3. **Phase 3: Retrospective Longitudinal Repository Studies** Phase 3 studies assess how well a biomarker can be used for early disease detection by examining whether levels of the biomarker in clinical specimens differ significantly between disease cases and healthy controls during the time period before the cases were diagnosed. Phase 3 studies can be used to define criteria for a screening test, which is evaluated in future phases.
4. **Phase 4: Prospective Screening Studies** Phase 4 prospective studies evaluate the performance and determine the operating characteristics (see Sect. 3.6) of a screening test. Patients are screened with the proposed test, and true disease status is ascertained with a "gold standard" diagnostic test.
5. **Phase 5: Disease Control Studies** Phase 5 confirmatory randomized trials address whether biomarker-based screening reduces the actual burden of disease. There is a distinction between success in phases 4 and 5: a biomarker may screen for disease effectively but not lead to a decrease in mortality due to other factors, such as lack of appropriate treatment.

While we have presented these phases as a straightforward progression, not all prognostic biomarkers will progress linearly through the five phases, and some study designs will combine elements of multiple phases.

Predictive biomarkers are typically incorporated into pivotal phase III trials of experimental treatments. The reason is twofold. First, predictive biomarkers assist in determining which of several treatments is likely to be more effective for a given patient; this information can help clarify the treatment effect that a phase III trial intends to estimate. Second, predictive biomarkers are causal in nature, and the setting of a randomized clinical trial provides the most compelling evidence to support claims of causation. Two simple questions can assist in selecting the correct phase III biomarker design: how many candidate biomarkers are in consideration, and how strong is the evidence that supports them?

Trials that incorporate one biomarker supported by strong evidence often take the form of biomarker-enriched, biomarker-stratified, or biomarker-strategy studies [16,17]. In all three cases, the study population is assayed for the biomarker of interest before randomization. In biomarker-enriched trials, only patients testing positive for the biomarker proceed to randomization; this scheme is particularly appropriate when biological evidence suggests that the test-negative population will not benefit from the treatment, raising concerns of ethics and efficiency [18,19]. In biomarker-strategy trials, patients are randomized into either a biomarker-directed arm, in which their treatment is dictated by the biomarker, or a control arm, where all patients receive control treatment; this scheme may be preferable when the biomarker-directed treatment strategy is complex [16]. In biomarker-stratified trials, patients are split into two groups, test-positive and test-negative, and then randomized normally within these groups; biomarker-stratified designs, when logistically and ethically appropriate, offer a great deal of efficiency [16,17]. These designs can be combined to address complex research questions—for instance, when a complex experimental therapy is enriched by multiple biomarkers at once [17].

Extensions of these methods can accommodate weaker assumptions on the biomarkers of interest by performing inference on biomarker properties in tandem with estimation of treatment effect. Adaptive threshold designs use a single biomarker without a pre-specified test-positive threshold, which reduces reliance on phase II studies to correctly determine the threshold [20]. Adaptive biomarker designs consider a relatively small pool of candidate biomarkers rather than a single biomarker, selecting the most promising biomarker or biomarkers during the course of the trial [18,20].

Even in the most restrictive setting, where investigators have a large pool of candidate biomarkers with little to no prior evidence supporting them, clever study designs enable valid statistical inference. One such design, the adaptive signature design, employs two outcome stages [21]. The first outcome stage tests for treatment efficacy at the α_1 significance level in the overall population of size N; if this stage is successful, the drug is considered generally useful. If the first stage does not find overall efficacy, the second stage uses the first N_1 accrued patients to train a machine learning classifier that divides the final $N_2 = N - N_1$ patients into two groups: those who are likely to benefit from the experimental treatment, E, and those who are not likely to, C. Then treatment efficacy is tested at the α_2 significance level in the promising group E. If efficacy is shown in phase 2, the drug is considered effective for the biomarker-selected group, and the machine learning classifier can be used to predict group status for future patients. Choosing $\alpha_1 + \alpha_2 = \alpha$ controls type I error at the α level; see Sect. 3.4 for more details. Adaptive signature designs were proposed with a simple machine learning classifier that aptly handled a variety of simulation settings [21], but any number of the more sophisticated methods discussed in Sect. 3.3 may prove useful in extending adaptive signature designs.

The incorporation of biomarkers poses its fair share of challenges to common considerations in phase III trials. For one, biomarker-based designs may complicate interim analyses, encouraging flexible stopping rules over rigid ones [16]. For another, biomarkers may define subgroups of scientific interest to test as secondary outcomes, making multiple comparisons adjustments (see Sect. 3.4) especially relevant [18].

In addition, several study designs address the task of discovering predictive biomarkers outside of phase III trials. Sequential multiple assignment randomized trial (SMART) designs offer a framework for applying predictive biomarkers to dynamic treatment regimes, often in phase II trials [22]. Electronic health record data, used in concert with causal inference, could give rise to efficient observational and other non-randomized predictive biomarker studies [3,23].

3.2 Ensuring Data Quality

Unlike in the myth of Athena's birth, which depicts the goddess leaping from Zeus's forehead fully formed and armed for battle, a well-executed study yielding reliable results does not spontaneously arise from a well-designed study. Data management is a crucial step of a successful study—mishandling a study's data threatens the validity of everything that follows.

Often, when errors creep into a dataset, they do so at the phase of data collection. Although human and measurement error will always lie outside an investigator's control, investigators can limit the impact of these factors. A detailed study protocol that lists how data collection should be carried out reduces ambiguity and lessens reliance on subjective judgments. Studies that utilize multiple data collection sites carry an additional burden: measurements must be consistent not only within sites, but across sites. For a much more thorough treatment of the topic, see the Data Acquisition section of the Society for Clinical Data Management's GCDMP 4.0 [24].

Investigators must also pay close attention to how their data are stored and linked. The optimal data management plan will vary from study to study based on numerous factors, including the physical and institutional proximity of collaborators, the volume and frequency of data collected, and the data use guidelines put in place by participating institutions. Extra care must be taken with "big data," which may tax the computing resources available to a research team. What should not vary is the investigators' approach to data management: data management requires a clearly stated plan and thorough documentation of all steps taken throughout the process. A data flow diagram may help clarify the steps of data collection, processing, and storage, and potentially aid in identifying problems [25]. Overall, investigators should balance two guiding principles: ease of access and protection of privacy.

While the first of these principles is intuitively clear, the second deserves some elaboration. In the course of data collection, investigators will have access to sensitive personal information, and investigators have a solemn obligation to protect the privacy of their participants to the greatest extent possible. This obligation may be legal in addition to ethical, thanks to privacy-protecting statutes such as HIPAA [26]. Investigators should familiarize themselves with statutes that apply to their study and make sure their methods of data collection and storage comply with all relevant guidelines.

Investigators should also be wary of losing sight of what their data mean functionally—they should be able to describe the information contained in every column of every dataset. Informative file and variable names can help, but they are not enough. As standard practice, investigators should draw up a data dictionary that explains each dataset and each variable the datasets contain.

3.3 Statistical Methods for Biomarkers

In this section, we provide a brief overview of statistical methods appropriate for the analysis of biomarker data. We pay particular attention to machine learning methods, which offer an attractive combination of flexibility and desirable statistical properties.

While we present a variety of methods for both supervised and unsupervised learning below, we wish to emphasize that the two are rarely as disjoint as they may appear in this section. They are often used in concert: covariates are often pre-processed through an unsupervised method before being employed in a supervised method, for instance. The matter is further complicated by latent supervised learning, which posits intermediate ground between supervised and unsupervised methods based on latent subgroups [27], and semi-supervised learning, which trains a model on both data where the outcome variable is observed and data where it is not [28].

Supervised Methods. The taxonomy of supervised methods is expansive—supervised methods can accommodate data from a truly staggering variety of studies. While the details of a specific biomarker study and data type are invaluable in selecting the correct method, the search for the appropriate method in any study can be aided by two general questions. First, what is the goal of the method? Second, what type of information does the method need to provide? The questions are clearly related, and together they often point directly to a small class of methods. For instance, if the investigators primarily care about prediction of future values of the outcome, and they do not particularly care about interpreting the effect of covariates, a nonparametric machine learning method may prove their best option; but if their primary research question is quantifying the relationship between a biomarker of interest and the outcome, a parametric or semiparametric model will likely serve them better. The spectrum of supervised methods offers a trade-off between flexibility and interpretability, between what Kosorok (2009) [29] calls "the ability to discover and the ability to generalize."

1. **Parametric Methods** Parametric methods assume that the data are generated by a known probability distribution with a small, fixed number of parameters (e.g. the mean and variance of a Gaussian random variable, or the rate of an exponential). The parameters of that distribution provide a concise way to summarize and interpret the data, and they serve as the target of statistical inference. Another attractive property of parametric methods is their efficiency: when the assumptions for a parametric method are truly met, the estimates that method provides are highly precise.

   Non-Penalized Methods Non-penalized methods estimate the parameters directly from the form of the probability distribution, or likelihood function, by finding the parameter values that maximize the likelihood. Several popular and widely-used methods belong to the class of non-penalized parametric methods, among them linear regression, logistic regression, and the accelerated failure time model for survival analysis.

   Accelerated Failure Time (AFT) Model The AFT model poses a regression model on the scale of the hazard function, λ, of the failure time T. Let Z denote the (potentially time-varying) covariates, and let $\lambda(t|Z)$ denote the hazard function at time t conditional on the covariates. Then the AFT model is given by $\lambda(t|Z) = e^{-\beta' Z(t)} \lambda_0 \left(e^{-\beta' Z(t)} t \right)$ where λ_0 represents the unobserved baseline hazard function of T when all covariates equal zero. When λ_0's parametric distribution is specified in advance, the AFT model is fully parametric [30]; when λ_0 is estimated nonparametrically, the AFT model is semiparametric [31]. The parameter β is the target of inference, as it describes the effect of the covariates on survival time. As an example, Altstein and Li (2013) [31] used the AFT model to discover biomarker-based latent subgroups in a melanoma trial.

Penalized Methods Penalized methods estimate model parameters by maximizing a likelihood function that is modified by a penalty term. The penalty term is added in to regularize parameter estimates, which can reduce overfitting and aid the model's performance in prediction. Many penalty terms can be chosen, each of which offer their own benefits; we present only one in this chapter. For a more thorough treatment of penalized methods, see chapters 3 and 4 of Hastie, Tibshirani, and Friedman (2008) [32].

LASSO The least absolute shrinkage and selection operator (LASSO) is among the most popular penalized methods, and is particularly useful for high-dimensional data where the number of variables is much larger than the number of data points. A primary reason is that the LASSO, in addition to regularizing parameter estimates, also sets the estimates of many coefficients exactly equal to zero—hence, the LASSO performs both regularization and variable selection. If we let Y_i denote the continuous outcome for patient i and X_i denote that patient's covariates, then the LASSO estimate of β minimizes the function $\sum_{i=1}^{n} (Y_i - \beta' X_i)^2 + \lambda \sum_{j=1}^{p} |\beta_j|$, where $\beta = (\beta_1, ..., \beta_p)$ and $\lambda \geq 0$ is an L_1-constrained penalty parameter. When λ is small, the LASSO estimate of β resembles the result from ordinary least squares, but as λ grows, increasingly many components of β are set equal to zero. Cross-validation is typically used to specify the value of λ. Once λ is chosen, the optimization problem simplifies to a quadratic programming problem, which can be solved through an efficient sequential algorithm [33]. There are many extensions of the LASSO which accommodate categorical data [33,34], survival data [35], study designs with interactions [36], and mixed models [37,38].

2. **Nonparametric Methods** Nonparametric methods assume that the data are not generated by a probability distribution with a fixed number of parameters—rather, the number of parameters needed to explain the data is allowed to grow to infinity as the sample size grows. While some nonparametric methods are complex and computationally intensive, a number of convenient nonparametric methods are available for data analysis. Many **machine learning techniques**, which perform well at a variety of difficult prediction tasks and are becoming increasingly well-studied from a statistical perspective, fall under the umbrella of nonparametric methods.

Random Forests Random forest approaches, which are fully nonparametric machine learning tools, offer great predictive power in both regression and classification. The technical details underlying random forests are rather complex, and a full treatment of them is beyond the scope of this chapter; we simply mention that they combine the strengths of two well-known techniques, decision trees and bootstrap aggregation [39]. Random forests offer a measure of covariate importance, albeit a much less interpretable measure than a regression coefficient in a parametric model. Random forests have inspired many extensions. Among them are Bayesian additive regression trees (BART), which marry the random forest and Bayesian nonparametric approaches [40], and reinforcement learning trees (RLT), which use reinforcement learning to select important variables while muting unimportant ones [41]. RLTs appear particularly promising, as several results about their statistical inference properties have been shown [41]. As an example, Gray et al. (2013) used random forests to classify patients into subgroups of Alzheimer's disease based on a variety of biomarkers, including MRI volumes, cerebrospinal fluid measures, and genetic markers [42].

Deep Learning Deep learning methods have proven quite powerful in prediction, both in the regression and classification setting, in a variety of difficult prediction contexts, such as speech recognition [43] and image processing [44]. The most commonly used deep learning methods are deep neural networks, which posit that the covariates are related to the outcome through multiple hidden layers of weighted sums and nonlinear transformations. Some deep neural networks, such as convolutional neural networks, build a spatial dependency into the structure of the hidden layers. Deep neural networks can be plagued by overfitting; the introduction of dropout, which reduces dependencies among nodes in the hidden layers, appears to greatly reduce this weakness [45]. Although deep learning techniques have met with great success in application, their inferential properties are, as of yet, not well-studied, though research in this area is currently active. As an example, Xiong et al. (2015) used deep neural networks to predict disease status based on alternative genetic splicing [46].

Support Vector Machine Another popular machine learning method for nonparametric classification is the support vector machine (SVM). The support vector machine considers each observation of covariates X_i as a point in d-dimensional space with a class label $Y_i \in \{-1, 1\}$. The SVM sets up a classification rule by finding the $d - 1$-dimensional hyperplane that optimally separates points with $Y_i = 1$ and $Y_i = -1$. This problem can be formulated as a constrained optimization problem and analytically solved; for details, see chapter 7 of Cristianini and Taylor (2000) [47]. The SVM can be extended to nonlinear classification using reproducing kernel Hilbert spaces [48] and regression settings using support vector regression [49].

Q-Learning Q-learning is a regression-based method for estimating an optimal personalized treatment strategy, which consists of a sequence of clinical decisions over time. Q-learning estimates a set of time-varying Q-functions, Q_t, $t = 1, \ldots, T$, which take the current patient state S_t and the clinical decision D_t as inputs and give the value, which is based on the clinical outcome of interest, as an output. When the Q-functions have been estimated, the only information we need to determine the optimal future treatment is the patient's current state. Estimates of the Q-functions, $\{\hat{Q}_1, \ldots, \hat{Q}_T\}$, are obtained through a backwards iterative algorithm [50]. The estimated Q-functions allow us to estimate the optimal treatments:

$$\hat{\pi}_t = \underset{d_t}{\arg\max}\, \hat{Q}_t(s_t, d_t) \qquad \text{for } t = 1, \ldots, T,$$

That is, we select the treatment sequence $\{\hat{\pi}_1, \ldots, \hat{\pi}_T\}$ that maximizes the sequence of Q-functions. Q-learning can be applied to complex, multi-stage trials, such as sequential multiple assignment randomized trials [51].

G-Estimation Predictive biomarkers are often used to provide information for several decisions over a period of time. Suppose that we are interested in discovering a causal relationship between an exposure and an outcome over time. If any time-varying confounder is also related to future exposure, standard methods for adjusting for confounders will fail. G-estimation, a method for estimating a causal effect in structural nested models while accounting for both confounders and mediators [52], is useful in this setting [53,54]. G-estimation has been applied in a number of settings where time-varying covariates are of interest, such as cardiovascular disease [55] and AIDS [56]. Vansteelandt et al. (2014) [52] give a more thorough overview of G-estimation and structural nested models.

Outcome Weighted Learning (OWL) OWL offers a method for identifying predictive biomarkers in a randomized trial or observational study testing binary treatments which have substantial treatment heterogeneity [57]. OWL estimates the optimal individualized treatment rule by formulating it as a weighted classification problem, which can be solved through a computationally efficient algorithm. For ease of notation, we present the case of a two-arm randomized trial in this chapter. Suppose we have a binary treatment $A \in \{-1, 1\}$, and that the p biomarkers of the n patients are recorded in the $n \times p$ covariate matrix X. Let R denote the clinical outcome, or reward, that we wish to maximize. In this framework, an individualized treatment rule (ITR) is a function that takes the covariates as an input and recommends one of the two treatments as an output. The optimal ITR, then, is the function that satisfies

$$\mathcal{D}^*(x) = \underset{\mathcal{D}}{\arg\min}\left\{ E\left(\frac{R \cdot 1\{A \neq \mathcal{D}(X)\}}{\Pr(A)} \right) \right\}, \tag{1}$$

where $\Pr(A)$ is the prime probability of being assigned to treatment A [58]. Essentially, OWL finds the optimal ITR by matching the treatments of patients with a high reward and mismatching patients who have small rewards. Equation 1 with 0–1 loss yields an optimization problem that is non-deterministic polynomial-time (NP) hard, and can be quite computationally intensive to solve. To alleviate this difficulty, OWL employs the hinge loss used in the Support Vector Machine. In addition, OWL uses regularization to stabilize the estimate of the ITR based on the observed sample (x_i, a_i, r_i),

$i = 1, \cdots, n$. Hence, OWL searches for the decision rule f that minimizes the regularized optimization problem

$$\frac{1}{n} \sum_{i=1}^{n} \frac{r_i}{\Pr(a_i)} \left(1 - a_i f(x_i)\right)_+ + \lambda ||f||^2, \tag{2}$$

where $||f||^2$ is the squared L_2-norm of f and λ is a tuning parameter used to balance model accuracy and complexity. Once we have estimated f, the OWL ITR is simply $\hat{\mathcal{D}}(X) = \text{sign}(f)$. OWL has many attractive inferential properties, including results for Fisher consistency and risk bounds [57].

Several methods extend the capabilities of OWL. Zhou et al. (2015) [59] improve OWL model accuracy by fitting the reward function with the covariates ahead of time and plugging the residuals into Eq. 2 instead of the reward. Xu et al. (2015) [60] add an L_1 penalty term to OWL, allowing OWL to perform variable selection. Zhao et al. (2015) [61] extend OWL from a single-stage trial, as described above, into multiple-stage clinical trials, allowing OWL to inform optimal dynamic treatment regimes.

OWL is not the only approach to finding predictive biomarkers in trials with treatment heterogeneity. Other approaches examine the interaction between treatment and candidate predictive biomarkers, including recent work in tree-based methods that provide flexible models for determining variable importance [62]. Zhang et al. (2012) take a similar approach based on a semiparametric model that uses inverse-probability weighting to analyze observational studies [63]. Tian et al. (2014) [64] model the interactions between the treatment and modified covariates in a variety of settings, including the setting with a large pool of biomarkers about which little is known and only a subset of patients expected to benefit from treatment.

3. **Semiparametric Methods** Semiparametric methods contain a parametric piece and a nonparametric piece, offering a trade-off between the flexibility offered by nonparametric methods and the efficiency offered by parametric methods. Although some semiparametric models are in wide use, others which offer the same attractive balance have found adoption much slower. In this section, we only discuss the most commonly used semiparametric model: the Cox proportional hazards model.

Cox proportional hazards model The Cox proportional hazards model, like the AFT model, poses a regression model on the scale of the hazard function [65]. If we let Z denote the potentially time-varying covariates, and we let $\lambda(t|Z)$ denote the hazard function at time t conditional on the covariates, the Cox model can be expressed as $\lambda(t|Z) = \lambda_0(t)e^{\beta'Z(t)}$, where λ_0 denotes the unobserved baseline hazard function, which can be estimated nonparametrically or assumed to follow a parametric distribution. The former is more common, and leads to a semiparametric model. The parametric piece of the Cox model is $e^{\beta'Z(t)}$, and β is estimated through maximum partial likelihood. As an example, Kalantar-Zadeh et al. (2007) used the Cox model to show an association between levels of A1C and mortality risk after controlling for several demographic characteristics [66].

Latent Supervised Learning. Latent supervised learning, a novel approach that exists in the middle ground between supervised and unsupervised learning, simultaneously handles parameter estimation and the problem of unlabeled subgroups. To illustrate: suppose that the patient population in a clinical trial consists of several underlying subgroups, and treatment efficacy differs according to these latent subgroups. Ignoring these subgroups can cause a supervised method to produce poor estimates [27]. Let Y denote the outcome and X denote the covariates. Wei and Kosorok (2013) proposed the following model for binary classification using latent supervised learning [27]:

$$Y = \mu_{1,0}1\{\omega_0^T X - \gamma_0 \geq 0\} + \mu_{2,0}1\{\omega_0^T X - \gamma_0 < 0\} + \epsilon$$

The model posits that an unknown linear function of the covariates determines the mean value of the outcome—patients with different signs of $\omega_0^T X - \gamma_0$ have different means ($\mu_{1,0}$ vs. $\mu_{2,0}$). The underlying subgroup structure is assumed to be linear. When ϵ is Gaussian, model parameters can be estimated through maximum likelihood [27]. These model parameters provide not only an estimate of the treatment effect, but also subgroup predictions based on covariates.

The assumption of latent subgroups that depend on biomarkers is not only reasonable, but often of primary scientific interest. Methods that can accommodate this assumption and simultaneously provide estimates of its effect, as the emerging field of latent supervised learning does, offer a great deal of promise for future research.

Unsupervised Methods. In some settings, it may be impractical to observe the outcome due to logistics or cost, or the exact nature of the outcome may not be known. More commonly, investigators may wish to perform some sort of data pre-processing before plugging their data into a supervised method. In these settings, **unsupervised learning** techniques assist in conducting statistical inference about the underlying structure of the data. Identifying the underlying structure can provide valuable insight into different classes that exist among the data, and which subset of variables determines those classes [67].

Dimension reduction reduces the number of effective covariates and brings data into a lower-dimension space that is easier to analyze. The most commonly used dimension reduction techniques are principal component analysis (PCA), linear discriminant analysis (LDA), and classical multidimensional scaling (MDS). While these methods are widely used, they may fail to capture the underlying structure of complex data. In these situations, nonlinear dimension reduction methods may prove more fruitful. Isometric feature mapping, or Isomap, builds a weighted graph using data points as nodes and calculates the geodesic distance between data points as the sum of weights along the shortest path between points. The geodesic distance is then used in place of Euclidean distance in MDS, which allows for Isomap to handle points that lie on a nonlinear manifold [68]. Another popular technique is t-Stochastic Neighbor Embedding, or t-SNE, which finds a low dimensional mapping to minimize the Kullback–Leibler divergence between the distributions of the data in low and high dimensional spaces [69]. t-SNE commonly employs a normal distribution in the high dimensional space and a t-distribution in the low dimensional space. Many other nonlinear dimension reduction methods are available, such as Locally Linear Embedding (LLE) [70] and diffusion maps [71].

Traditional clustering methods, such as k-means and hierarchical clustering, treat covariates of interest as a monolithic collection, which proves ineffective if only a subset of the covariates is truly informative. **Biclustering** methods address this issue by considering clusters among both subjects and covariates simultaneously. We present several methods for biclustering.

Let X denote the overall data matrix. Large Average Submatrix (LAS) finds K constant, potentially overlapping submatrices of X via maximum likelihood, then poses X as the sum of these submatrices and random noise [72]. Sparse clustering imposes a Gaussian likelihood on the biclusters of X, where the biclusters have unique means and common variance. The means are estimated through L_1-penalized least squares, which sets many bicluster means identical to zero, inducing sparsity [73].

Several biclustering methods use **singular value decomposition (SVD)** for dimension reduction. Sparse SVD (SSVD) additionally shrinks small nonzero singular vectors to zero through an L_1 penalty on the squared Frobenius norm of X, meaning only a checkerboard pattern of influential rows and columns remains nonzero [14]. Heterogeneous sparse SVD (HSSVD) functions in the case where biclusters vary in both mean and variance. HSSVD has the advantages of scale and rotation invariance, and has an improved capacity for detecting overlapping biclusters compared to classic SVD, as well as improved performance relative to several methods even in the case where the biclusters have homogeneous variance [74]. Currently, HSSVD has limited utility in handling count data and data that arise from more than one "-omics" platform.

Example: The following example comes from a lung cancer dataset with the expression levels of 12,625 genes from 56 patients discussed in [74]. The investigators performed HSSVD, classifying patients' lung cancer subtype (normal lung, pulmonary carcinoid tumors, colon metasteses, and small-cell carcinoma). They then compared the results of HSSVD with those of FIT-SSVD, LSHM, and SVD. The comparison is visualized in the checkerboard plots in Fig. 1. Successful biclustering is expected to produce the checkerboard appearance exhibited by HSSVD and FIT-SSVD, but not LSHM and SVD. The biclusters are identified as the rows divided by the white lines.

3.4 Power

Machine learning techniques appear prominently in biomarker discovery studies, especially in genomics settings [75, 76]. While machine learning techniques are well-suited to analyzing large, heterogeneous datasets, many core statistical concepts—such as power calculations—are essentially absent from the machine learning literature [77]. In this section, we emphasize that power should play a central role in any biomarker study, regardless of the analysis method selected.

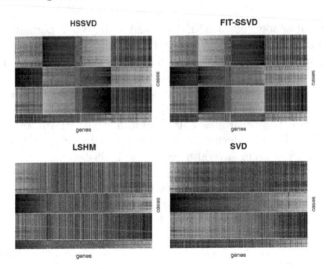

Fig. 1. Checkerboard plots produced by four different SVD biclustering methods on 12,625 genes from 56 patients with four levels of lung cancer [74].

The exact definition of power relevant to a biomarker study depends on the study's goal. Phase III trials incorporating predictive biomarkers revolve around one or more hypothesis tests that address whether the experimental treatment has a significant effect. In this setting, the traditional definition of power—the probability that, if the null hypothesis is truly false, it will be rejected—is appropriate. Trials evaluating a screening test based on a prognostic biomarker require a modified definition of power: the probability that the screening test correctly classifies a high proportion of patients, e.g. 90%. It is immediately apparent that both formulations of power are eminently desirable—without power, an unacceptably high number of results are likely to be false positives. Sample size is one of the drivers of power; in a typical study, investigators should aim for a sample size that enables at least 80% power.

Unacceptably high rates of false positives, or type I errors, threaten the validity of a study's conclusions. This concern is especially relevant when many hypotheses are tested simultaneously, as multiple comparisons inflate the type I error if they are not controlled for. Investigators can choose between many well-studied methods to limit type I error rate to a low level, conventionally 5%, in the presence of multiple tests, most commonly family-wise error rate (FWER) or false discovery rate (FDR). The FWER is the probability that we incorrectly reject even one true null hypothesis. FDR, meanwhile, is the expected proportion of falsely rejected hypotheses. FWER offers a stronger control than FDR, in the sense that if we control FWER at a certain level, we automatically also control FDR at that level. FWER and FDR may be preferred in different settings: FWER is used in many confirmatory studies [78], while FDR may be more logical in exploratory and other settings [79]. The most popular procedure for control of FWER is the Bonferroni correction [80]; despite this method's numerical simplicity, however, it is not recommended in light of Holm's step-down procedure [81], which is uniformly more powerful than the Bonferroni correction at the same level of control. The Benjamini-Hochberg step-up procedure offers control of FDR [82,83]. For a more detailed overview of multiple comparisons, we direct the reader to Dudoit and van der Laan's book [84].

We now present a general algorithm for calculating sample size in biomarker studies via simulation. The crux of the algorithm is the generation of *realistic data scenarios*, simulated datasets that incorporate information about the study design, method, and biomarkers in question. Information needed for all study designs includes the maximum allowable type I error rate, α, the multiple comparisons adjustment method, the desired power, β, the number of simulations to be run, B, an initial guess of the sample size, n_0, and the study's *minimal clinical measure of importance*. The specific measure of importance will vary by study. In a biomarker-stratified study, for instance, the measure of importance would be the expected change in effect size for the experimental treatment from the biomarker-positive to biomarker-negative groups. In an adaptive signature study, the measure of importance would be the change in effect size between overall and biomarker-specific groups, and additional necessary information would include the expected proportion of biomarkers that are true predictive biomarkers (likely below 1%). In a phase 4 prospective study of a screening test based on a prognostic biomarker, the measure of importance would be the misclassification proportion of the test compared to gold standard (e.g. 10%), and other necessary information would include the expected operating characteristics of the test, which may be based on information from a phase 3 prognostic biomarker study. While the details vary, the philosophy remains constant: investigators should not be excessively optimistic when generating realistic data scenarios. Most values should represent a worst-case scenario—e.g., the minimum effect size the investigators could observe and still conclude that a drug has a meaningful effect worth pursuing.

Algorithm 1. Power calculations through simulation

1 Run B simulations adjusting for a type I error rate of at most α, under a realistic data scenario with sample size n_0. This will entail simulating the correct number of biomarkers necessary for the study, under the assumption that they attain only the minimum clinical measure of importance.

2 Calculate the proportion of times the simulated biomarkers were detected and/or the hypotheses of interest were correctly rejected. This proportion is the estimated power of the test.

3 If the estimated power is ϵ less (or more) than the prespecified β, then increase (or decrease) n_0 by 1 and go back to step **1**.

4 Otherwise, stop the algorithm and the desired sample size is n_0.

3.5 Validation

When candidate biomarkers have been identified, they must be validated through an external dataset. At times, it is appropriate to consider truly exogenous data—data from a previous study that have evaluated the same outcome and biomarkers, for instance. At other times, this is infeasible or inappropriate; in these cases, researchers should plan to collect a secondary dataset. Researchers should consider the same issues listed above when determining the sample size for the validation set, but the set of assumptions should be less restrictive—namely, the number of biomarkers will be smaller and the proportion of biomarkers believed to be true will be higher. Algorithm 1 once again provides a convenient way to calculate sample size under these new assumptions.

3.6 Evaluation

In most real-world applications, it is not enough for a candidate biomarker to exist—it must also be useful. Once researchers have identified and validated a candidate biomarker, they can turn their attention to the issue of evaluating a biomarker's utility, whether that utility is in diagnosis, risk prediction, or any of a variety of functions in clinical practice. There are many statistical methods available for evaluating both the relationship between a biomarker and the disease area of interest and the usefulness of a biomarker when applied to specific populations; we outline only a few of these methods. Researchers should choose evaluation methods based on the specifics of their experiment while putting together their analysis plan, before data are collected. For a more in-depth introduction to some of the techniques mentioned in this section, see Pepe (2003) [85].

Measures of Accuracy. Biomarkers are often used in diagnostic medicine to classify patients as diseased or non-diseased. In this setting, evaluating the performance of a candidate biomarker is informed by the typical measures of accuracy for any diagnostic test. Let X be a candidate biomarker, and let $Y = 1\{X > c\}$ be an indicator equal to one when the biomarker exceeds a certain threshold, c, and zero otherwise. Suppose that a researcher intends to diagnose disease based on Y. Let D be an indicator of disease, so that D is equal to one for diseased subjects and zero otherwise. We define the **sensitivity** of Y as $se = \Pr(Y = 1 | D = 1)$. The **specificity** of Y is $sp = \Pr(Y = 0 | D = 0)$. Sensitivity is also referred to as the true positive fraction (TPF) and one minus specificity as the false positive fraction (FPF). Sensitivity and specificity give the probability of correct classification, conditional on disease status.

Two additional accuracy measures are the positive predictive value (PPV) and negative predictive value (NPV), given by $\mathrm{PPV} = \Pr(D = 1 | Y = 1)$ and $\mathrm{NPV} = \Pr(D = 0 | Y = 0)$. That is, the positive and negative predictive values give the probability of correct disease classification, conditional on test result. Although PPV and NPV are related to sensitivity and specificity, there is an important distinction between them. Sensitivity and specificity are functions of the test alone—they do not vary when the test is applied to different populations. Positive and negative predictive values, on the other hand, are highly dependent on the disease prevalence in the population the test is applied to: the same test may have wildly different positive and negative predictive values when applied to different populations. As such, the positive and negative predictive values cannot be estimated using data from studies that lack an estimate of disease prevalence, such as case-control studies. Accuracy measures are typically estimated empirically, and confidence regions for these measures can be constructed using the methods outlined in chapter 2 of Pepe (2003) [85].

Receiver Operating Characteristic Curves. Often, investigators will wish to evaluate a continuous biomarker. Receiver operating characteristic (ROC) curves are frequently used to do so, and they can be applied to a wide variety of tasks: comparing two biomarkers, constructing single-number summaries of biomarker performance, and selecting the screen positive threshold, c, among others. Roughly speaking, the ROC curve for a biomarker, X, is a plot of the true positive fractions and false positive fractions as functions of the threshold c. That is, if $\text{TPF}(c)$ and $\text{FPF}(c)$ are the true and false positive fractions for the test $1\{X > c\}$, respectively, then $\text{ROC}(\cdot) = \{(\text{FPF}(c), \text{TPF}(c)), -\infty < c < \infty\}$. If we let S_D and $S_{\bar{D}}$ denote the survival functions for X in the diseased and non-diseased populations, respectively, then the ROC curve can be equivalently defined as $\text{ROC}(t) = S_D(S_{\bar{D}}(t))$ for $0 < t < 1$. ROC curves boast well-developed theory, and the literature contains many procedures for ROC curve estimation and inference, both parametric and semiparametric [86–90]. Pepe (2000) [91] proposes a method to adjust ROC curves for covariates.

An advantage of the ROC framework is the ability to construct single number summaries that can be used to evaluate biomarkers. One such summary is the area under the ROC curve (AUC). A test that classifies perfectly yields AUC = 1, while a test that is no better than random chance has AUC= 0.5. If we let X_D and $X_{\bar{D}}$ denote observed biomarkers from the diseased and non-diseased populations, respectively, then AUC has an attractive interpretation as the probability of correctly ordered biomarkers—that is, $\text{AUC} = \Pr(X_D > X_{\bar{D}})$. Two candidate biomarkers can be compared by testing whether the corresponding AUCs differ, as in chapter 5 of Pepe (2003) [85].

Alternative Methods. While AUC is often a useful summary of a biomarker's performance, other methods may be more relevant for risk prediction models. Consider a risk prediction model that contains several biomarkers, and suppose we add a new biomarker to the model. Ware (2006) [92] observed that doing so may result in many subjects being placed in new risk categories, even if the change in AUC is small. Pencina et al. (2008) [93] propose using reclassification statistics to more adequately capture the effect of the new biomarker. Specifically, net reclassification improvement (NRI) measures how much an additional biomarker improves model-predicted probabilities of disease. When a strongly predictive biomarker enters the model, subjects with disease are reclassified into higher risk categories while subjects without disease are reclassified into lower risk categories, resulting in a large NRI. Pencina et al. (2011) [94] present a number of extensions to reclassification statistics.

Pencina et al. (2008) [93] propose a second alternative to AUC for evaluating biomarkers called integrated discrimination improvement (IDI). IDI measures how much a new biomarker increases the values of sensitivity and specificity, integrated over all possible thresholds. IDI also has a useful interpretation as the change in average TPF corrected for any increase in average FPF.

Predictive Biomarkers. The evaluation of predictive biomarkers requires special care. Predictive biomarkers are often evaluated by considering the interaction between the biomarker and treatment in a regression analysis [95,96]. While a strong interaction between a biomarker and treatment is consistent with the role of a predictive biomarker, it is not sufficient: predictive biomarkers are causal in nature, and causal evidence is needed to truly support them. The potential outcomes framework may help overcome this pitfall. Huang et al. (2012) [97] use the potential outcomes framework to evaluate a predictive biomarker under the assumption of monotone treatment effect, while Zhang et al. (2014) [98] propose a method that relaxes the assumption of monotonicity. For a general discussion of the evaluation of predictive biomarkers, see Polley et al. (2013) [99].

3.7 Reproducibility

"Non-reproducible single occurrences are of no significance to science."

- Karl Popper

Reproducibility is not just a criterion for a research study or manuscript to be accepted—it is a central, guiding tenet of the scientific method, an aim that every study should seek to attain. The Oxford English Dictionary defines reproducibility as "the extent to which consistent results are obtained when produced repeatedly." Applied to the setting of biomarker studies, reproducibility is the principle that experiments conducted under similar conditions should give similar results. Reproducibility is a crucial goal: if a study is not reproducible, its results will be difficult, and perhaps inappropriate, to apply to other settings.

In practice, to validate whether results can be reproduced, researchers may carry out a new experiment under similar conditions. The results of the new experiment can be compared to those of the original using a variety of methods, such as the Pearson correlation coefficient, the paired t-test, the intraclass correlation coefficient or the concordance correlation coefficient (CCC) [100]. When researchers wish to compare multiple outcomes, they should be careful to correct for multiple comparisons, as described in Sect. 3.4.

To clarify a subtle point: there is a distinction between reproducibility and replicability. An experiment need not be exactly replicated to qualify as reproducible–in fact, it may be very difficult to achieve perfect replication. A reproducible study's results can recur, or be reaffirmed, under similar but not identical settings–researchers at different labs testing the same biomarker, for instance [101]. A replicable study, on the other hand, would lead to identical results when it is conducted under the same conditions [102]. Whether strict replicability is necessary or not is currently the topic of some debate. To return to the biomarker example, Drummond [101] notes that such experiments can easily be affected by gene-deficient variants of the biomarkers in question, as these could lead independently synthesized gene segments to have significantly differing effects. As a consequence, it is unlikely for researchers to achieve a precise replication of the original experiment–but it may be unimportant to do so as long as the results of the experiments are consistent.

A natural question to ask is how many times an experiment should be repeated before it is considered trustworthy enough to publish. The answer to this question depends on expense and ethical considerations. Generally speaking, an experiment should be repeated several times before it is reported. This recommendation can be relaxed in some settings when it would prove overly restrictive, for instance when replication is excessively costly or when a repeated experiment's ethics would be questionable [102]. An illustration of the latter comes from the guidelines for experimentation on vertebrate animals, which discourages the use of unnecessary duplication. Casadevall [102] and Laine [103] suggest that, in order to make full use of each experiment, researchers "strive for reproducibility instead of simple replicability." For example, if the original experiment tests the efficacy of a drug on controlling glucose level in a certain time period, a second experiment could test for a dose-response relationship while simultaneously confirming the original conclusion of efficacy.

While external confirmation is the gold standard for establishing the reproducibility of a result, investigators can ensure substantial levels of reproducibility simply by choosing appropriate methods. The inferential properties of a statistical method, such as consistency and power (see Sect. 3.4), are directly connected to the reproducibility of that method's results. Large, well-designed studies, equipped with inferentially sound methods and powered appropriately for the questions of scientific interest, are inherently highly reliable. Investigators can save a great deal of time and effort by striving for such studies initially.

4   Clinical Interpretation

Ultimately, statistical validation and evaluation of a biomarker can only go so far. A biomarker's long-term worth depends heavily on its clinical interpretation and utility. Investigators should also take care not to dramatically depart from standardized, consistent definitions and properly executed methods. Inconsistencies across studies can hinder research producing robust conclusions.

In many instances, biomarkers are used as substitutes, or surrogates, for clinical endpoints. Surrogates may improve the feasibility of a trial through reduction in sample size or trial duration, and they are especially attractive when there are ethical concerns with the clinical endpoint, such as invasive procedures. Determining whether or not a biomarker is an appropriate surrogate endpoint relies on knowledge of the disease process and the causal pathways the biomarker lies in. However, disorders are often complex, clinically heterogeneous, and subject to large inter-individual variation, with the same disorder appearing drastically different at distinct points along the continuum between severe pathology and non-disease state. As such, investigators should be wary of jumping to belief of a causal link between a biomarker and a clinical outcome, even when they find a statistical and temporal association: the biomarker may affect a causal pathway present in only a small number of patients, or may not play a role in the relevant causal pathway at all [104]. Even when the biomarker is in the correct causal pathway, its effect on the biological process may be of insufficient size or duration to significantly affect the clinical outcome [104]. Hence, while surrogate biomarkers can be useful tools, relying solely on surrogates may lead to misleading conclusions and even harm to patients. For example, the use of ventricular premature depolarization (VPD) suppression as a primary outcome in clinical trials had led to the approval of antiarrhythmic drugs for patients with myocardial infarction [105]. Subsequent studies, however, found that, despite being effective in suppressing VPD, some antiarrhythmics actually increased mortality [106]. Prentice (1989) proposes an operational criterion to validate surrogate endpoints in clinical trials comparing two or more interventions: the surrogate endpoint should fully capture the net effect of the intervention on the clinical endpoint conditional on the surrogate endpoint [107]. The Prentice criterion is not universally accepted: some argue that it does not allow for valid inference on the effect of the intervention on the clinical endpoint [108].

Similarly, biomarkers that perform well in a narrow context may not be applicable to other settings [109]. Patient heterogeneity is among the most important factors to account for in biomarker studies; we recommend employing matching or stratification based on relevant characteristics, such as age, race/ethnicity, or body mass index, to help account for it. For example, there are consistent gender differences in patients with acute myocardial infarction: elevation of troponins are less common and lower in women than in men, while natriuretic peptides and C-reactive protein are more elevated in women than men [110]. The heterogeneity in symptoms between genders may contribute to the poorer prognosis of myocardial infarction in women, as well as demonstrating a facet of the "Yentl syndrome," the gender bias against women in the identification and management of coronary heart disease [111].

Finally, whether a biomarker is used for clinical prediction and screening should be based heavily on the benefits and risks involved. For example, the utility of prostate cancer screening that relies on the prostate-specific antigen (PSA) is controversial [112]. A substantial proportion of PSA-detected cancers are benign enough that they would not cause clinical problems during a man's lifetime. In these cases, the potential benefits of PSA testing may not outweigh the harms of the invasive diagnostic procedures and unnecessary treatment, including urinary, sexual, and bowel complications [112].

5   Limitations

This chapter was constructed to be general enough to appeal to a wide audience of researchers working in biomarker discovery. Moreover, we are attempting to provide an overall pipeline. As such, we could not address individual parts of this pipeline in sufficient detail, and we may have left out some important specifics. This section is meant primarily to serve as a safeguard for readers against known potential issues so they can avoid errors in advance.

While having a data management plan and protocol is necessary, it is rarely completely sufficient—issues always arise during data cleaning and management that were not anticipated by the plan. For this reason, we recommend having a research team member specializing in data management, whose expertise can help tackle unexpected issues.

While we have suggested several supervised and unsupervised methods for biomarker discovery, this review only scratches the surface of the sum total of methods available. Domain expertise is necessary to select appropriate methods; such knowledge is not provided in this chapter (due to limited space).

Power analysis was defined in very general terms, and we provided an all-purpose algorithm for its calculation through simulation. Our exposition may leave readers with the false impression that power calculations are an easy business with few complications. Nothing could be farther from the truth. Power calculations should, if possible, be left to a senior statistician well-versed in multiple comparisons, and adequate time should be allowed for them.

While sensitivity, specificity, and ROC curves are useful methods for biomarker evaluation, great care needs to be taken when specifying what magnitude of improvement is useful. Biomarkers might lead to an incremental improvement in the operating characteristics we have presented, but only at the expense of prohibitive cost. We recommend consulting with a physician with expertise on the particular application when considering this trade-off.

6   Conclusion

The rapid increase of available data—a process that is only accelerating—provides immense opportunities for improving the health of both individuals and populations. Fields that can harness "big data" to make health care decisions that take patient heterogeneity into account, as precision medicine seeks to do, have the potential to advance human health dramatically. However, the rise of "big data" presents not only opportunities, but a whole host of complications and challenges. The discovery and validation of biomarkers that can guide treatment decisions is more relevant than it has ever been, and methodologies that accomplish this task in a reliable, reproducible, and statistically rigorous way are of utmost necessity.

The discovery and validation of biomarkers is a complex process. Statistical issues are inherent to every step of the process, and they must be carefully considered as they are encountered. We propose the following master pipeline to help ensure the reproducibility of research related to biomarker discovery. For each step in the pipeline, we provide questions that researchers should answer affirmatively before proceeding.

1. Consider research goals to choose an appropriate design. *Does the study design reflect the role the biomarkers are expected to play in a clinical setting? Is the study design consistent with the current state of knowledge for the biomarkers being analyzed?*
2. Design data analysis plan. Consider both supervised and unsupervised statistical methods. *Are the method's assumptions consistent with the study design? Is the method suited to the research question at hand?*
3. Conduct power calculations to determine the appropriate sample size. *Did you correctly define a minimum clinical measure for calculating power? Is your minimum clinical measure chosen to represent a worst case scenario? Did the power calculation adjust for multiple comparisons? Did the power calculation incorporate prior knowledge effectively?*
4. Collect and curate data. *Are the data collected consistently and reliably? Are the data stored and linked in a way that respects patients' privacy?*
5. Conduct planned analyses and validate on an external data set. *Were the candidate biomarkers discovered in the initial analysis confirmed by the validation analysis?*
6. Evaluate the usefulness of the biomarker in practice. *Do the biomarkers offer a clinically relevant improvement in TPF and FPF?*
7. Consider clinical implications. *Is the cost of the proposed biomarker justified by its benefits?*

The above pipeline will need to be modified on a case-by-case basis, but it should provide a useful guide for any researcher and starting point for any study in the biomarker discovery field.

Many areas of research pertaining to the discovery of biomarkers are fervently active. The optimal approach for incorporating predictive biomarkers into modern, multi-stage study designs, such as SMARTs, is an area of open research, as is the proper use of electronic health record data and causal inference for observational and other non-randomized biomarker studies. The development of machine learning techniques with desirable inferential properties is an ongoing task, as is the use of these inferential properties to derive formal power calculations. Note that automatic approaches, such as many of the approaches described above, greatly benefit from "big data" with large training sets. However in some health informatics settings, we can be confronted with a small amount of data and/or rare events, where completely automatic approaches may suffer from insufficient training data. In these settings, interactive machine learning (iML) may be applicable, where a "doctor-in-the-loop" can help to refine the search space through heuristic selection of samples. Therefore, what would otherwise be an almost intractable problem, reduces greatly in complexity through the input and assistance of a human agent involved in the learning phase [113]. In all of these developments, proper attention to statistical considerations will enhance the ability of biomarker discovery studies to demonstrably improve clinical care through precision medicine.

References

1. Oldenhuis, C., Oosting, S., Gietema, J., De Vries, E.: Prognostic versus predictive value of biomarkers in oncology. Eur. J. Cancer **44**(7), 946–953 (2008)
2. National Institutes of Health: Precision Medicine Initiative Cohort Program (2016). Accessed 25 Feb 2016
3. Poste, G.: Bring on the biomarkers. Nature **469**(7329), 156–157 (2011)
4. Preedy, V.R., Patel, V.B.: General Methods in Biomarker Research and Their Applications. Springer, Netherlands (2015)
5. Novelli, G., Ciccacci, C., Borgiani, P., Papaluca Amati, M., Abadie, E.: Genetic tests and genomic biomarkers: regulation, qualification and validation. Clin. Cases Min. Bone Metab. **5**(2), 149–154 (2008)
6. Sun, Q., Van Dam, R.M., Spiegelman, D., Heymsfield, S.B., Willett, W.C., Hu, F.B.: Comparison of dual-energy x-ray absorptiometric and anthropometric measures of adiposity in relation to adiposity-related biologic factors. Am. J. Epidemiol. kwq306 (2010)
7. Flegal, K.M., Graubard, B.I.: Estimates of excess deaths associated with body mass index and other anthropometric variables. Am. J. Clin. Nutr. **89**(4), 1213–1219 (2009)
8. Task Force of the European Society of Cardiology and the North American Society of Pacing Electrophysiology: Heart rate variability: standards of measurement, physiological interpretation and clinical use. Circulation **93**(5), 1043–1065 (1996)
9. Huikuri, H.V., Stein, P.K.: Heart rate variability in risk stratification of cardiac patients. Prog. Cardiovasc. Dis. **56**(2), 153–159 (2013)
10. Association, A.D., et al.: Standards of medical care in diabetes - 2015 abridged for primary care providers. Clin. Diab. **33**(2), 97–111 (2015)
11. Larsen, M.L., Hørder, M., Mogensen, E.F.: Effect of long-term monitoring of glycosylated hemoglobin levels in insulin-dependent diabetes mellitus. N. Engl. J. Med. **323**(15), 1021–1025 (1990)
12. Karapetis, C.S., Khambata-Ford, S., Jonker, D.J., O'Callaghan, C.J., Tu, D., Tebbutt, N.C., Simes, R.J., Chalchal, H., Shapiro, J.D., Robitaille, S., et al.: K-ras mutations and benefit from cetuximab in advanced colorectal cancer. N. Engl. J. Med. **359**(17), 1757–1765 (2008)
13. Miki, Y., Swensen, J., Shattuck-Eidens, D., Futreal, P.A., Harshman, K., Tavtigian, S., Liu, Q., Cochran, C., Bennett, L.M., Ding, W., et al.: A strong candidate for the breast and ovarian cancer susceptibility gene BRCA1. Science **266**(5182), 66–71 (1994)
14. Lee, M., Shen, H., Huang, J.Z., Marron, J.: Biclustering via sparse singular value decomposition. Biometrics **66**(4), 1087–1095 (2010)
15. Pepe, M.S., Etzioni, R., Feng, Z., Potter, J.D., Thompson, M.L., Thornquist, M., Winget, M., Yasui, Y.: Phases of biomarker development for early detection of cancer. J. Natl Cancer Inst. **93**(14), 1054–1061 (2001)
16. Sargent, D.J., Conley, B.A., Allegra, C., Collette, L.: Clinical trial designs for predictive marker validation in cancer treatment trials. J. Clin. Oncol. **23**(9), 2020–2027 (2005)

17. Freidlin, B., McShane, L.M., Korn, E.L.: Randomized clinical trials with biomarkers: design issues. J. Natl Cancer Inst. **102**(3), 152–160 (2010)
18. Simon, R.: Clinical trial designs for evaluating the medical utility of prognostic and predictive biomarkers in oncology. Personalized Med. **7**(1), 33–47 (2010)
19. Mandrekar, S.J., Sargent, D.J.: Clinical trial designs for predictive biomarker validation: one size does not fit all. J. Biopharm. Stat. **19**(3), 530–542 (2009)
20. Jiang, W., Freidlin, B., Simon, R.: Biomarker-adaptive threshold design: a procedure for evaluating treatment with possible biomarker-defined subset effect. J. Natl Cancer Inst. **99**(13), 1036–1043 (2007)
21. Freidlin, B., Simon, R.: Adaptive signature design: an adaptive clinical trial design for generating and prospectively testing a gene expression signature for sensitive patients. Clin. Cancer Res. **11**(21), 7872–7878 (2005)
22. Murphy, S.A.: An experimental design for the development of adaptive treatment strategies. Stat. Med. **24**(10), 1455–1481 (2005)
23. Denny, J.C.: Mining electronic health records in the genomics era. PLoS Comput. Biol. **8**(12), e1002823 (2012)
24. Society for Clinical Data Management, I: Good Clinical Data Management Practices (2005). Accessed 25 Feb 2016
25. Bruza, P.D., Van der Weide, T.P.: The semantics of data flow diagrams. University of Nijmegen, Department of Informatics, Faculty of Mathematics and Informatics (1989)
26. U.S. Department of Health & Human Services: HIPAA Administrative Simplification (2013). Accessed 25 Feb 2016
27. Wei, S., Kosorok, M.R.: Latent supervised learning. J. Am. Stat. Assoc. **108**(503), 957–970 (2013)
28. Chapelle, O., Schölkopf, B., Zien, A., et al.: Semi-supervised learning (2006)
29. Kosorok, M.R.: What's so special about semiparametric methods? Sankhya. Ser. B [Methodol.] **71**(2), 331–353 (2009)
30. Wei, L.: The accelerated failure time model: a useful alternative to the Cox regression model in survival analysis. Stat. Med. **11**(14–15), 1871–1879 (1992)
31. Altstein, L., Li, G.: Latent subgroup analysis of a randomized clinical trial through a semiparametric accelerated failure time mixture model. Biometrics **69**(1), 52–61 (2013)
32. Hastie, T., Tibshirani, F.: The Elements of Statistical Learning (2001)
33. Tibshirani, R.: Regression shrinkage and selection via the lasso. J. Roy. Stat. Soc.: Ser. B (Methodol.) **58**(1), 267–288 (1996)
34. Meier, L., Van De Geer, S., Bühlmann, P.: The group lasso for logistic regression. J. Roy. Stat. Soc.: Ser. B (Methodol.) **70**(1), 53–71 (2008)
35. Tibshirani, R., et al.: The lasso method for variable selection in the Cox model. Stat. Med. **16**(4), 385–395 (1997)
36. Bien, J., Taylor, J., Tibshirani, R.: A lasso for hierarchical interactions. Ann. Stat. **41**(3), 1111 (2013)
37. Bondell, H.D., Krishna, A., Ghosh, S.K.: Joint variable selection for fixed and random effects in linear mixed-effects models. Biometrics **66**(4), 1069–1077 (2010)
38. Ibrahim, J.G., Zhu, H., Garcia, R.I., Guo, R.: Fixed and random effects selection in mixed effects models. Biometrics **67**(2), 495–503 (2011)
39. Breiman, L.: Random forests. Mach. Learn. **45**(1), 5–32 (2001)
40. Chipman, H.A., George, E.I., McCulloch, R.E.: BART: Bayesian additive regression trees. Ann. Appl. Stat. **4**(1), 266–298 (2010)
41. Zhu, R., Zeng, D., Kosorok, M.R.: Reinforcement learning trees. J. Am. Stat. Assoc. **110**(512), 1770–1784 (2015)

42. Gray, K.R., Aljabar, P., Heckemann, R.A., Hammers, A., Rueckert, D., Initiative, A.D.N., et al.: Random forest-based similarity measures for multi-modal classification of Alzheimer's disease. NeuroImage **65**, 167–175 (2013)

43. Hinton, G., Deng, L., Yu, D., Dahl, G.E., Mohamed, A.R., Jaitly, N., Senior, A., Vanhoucke, V., Nguyen, P., Sainath, T.N., et al.: Deep neural networks for acoustic modeling in speech recognition: the shared views of four research groups. IEEE Sig. Process. Mag. **29**(6), 82–97 (2012)

44. Krizhevsky, A., Sutskever, I., Hinton, G.E.: Imagenet classification with deep convolutional neural networks. In: Advances in Neural Information Processing Systems, pp. 1097–1105 (2012)

45. Hinton, G.E., Srivastava, N., Krizhevsky, A., Sutskever, I., Salakhutdinov, R.R.: Improving neural networks by preventing co-adaptation of feature detectors. arXiv preprint (2012). arXiv:1207.0580

46. Xiong, H.Y., Alipanahi, B., Lee, L.J., Bretschneider, H., Merico, D., Yuen, R.K., Hua, Y., Gueroussov, S., Najafabadi, H.S., Hughes, T.R., et al.: The human splicing code reveals new insights into the genetic determinants of disease. Science **347**(6218), 1254806 (2015)

47. Cristianini, N., Shawe-Taylor, J.: An Introduction to Support Vector Machines and Other Kernel-Based Learning Methods. Cambridge University Press, Cambridge (2000)

48. Boser, B.E., Guyon, I.M., Vapnik, V.N.: A training algorithm for optimal margin classifiers. In: Proceedings of the Fifth Annual Workshop on Computational Learning Theory, pp. 144–152. ACM (1992)

49. Smola, A., Vapnik, V.: Support vector regression machines. Advances in Neural Information Processing Systems, vol. 9, pp. 155–161 (1997)

50. Zhao, Y., Kosorok, M.R., Zeng, D.: Reinforcement learning design for cancer clinical trials. Stat. Med. **28**(26), 3294–3315 (2009)

51. Zhao, Y., Zeng, D., Socinski, M.A., Kosorok, M.R.: Reinforcement learning strategies for clinical trials in nonsmall cell lung cancer. Biometrics **67**(4), 1422–1433 (2011)

52. Vansteelandt, S., Joffe, M., et al.: Structural nested models and G-estimation: The partially realized promise. Stat. Sci. **29**(4), 707–731 (2014)

53. Robins, J.: A new approach to causal inference in mortality studies with a sustained exposure period-application to control of the healthy worker survivor effect. Math. Model. **7**(9), 1393–1512 (1986)

54. Robins, J.M.: The analysis of randomized and non-randomized AIDS treatment trials using a new approach to causal inference in longitudinal studies. Health Service Res. Methodol.: A Focus on AIDS **113**, 159 (1989)

55. Witteman, J.C., D'Agostino, R.B., Stijnen, T., Kannel, W.B., Cobb, J.C., de Ridder, M.A., Hofman, A., Robins, J.M.: G-estimation of causal effects: isolated systolic hypertension and cardiovascular death in the Framingham Heart Study. Am. J. Epidemiol. **148**(4), 390–401 (1998)

56. Robins, J.M., Blevins, D., Ritter, G., Wulfsohn, M.: G-estimation of the effect of prophylaxis therapy for pneumocystis carinii pneumonia on the survival of AIDS patients. Epidemiology **3**, 319–336 (1992)

57. Zhao, Y., Zeng, D., Rush, A.J., Kosorok, M.R.: Estimating individualized treatment rules using outcome weighted learning. J. Am. Stat. Assoc. **107**(449), 1106–1118 (2012)

58. Qian, M., Murphy, S.A.: Performance guarantees for individualized treatment rules. Ann. Stat. **39**(2), 1180–1210 (2011)

59. Zhou, X., Mayer-Hamblett, N., Khan, U., Kosorok, M.R.: Residual weighted learning for estimating individualized treatment rules. J. Am. Stat. Assoc., October 2015

60. Xu, Y., Yu, M., Zhao, Y.Q., Li, Q., Wang, S., Shao, J.: Regularized outcome weighted subgroup identification for differential treatment effects. Biometrics **71**(3), 645–653 (2015)

61. Zhao, Y.Q., Zeng, D., Laber, E.B., Kosorok, M.R.: New statistical learning methods for estimating optimal dynamic treatment regimes. J. Am. Stat. Assoc. **110**(510), 583–598 (2015)

62. Su, X., Meneses, K., McNees, P., Johnson, W.O.: Interaction trees: exploring the differential effects of an intervention programme for breast cancer survivors. J. Roy. Stat. Soc. C (Appl. Stat.) **60**(3), 457–474 (2011)

63. Zhang, B., Tsiatis, A.A., Laber, E.B., Davidian, M.: A robust method for estimating optimal treatment regimes. Biometrics **68**(4), 1010–1018 (2012)

64. Tian, L., Alizadeh, A.A., Gentles, A.J., Tibshirani, R.: A simple method for estimating interactions between a treatment and a large number of covariate. J. Am. Stat. Assoc. **109**(508), 1517–1532 (2014)

65. Cox, D.: Regression models and life tables (with discussion). J. Roy.Stat. Soc, B **34**, 187–220 (1972)

66. Kalantar-Zadeh, K., Kopple, J.D., Regidor, D.L., Jing, J., Shinaberger, C.S., Aronovitz, J., McAllister, C.J., Whellan, D., Sharma, K.: A1C and survival in maintenance hemodialysis patients. Diab. Care **30**(5), 1049–1055 (2007)

67. Kyan, M., Muneesawang, P., Jarrah, K., Guan, L.: Unsupervised Learning: A Dynamic Approach. IEEE Press Series on Computational Intelligence, pp. 275–276

68. Tenenbaum, J.B., De Silva, V., Langford, J.C.: A global geometric framework for nonlinear dimensionality reduction. Science **290**(5500), 2319–2323 (2000)

69. Van der Maaten, L., Hinton, G.: Visualizing data using t-SNE. J. Mach. Learn. Res. **9**(2579–2605), 85 (2008)

70. Roweis, S.T., Saul, L.K.: Nonlinear dimensionality reduction by locally linear embedding. Science **290**(5500), 2323–2326 (2000)

71. Coifman, R.R., Lafon, S., Lee, A.B., Maggioni, M., Nadler, B., Warner, F., Zucker, S.W.: Geometric diffusions as a tool for harmonic analysis and structure definition of data: diffusion maps. Proc. Natl. Acad. Sci. U.S.A. **102**(21), 7426–7431 (2005)

72. Shabalin, A.A., Weigman, V.J., Perou, C.M., Nobel, A.B.: Finding large average submatrices in high dimensional data. Ann. Appl. Stat. **3**(3), 985–1012 (2009)

73. Tan, K.M., Witten, D.M.: Sparse biclustering of transposable data. J. Comput. Graph. Stat. **23**(4), 985–1008 (2014)

74. Chen, G., Sullivan, P.F., Kosorok, M.R.: Biclustering with heterogeneous variance. Proc. Natl. Acad. Sci. **110**(30), 12253–12258 (2013)

75. Cruz, J.A., Wishart, D.S.: Applications of machine learning in cancer prediction and prognosis. Cancer Inform. **2**, 59–78 (2006)

76. Swan, A.L., Mobasheri, A., Allaway, D., Liddell, S., Bacardit, J.: Application of machine learning to proteomics data: classification and biomarker identification in postgenomics biology. OMICS **17**(12), 595–610 (2013)

77. Libbrecht, M.W., Noble, W.S.: Machine learning applications in genetics and genomics. Nat. Rev. Genet. **16**(6), 321–332 (2015)

78. Bender, R., Lange, S.: Adjusting for multiple testing? when and how? J. Clin. Epidemiol. **54**(4), 343–349 (2001)

79. Glickman, M.E., Rao, S.R., Schultz, M.R.: False discovery rate control is a recommended alternative to Bonferroni-type adjustments in health studies. J. Clin. Epidemiol. **67**(8), 850–857 (2014)

80. Westfall, P.H., Young, S.S.: Resampling-based multiple testing: examples and methods for p-value adjustment, vol. 279. John Wiley & Sons, New York (1993)

81. Holm, S.: A simple sequentially rejective multiple test procedure. Scand. J. Stat. **6**, 65–70 (1979)

82. Benjamini, Y., Hochberg, Y.: Controlling the false discovery rate: a practical and powerful approach to multiple testing. J. Roy. Stat. Soc.: Ser. B (Methodol.) **57**(1), 289–300 (1995)

83. Efron, B.: Large-Scale Inference: Empirical Bayes Methods for Estimation, Testing, and Prediction, vol. 1. Cambridge University Press, Cambridge (2012)

84. Van der Laan, M.J.: Multiple Testing Procedures with Applications to Genomics. Springer Series in Statistics. Springer, Heidelberg (2008)

85. Pepe, M.S.: The statistical evaluation of medical tests for classification and prediction. Oxford University Press, USA (2003)

86. Pepe, M.S.: A regression modelling framework for receiver operating characteristic curves in medical diagnostic testing. Biometrika **84**(3), 595–608 (1997)

87. Cai, T., Pepe, M.S.: Semiparametric receiver operating characteristic analysis to evaluate biomarkers for disease. J. Am. Stat. Assoc. **97**(460), 1099–1107 (2002)

88. Chrzanowski, M.: Weighted empirical likelihood inference for the area under the ROC curve. J. Stat. Plan. Infer. **147**, 159–172 (2014)

89. Cai, T., Dodd, L.E.: Regression analysis for the partial area under the ROC curve. Statistica Sin. **18**, 817–836 (2008)

90. Cai, T., Moskowitz, C.S.: Semi-parametric estimation of the binormal ROC curve for a continuous diagnostic test. Biostatistics **5**(4), 573–586 (2004)

91. Pepe, M.S.: An interpretation for the ROC curve and inference using GLM procedures. Biometrics **56**(2), 352–359 (2000)

92. Ware, J.H.: The limitations of risk factors as prognostic tools. N. Engl. J. Med. **355**(25), 2615–2617 (2006)

93. Pencina, M.J., D'Agostino, R.B., Vasan, R.S.: Evaluating the added predictive ability of a new marker: from area under the ROC curve to reclassification and beyond. Stat. Med. **27**(2), 157–172 (2008)

94. Pencina, M.J., D'Agostino, R.B., Steyerberg, E.W.: Extensions of net reclassification improvement calculations to measure usefulness of new biomarkers. Stat. Med. **30**(1), 11–21 (2011)

95. Gail, M., Simon, R.M.: Testing for qualitative interactions between treatmenteects and patient subsets. Biometrics **41**(2), 361–372 (1985)

96. Russek-Cohen, E., Simon, R.M.: Evaluating treatments when a gender by treatment interaction may exist. Stat. Med. **16**(4), 455–464 (1997)

97. Huang, Y., Gilbert, P.B., Janes, H.: Assessing treatment-selection markers using a potential outcomes framework. Biometrics **68**(3), 687–696 (2012)

98. Zhang, Z., Nie, L., Soon, G., Liu, A.: The use of covariates and random effects in evaluating predictive biomarkers under a potential outcome framework. Ann. Appl. Stat. **8**(4), 2336 (2014)

99. Polley, M.Y.C., Freidlin, B., Korn, E.L., Conley, B.A., Abrams, J.S., McShane, L.M.: Statistical and practical considerations for clinical evaluation of predictive biomarkers. J. Natl. Cancer Inst. **105**(22), 1677–1683 (2013)

100. Lawrence, I., Lin, K.: A concordance correlation coefficient to evaluate reproducibility. Biometrics **45**, 255–268 (1989)

101. Drummond, C.: Replicability is Not Reproducibility: Nor is it Good Science (2009)
102. Casadevall, A., Fang, F.C.: Reproducible science. Infect. Immun. **78**(12), 4972–4975 (2010)
103. Laine, C., Goodman, S.N., Griswold, M.E., Sox, H.C.: Reproducible research: moving toward research the public can really trust. Ann. Intern. Med. **146**(6), 450–453 (2007)
104. Fleming, T.R., DeMets, D.L.: Surrogate end points in clinical trials: are we being misled? Ann. Intern. Med. **125**(7), 605–613 (1996)
105. Connolly, S.J.: Use and misuse of surrogate outcomes in arrhythmia trials. Circulation **113**(6), 764–766 (2006)
106. Weir, M., Investigators, C.A.S.T., et al.: The cardiac arrhythmia suppression trial investigators: Preliminary report: Effect of encainide and flecainide on mortality in a randomized trial of arrhythmia suppression after myocardial infarction. Cardiopul. Phys. Ther. J. **1**(2), 12 (1990)
107. Prentice, R.L.: Surrogate endpoints in clinical trials: definition and operational criteria. Stat. Med. **8**(4), 431–440 (1989)
108. Berger, V.W.: Does the prentice criterion validate surrogate endpoints? Stat. Med. **23**(10), 1571–1578 (2004)
109. Strimbu, K., Tavel, J.A.: What are biomarkers? Curr. Opin. HIV AIDS **5**(6), 463 (2010)
110. Sbarouni, E., Georgiadou, P., Voudris, V.: Gender-specific differences in biomarkers responses to acute coronary syndromes and revascularization procedures. Biomarkers **16**(6), 457–465 (2011)
111. Healy, B.: The yentl syndrome. N. Engl. J. Med. **325**(4), 274–276 (1991)
112. Hoffman, R.M.: Screening for prostate cancer. N. Engl. J. Med. **365**(21), 2013–2019 (2011)
113. Holzinger, A.: Interactive machine learning for health informatics: When do we need the human-in-the-loop? Brain Inform. **3**(2), 119–131 (2016)

Machine Learning Solutions
in Computer-Aided Medical Diagnosis

Smaranda Belciug[(✉)]

Faculty of Sciences, Department of Computer Science,
University of Craiova, A.I. Cuza street, 200585 Craiova, Romania
smaranda.belciug@inf.ucv.ro

Abstract. The explosive growth of medical databases and the widespread development of high performance machine learning (ML) algorithms led to the search for efficient computer-aided medical diagnosis (CAMD) techniques. Automated medical diagnosis can be achieved by building a model of a certain disease under surveillance and comparing it with the real time physiological measurements taken from the patient. If this practice is carried out on a regular basis, potential risky medical conditions can be detected at an early stage, thus making the process of fighting the disease much easier. With CAMD, physicians can trustfully use the "second opinion" of the 'digital assistant' and make the final optimum decision. The recent development of intelligent technologies, designed to enhance the process of differential diagnosis by using medical databases, significantly enables the decision-making process of health professionals. Up-to-date online medical databases can now be used to support clinical decision-making, offering direct access to medical evidence. In this paper, we provide an overview on selected ML algorithms that can be applied in CAMD, focusing on the enhancement of neural networks (NNs) by hybridization, partially connectivity, and alternative learning paradigms. Particularly, we emphasize the benefits of using such effective algorithms in breast cancer detection and recurrence, colon cancer, lung cancer, liver fibrosis stadialization, heart attack, and diabetes. Generally, the aim is to provide a theme for discussions on ML-based methods applied to medicine.

Keywords: Data mining · Machine learning · Biomedical informatics · Computer-aided medical diagnosis

1 Introduction and Motivation

Establishing a medical diagnosis, more precisely, a differential diagnosis (DF) is a process of differentiating among different possible diseases presenting more or less similar symptoms. From a medical point of view, this process resides in highlighting the connection between a certain disease and the patient's history (patient file), physical examinations, tests, clinical, radiological and laboratory data, etc. From a biomedical informatics point of view, DF assumes a classification procedure involving a decision-making process based on the available medical data processed by an "intelligent" system (IS) borrowed from the information technology. In this way, IS directly

© Springer International Publishing AG 2016
A. Holzinger (Ed.): ML for Health Informatics, LNAI 9605, pp. 289–302, 2016.
DOI: 10.1007/978-3-319-50478-0_14

assists the DF process, representing a clinical decision-support system (CDSS) [1]. Physicians have thus access to a wide range of Data Mining (DM) methods (e.g., NNs, genetic algorithms (GAs), support vector machines (SVMs), etc.), from which to choose the most appropriate one to the given situation [3]. Hence, the nowadays widespread use of computer technology takes advantage of the huge computational power and the fast processing speed as compared to that of the humans, in order to minimize the possible physician's error when using a huge amount of data.

The motivation for this study is the tremendous opportunity for ML methods, within the DM field, to assist the physician deal with the flood of patient information and scientific knowledge. Its primary goal is to draw attention to the applications and challenges faced by this approach, and, secondly, to highlight its strong potential in helping to optimally solve medical decision problems. The chapter is meant for all those working in the medical field, who wish to use modern and efficient computerized tools, and, at the same time, to all researchers in the health informatics domain, who develop such "intelligent" tools.

2   Glossary and Key Terms

Biomedical Informatics: in the classical definition: "the study of biomedical information and its use in decision making…" [1];

Data Mining: "the automatic search of patterns in huge databases, using computational techniques from statistics, machine learning, and pattern recognition" [3];

Machine Learning: "the field of machine learning is concerned with the question of how to construct computer programs that automatically improve with experience" [4];

Artificial Intelligence: "learning symbolic representation of concepts. Using prior knowledge together with training data to guide learning" [4];

Supervised learning: "the process of establishing a correspondance (function) using a training set, seen as a 'past experience' of the model" [3];

Unsupervised learning: "the model is adapted to observations, being distinguished by the fact that there is no *a priori* output" [3];

Neural Networks: "represent non-programmed (non-algorithmic) adaptive information processing systems" [3];

Genetic Algorithms: "provide a learning method motivated by an analogy to biological evolution" [4];

SVMs: "is a linear machine, equipped with special features, and based on the structural risk minimization method and the statistical learning theory" [3];

Feature selection: "is used to eliminate irrelevant and redundant features, possibly causing confusion, by using specific methods" [3];

Clustering: "the method to divide a set of data (records/tuples/vectors/instances/objects/sample) into several groups (clusters), based on certain predetermined similarities" [3].

3   State-of-the-Art of ML Solutions in CAMD

The basic paradigm underlying IS can be summarized as follows. The input consists of different attributes (symptoms), while the output consists of possible diseases caused by them. After comparing a certain data corresponding to a yet undiagnosed patient with the observations and corresponding diagnoses contained in the medical database (medical data of patients), IS will provide the most probable diagnosis based on the human knowledge embedded in that database.

The use of medical datasets belonging to large data repository, such as UCI Machine Learning Repository (http://archive.ics.uci.edu/ml/), requires state-of-the-art ML techniques [1, 2]. In this context, NNs have become a popular tool for solving such tasks [5]. Belciug & El-Darzi [6] present a partially connected NN-based approach with application to breast cancer detection and recurrence. A hybrid NN/GA model is developed by Belciug & Gorunescu [7] for the same task. Andersson et al. [8] use NNs to predict severe acute pancreatitis at admission to hospital. Gorunescu et al. [9] present a competitive/collaborative neural computing system for pancreatic cancer detection. Kalteh et al. [10] present a research regarding the use of NNs to breast cancer detection. A swarm optimized NN has been used by Dheeba & Selvi [11] for micro-classification in mammograms. A novel evolutionary strategy to develop learning-based decision systems applied to breast cancer and liver fibrosis stadialization has been developed by Gorunescu & Belciug [12]. Gorunescu & Belciug [13] has proposed a new learning technique for NN, based on the Bayesian paradigm, with applications to automated diagnosis of breast cancer, lung cancer, heart attack, and diabetes. Holzinger [14] presents the interactive machine learning paradigm, which has its roots in reinforcement learning and active learning. In Holzinger et al. [15], an experimental proof of the interactive machine learning paradigm is proposed, by applying ant colony algorithms in solving the traveling salesman problem with the human-in-the-loop approach. Girardi et al. [16] use the interactive knowledge discovery with the doctor-in-the-loop in cerebral aneurysms research. Hund et al. [17] propose an interactive tool to visually explore subspace clusters from different perspectives, thus using the doctor-in-the-loop for complex patient datasets.

4   Towards Finding Solutions: The CAMD Approach

Over the last years, recent advances in DM/ML fields provided highly efficient algorithms for CAMD, with a huge impact in the health care domain. A gain in applying them lies in improving the diagnosis of different diseases, and in reducing the time pressure on physicians and nurses. Among the most common algorithms used in CAMD, one can mention NNs, SVMs, GAs, etc. This paper focuses mainly on neural computing, with the primary purpose of drawing attention to the challenges faced by this approach, and, secondary, in highlighting the strong potential of these models in supporting solutions to these medical decision problems. Figure 1 synthesizes the CAMD 'picture' "robot doctor".

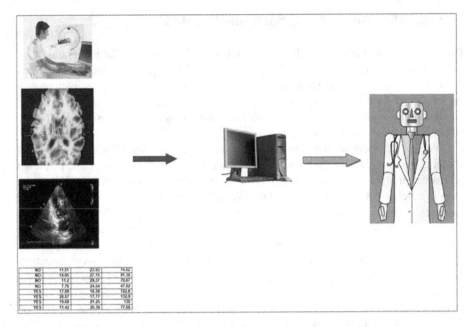

Fig. 1. Illustration of the CAMD paradigm

4.1   Area 1: Neural Networks

NN is an information-processing paradigm inspired by the way the human brain processes information. Its complex architecture consists of a large number of highly interconnected processing elements (neurons) working together to solve specific problems. The multi-layer perceptron (MLP) represents the most popular NN architecture in use today, typically consisting of a set of source units (input layer), one or more hidden layers of neurons, an output layer, and the back-propagation algorithm (BP) as learning algorithm. The radial-basis function (RBF) represents an equally appealing and intuitive alternative, consisting of a hidden layer of radial units, each actually modeling a Gaussian response surface. The probabilistic neural network (PNN) represents a completely different NN structure, the network actually learning to estimate a probability density function using the Bayes strategy and a sum of small multivariate Gaussian distributions as the activation function.

4.1.1   Area 2: Partially-Connected Neural Network (PCNN)

In paper "*A partially connected neural network-based approach with application to breast cancer detection and recurrence*", Belciug & El-Darzi [6] assess the effectiveness of a partially connected neural network (PCNN) used to detect breast cancer and recurrence. The PCNN architecture is based on a traditional MLP, trained with the BP algorithms, with the sum of squared errors (SSE) as *error (loss) function*, and using the *winner-takes-all* rule to compute the network output. The key idea behind this model is that the weights that did not suffer major modifications, i.e., did not surpass a certain threshold τ after a certain number of training samples presented to the network, are erased from the network's architecture, being inhibited.

Experimental results using four publically available breast cancer datasets from UCI Machine Learning Repository have shown that the simplified MLP architecture have proven classification performance consistent with some of the highest results obtained by using sophisticated and expensive medical imaging, such as MRI/PET methods. Compared to a fully connected NN, the results have been similar or even better, with a slight gain in CPU time.

4.1.2   Area 3: Hybrid NN-GA Algorithm (MLP-GA)

In paper "*A hybrid neural network/genetic algorithm system applied to the breast cancer detection and recurrence*", Belciug & Gorunescu [7] propose a GA-based routine to set the synaptic weights of a MLP, and use this algorithm to detect breast cancer and recurrence. While MLP has a standard architecture (SSE as *error function*, and *winner-takes-all* rule to compute the network output), a GA was especially designed to optimize the MLP weights, substituting the classical BP algorithm. In this evolutionary-based training paradigm, a weight vector is represented through a chromosome, which contains a number of genes equaling the number of neurons from the input layer multiplied by the number of neurons from the hidden layer. The weights between input units and hidden units were read off the network from top to bottom, representing the components of the weight vector $w = (w_{(x_1)1}, w_{(x_2)1}, w_{(x_3)1}, \ldots, w_{(x_n)1}, w_{(x_1)2}, w_{(x_2)2}, w_{(x_3)2}, \ldots, w_{(x_n)2})$. The model hyper-parameters, as population size, number of generations, mutation rate, etc. have been set heuristically, in order to obtain optimal performance. The classical sigmoid $f(x) = \frac{1}{(1+e^{-x})}$ has been chosen as activation function, 40% of the existing chromosomes (the best ones) have been kept for reproduction and mutation. The *arithmetic crossover/BLX-α*, the *linear BGA crossover*, the *Wright's heuristic crossover*, and the *uniform crossover* have been used as crossover operators, while the process of mutation contained two steps. Firstly, a number between 0 and 1 has been randomly generated. If the number was smaller than the standard default threshold 0.5, a subtraction has been made, otherwise an addition. Then, using the *chromosome_error* $= \frac{(100 - chromosome\_accuracy)}{100}$, each gene has been mutated according to the previous step. Applied to the four publically available breast cancer datasets mentioned above, the hybrid MLP-GA model has proven a classification accuracy that exceeded the performance of most other ML algorithms (MLP, RBF, PNN), and similar to PCNN.

4.1.3   Area 4: Radial Basis Function Network

In paper "*Radial Basis Function network-based diagnosis for liver fibrosis estimation*" Gorunescu et al. [18] assess the effectiveness of a RBF-based approach in the special case of liver fibrosis stadialization. Using data obtained by the relatively novel non-invasive technique represented by Fibroscan (Fibroscan® -Echosens, Paris, France), the study proved both the suitability of the RBF approach for the classification of liver fibrosis stages, and also highlighted the role of the Fibroscan use in liver fibrosis evaluation.

4.1.4   Area 5: Competitive/Collaborative Neural Computing System

In paper "*Competitive/Collaborative Neural Computing System for Medical Diagnosis in Pancreatic Cancer Detection*" Gorunescu et al. [9] have developed a competitive/collaborative neural computing system designed to support the medical decision process using medical imaging databases, with a concrete application in the differential diagnosis of chronic pancreatitis and pancreatic cancer. The neural computing system consists of a set of five neural network algorithms (linear neural network (LNN), MLP (3-layer/4-layer), RBF, and PNN) working in both competitive and collaborative way. In the competitive phase, the NN algorithms have been applied to the same medical dataset regarding pancreatic cancer, and they have been statistically evaluated by using differences in mean tests (*t*-test for independent samples, Mann & Whitney U test), comparing proportions (two-sided *t*-test), comparing agreements (Cohen's kappa test), and comparing performances through the area under the ROC (receiver operating characteristic) curve. Based on the statistical assessment, they have been ranked in descending order regarding their effectiveness, and the first three of them (i.e., MLP (4-layer), MLP (3-layer), and RBF) have been retained for the next stage. In the collaborative phase, using a weighted voting system (WVS), the output diagnosis of the ensemble of NNs represented the weighted vote of the computing system components. Finally, the effectiveness of such an approach in comparison to separate standalone networks has been proven by a concrete example consisting in three different testing cases (i.e., three new, unknown, patients).

4.1.5   Area 6: Tandem Feature Selection/Evolutionary-Driven NN

In paper "*Intelligent decision-making for liver fibrosis stadialization based on tandem feature selection and evolutionary-driven neural network*" Gorunescu et al. [19] propose a tandem feature selection mechanism and evolutionary-driven neural network (MLP/GA) as a computer-based support for liver fibrosis stadialization in chronic hepatitis C, using the Fibroscan device. A synergetic system, based on both specific statistical tools (discriminant function analysis-DFA, multiple linear regression (forward and backward stepwise approaches), and analysis of correlation matrix), and the sensitivity analysis provided by five neural networks (LNN, PNN, RBF, 3-MLP, and 4-MLP), has been used for reducing the dimension of the database from twenty-five to just six attributes. The experimental results have shown that the proposed tandem system has provided a significantly better accuracy than its competitors (PNN, MLP, RBF, and SVM), a relatively high computational speed, and the ability to detect the most important liver fibrosis stages, i.e., F1 -disease starting stage, and F4 -cirrhosis.

4.1.6   Area 7: Alternative Network Learning Using the Bayesian Paradigm

In paper "*Error-correction learning for artificial neural networks using the Bayesian paradigm: Application to automated medical diagnosis*", Gorunescu & Belciug [13] present an alternative to the BP learning algorithm based on the Bayesian paradigm. Thus, the Bayesian paradigm has been used to learn the weights in NNs, by considering the concept of subjective probability instead of objective probability. Based on the standard architecture of a feed-forward network (3-MLP), this approach replaces the standard updating technique of weights by using the Bayesian model. The weights are updated using their posterior probability distribution given the error function through the non-parametric Goodman-Kruskal Γ rank correlation. Technically, the rank correlation Γ between attributes and decision classes was used for the synaptic weights initialization. Next, the updating process was based on the Bayes' theorem. The synaptic weights were considered as posterior probabilities, the probabilities corresponding to a partition of the weight space were considered as prior probabilities, the probabilities of the error conditioned by the partition of the weight space represented the likelihood, and the error probability represented the evidence. The rank correlation Γ was used to estimate the above mentioned probabilities. The model assessment has been achieved through the standard 10-fold cross-validation, and the training process stopped after a fixed number of iterations. The model has been applied on six real-world publically available datasets regarding breast cancer, lung cancer, heart attack, and diabetes, and the experimental results showed that this model provided performance equaling or exceeding the results reported in literature.

4.1.7   Area 8: Cooperative Co-evolution for Classification (CCEA)

In paper *"Evolution of cooperating classification rules with an archiving strategy to underpin collaboration"*, Stoean & Stoean [20, 21] propose an evolutionary algorithm (EA)-based approach to encode rules to model the partition of the samples into categories. A typical EA would conduct to one global or local optimum, so instead a methodology to maintain several basins is put forward. The solution for the classification problem is regarded as a set of rules. This is decomposed into components (rules) and a different EA deals with the discovery of a rule. The evolution of each population is separate with the only exception of the fitness evaluation. In order to evaluate an individual (that corresponds to a rule), collaborators have to be selected from all the other populations and thus a complete set of rules is reached, which is applied on the training set and the obtained accuracy represents the evaluation. In order to conserve a diverse selection of rules, after each generation, a fixed number of best collaborators from the current population and the previous archive (chosen such that there are no two rules alike) is retained in an archive. When the evolutionary process ends, the archive represents the actual found rule set and is applied on the test set. A methodology that is endowed with feature selection is presented in [21]. The average accuracy for the breast cancer dataset is of 95.52% and the standard deviation is of 1.56%.

4.1.8   Area 9: Clustering-Based Approach

In paper *"Clustering-based approach for detecting breast cancer recurrence"*, Belciug et al. [23] assess the effectiveness of three different clustering algorithms used to detect breast cancer recurrent events. The performance of the traditional k-means algorithm has been compared with a Self-Organizing Map (SOM-Kohonen network) and with a cluster network (CN), illustrated in Fig. 2.

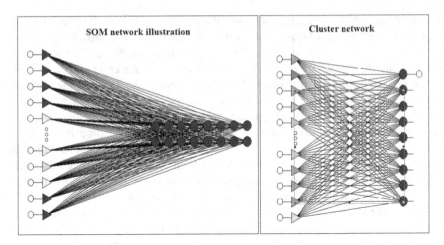

Fig. 2. Illustration of SOM and CN topologies

Using a real-world breast cancer dataset (Wisconsin Recurrence Breast Cancer) from UCI Machine Learning Repository, the experimental results have shown that, in this particular case, the CN performance, equaling 78%, was is in accordance to the reported modern medical imaging experience, while SOM provided good enough diagnosis accuracy (67%), followed by the standard k-means algorithm (62%). To conclude, from this simple experiment it came out that the three clustering models have proved a diagnosing performance comparable to the standard medical experience, but much cheaper and faster.

4.1.9   Area 10: Supervised vs. Unsupervised Neural Networks

In paper "*Assessing performances of unsupervised and supervised neural networks in breast cancer detection*" Belciug et al. [24] compare the performance of three supervised NNs (3 layer-MLP), RBF, and PNN) with the unsupervised SOM network, using the Wisconsin Prognostic Breast Cancer dataset from Machine Learning Repository. In the concrete problem regarding the breast cancer detection, the SOM model has proved a diagnosing performance comparable to the application of standard NNs. In addition, the diagnosis accuracy of SOM was in accordance with the reported modern medical imaging experience. Thus, beyond the debate that the traditional supervised NNs, and not only, are not enough biological plausible, the concept of self-organizing networks became a point of interest among researchers.

4.2   Area 11: Comparing Algorithms: A Statistical Approach

Most of the papers that are dealing with DM or ML algorithms suffer from a lack of rigor in terms of assessing their performance. Usually, the vast majority of studies regarding the application of DM/ML algorithms in health care are limited to reporting the classification accuracy along with the corresponding standard deviation. In addition, the decision summary statistics presents the total number of cases in each class, cases of each class that were correctly (and incorrectly) classified, and cases of that class which could not be classified at all (unknown cases). The most evolved of them report the following performance measures (binary classification case): confusion matrix, sensitivity and specificity, positive and negative predictive values, or even the area under the ROC curve [3]. For this reason, we present hereinafter a solution to this problem, based on a statistical analysis of the data regarding the algorithms performance.

The vast majority of ML algorithms are of stochastic nature, so they have to be independently run a sufficient number of times in order to obtain a reliable result regarding both their robustness and effectiveness. From a statistical point of view, the testing classification accuracy obtained during the multiple independent computer runs constituted a sample of decision performance. Since most of the medical databases used in experiments have a rather small size, the 10-fold cross-validation is commonly used as testing method. The classification accuracy is computed 10 times, each time leaving out one of the sub-samples and using that sub-sample as a test sample for cross-validation; therefore, each sub-sample is used 9 times as training sample and just once as testing sample. The algorithm correct classification rates, computed for each of the 10 runs of the model, are then averaged to give the 10-fold estimate of the classification accuracy. This procedure is repeated 10 times to complete a cross-validation cycle, consisting of the 10 runs of the model. It is noteworthy that, in case of relatively large databases, the holdout cross-validation is used instead of 10-fold cross-validation. In this regard, 2/3 of data form the training set, while the rest of 1/3 represents the testing set, and the process is repeated, with a random choice of samples regarding each dataset.

The benchmarking process of the algorithms involved in the study is assessed by statistical means, seen as an objective quality procedure. As mention above, the data statistically analyzed consist of samples concerning training and testing performances of each ML model, run in a certain number of complete cross-validation cycles. The benchmarking process usually envisages three aspects:

- *Data screening*, involving the suitability of the data for the type of statistical analysis that is intended;
- *Hypotheses testing*, involving the comparison between the testing performances obtained in the diagnosing process;
- *Over-learning control*, involving the analysis of the correlation between training and testing performances, enabling the statistical investigation of the model ability to generalize well on new cases.

An *a priori* statistical power analysis (*two-tailed* type of null hypothesis) is usually performed in advance with the aim to determine the appropriate sample size, i.e., the appropriate number of independent computer runs for each algorithm, in order to achieve adequate statistical power.

Data screening consists in applying classical normality tests (i.e., *Kolmogorov-Smirnov & Lilliefors* test, and *Shapiro-Wilk W* test) and the homogeneity of variances test (*Levene*'s test).

Hypotheses testing consists in using different statistical comparison tests, such as:

- *t*-test for independent samples or/and its non-parametric alternative of *Mann-Whitney U* test, *Kolmogorov-Smirnov* two-sample test (K-S), and *Wald-Wolfowitz* runs test (W-W), in case of non-normal distributions;
- Two-sided test (*z*-value) to compare the average proportions of correctly classified cases/two means;
- Cohen's *kappa* test to compare the agreement between ML models, seen as independent 'raters';
- Classical one-way ANOVA technique along with the Tukey's honestly significant difference (Tukey HSD) *post-hoc* test in order to quantify the magnitude of the contrast between the corresponding performances (more than two 'competitors').

5   Advantages and Disadvantages of CAMD

In paper "*Intelligent decision systems in medicine -a short survey on medical diagnosis and patient management*" Gorunescu [22] presents a short review regarding the applications of ML algorithms in health care. A special attention has been paid to the 'Ups and Downs' of this domain. Thus, it is noteworthy that:

- Medical diagnosis is 'subjective' and depends both on available data, and on the experience of the physician;
- Specific requirements for the ML algorithms are: (*i*) good performance (*ii*) handling missing/noisy data, (*iii*) transparency of diagnosis knowledge despite the "black-box" property of certain algorithms, (*iv*) ability to explain new patient diagnosis, (*v*) reduction of the amount of data needed/feature selection ability;
- In many cases, various classifiers perform roughly the same. However, there are significant differences between them, mostly depending on the database and data type;
- When choosing between ML techniques, physicians prefer those with high explanation ability (e.g., Bayesian decision, classification tree);
- Instead of using standalone algorithms, a better idea is to use a committee-machine approach;
- ML-based diagnosis (automated diagnosis) remains just another source of possibly useful information that helps to improve the diagnostic accuracy. The final responsibility whether to accept or reject this information belongs to the physician.

Remark. It is noteworthy that the most misplaced expectation is the idea that CAMD is intended to replace doctors in the medical decision process. On the contrary, physicians are necessarily required to make the final decision based on the computer support.

Let us also mention that the ML algorithms used within CAMD are often based on heuristics. Therefore, despite their well-known effectiveness and easy-to-use in clinical research, one can be cautious with their decision, which should always be censored by the human specialist.

5.1 Area 1: Note on Privacy

In CAMD, it is mandatory to consider possible implications regarding privacy when using medical datasets. Medical records contain personal information that can be used for unethical purposes. For this reason, in all developed countries, the respective governments and other official institutions have considered strict regulations regarding the use of such data.

In paper "*Ethical issues in electronic health records; A general overview*", Ozair et al. [25] discuss various ethical issues faced by the wide nowadays use of medical data obtained from electronic health records.

In paper "*Privacy-preserving data publishing: a survey of recent developments*", Fung et al. [26] systematically summarize and evaluate different approaches regarding privacy-preserving data publishing, and analyse challenges in practical data publishing and other issues related to the use of collections of digital information.

In paper [27] "*The right to be forgotten: Towards Machine Learning on perturbed knowledge bases*" it is disscused the effect of the perturbed/anonymized knowledge on the results of four machine learning techniques.

6 Conclusion and Future Outlook

Clinical databases store large amounts of information of all kinds about patients and their medical conditions. State-of-the-art ML techniques are designed to deal with this information in order to discover relationships and patterns which are helpful in studying the progression and the management of diseases.

In this context, it is noteworthy to mention the existence of powerful research groups within well-established universities, working in developing effective intelligent decision systems, based on ML technologies, for medical decision-making. Among well-known examples of such groups, we mention the research group *Clinical Decision Making*, within the *Computer Science and Artificial Intelligence Laboratory*, Massachusetts Institute of Technology-MIT, USA, "dedicated to exploring and furthering the application of technology and artificial intelligence to clinical situations" - https://www.csail.mit.edu/, http://groups.csail.mit.edu/medg/. In addition, one can mention *Human-Computer Interaction and Knowledge Discovery/Data Mining*-http://hci-kdd. org/, *Image Sciences Institute*-http://www.isi.uu.nl/Research/Themes/CAD/, and *Cornell University Vision and Image Analysis Group* - http://www.via.cornell.edu/research/.

Some of the most important research themes approached in about thirty years of using Artificial Intelligence tools in health care are reviewed in [28]. The conclusion of this survey is that "There has been a major shift from knowledge-based to data-driven methods, while the interest for other research themes such as uncertainty management, image and signal processing, and natural language processing has been stable since the early 1990s".

Nowadays, researchers have to cope with collections of large and complex datasets, difficult to be processed with traditional tools. In this context, by "big data" we commonly understand the tools, processes, and techniques enabling to create, manipulate and manage very large datasets. In the "big data" era, health care informatics has been significantly grown, and a large amount of digital health care and medical data is produced [29].

To conclude, there are many challenges in dealing with big data. The ultimate goal of future research in this domain is to bridge physicians, DM/ML and medical informatics communities to foster interdisciplinary studies between the three research groups.

References

1. Shortliffe, E., Cimino, J. (eds.): Biomedical Informatics: Computer Applications in Health Care and Biomedicine, 4th ed. Springer, London (2014)
2. Holzinger, A.: Biomedical Informatics: Discovering Knowledge in Big Data. Springer, New York (2014). doi:10.1007/978-3-319-04528-3
3. Gorunescu, F.: Data Mining: Concepts, Models and Techniques. Springer, Heidelberg (2011/2013)
4. Mitchell, T.M.: Machine Learning. McGraw-Hill, Boston (1997)
5. Amato, F., Lopez, A., Pena-Mendez, E.M., et al.: Artificial neural networks in medical diagnosis. J. Appl. Biomed. 11, 47–58 (2013)
6. Belciug, S., El-Darzi, E.: A partially connected neural network-based approach with application to breast cancer detection and recurrence. In: Proceedings of the 5th IEEE Conference on Intelligent Systems-IS, 7–9 July 2010, London, UK, pp. 191–196 (2010)
7. Belciug, S., Gorunescu, F.: A hybrid neural network/genetic algorithm system applied to the breast cancer detection and recurrence. Expert Syst. 30(3), 243–254 (2013)
8. Andersson, B., Andersson, R., Ohlsson, M., Nilsson, J.J.: Prediction of severe acute pancreatitis at admission to hospital using artificial neural networks. Pancreatology 11, 328–335 (2011)
9. Gorunescu, F., Gorunescu, M., Saftoiu, A., Vilmann, P., Belciug, S.: Competitive/collaborative neural computing system for medical diagnosis in pancreatic cancer detection. Expert Syst. 28(1), 33–44 (2011)
10. Kalteh, A.A., Zarbakhsh, P., Jirabadi, M., Addeh, J.: A research about breast cancer detection using different neural networks and K-MICA algorithm. J. Cancer Res. Ther. 9(3), 456–466 (2013)
11. Dheeba, J., Selvi, S.T.: A swarm optimized neural network system for classification of microcalcification in mammograms. J. Med. Syst. 36(5), 3051–3061 (2012)

12. Gorunescu, F., Belciug, S.: Evolutionary strategy to develop learning-based decision systems. Application to breast cancer and liver fibrosis stadialization. J. Biomed. Inform. **49**, 112–118 (2014)
13. Gorunescu, F., Belciug, S.: Error-correction learning for artificial neural networks using the Bayesian paradigm. Application to automated medical diagnosis. J. Biomed. Inform. **52**, 329–337 (2014)
14. Holzinger, A.: Interactive Machine Learning for Health Informatics: when do we need the human-in-the-loop? Springer Brain Inform. (BRIN) **3**(2), 119–131 (2016). doi:10.1007/s40708-016-0042-6
15. Holzinger, A., Plass, M., Holzinger, K., Crişan, G.C., Pintea, C.-M., Palade, V.: Towards interactive Machine Learning (iML): applying ant colony algorithms to solve the traveling salesman problem with the human-in-the-loop approach. In: Buccafurri, F., Holzinger, A., Kieseberg, P., Tjoa, A.M., Weippl, E. (eds.) CD-ARES 2016. LNCS, vol. 9817, pp. 81–95. Springer, Heidelberg (2016). doi:10.1007/978-3-319-45507-5_6
16. Girardi, D., Kung, J., Kleiser, R., Sonnberger, M., Csillag, D., Trenklwe, J., Holzinger, A.: Interatcive knowledge discovery with the doctor-in-the-loop: a practical example of cerebral aneurysms research. Brain Inform. **3**, 1–11 (2016). doi:10.1007/s40708-016-0038-2
17. Hund, M., Bohm, D., Sturm, W., Sedlmair, M., Schreck, T., Ullrich, T., Keim, D.A., Majnaric, L, Holzinger, A.: Visual analytics for concept exploration in subspaces of patient groups: Making sense of complex datasets with the Doctor-in-the loop. Brain Inform., 1–15 (2016). doi:10.1007/s40708-016-0043-5
18. Gorunescu, F., Belciug, S., Gorunescu, M., Lupsor, M., Badea, R., Ştefanescu, H.: Radial basis function network-based diagnosis for liver fibrosis estimation. In: Proceedings of the 2nd International Conference on e-Health and Bioengineering-EHB 2009, 17–18th September, 2009, IaşiConstanţa, Romania, Ed. UMF "Gr.T. Popa" Iasi, pp. 209–212 (2009)
19. Gorunescu, F., Belciug, S., Gorunescu, M., Badea, R.: Intelligent decision-making for liver fibrosis stadialization based on tandem feature selection and evolutionary-driven neural network. Expert Syst. Appl. **39**(17), 12824–12832 (2012)
20. Stoean, C., Stoean, R.: Evolution of cooperating classification rules with an archiving strategy to underpin collaboration. In: Teodorescu, H.N., Watada, J., Jain, L. (eds.) Intelligent Systems and Technologies - Methods and Applications. SCI, vol. 217, pp. 47–65. Springer, Heidelberg (2009)
21. Stoean, C., Stoean, R., Lupsor, M., Stefanescu, H., Badea, R.: Feature selection for a cooperative coevolutionary classifier in liver fibrosis diagnosis. Comput. Biol. Med. **41**(4), 238–246 (2011)
22. Gorunescu, F.: Intelligent decision systems in Medicine -a short survey on medical diagnosis and patient management (*keynote speech*). In: Proceedings of the 5th IEEE International Conference on "E-Health and Bioengineering"-EHB 2015, 19–21 November 2015, Iasi, Romania, pp. 1–8 (2015)
23. Belciug, S., Gorunescu, F., Gorunescu, M., Salem, AB.: Clustering-based approach for detecting breast cancer recurrence. In: Proceedings of the 10th IEEE International Conference on Intelligent Systems Design and Applications-ISDA10, 29 November–1 December 2010, Cairo, pp. 533–538 (2010)
24. Belciug, S., Gorunescu, F., Gorunescu, M., Salem, A., B.: Assessing performances of unsupervised and supervised neural networks in breast cancer detection. In: Proceedings of the 7th IEEE International Conference on Informatics and Systems-INFOS 2010. Advances in Data Engineering and Management-ADEM, 28–30 March 2010, Cairo, pp. 80–87 (2010)
25. Ozair, F., Jamshed, N., Sharma, A., Aggarwal, P.: Etical issues in electronic health records: A general overview. Perspect. Clin. Res. **6**(2), 73–76 (2015)

26. Fung, B., Wang, K, Chen, R., Yu, P.: Privacy-preserving data publishing: a survey of recent developments. ACM Comput. Surv. **42**(4), 14:1–14:53 (2010)
27. Malle, B., Kieseberg, P., Weippl, E., Holzinger, A.: The right to be forgotten: towards machine learning on perturbed knowledge bases. In: Buccafurri, F., Holzinger, A., Kieseberg, P., Tjoa, A.M., Weippl, E. (eds.) CD-ARES 2016. LNCS, vol. 9817, pp. 251–266. Springer, Heidelberg (2016). doi:10.1007/978-3-319-45507-5_17
28. Peek, N., Combi, C., Marin, R., Bellazzi, R.: Thirty years of artificial intelligence in medicine (AIME) conferences: a review of research themes. Artif. Intell. Med. **65**(1), 61–73 (2015)
29. Yang, C., Veltri, P.: Intelligent healthcare informatics in big data era. Artif. Intell. Med. **65**(2), 75–77 (2015)

Processing Neurology Clinical Data for Knowledge Discovery: Scalable Data Flows Using Distributed Computing

Satya S. Sahoo[1,2(✉)], Annan Wei[2], Curtis Tatsuoka[3],
Kaushik Ghosh[4], and Samden D. Lhatoo[3]

[1] Division of Medical Informatics, Department of Epidemiology
and Biostatistics, School of Medicine, Case Western Reserve University,
Cleveland, OH, USA
satya.sahoo@case.edu
[2] Department of Electrical Engineering and Computer Science,
School of Engineering, Case Western Reserve University, Cleveland, OH, USA
annan.wei@case.edu
[3] Department of Neurology, Epilepsy Center, University Hospitals Case
Medical Center, Cleveland, OH, USA
curtis.tatsuoka@case.edu,
Samden.Lhatoo@uhhospitals.org
[4] Department of Mathematical Sciences, University of Nevada,
Las Vegas, NV, USA
kaushik.ghosh@unlv.edu

Abstract. The rapidly increasing capabilities of neurotechnologies are generating massive volumes of complex multi-modal data at a rapid pace. This neurological big data can be leveraged to provide new insights into complex neurological disorders using data mining and knowledge discovery techniques. For example, electrophysiological signal data consisting of electroencephalogram (EEG) and electrocardiogram (ECG) can be analyzed for brain connectivity research, physiological associations to neural activity, diagnosis, and care of patients with epilepsy. However, existing approaches to store and model electrophysiological signal data has several limitations, which make it difficult for signal data to be used directly in data analysis, signal visualization tools, and knowledge discovery applications. Therefore, use of neurological big data for secondary analysis and potential development of personalized treatment strategies requires scalable data processing platforms. In this chapter, we describe the development of a high performance data flow system called Signal Data Cloud (SDC) to pre-process large-scale electrophysiological signal data using open source Apache Pig. The features of this neurological big data processing system are: (a) efficient partitioning of signal data into fixed size segments for easier storage in high performance distributed file system, (b) integration and semantic annotation of clinical metadata using an epilepsy domain ontology, and (c) transformation of raw signal data into an appropriate format for use in signal analysis platforms. In this chapter, we also discuss the various challenges being faced by the biomedical informatics community in the context of Big Data, especially the increasing need to ensure data quality and scientific reproducibility.

© Springer International Publishing AG 2016
A. Holzinger (Ed.): ML for Health Informatics, LNAI 9605, pp. 303–318, 2016.
DOI: 10.1007/978-3-319-50478-0_15

Keywords: Electrophysiological signal data · Epileptic seizure networks · Neurology · Clinical research · Apache pig · Distributed computing

1   Introduction and Motivation

The Brain Research through Advancing Innovative Neurotechnologies (BRAIN) initiativeannounced by the US President in 2013 has defined an ambitious vision to understand how individual neural cells and complex neural networks interact to accelerate neuroscience research [1]. The BRAIN initiative aims to undertake a comprehensive effort similar to the Human Genome Project (HGP) to facilitate new discoveries in neuroscienceand potentially facilitatedevelopment of new treatment mechanisms for a range of neurological disorders. The rapid increase in the capabilities of neurotechnologies is enabling us to collect neuroscience data at unprecedented levels of granularity, for example real time functional Magnetic Resonance Imaging (fMRI) and intracranial electroencephalogram (EEG) provide high quality data corresponding to complexbrain activities [2, 3]. One of the key advantages of this neuroscience "Big Data" is the ability to derive actionable information from analysis of statistically significant volumes of data that can also support knowledge discovery applications [2, 4]. However, the large volume and rapid rate of multi-modal neuroscience data generation has made it difficult to process and analyze these datasets using existing neuroscience data processing tools [5]. The limitations of existing data processing tools make it difficult to define new data-driven research techniques for variety of neuroscience applications, for example mapping brain activities derived from fMRI to task complexities using adaptive testing, computing anatomical connections between different brain regions using diffusion MRI [6], and computing brain connectivity measures from EEG data [7].

Computing functional connectivity measures is important for characterizingthe extent of seizure networks in epilepsy patients. Epilepsy is one of the most common serious neurological disease affecting more than 50 million persons worldwide with 200,000 new cases diagnosed each year [8]. Patients with epilepsy suffer from repeated "seizures" that are caused by abnormal electrical activity, which arerecorded as EEG recordings using electrodes implanted on the brain surface (scalp electrodes) or within the brain (intracranial electrodes). Electrophysiological signal data are interpreted by signal processing algorithms to detect important events, such as the start or end of epileptic seizures, and are also manually reviewed by domain experts to characterize the extent of the "seizure network" [9]. Accurate characterization ofthe spatial and temporal characteristics of seizure networks is important for diagnosis and treatment of epilepsy patients, including prescribing anti-epileptic medication and making appropriate decisions related to surgical interventions [10]. In addition to epilepsy, the growing role of signal data analysis in evaluating brain trauma, for example concussions in sports medicine, and imaging data for brain function tests in neurodegenerative diseases (e.g. Alzheimer's disease) make it important to develop efficient data processing pipelines to support neuroscience Big Data applications [11].

However, there are several key data processing challenges that impede the effective use of large-scale signal data for computing brain connectivity measures. For example, signal data is often stored in European Data Format (EDF) files that collate signal data in a contiguous order corresponding to all recording channels [12], which makes it difficult to efficiently extract specificsegment of signal data for secondary analysis. In addition, an EDF file stores all data recorded during a recording session as a single unit, which makes it difficult for analysis applications to process and interpret specific segments of data. The rapidly increasing volume of signal data, which is highlighted by the more than 32 TB of signal data collected at the University Hospitals of Cleveland (USA) Epilepsy Center, makes it extremely difficult for existing data processing tools to efficiently store and retrieve signal data for visualization or analysis. Specific neuroscience applications, for example computation of functional connectivity measures using phase synchronization, generalized synchronization or regression methods [7] requires efficient and scalable data processing techniques. In our ongoing research project, we are using non-linear correlation coefficient measures to compute functional connectivity between different brain regions involved in onset and propagation of epilepsy seizures.

To compute correlation measures between two channels requires several pre-processing steps to address the limitations of the default format of EDF files used to store signal data, including:

1. Data corresponding to specific signal channels (e.g., data recorded from two brain locations Gx and Gy) need to be extracted from an EDF record that stores signal data from all channels contiguously;
2. Segments of signal data corresponding to seizure eventsneed to be extracted for computing the connectivity measures during seizures;
3. The EDF file stores signal values as "raw" binary values that need to be transformed into appropriate numeric values;
4. Finally, the clinical events detected by physicians in the signal data (e.g., occurrence of an epilepsy seizure) are stored separately from an EDF file. Therefore, the clinical annotations need to be integrated with the signal data for subsequent analysis.

However, processing large volumes of EDF files and computing correlation coefficient values over large EDF files (e.g., 3 GB files) with more than 170 signal channels with large number of combinatorial selections is a complex taskand cannot be done manually by neuroscience researchers. Therefore, we have developed a two-phase data processing approach to address these challenges, which consists of: (1) development of a new JSON-based signal data representation format that supports partitioning signal data into smaller segments with integrated clinical annotations describing seizure-related events; and (2) development of highly scalable data pre-processing pipeline using Apache Pig that can leverage commodity hardware for distributed data processing.

Our two-phasedata flowaims toenable neuroscience researchers to effectively leverage the growing volume of signal data for brain connectivity research in various research applications. We developed and evaluated our two-phase data processing pipeline using de-identified SEEG data, which was collected in the epilepsy center at the University Hospitals of Cleveland.The performance of the data processing pipeline was evaluated using more than 700 GB of data to simulate real world scenario [13].

The different computational functions of the two-phase data flow wereevaluated to demonstrate the scalability of our implementation by effectively leveraging the capabilities of a multi-node Hadoop cluster.The Apache Pig system features high level programming constructs defined using the Pig Latin language to describe complex data processing tasks, which are automatically compiled into MapReduce tasks by the Pig compiler [14]. Each MapReduce task corresponds to the well-known two-step distributed computing programming approach developed by Google for extremely large volumes of data [15].

Apache Pig is an open source system that features a set of built-in data processing tasks and User Defined Functions (UDF), which allows users to develop customized data processing functions. The primary advantage of Apache Pig is that it allows users to define scalable and customized data processing pipelines for various domains, for example neuroscience signal processing. Our two-phase scalable signal data processing pipeline can be readily integrated with multiple functional connectivity computation workflows that aim to analyze specific segments of signal data using different functional connectivity measures. We note that functional connectivity measures can be computed using other neuroscience data modalities, including functional Magnetic Resonance Imaging (fMRI) for real time adaptive evaluation. Although the current version of our approach does not support other data modalities, weare extending our data processing pipeline to compute functional connectivity using fMRI data as part of ongoing research. This will allow researchers with limited programming experienceto easily construct scalable data processing pipelinesusing high-level programming constructs defined in Apache Pig.

2 Glossary and Key Terms

Brain Connectivity: represents connections between different locations of the brain that are derived from various brain activities (also called functional connectivity) or anatomical connections (also called structural connectivity) [16];

Functional connectivity: Functional connectivity represents correlated brain activity recorded from different brain regions using different modalities, for example SEEG and fMRI [17, 18];

Electrophysiological Signal Data: record the electrical signals produced in biological systems, for example signal data recorded as electroencephalogram (EEG) data using scalp or intracranial electrodes implanted in brain [17];

European Data Format (EDF): is a widely used file format for storage of electrophysiological signal data. EDF files store information corresponding to predefined metadata fields (both study and channel-specific record) and raw signal data in binary format [12];

Biomedical Ontology: is a formal representation of biomedical information using knowledge representation languages such as the Web Ontology Language (OWL) that can be consistently and accurately interpreted by software tools [19];

Epilepsy: is a serious neurological disorder characterized by abnormal electrical brain signalsthat cause repeated seizures and manifest as physical or behavioral changes. Epilepsy affects more than 50 million persons worldwide [20];

Epilepsy Seizure Network: consists of different brain regions that participate in epileptic seizures and are characterized by coupling or synchronization [17];

Neuroscience Big Data: is characterized by the growing volume of multi-modal neuroscience data being generated at a rapid rate bya new generation of neurotechnologies, which record data at high level of granularity [5];

Apache Hadoop: is an open source implementation of the Google MapReduce distributed computing approach consisting of repeated two steps of Map and Reduce to process extremely large volumes of data [21];

Apache Pig: is a dataflow system consisting of data manipulation functions using Pig Latin program that are used to describe data processing steps. Apache Pig functions are converted into MapReduce programs by the Pig compiler [14];

Hadoop Cluster: consists of multiple computing nodes that are physically connected with built-in support for redundancy and load balancing to enable distributed analysis of large-scale data.

3   Related Work: Processing Neurological Data for Brain Connectivity Research

High performance distributed computing approaches are being increasingly used to process and analyze neuroscience data, for example use of Apache Spark for mapping brain activity in model organisms [22]. Clusters of Graphical Processing Unit (GPU) have been used to process large volumes of EEG data [23, 24] and data analysis [25]. GPU and Apache Spark algorithms are also being used to process and analyze neuroimaging datasets generated in the Human Connectome Project (HCP) [26]. The HCP is a multi-institutional initiative to map both functional and structural networks of human brain using advanced imaging techniques that provide extremely high spatial resolution with faster imaging frequency [3]. To process the extremely large volume of neuroimaging data, the HCP researchers have developed scalable pipelines to compute functional connectivity using fMRI data stored in the Neuroimaging Informatics Technology Initiative (NIfTI) format. The pipeline uses a distributed NIfTI reader written in Scala for Apache Spark that can be subsequently analyzed using the GraphX library [26].

Network analysisis an intuitive approach for modeling brain connectivity structures with brain regions represented as nodes and structural or functional connections between the nodes represented as edges [17]. Brain connectivity researchers use various measures to evaluate functional networks, for example the number of edges between nodes, number of edge hops connecting two nodes and even clustering coefficient measures corresponding to total number of triangles in a network. In epilepsy seizure network-related research, three primary networks are usually used namely, "regular networks" with high path density between brain regions, "random networks" with paths connecting brain regions with some probability, and "small-world network" that have short paths and high clustering coefficients [27]. Research in functional connectivity measures, which are derived from EEG data, aim to accurately characterize the spatial and temporal properties of seizure networks in epilepsy neurological disorder.

In patients with "focal epilepsy", abnormal electrical activity called seizures originate in specific brain regions and may or may not involve other brain regions over a period of time. The brain regions involved in the initial and subsequent stages of the seizures constitute a seizure network with brain regions represented as nodes and propagation paths of seizures represented as edges. An important neuroscience challenge is to precisely localize the origin of seizure and its subsequent propagation using spatial and temporal properties of electrical activity recorded across different brain regions [9, 27]. The accurate characterization of seizure network is important to identify brain tissues responsible for epileptic seizures and to subsequently remove them during surgery to help patients who do not respond to anti-epileptic drugs [7]. Our research is focused on using high resolution SEEG that precisely records electrical activity in specific brain region to characterize seizure networks and facilitate accurate identification of brain regions involved in seizures [28].

Our work in the development of distributed and parallel data processing pipelines for multi-modal neuroscience data is related to the general approach of using high performance computing techniques deployed over commodity hardware. However, our data processing pipeline effectively uses new data partitioning techniques for segmenting electrophysiological datainto smaller fragments that can be processed and analyzed in parallel for scalability. At present, we are not aware of any existing work that uses distributed computing approaches with data partitioning techniquesto process and analyze signal data for computing functional connectivity using Apache Pig. Another key feature of our data processing pipeline is the use an Epilepsy and Seizure Ontology (EpSO) [29] as standardized terminological system for clinical events detected in signal data. EpSO is a domain ontology modeled using the description logic-based W3C Web Ontology Language (OWL2) [30] to represent the well-known four-dimensional classification system of epilepsy together with brain anatomy, drug information, and genetic information. The use of EpSO for annotating SEEG data allows easier retrieval of specific signal segments annotated with relevant clinical events and facilitates data integration of signal data generated from multiple sources.

4 A Modular and Scalable Data Flow for Processing Neuroscience Data

To develop our two-phase data processing pipeline, we used de-identified signal data from a 44 years old female epilepsy patient with intractable focal epilepsy (patient did not respond to anti-epileptic medications) as test case. The patient was evaluated for surgical intervention using stereotactically placed symmetric depth electrodes in both left and right insular region of the patient's brain [31]. The SEEG signal data was de-identified to remove protected health information (PHI) and eight EDF files were created with each file corresponding to an occurrence of seizure in the patient. The two-fold objectives of the data flow development process were to identify data processing bottlenecks in the pipeline and to address these bottlenecks using distributed computing techniques. The output of the data processing pipeline was used as input data to thedata flow for computing functional connectivity measures using non-linear correlation coefficient. The complete data processing and analysis pipeline consists of three distinct steps (illustrated in Fig. 1):

1. **Step 1: Pre-processing of SEEG data** to partition signal data in an EDF file into smaller time segments (default of 30 s), integrate the clinical annotations stored in a separate file with the signal data, transform the layout of signal data corresponding to channel-oriented structure and compute numeric values from raw binary signal data;
2. **Step 2: Transform and aggregate channel-specific data** to allow computation of the nonlinear correlation coefficient and store them as Javascript Object Notation (JSON) files;
3. **Step 3: Compute the degree of co-occurrence of signals at two locations Gx and Gy** representing functional connectivity to facilitate characterization of the spatial and temporal characteristics of seizure networks. These functional connectivity measures will help identify candidate brain locations for surgery in focal epilepsy patients who do not respond to anti-epileptic medications.

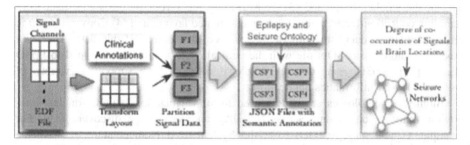

Fig. 1. The three steps constituting the data processing and analysis pipeline for SEEG data to compute functional connectivity measure

4.1   Computing Functional Connectivity Measures

Nonlinear correlation coefficientis used to compute the degree of co-occurrence between signals X(t) and Y(t) recorded at two brain locations Gx and Gy [7]. The equation:

$$h_{XY}^2(\tau) = 1 - Var(Y\,(t\,+\,\tau)\,|\,X\,(t) \div Var\,(Y\,(t\,+\,\tau))$$

gives the non-linear measure of association between the two signals at time lag of τ in the direction of Gx to Gy. The maximum of this nonlinear measure computed over all possible lag values of τgives the overall measure of association from region Gx to Gy and is computed as follows:

$$h_{XY}^2 = \max \tau_{min} < \tau < \tau_{max} h_{XY}^2(\tau)$$

The resulting h^2_{XY} value is called the nonlinear correlation coefficient in the direction from Gx to Gy. The value of h^2_{XY} varies from 0 to 1, where 0 represents no association between signal recorded at G_X, Gy and 1 represents perfect correlation between the signals recorded at the two locations.

To identify the performance bottlenecks of the functional connectivity pipeline, we processed and analyzed all the twelve EDF files generated from the insular epilepsy patient. The results of the evaluation demonstrated thatStep 1 and Step 2 required-significantly more time to process signal data as compared to Step 3. For example, it requires nearly 40 min to process a single 1.26 GB EDF file and approximately 30 min to process a smaller 830 MB sized EDF file (a detailed description of the evaluation results for various sizes of signal data is presented in our paper [13]). Clearly, this is a significant bottleneck to rapidly process and analyze large volumes of signal data for computing functional connectivity. Therefore, there is a clear need to address the computational bottleneck in Step 1and Step 2 to process large volumes of signal data.

We have developed a scalable data processing pipeline for signal data consisting of four modules that support the following functionalities: (1) Partitioning the signal data in an EDF file into smaller segments, (2) Integration of clinical annotations with signal data in the smaller segments, (3) Transforming the layout of the signal data from sampling collection-based layout to channel-oriented layout, and (4) Conversion of the binary raw signal data into numeric values. The final output of this data processing pipeline is stored asa JSON file with the clinical event annotations mapped to EpSO classes [29]. EpSO is a domain ontology developed to support a variety of epilepsy-focused informatics applications.

Biomedical ontologies are widely used in informatics applications for data integration, ontology-based data access (OBDA), and knowledge discovery [19]. For example, Gene Ontology (GO) [32], the Systematized Nomenclature of Medicine Clinical Terms (SNOMED CT) [33], and the Human Phenotype Ontology (HPO) [34] are widely used in biomedical informatics applications as common reference terminological systems. The use of EpSO classes to semantically annotate clinical events in signal data allows the data processing pipeline toreconcile terminological heterogeneity in signal data collected from different sources (for example in multi-center clinical research projects). The use of OWL2 to model epilepsy-related terms in EpSO also allows software tools to use reasoning rules during query and retrieval of signal data segments corresponding to specific clinical events [29].

The use of EpSO to annotate signal data highlights the key role of common terminology in biomedical data processing pipeline. In addition to signal data, there has been extensive work in use of biomedical ontologies to annotate gene expression data [35], protein function data [36], and the increasing use of SNOMED-CT to annotate clinical research data extracted from Electronic Health Records (EHR). The use of EpSO classes significantly improves data harmonization in neuroinformatics applications, however the data processing bottleneck identified in Step 1 and Step 2 requires the use of distributed computing techniques. We describe this Apache Pig-based scalable data processing pipeline in the next section.

4.2   Scalable Data Processing Using Apache Pig

Various components of the Hadoop technology stack are being increasingly used in scientific applications to develop highly scalable data flow pipelines that can effectively leverage distributed computing techniques. The Hadoop MapReduce programming approach parallelizes data processing and analysis tasks over hundred or thousands of computing nodes to help address the challenges of data and compute intensive tasks in the scientific community [15]. Apache Pig is an open source dataflow system that allows users to use high-level programming constructs to compose data processing functions into a multi-step pipeline [14]. Apache Pig is a component of the Hadoop technology stack. We use the Apache UDF feature (described earlier in Sect. 1) to define customized functions for processing signal data. These signal data-specific UDFs, which are part of the NeuroPigPen toolkit [13], are automatically compiled into MapReduce tasks by the Pig compiler [14].

The NeuroPigPen toolkit consists of five modules that are customized to support loading, parsing, processing, and partitioning signal data:

1. **PigSignalLoad:** The PigSignalLoadmoduleextends the Hadoop *InputFormat* and *RecordReader* Application Programming Interface (API) for reading and parsing EDF files. The load module locates and integrates the clinical event annotation files, which are stored separately from the EDF file, into a single file.
2. **PigSignalReader:** The PigSignalReader module supports the extraction of meta-data values associated with signal data, for example sampling rate of each signal channel, the specific category of electrode used to record the signal data, the physical and digital minimum as well as maximum values. The PigSignalReader module can be used as a standalone tool to read and process signal data.
3. **PigSignalPartitioner:** The PigSignalPartitioner module addresses the need to partition large volumes of signal data stored in an EDF file into smaller segments, which can be processed and analyzed in a distributed computing infrastructure. This module partitions the signal data into smaller segments with the size of each segment configured as a user-defined parameter in terms of time duration (for example, 30 s duration). After partitioning the data into smaller segments, this module adds the signal metadata information together with clinical annotations extracted by the PigSignalReader module. The output of this module is processed in the next step of the data flow pipeline by the PigSignalProcessor module.
4. **PigSignalProcessor:** The PigSignalProcessor module transforms the layout of the signal data from the default EDF file format, which stores the signal data as contiguous values recorded from all channels, into channel-oriented layout. The channel-oriented layout stores all the data recorded from a single channel contiguously. The PigSignalProceesor module also transforms the signal data from a binary format into numeric format and "digital values" to "physical values" [12] to allow functional connectivity tools to directly use the signal data without the need for additional processing.
5. **PigSignalCSFGenerator:** The PigSignalCSFGenerator module generates the JSON files corresponding to the partitioned and transformed signal data, which

contains appropriate metadata information to allow these file segments to be self-descriptive. These JSON files correspond to a new format called Cloudwave Signal Format (CSF) developed in our previous work [37] to support signal data processing in a distributed computing environment as well as used by different neuroscience research applications.

The NeuroPigPen toolkit was designed to be a highly scalable data processing pipeline with support for deployment in Hadoop clusters with different number of computing nodes. To evaluate the performance of this data processing pipeline, we processed the twelve de-identified EDF files (described earlier in Sect. 1) using a sequential data processing approach and Apache Pig. The data was processed over a 31-node Hadoop cluster at our High Performance Computing Cluster (HPCC) using Cloudera CDH 5.4 distribution. Each Data node in the Hadoop cluster has a dual Xeon E5450 3.0 GHz processor with 8 cores per processor, 16 GB memory, and 2 TB disk storage. The Hadoop Name node has a dual Xeon 2.5 GHz E5-2450 processor with 16 cores, 64 GB memory, and 1 TB disk storage. The nodes are connected by 10 gigabits network connection. We used a HDFS replication factor of three to store the datasets in the HPCC cluster. The results reported in this section are the average value of three executions on the HPCC cluster.

The results (Fig. 2) clearly show a significant gain in time performance for the 12 EDF files, which vary in size from 362.8 MB to 1.36 GB. The Apache Pig implementation reduces the time taken to process the data from 36.28 min to 1.54 min for the largest EDF file with size of 1.36 GB, which is 40 times faster as compared to the sequential data processing implementation. We note that there is significant improvement in time performance even for the smallest EDF file with size of 362.8 MB from 11.22 min to 0.96 min, which is 11 times faster as compared to the sequential implementation. We demonstrated the scalability of the data processing pipeline in our

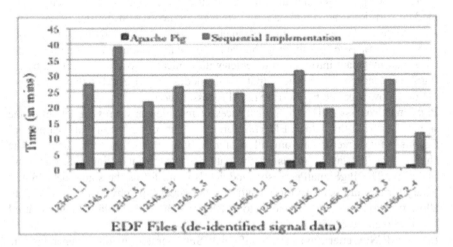

Fig. 2. A comparative evaluation of processing time for 12 EDF files with different sizes using Apache Pig and sequential evaluation demonstrates the significant improvement in data processing time.

previous work using more than 700 GB of de-identified signal data [13]. We used EDF files with different sizes ranging from 248 MB to 19.6 GB and clustered them into five datasets with sizes 1 GB, 50 GB, 100 GB, 500 GB, and 750 GB. The NeuroPigPen was also evaluated using five different configurations of Hadoop consisting of 3, 6, 12, 18, 24, and 30 Data nodes. The results from these evaluations demonstrated that the NeuroPigPen toolkit met its design objectives.

As part of our ongoing research, we are exploring the use of distributed computing approaches to compute the functional connectivity measure also. The NeuroPigPen toolkit is a real world and practical example of multi-modal data processing pipelines being developed in biomedical informatics using distributed computing techniques to address the challenges of biomedical Big Data. In the next section, we discuss some of the existing and future challenges in biomedical data processing that requires the development of new data flows that support various data mining and knowledge discovery applications in biomedical research [38–40].

5 Current and Future Challenges

The unprecedented growth in the volume and variety of neuroscience data is opening new avenues for researchers to address the societal grand challenge of understanding the complex dynamics of human brain. High-resolution multi-modal data ranging from imaging to multi-channel electrophysiology signal data are providing unique new insights into the structure and functions of human brain. Integrative analysis of structural and functional brain connectivity network data has the potential to make critical advances in understanding the role of brain connectivity in complex neurological disorders affecting millions of persons worldwide. However, neuroscience researchers face critical challenges in effectively leveraging this new paradigm of neuroscience Big Data due to lack of scalability of existing neuroinformatics tools. This is clearly demonstrated in the domain of epilepsy seizure network research that requires the analysis of extremely large volumes of high-resolution signal data collected using multiple electrodes implanted in human brain during pre-surgical evaluation of epilepsy patients. Results from our research project demonstrate that many challenges posed by biomedical Big Data can be effectively addressed through use of new distributed computing techniques. However, there are several existing challenges that need to be addressed by the biomedical informatics research community and we discuss some of these challenges in the next few sections.

5.1 Towards Effective Secondary Use of Biomedical Data: Challenges in Sharing and Integration of Data

Biomedical research projects often involve multiple research centersand data from each center needs to be aggregated and integrated into a common repository for query and analysis by the project team members. In addition to multi-center research projects, there is a growing need to integrate data collected across different projects into publicly accessible repositories to allow the biomedical research community to leverage the large volume of existing study data [41]. For example, the US National Institutes of Health (NIH) has funded the development of one of the largest data repositories for sleep medicine research called the National Sleep Research Resource (NSRR) that aims to aggregate and integrate study data from 50,000 studies [42]. Integration of large volumes of disparate datasetsrequires processing the source data and using common terminology for subsequent querying. However, there are no existing best practices that can easily define mappings for domain-specific data collected from different sources. Therefore, there is a clear need to develop scalable data processing and integration tools for managing large biomedical datasets for data repositories such as NSRR.

Biomedical ontologies can play a significant role in development of data processing and integration tools for large-scale datasets, which was demonstrated in our neuroinformatics project through the use of EpSO. However, the development of appropriate domain ontologies to support large-scale data integration requires significant time and effort with close collaboration between computer science and biomedical domain experts. This bottleneck can be effectively addressed through re-use of terms from existing biomedical ontologies, for example SNOMED CT is comprehensive with wide coverage of the clinical research domain that may be used for integrating large datasets. In addition to biomedical ontologies, controlled vocabularies with simpler structure and minimal formal semantics can also be used for processing and integrating data. For example, the US NIH has initiated a project to develop Common Data Elements (CDE) to facilitate uniform data collection and storage in research project. Although CDEs can help address some of the challenges associated with integrating disparate datasets, they require additional data processing steps to reconcile data heterogeneity in comparison to biomedical ontologies.

5.2 Provenance Metadata-Aware Biomedical Data Processing for Scientific Reproducibility

Provenance metadata describes the history or origin of data and it plays an important role in ensuring data quality and supporting scientific reproducibility [43]. Collecting and integrating provenance information with biomedical data processing pipeline is important to ensure that researchers using integrated biomedical data repositories can access information describing the techniques used to collect biomedical data in the original study. Provenance metadata is often represented using the W7 model consisting of information describing "who", "where", "why", "which", "what", "how", and "when" [44]. There has been extensive work in use of provenance metadata in scientific workflow systems used to process and analyze scientific data, including biomedical datasets [45]. There is an increasing need to incorporate provenance information in biomedical data processing pipeline especially in healthcare and clinical research applications. The development of the World Wide Web Consortium (W3C) PROV specifications has allowed the use of a common provenance model, which can be extended to represent domain-specific provenance information, to facilitate interoperability [43].

Provenance information describing the context of the biomedical data needs to be propagated together with the data through the various stages of data processing. The size and heterogeneity of the provenance information collected by different centers or sourced from different projects increases the computational complexity of data processing pipelines. As the volume of biomedical data increases, the size of provenance information associated with data also increases to incorporate detailed description of the dataset (also called fine-level provenance versus coarse-level provenance). Therefore, it is important to design and implement scalable data processing pipeline that can be extended to incorporate provenance metadata. The role of provenance metadata in supporting scientific reproducibility is an area of active research that has led to development of clinical research-focused provenance models [37].

5.3   Privacy of Patients in Context of Biomedical Data Processing and Analysis

The widespread adoption of electronic health records in the US and other countries has highlighted the need to protect patient privacy [41]. Data processing pipeline need to be aware of the critical importance of preserving privacy and security of protected health information (PHI) of patients. Removal of PHI from healthcare and biomedical dataset that is used outside of the original research study is an essential part of the data-processing pipeline. The accurate identification and removal of PHI using automated tools is an area of active research in biomedical informatics due to the challenges associated with identifying PHI related data in unstructured or semi-structured datasets. Many data processing pipelines used for biomedical data with PHI requires manual validation, which may be bottleneck for Big Data applications.

Many biomedical data integration applications often rely on an "honest broker" to access medical record information and remove identifiable information to generate de-identified data for use by researchers. Big Data applications require the development of new approaches that scale with the increasing volume of biomedical data while ensuring the privacy of patients. The design of effective biomedical data processing pipeline needs to incorporate privacy preserving features without adding to the complexity of processing and integrating large data.

6   Conclusion

In this chapter, we describe the development of a scalable data processing pipeline for neuroscience data to support brain connectivity research. The data processing pipeline transforms electrophysiological signal data collected from epilepsy patients into appropriate format to allow computation of functional connectivity measures between different brain regions. The functional connectivity measures, which are derived from EEG data, are used to characterize the spatio-temporal properties of epilepsy seizure networks. The signal data-processing pipeline is implemented using Apache Pig, which is an open source high-level distributed computing system, to process large scale signal data. The data processing pipeline has been systematically evaluated using more than 700 GB of signal data. The data processing pipeline uses an epilepsy domain ontology called EpSO to semantically annotate signal data, which allow easier querying and retrieval of signal data. We also discuss some of the challenges faced in development of biomedical data processing systems, for example the role of biomedical ontologies for data integration, provenance metadata to ensure data quality and scientific reproducibility, and the challenges associated with preserving privacy of patients during processing of biomedical data.

Acknowledgements. This work is supported in part by the National Institutes of Biomedical Imaging and Bioengineering (NIBIB) Big Data to Knowledge (BD2 K) grant (1U01EB020955) and the National Institutes of Neurological Disorders and Stroke (NINDS) Center for SUDEP Research grant (1U01NS090407-01).

References

1. Brain Research through Advancing Innovative Neurotechnologies (BRAIN). The White House, Washington, D.C. (2013)
2. Bargmann, C., Newsome, W., Anderson, D., et al.: BRAIN 2025: a scientific vision. US National Institutes of Health 2014
3. Marcus, D.S., Harwell, J., Olsen, T., Hodge, M., Glasser, M.F., Prior, F., Jenkinson, M., Laumann, T., Curtiss, S.W., Van Essen, D.C.: Informatics and data mining tools and strategies for the human connectome project. Front. Neuroinformatics 5 2011
4. Agrawal, D., Bernstein, P., Bertino, E., Davidson, S., Dayal, S., Franklin, M., Gehrke, J., Haas, L., Halevy, A., Han, J., Jagadish, H.V., Labrinidis, A., Madden, S., Papakonstantinou, Y., Patel, J.M., Ramakrishnan, R., Ross, K., Shahabi, C., Suciu, D., Vaithyanathan, S., Widom, J.: Challenges and Opportunities with Big Data. Purdue University 2011
5. Sejnowski, T.J., Churchland, P.S., Movshon, J.A.: Putting big data to good use in neuroscience. Nature Neurosci. **17**, 1440–1441 (2014)
6. Hagmann, P., Jonasson, L., Maeder, P., Thiran, J.P., Wedeen, V.J., Meuli, R.: Understanding diffusion MR imaging techniques: from scalar diffusion-weighted imaging to diffusion tensor imaging and beyond. RadioGraphics **26**, 205–223 (2006)
7. Wendling, F., Ansari-Asl, K., Bartolomei, F., Senhadji, L.: From EEG signals to brain connectivity: a model-based evaluation of interdependence measures. J. Neurosci. Methods **183**, 9–18 (2009)
8. Epilepsy Foundation. http://www.epilepsyfoundation.org/aboutepilepsy/whatisepilepsy/statistics.cfm. Accessed May 3, 2016
9. Wendling, F., Bartolomei, F., Senhadji, L.: Spatial analysis of intracerebral electroencephalographic signals in the time and frequency domain: identification of epileptogenic networks in partial epilepsy. Philos. Tansa. Maths Phys. Eng. Sci. **367**, 297–316 (2009)
10. Fisher, R.S.: Emerging antiepileptic drugs. Neurology **43**, 12–20 (1993)
11. Wagenaar, J.B., Brinkmann, B.H., Ives, Z., Worrell, G.A., Litt, B.: A multimodal platform for cloud-based collaborative research. In: Presented at the 6th International IEEE/EMBS Conference on Neural Engineering (NER), San Diego, CA (2013)
12. Kemp, B., Olivan, J.: European data format 'plus' (EDF+), an EDF alike standard format for the exchange of physiological data. Clin. Neurophysiol. **114**, 1755–1761 (2003)
13. Sahoo, S.S., Wei, A., Valdez, J., Wang, L., Zonjy, B., Tatsuoka, C., Loparo, K.A., Lhatoo, S.D.: NeuroPigPen: a data management toolkit using hadoop pig for processing electrophysiological signals in neuroscience applications. Front. Neuroinformatics (2016)

14. Gates, A.F., Natkovich, O., Chopra, S., Kamath, P., Narayanamurthy, S.M., Olston, C., Reed, B., Srinivasan, S., Srivastava, U.: Building a high-level dataflow system on top of Map-Reduce: the Pig experience. In: 35th International Conference on Very Large Data Bases, Lyon, France, pp. 1414–1425 (2009)
15. Dean, J., Ghemawat, S.: MapReduce: a flexible data processing tool. Commun. ACM **53**, 72–77 (2010)
16. Friston, K.J.: Functional and effective connectivity: a review. Brain Connectivity **1**, 13–36 (2011)
17. Kramer, M.A., Cash, S.S.: Epilepsy as a disorder of cortical network organization. Neuroscientist **18**, 360–372 (2012)
18. Rogers, B.P., Morgan, V.L., Newton, A.T., Gore, J.C.: Assessing functional connectivity in the human brain by fMRI. Magn. Reson. Imaging **25**, 1347–1357 (2007)
19. Bodenreider, O., Stevens, R.: Bio-ontologies: Current trends and future directions. Briefings Bioinform. **7**, 256–274 (2006)
20. Fisher, R.S., Boas, W.E., Blume, W., Elger, C., Genton, P., Lee, P.Engel, Jr., J.: Epileptic Seizures and epilepsy: definitions proposed by the international league against epilepsy (ILAE) and the international bureau for epilepsy (IBE). Epilepsia **46**, 470–472 (2005)
21. Dean, J.: Challenges in building large-scale information retrieval systems. In: Invited Talk, ed. ACM International Conference on Web Search and Data Mining (WSDM) (2009)
22. Freeman, J., Vladimirov, N., Kawashima, T., Mu, Y., Sofroniew, N.J., Bennett, D.V., Rosen, J., Yang, C.T., Looger, L.L., Ahrens, M.B.: Mapping brain activity at scale with cluster computing. Nat. Methods **11**, 941–950 (2014)
23. Chen, D., Wang, L., Ouyang, G., Li, X.: Massively parallel neural signal processing on a many-core platform. Comput. Sci. Engg. **13**, 42–51 (2011)
24. Wang, L., Chen, D., Ranjan, R., Khan, S.U., KolOdziej, J., Wang, J.: Parallel processing of massive EEG data with MapReduce. presented at the ICPADS (2012)
25. Wu, Z., Huang, N.E.: Ensemble empirical mode decomposition: a noise-assisted data analysis method. Adv. Adapt. Data Anal. **1**, 1–41 (2009)
26. Boubela, R.N., Kalcher, K., Huf, W., Našel, C., Moser, E.: Big data approaches for the analysis of large-scale fMRI data using apache spark and GPU processing: a demonstration on resting-state fMRI data from the human connectome project. Front. Neurosci. 9 (2016)
27. Guye, M., Bettus, G., Bartolomei, F., Cozzone, P.J.: Graph theoretical analysis of structural and functional connectivity MRI in normal and pathological brain networks. Magn. Reson. Mater. Phys., Biol. Med. **23**, 409–421 (2010)
28. Yang, S., Tatsuoka, C., Ghosh, K., Lacuey-Lecumberri, N., Lhatoo, S.D., Sahoo, S.S.: Comparative Evaluation for Brain Structural Connectivity Approaches: Towards Integrative Neuroinformatics Tool for Epilepsy Clinical Research. In: Presented at the AMIA 2016 Joint Summits on Translational Science, San Francisco, CA (2016)
29. Sahoo, S.S., Lhatoo, S.D., Gupta, D.K., Cui, L., Zhao, M., Jayapandian, C., Bozorgi, A., Zhang, G.Q.: Epilepsy and seizure ontology: towards an epilepsy informatics infrastructure for clinical research and patient care. J. Am. Med. Inform. Assoc. **21**, 82–89 (2014)
30. Hitzler, P., Krötzsch, M., Parsia, B., Patel-Schneider, P.F., Rudolph, S.: OWL 2 web ontology language primer. In: World Wide Web Consortium W3C2009
31. Lacuey, N., Zonjy, B., Kahriman, E.S., Marashly, A., Miller, J., Lhatoo, S.D., Lüders, H.O.: Homotopic reciprocal functional connectivity between anterior human insulae. Brain Struct. Funct. **221**, 1–7 (2015)

32. Ashburner, M., Ball, C.A., Blake, J.A., Botstein, D., Butler, H., Cherry, J.M., Davis, A.P., Dolinski, K., Dwight, S.S., Eppig, J.T., Harris, M.A., Hill, D.P., Issel-Tarver, L., Kasarskis, A., Lewis, S., Matese, J.C., Richardson, J.E., Ringwald, M., Rubin, G.M., Sherlock, G.: Gene ontology: tool for the unification of biology. The gene ontology consortium. Nat. Genet. **25**, 25–29 (2000)

33. Rector, A.L., Brandt, S., Schneider, T.: Getting the foot out of the pelvis: modeling problems affecting use of SNOMED CT hierarchies in practical applications. J. Am. Med. Inform. Assoc. **18**, 432–440 (2011)

34. Köhler, S., Doelken, S.C., Mungall, C.J., et al.: The human phenotype ontology project: linking molecular biology and disease through phenotype data. Nucleic Acids Res. **42**, 966–974 (2014)

35. Diehn, M., Sherlock, G., Binkley, G., Jin, H., Matese, J.C., Hernandez-Boussard, T., Rees, C.A., Cherry, J.M., Botstein, D., Brown, P.O., Alizadeh, A.A.: SOURCE: a unified genomic resource of functional annotations, ontologies, and gene expression data. Nucleic Acids Res. **31**, 219–223 (2003)

36. Xie, H., Wasserman, A., Levine, Z., Novik, A., Grebinskiy, V., Shoshan, A., Mintz, L.: Large-scale protein annotation through gene ontology. Genome Res. **12**, 785–794 (2002)

37. Jayapandian, C., Wei, A., Ramesh, P., Zonjy, B., Lhatoo, S.D., Loparo, K., Zhang, GQ, Sahoo, S.S.: A scalable neuroinformatics data flow for electrophysiological signals using MapReduce. Front. Neuroinformatics 9 (2015)

38. Yildirim, P., Majnaric, L., Ekmekci, I.O., Holzinger, A.: Knowledge discovery of drug data on the example of adverse reaction prediction. BMC Bioinform. **15**, S7 (2014)

39. Holzinger, A.: Trends in interactive knowledge discovery for personalized medicine: cognitive science meets machine learning. IEEE Intell. Inf. Bull. **15**, 6–14 (2014)

40. Preuß, M., Dehmer, M., Pickl, S., Holzinger, A.: On terrain coverage optimization by using a network approach for universal graph-based data mining and knowledge discovery. In: Ślezak, D., Tan, A.-H., Peters, James, F., Schwabe, L. (eds.) BIH 2014. LNCS (LNAI), vol. 8609, pp. 564–573. Springer, Heidelberg (2014). doi:10.1007/978-3-319-09891-3_51

41. Holdren, J.P., Lander, E.: Realizing the full potential of health information technology to improve healthcare for americans: the path forward. PCAST Report, Washington, D.C. (2010)

42. Dean, D.A., Goldberger, A.L., Mueller, R., Kim, M., Rueschman, M., Mobley, D., Sahoo, S.S., Jayapandian, C.P., Cui, L., Morrical, M.G., Surovec, S., Zhang, G.Q., Redline, S.: Scaling up scientific discovery in sleep medicine: the National Sleep Research Resource. Sleep **39**, 1151–1164 (2016)

43. Lebo, T., Sahoo, S.S., McGuinness, D.: PROV-O: The PROV Ontology. World Wide Web Consortium W3C2013

44. Goble, C.: Position statement: musings on provenance, workflow and (semantic web) annotations for bioinformatics. In: Workshop on Data Derivation and Provenance, Chicago (2002)

45. Missier, P., Sahoo, S.S., Zhao, J., Goble, C., Sheth, A.: Janus: from Workflows to semantic provenance and linked open data. In: Presented at the IPAW 2010, Troy, NY (2010)

Network-Guided Biomarker Discovery

Chloé-Agathe Azencott[1,2,3(✉)]

[1] CBIO-Centre for Computational Biology, MINES ParisTech,
PSL-Research University, 35 rue St Honoré, 77300 Fontainebleau, France
chloe-agathe.azencott@mines-paristech.fr
[2] Institut Curie, 75248 Paris Cedex 05, France
[3] INSERM, U900, 75248 Paris Cedex 05, France

Abstract. Identifying measurable genetic indicators (or biomarkers) of a specific condition of a biological system is a key element of precision medicine. Indeed it allows to tailor diagnostic, prognostic and treatment choice to individual characteristics of a patient. In machine learning terms, biomarker discovery can be framed as a feature selection problem on whole-genome data sets. However, classical feature selection methods are usually underpowered to process these data sets, which contain orders of magnitude more features than samples. This can be addressed by making the assumption that genetic features that are linked on a biological network are more likely to work jointly towards explaining the phenotype of interest. We review here three families of methods for feature selection that integrate prior knowledge in the form of networks.

Keywords: Biological networks · Structured sparsity · Feature selection · Biomarker discovery

1 Introduction and Motivation

Therapeutic development today is largely based on large-scale clinical trials and the average responses of thousands of people. However, a large number of medical conditions have no satisfactory treatment, and when treatment is available, many patients either do not respond or experience unacceptable side effects [1]. This is explained both by variations in environment and life styles between individuals, and by their genetic differences. As a consequence, precision medicine, which aims at tailoring preventive and curative treatments to patients based on their individual characteristics, is gaining considerable momentum. At its core, it relies on identifying features, genetic or otherwise, that correlate with risk, prognosis or response to treatment. Here we are interested in the identification, from large whole-genome dataset, of *genetic* features associated with a trait of interest. Such features, which can be used to aid diagnostic, prognostic or treatment choice, are often refered to as *biomarkers.*

Biomarker discovery, which can be framed as a *feature selection* problem, depends on collecting considerable amounts of molecular data for large numbers of individuals. This is being enabled by thriving developments in genome

© Springer International Publishing AG 2016
A. Holzinger (Ed.): ML for Health Informatics, LNAI 9605, pp. 319–336, 2016.
DOI: 10.1007/978-3-319-50478-0_16

sequencing and other high-throughput experimental technologies, thanks to which it is now possible to accumulate tens of millions of genomic descriptors (such as single-nucleotide polymorphisms or copy number variations of the DNA, gene expression levels, protein activities, or methylation status) for thousands of individuals [2]. However, these technological advances have not yet been accompanied by similarly powerful improvements in the methods used to analyze the resulting data [3].

One of the major issues we are facing is that feature selection methods suffer from a small sample size problem: they are statistically underpowered when the dimensionality of the data (the number of biomarkers to investigate) is orders of magnitude larger than the number of samples available. This is one of the reasons behind the relative failure of genome-wide association studies to explain most of the genetic heredity of many complex traits [4].

This problem can be addressed by using *prior biological knowledge*, which reduces the space of possible solutions and helps capturing relevant information in a statistically sound fashion. When a human expert is available, this is a typical application case for interactive machine learning [5], where a domain expert drives a heuristic procedure to reduce the complexity of the search space. This type of "doctor-in-the-loop" approach has recently been successfully applied in the clinic [6]. However, such analyses are currently restricted to relatively small numbers of a variables (61 in the example cited above) and it is not always possible to involve an expert directly. Hence, we will focus on using prior knowledge compiled in databases.

Because genes do not work in isolation, but rather cooperate through their interaction (physical, regulatory, or through co-expression) in cellular pathways and molecular networks, this prior biological knowledge is often available in a structured way, and in particular under the form of networks. Examples include the STRING database [7], which contains physical and functional interactions, both computationally predicted and experimentally confirmed, for over 2,000 organisms, or BioGRID [8], which includes interactions, chemical associations, and post-translational modifications from the literature. In addition, systems biologists are building specialized networks, focused on the pathways involved in a particular disease. One example of such networks is ACSN [9], a comprehensive map of molecular mechanisms implicated in cancer. These gene-gene interaction networks can be used to define networks between genomic descriptors, by mapping these descriptors to genes, using for instance in the case of SNPs a fixed-size window over the genetic sequence, and connecting together all descriptors mapped to the same gene, and all descriptors mapped to either of two interacting genes [10]. We will here make the assumption that genetic features that are linked on such a network are more likely to work jointly towards explaining the phenotype of interest, and that such effects would otherwise be missed when considering them individually.

This chapter focuses on methods for feature selection that integrate prior knowledge as networks. Compared to pathway-based approaches, which assess whether predefined sets of genes are associated with a given trait, network-based approaches introduce flexibility in the definition of associated gene sets. We will review three families of approaches, namely post-hoc analyses, regularized regression and penalized relevance, before presenting their multi-task versions and discussing open problems and challenges in network-guided biomarker discovery.

2 Glossary and Key Terms

Feature selection: In machine learning, feature selection [11] aims at identifying the most important features in a data set and discarding those that are irrelevant or redundant. This framework is clearly well-suited to the identification of biologically relevant features.

Sparsity: A model is said to be sparse when it only contains a small number of non-zero parameters, with respect to the number of features that can be measured on the objects this model represents [12]. This is closely related to feature selection: if these parameters are weights on the features of the model, then only the few features with non-zero weights actually enter the model, and can be considered selected.

Genome-Wide Association Study (GWAS): GWAS are one of the prevalent tools for detecting genetic variants associated with a phenotype. They consist in collecting, for a large cohort of individuals, the alleles they exhibit across of the order of $250,000$ to several millions of Single Nucleotide Polymorphisms (SNPs), that is to say, individual locations across the genome where nucleotide variations can occur. The individuals are also phenotyped, meaning that a trait of interest (which can be binary, such as disease status, or continuous, such as age of onset) is recorded for each of them. Statistical tests are then run to detect associations between the SNPs and the phenotype. A recent overview of the classical GWAS techniques can be found in [13].

Graph/Network: A graph (network) $(\mathcal{V}, \mathcal{E})$ consists of a set of vertices (nodes) $\mathcal{V}$ and a set of edges (links) $\mathcal{E}$ made of pairs of vertices. If the pair is ordered, then the edge is directed; otherwise, it is undirected. A graph with no directed edge is called undirected; unless otherwise specified, this is the type of graph we consider here. We use the notation $i \sim j$ to denote that vertex i and vertex j form an edge in the graph considered.

Adjacency matrix: Given a graph $(\mathcal{V}, \mathcal{E})$, its adjacency matrix is a square matrix $W \in \mathbb{R}^{d \times d}$, where $d = |\mathcal{V}|$ is the number of vertices, and $W_{ij} \neq 0$ if and only if there is an edge between the i-th and the j-th elements of $\mathcal{V}$. $W_{ij} \in \mathbb{R}$ represents the weight of edge (i, j). If all non-zero entries of W are equal to 1, the graph is said to be unweighted.

Network module: Given a graph $G = (\mathcal{V}, \mathcal{E})$, a graph $G' = (\mathcal{V}', \mathcal{E}')$ is said to be a subgraph of G if and only if $\mathcal{V}'$ is a subset of $\mathcal{V}$ and $\mathcal{E}'$ is a subset of $\mathcal{E}$. In systems biology, the term "network module" refers to a subgraph of a biological network whose nodes work together to achieve a specific function. Examples of modules include transcriptional modules, which are sets of co-regulated genes that share a common function, or signaling pathways, that is to say chains of interacting proteins that propagate a signal through the cell. In the context of biomarker discovery, we are interested in finding modules of a given biological network that are associated with the phenotype under study.

Graph Laplacian: Given a graph G of adjacency matrix $W \in \mathbb{R}^{d \times d}$, the Laplacian [14] of G is defined as $L := D - W$, where D is a $d \times d$ diagonal matrix with diagonal entries $D_{ii} = \sum_{j=1}^{d} W_{ij}$. The graph Laplacian is analog to the Laplacian operator in multivariable calculus, and similarly measures to what extent a graph differs at one vertex from its values at nearby vertices. Given a function $f : \mathcal{V} \mapsto \mathbb{R}$, $f^{\top} L f$ quantifies how "smoothly" f varies over the graph [15].

Submodularity: Given a set $\mathcal{V}$, a function $\Phi : 2^{\mathcal{V}} \to \mathbb{R}$ is said to be submodular if for any $\mathcal{S}, \mathcal{T} \subseteq \mathcal{V}$, $\Phi(\mathcal{S}) + \phi(\mathcal{T}) \geq \Phi(\mathcal{S} \cup \mathcal{T}) + \Phi(\mathcal{S} \cap \mathcal{T})$. This property is also referred to as that of diminishing returns. Given a graph G and its adjacency matrix W, an example of submodular function is the function $\Phi : \mathcal{S} \mapsto \sum_{p \in \mathcal{S}} \sum_{q \notin \mathcal{S}} W_{pq}$. In the case of equality, i.e. $\Phi(\mathcal{S}) + \phi(\mathcal{T}) = \Phi(\mathcal{S} \cup \mathcal{T}) + \Phi(\mathcal{S} \cap \mathcal{T})$ for any $\mathcal{S}, \mathcal{T} \subseteq \mathcal{V}$, Φ is said to be *modular*. In this case, the value of Φ over a set is equal to the sum of its values over items of that set. The cardinality function $\Phi : \mathcal{S} \mapsto |\mathcal{S}|$ is a simple example of a modular function. Submodular functions play an important role in optimization [16] and machine learning [17].

3   State of the Art

3.1   Network-Based Post-analysis of Association Studies

We start by describing methods that have been developed for the network-based analysis of GWAS outcomes; these methods can easily be extended to other type of biomarkers. These approaches start from a classical, single-SNP GWAS, in which the association of each SNP with the phenotype is evaluated thanks to a statistical test. This makes it possible to leverage state-of-the-art statistical tests that, for example, account for sample relatedness [18], address issues related to correlation between markers (linkage disequilibrium) [19], or are tailored to the discovery of rare variants [20]. In addition, they can easily be applied without access to raw data, only on the basis of published summary statistics. Their goal is to find modules of a given gene-gene network that concentrate more small p-values than would be expected by chance.

The first step is to map all SNPs from the dataset to genes, and to summarize the p-values of all SNPs mapped to a given gene as a unique gene p-value. This summary can be based for example on the minimum, maximum, or average p-value. A popular alternative consists in using VEGAS, which accounts for linkage disequilibrium between markers [21].

Several search methods have been proposed to find modules of significantly associated genes from such data. In dmGWAS [22], the authors use a dense module searching approach [23] to identify modules that locally maximize the proportion of low p-value genes. This search algorithm is greedy. It considers each gene in the network as a starting seed, from which it grows modules by adding neighboring genes to the set as long as adding them increases the module's score by a given factor.

An alternative approach, first proposed in [24] and refined in PINBPA [25], relies on a simulated annealing search called JActiveModule and first proposed for the discovery of regulatory pathways in protein-protein interaction networks [26].

Finally, GrandPrixFixe [27] uses a genetic algorithm for its search strategy.

Limitations. Because exact searches are prohibitively expensive in terms of calculations, these approaches rely on heuristic searches that do not guarantee that the top-scoring module is found. Let us note however that any highly scoring module that is detected with such an approach is bound to be, if not biologically, at least statistically interesting. Methods exist to identify top-scoring sub-networks exactly, but they are too computationally intensive to have been applied to GWAS at this point [28]. An other way to mitigate this issue is to predefine potential modules of interest [29], but this strongly limits the flexibility offered by the use of networks rather than of predefined gene sets. Finally, these computational issues limit their application to networks defined over genes rather than directly over biomarkers.

More importantly, such methods rely on single-locus association studies, and are hence unsuited to detect interacting effects of joint loci. The failure to account for such interacting effects is advanced as one of the main reasons why classical GWAS often does not explain much of the heritability of complex traits [4,30].

3.2   Regularized Linear Regression

So-called embedded approaches for feature selection [11] offer a way to detect combinations of variants that are associated with a phenotype. Indeed, they learn which features (biomarkers here) contribute best to the accuracy of a machine learning model (a classifier in the case of case/control studies, or a regressor in the case of a quantitative phenotype) while it is being built.

Regularization. Within this framework, the leading example is that of linear regression [31]. Let us assume the available data is described as $(X, \boldsymbol{y}) \in \mathbb{R}^{n \times m} \times \mathbb{R}^n$, that is to say as n samples over a m biomarkers (X), together with their phenotypes ($\boldsymbol{y}$). A linear regression model assumes that the phenotype can be explained as a linear function of the biomarkers:

$$y_i = \sum_{p=1}^{m} X_{ip}\beta_p + \epsilon_i, \tag{1}$$

where the regression weights $\beta_1, \ldots, \beta_m$ are unknown parameters and ϵ_i is an error term. Note that we can equally assume that the mean of y is 0, or that the first of the m biomarkers is a mock feature of all ones that will serve to estimate the bias of the model. The least-squares methods provides estimates of $\beta_1, \ldots, \beta_m$ by minimizing the least-square objective function (or data-fitting term) given in matrix form by Eq. (2):

$$\underset{\beta \in \mathbb{R}^m}{\arg\min} \|X\beta - y\|_2^2. \tag{2}$$

When $m \gg n$, as it is the case in most genome-wide biomarker discovery datasets, Eq. (2) has an infinite set of solutions. In order to *regularize* the estimation procedure, one can add to the least-square objective function a *penalty term*, or *regularization term*, that will force the regression weights to respect certain constraints. A very popular regularizer is the l_1-norm of β, $\|\beta\|_1 = \sum_{p=1}^m |\beta_p|$, which has the effect of shrinking the β_p coefficients and setting a large number of them to zero, hence achieving feature selection: the features with zero weights do not enter the model and can hence be rejected. This results in the lasso [31], which estimates the regression weights by solving Eq. (3). The reason for using the l_1-norm, rather than the l_0-norm which counts the number of variables that enter the model and hence directly enforces sparsity, is that with the l_0-norm the resulting objective function would be non-convex, making its minimization very challenging computationally.

$$\underset{\beta \in \mathbb{R}^m}{\arg\min} \|X\beta - y\|_2^2 + \lambda \|\beta\|_1. \tag{3}$$

Here, $\lambda \in \mathbb{R}^+$ is a parameter which controls the balance between the relevance and the regularization terms.

Many other regularizers have been proposed, to satisfy a variety of constraints on the regression weights, and have led to many contributions for the analysis of GWAS data [32–36].

Network regularizers. In particular, it is possible to design regularizers that force the features that are assigned non-zero weights to follow a given underlying structure [37,38]. In the context of network-guided biomarker discovery, we will focus on regularizers $\Omega(\beta)$ that penalize solutions in which the selected features are not connected over a given network.

We are now assuming that we have access to a biological network over the biomarkers of interest. Such a network can usually be built from a gene interaction network [10].

A first example of such approaches is the Overlapping Group Lasso [39]. Supposing that the m markers are grouped into r groups $\{G_1, G_2, \ldots, G_r\}$, which can overlap, we denote by $\mathcal{V}_G$ the set of r-tuples of vector $v = (v_u)_{u=1, \cdots r}$ such that v_u is non-zero only on features belonging to group u. The Overlapping Group Lasso penalty, defined by Eq. (4), induces the choice of weight vectors β that can be decomposed in r weight vectors $v = (v_u)_{u=1, \cdots r}$ such that some of the v_u are equal to zero. This limits the non-zero weights to only some of the groups. If each network edge defines a group of two biomarkers, then this method can be applied to network-guided biomarker discovery, where it will encourage the selection of biomarkers belonging to the same group, i.e. linked by an edge.

$$\Omega_{\text{ogl}}(\boldsymbol{\beta}) = \inf_{v \in \mathcal{V}_\mathcal{G} : \sum_{u=1}^{r} v_u = \boldsymbol{\beta}} \sum_{u=1}^{r} ||v_u||_2 \,. \tag{4}$$

Another way to smooth regression weights along the edges of a predefined network, while enforcing sparsity, is a variant of the Generalized Fused Lasso [40]. The corresponding penalty is given by Eq. (5). The resulting optimization problem is typically solved using proximal methods such as the fast iterative shrinkage-thresholding algorithm (FISTA) [41]. While it has not been applied to biomarker discovery to the best of our knowledge, [42] successfully applied this approach to Alzheimer's disease diagnostic from brain images.

$$\Omega_{\text{gfl}}(\boldsymbol{\beta}) = \sum_{p \sim q} |\beta_p - \beta_q| + \eta \, ||\boldsymbol{\beta}||_1 \,. \tag{5}$$

Alternatively, based on work on regularization operators by Smola and Kondor [15], Grace [43,44] uses a penalty based on the graph Laplacian L of the biological network, which encourages the coefficients $\boldsymbol{\beta}$ to be smooth on the graph structure. This regularizer is given by Eq. (6), and yields a special case of the recently proposed Generalized Elastic Net [45]. It penalizes coefficient vectors $\boldsymbol{\beta}$ that vary a lot over nodes that are linked in the network. The corresponding optimization problem can be solved through a coordinate descent algorithm [46]. Grace was applied to gene-gene networks, but can theoretically be extended to other types of networks of biomarkers; the aGrace variant allows connected features to have effects of opposite directions.

$$\Omega_{\text{grace}}(\boldsymbol{\beta}) = \boldsymbol{\beta}^\top L \boldsymbol{\beta} = \sum_{p,q} W_{pq}(\beta_p - \beta_q)^2 \tag{6}$$

These approaches are rather sensitive to the quality of the network they use, and might suffer from bias due to graph misspecification. GOSCAR [47] was proposed to address this issue, and replaces the term $|\beta_p - \beta_q|$ in Eq. (5) with a non-convex penalty: $\max(|\beta_p|, |\beta_q|) = \frac{1}{2}(|\beta_p + \beta_q| + |\beta_p - \beta_q|)$. The authors solve the resulting optimization problem using the alternating direction method of multipliers (ADMM) [48,49].

Finally, while the previous approaches require to build a network over biomarkers, the Graph-Guided Group Lasso [50] encourages genes connected on the network to be selected in and out of the model together (graph penalty), and biomarkers attached to a given gene to be either selected together or not at all (group penalty). Supposing that the m biomarkers are grouped into r mutually exclusive genes $\{G_1, G_2, \ldots, G_r\}$, and calling $\boldsymbol{\beta}_{G_u}$ the coefficient vector $\boldsymbol{\beta}$ restricted to its entries in G_u, the Graph-Guided Group Lasso penalty is given by Eq. (7). As Grace's, this optimization problem can be solved with a coordinate descent algorithm.

$$\Omega_{\text{gggl}}(\boldsymbol{\beta}) = \sum_{u=1}^{r} \sqrt{|G_u|} \, ||\boldsymbol{\beta}_{G_u}||_2 + \eta_1 \, ||\boldsymbol{\beta}||_1 + \eta_2 \frac{1}{2} \sum_{\substack{p \in G_u, q \in G_v \\ G_u \sim G_v}} W_{uv}(\beta_p - \beta_q)^2. \tag{7}$$

Limitations. In practice, we found that the computational burden was a severe limitation to applying the Overlapping Group Lasso and Grace to the analysis of more than a hundred thousand markers [10]. On a similar note, the experiments presented in [47] used at most 8,000 genes; the graph-guided group lasso [50] used 1,000 SNPs only; and the work in [42] used 3,000 voxels to describe brain images. It is therefore unclear whether these methods can scale up to several hundreds of thousands of markers.

While these computational issues might be addressed by using more powerful solvers or parallel versions of the algorithms, these regularized linear regression approaches also suffer from their inability to guarantee their *stability* as feature selection procedures, meaning their ability to retain the same features upon minor perturbations of the data. These algorithms are typically highly unstable, often yielding widely different results for different sets of samples relating to the same phenotype [51]. There is hope that the use of structural regularizers, such as those we defined above, can address this phenomenon by helping the selection of "true" features, but ranking features based on t-test scores often still yields the most stable selection in practice [52,53].

Finally, it is interesting to note that biomarkers are often represented as categorical variables (such as the presence or absence of a mutation, or the number of minor alleles observed in the case of SNPs). Applying linear (or logistic) regressions in this context, although not entirely meaningless, can be considered an unsatisfying choice.

3.3 Penalized Relevance

Let us assume data is described over a set $\mathcal{V}$ of m features. The penalized relevance framework proposes to carry out feature selection by identifying the subset S of $\mathcal{V}$ that maximizes the sum of a data-driven *relevance function* and a domain-driven *regularizer*.

The relevance function $R : 2^{\mathcal{V}} \rightarrow \mathbb{R}$ quantifies the importance of a set of features with respect to the task under study. It can be derived from a measure of correlation, or a statistical test of association between groups of features and a phenotype.

Our objective is to find the set of features $S \subseteq \mathcal{V}$ that maximizes R under structural constraints, which we model, as previously, by means of a regularizer $\Phi : 2^{\mathcal{V}} \rightarrow \mathbb{R}$, which promotes sparsity patterns that are compatible with a priori knowledge about the feature space. A simple example of regularizer computes the cardinality of the selected set. More complex regularizers can be defined to enforce a specific structure on S, and in particular a network structure [10]. We hence want to solve the following problem:

$$\arg\max_{S \subseteq \mathcal{V}} R(S) - \lambda \Phi(S). \tag{8}$$

Here again, $\lambda \in \mathbb{R}^+$ is a parameter which controls the balance between the relevance and the regularization terms.

This formulation is close to that of the regularized linear regression presented in Sect. 3.2. However, Lasso-like approaches focus on the minimization of an empirical risk (or prediction error), while the penalized relevance framework shifts the emphasis to the maximization of feature importance with respect to the question under study. As with the approaches presented in Sect. 3.1, this formulation makes it possible to leverage a large body of work from statistical genetics to define relevance based on appropriate statistical tests. Moreover, in this framework, optimization is done directly over the power set of $\mathcal{V}$ (also noted as $2^{\mathcal{V}}$), rather than over $\mathbb{R}^m$. This presents the conceptual advantage of yielding sparsity formulations that can be optimized without resorting to convex relaxation, and offers better computational efficiency in very high dimension.

When relying on linear models, relevance functions are modular, meaning that the relevance of a set of biomarkers is computed as the sum of the relevances of the individual biomarkers in this set. Moreover, a number of submodular, structure-enforcing regularizers can be derived from sparsity-inducing norms [54]. Among them, the Laplacian-based graph regularizer, which encourages the selected features to be connected on a predefined graph defined by its adjacency matrix W, is very similar to Ω_{grace} in Eq. (6). It is given by

$$\Phi_{\text{Laplacian}} : \mathcal{S} \mapsto \sum_{p \in \mathcal{S}} \sum_{q \notin \mathcal{S}} W_{pq}. \tag{9}$$

The sum of submodular functions is submodular, hence if R is modular and Φ submodular, solving Eq. (8) becomes a submodular minimization problem and can be solved in polynomial time. Unfortunately, algorithms to minimize arbitrary submodular functions are slow ($\mathcal{O}(m^5 c + m^6)$ where c is the cost of one function evaluation [55]). However, faster algorithms exist for specific classes of submodular functions. In particular, *graph cut functions* can be minimized much more efficiently in practice with maximum flow approaches [56], a particularity that has long been exploited in the context of energy minimization in computer vision [57].

This property can be exploited in the specific case of penalized relevance implemented in SConES [10], where R is defined by linear SKAT [58] and Φ by the sum of a cardinality constraint $\eta|\mathcal{S}|$ and the Laplacian-based regularizer $\Phi_{\text{Laplacian}}$ defined above. SConES solves the optimization problem given by Eq. (10):

$$\arg\max_{\mathcal{S} \subseteq \mathcal{V}} \sum_{p \in \mathcal{S}} R(\{p\}) - \eta|\mathcal{S}| - \lambda \sum_{p \in \mathcal{S}} \sum_{q \notin \mathcal{S}} W_{pq}. \tag{10}$$

In this case, the submodular minimization problem can be cast as a graph-cut problem and solved very efficiently. Figure 1 shows the transformed s/t-graph for which finding a minimum cut is equivalent to solving Eq. (10). This approach is available as a Matlab implementation[1] as well as part of the `sfan` Python package[2].

---

[1] https://github.com/chagaz/scones.
[2] https://github.com/chagaz/sfan.

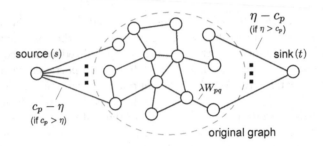

Fig. 1. This figure, taken from [10], shows a graph for which finding the minimum cut is equivalent to maximizing the objective function in Eq. (10). c_p denotes the relevance of biomarker p, and W_{pq} is the weight of the edge connecting biomarker p to biomarker q in the given network.

Limitations. An important aspect of both regularized regression and penalized relevance is the parameters (such as λ or η) that control the trade-off between the different terms and regularizers. While they afford these methods their flexibility, one needs to come up with appropriate ways to set them. This is typically done in an internal cross-validation setting, in which one explores several possible values for each of the parameters, and choose those leading to the best performance according to a given criterion. In biomarker discovery, this criterion can either be the predictivity of the selected biomarkers in a given model, or their stability [59]. Finding a good balance between both aspects is difficult, as approaches that either select all or none of the features will have high stability but poor predictivity – and little interest. In addition, exploring multiple parameter values increases the computational cost of these approaches.

While SConES is computationally more efficient than the regularized regression approaches, it also suffers from the limitation of relying on an additive model, in which the final phenotype is a function of a linear combination of the individual effects of each biomarker. Biology, however, is highly non-linear, and we expect the effect of a combination of biomarker to be more accurately approached by non-linear models. However, such models lead to optimization problems that are far more computationally expensive to solve.

3.4 Multi-task Extensions

Multi-task setting. The assumption that there are benefits to be gained from jointly learning on related tasks has long driven the fields of multi-task learning and multi-task feature selection. This also holds for biomarker discovery [60,61] For example, in toxicogenomics, where one studies the response of a population of cell lines to exposure to various chemicals [62], one could try to perform feature selection for each chemical separately, but jointly selecting features for all chemicals reduces the features-to-sample ratio of the data. eQTL studies, which try to identify the SNPs driving the expression level of various genes, also fall within this setting [63].

Multi-task regularized linear regression. Many multi-task variants of the lasso have been proposed [33, 64], and can be extended in spirit to various structural regularizers, such as Grace [65]. Assuming T tasks, each containing n_t training samples, and denoting by β_t the m-dimensional vector of regression weights for task t, the first of these approaches consists in solving the optimization problem defined by Eq. (11). The penalty term used enforces that the regression weights are both sparse and smooth across tasks.

$$\underset{\beta_1,\ldots,\beta_t \in \mathbb{R}^m}{\arg\min} \sum_{t=1}^{T} \frac{1}{n_t} \sum_{i=1}^{n_t} (X_i \beta_t - y_i)^2 + \lambda \sum_{t=1}^{T} ||\beta_t||_2 \,. \tag{11}$$

When a network structure is known over the *phenotypes*, the graph-fused Lasso can be used to smooth coefficients across tasks [66]. One could imagine combining this approach with a graph regularizer over the features. Although this has not been done with the graph-fused Lasso, the authors of [67] successfully used Laplacian-based regularizers both on the biomarkers and on the phenotypes to analyze associations between DNA methylation (about 15,000 CpG probes) and gene expression. In related work, the authors of [68] use a Laplacian-based penalty to discover the structure of the correlation between the traits.

Most of the multi-task approaches that have been proposed for regularized regression assume that the same features should be selected across all tasks. Indeed, while the multi-task lasso of [64] allows for different regression weights for the selected features, it imposes that the same features have non-zero weights across all tasks. While this is reasonable for some application domains, this assumption is violated in a number of biomarker discovery settings. For instance, lung diseases such as asthma and chronic obstructive pulmonary disease may be linked to a set of common mutations, but there is no indication that the exact same mutations are causal in both diseases. One way to address this problem is to decompose the regression weights in two components, one that is common to both tasks and one that is task specific, but this increases the computational complexity and is not yet amenable to hundreds of thousands of biomarkers [69, 70].

Moreover, to the best of our knowledge, none of the multi-task regularized regression methods that incorporate structured regularizers make it possible to consider different structural constraints for different tasks. However, we may for example want to consider different biological pathways for different diseases.

Multi-task penalized relevance. Because of the computational efficiency of graph-cut implementations, SConES can be extended to the multi-task setting in such a way as to address these issues. Multi-SConES [65] proposes a multi-task feature selection coupled with multiple network regularizers to improve feature selection in each task by combining and solving multiple tasks simultaneously.

The formulation of Multi-SConES is obtained by the addition of a regularizer across tasks. Assuming again T tasks, and denoting by $\triangle$ the symmetric difference between two sets, this formulation is given by Eq. (12).

$$\operatorname*{arg\,max}_{\mathcal{S}_1,\dots,\mathcal{S}_T \subseteq \mathcal{V}} \sum_{t=1}^{T} \left(\sum_{p \in \mathcal{S}_t} R(\{p\}) - \eta |\mathcal{S}_t| - \lambda \sum_{p \in \mathcal{S}_t} \sum_{q \notin \mathcal{S}_t} W_{pq} \right) - \mu \sum_{t<u} |\mathcal{S}_u \triangle \mathcal{S}_v|. \quad (12)$$

Limitations. The main challenges of current multi-task approaches for biomarker discoveries are linked to their computational complexity, which grows at best linearly with the number of tasks. Allowing different features to be selected across tasks, imposing different network constraints for different tasks, and leveraging prior knowledge on the correlation structure between tasks all increase the computational complexity of the model, which currently limits the applicability of existing methods to a handful of tasks at most.

4   Open Problems

The three main challenges in network-guided biomarker discovery today are: departing from linear models; guaranteeing stability; and evaluating the statistical significance of the detected modules.

Problem 1. **There is no method that incorporates network information and accounts for non-linear effects between genetic loci.** Non-additive epistatic effects are believed to play an important role in a number of human diseases, such as breast cancer [71], ovarian cancer [72], hypertension [73], or type-2 diabetes [74].

A large number of methods, reviewed in [75], have been proposed to perform exhaustive association tests between *pairs* of SNPs and a phenotype. A first step to address the lack of approaches relying on biological networks for the detection of non-linear interaction effects between SNPs and a phenotype would be to combine them with the approaches outlined above; the penalized relevance framework lends itself particularly well to this. However, this is still limited to interactions between two loci, but more might be at play, and models for higher-order interactions are required.

Embedded approaches for feature selection are not limited to linear algorithms. Several promising approaches have been proposed in recent years along those lines, based mostly on random forests [76,77], but also on Bayesian neural networks [78].

Alternatively, Drouin et al. [79] propose to use set covering machines [80] to learn conjunctions of disjunctions of short genomic sequences to predict bacterial resistance to antibiotics. Unlike random-forests-based approaches, this approach only consider specific types of biomarkers interactions (combinations of logical ANDs and ORs on their presence/absence), but it also has the potential to uncover epistatic interactions not detectable with the usual quadratic methods.

However, to the best of our knowledge, no approach exist that allows for the integration of prior knowledge as networks in these higher-order, non-linear interaction models, and this would be an exciting research avenue to pursue.

Problem 2. **There is no method to guarantee stable feature selection.** The *stability* (or *robustness*) of feature selection procedures, meaning their ability to retain the same features upon minor perturbations of the data, remains a major predicament in the high-dimensional, low sample-size setting. Current algorithms typically yield widely different results for different subsets of the same set of samples [51]. This high variability implies that they capture idiosyncrasies rather than truly relevant features. This casts doubts on the reliability of predictive algorithms built on the selected features and impedes interpreting these features to yield novel biological insights. However, this question has only recently started to come under investigation [81].

Most of the work in that domain has tried to yield lower-dimensional representations by grouping features together in meta-features, based either on the data or on prior knowledge [82,83]. Unfortunately, these groupings, if done wrongly, can confuse the feature selection procedure even more.

Alternatively, ensemble approaches are based upon the idea of ensemble learning methods to combine the strengths of multiple weak learners to form a stronger predictor. Bagging approaches, in which each of the selector is based on a subsample of the data, have been shown to be consistent in settings in which the procedure based on the full data was not [84,85].

Finally, variable-reduction approaches have led to schemes which reweight samples based on their suitability for the estimation of feature importance [86]. However, all these efforts are in their infancy and ranking features based on t-test scores often still yields the most stable selection in practice [52,53].

Problem 3. **There is no method to assess the statistical significance of the uncovered modules.** Very few methods can determine the statistical significance of the association between *multiple* biomarkers and a phenotype, despite it being key to the interpretation of biomarker discovery outcomes. A recent paper [87] proposes to do this for intervals of the genome. The extension of this work to network modules, however, is not trivial.

Work on confidence intervals on edge differences between brain imaging networks [88] solve a related problem. However, in the case of network-guided biomarker discovery, one is interested in evaluating the significance of node (and not edge) differences, and it is not obvious whether biological networks can be described with similar models as brain images.

5 Future Outlook

We can hardly hope to understand the biology underlying complex diseases without considering the molecular interactions that govern entire cells, tissues or organisms. The approaches we discussed offer a principled way to perform biomarker discovery in a systems biology framework, by integrating knowledge accumulated in the form of interaction networks into studies associating genomic features with a disease or response to treatment. While these methods are still in their infancy, in strong part because of the statistical and computational challenges outlined in Sect. 4, we believe that they can become powerful tools in the realization of precision medicine.

Future research directions for biomarker discovery include the development of (1) machine learning approaches for stable, non-linear, multi-task feature selection; (2) statistical techniques for the evaluation of the significance of the association detected by complex models; and (3) the refinement and choice of appropriate network data. While most network-guided biomarker discovery studies make use of generic gene-gene interaction networks such as STRING or BioGRID, many other possibilities are starting to open up. They include disease-specific networks such as ACSN, but we can also imagine using for example eQTL networks based on previous studies [89], or three-dimensional chromatin interaction networks [90]. Methods that integrate these multiple types of networks may be needed; that the regularized regression or penalized relevance methods we discussed can all accommodate weighted networks (either directly or through simple modifications) will facilitate these developments.

Finally, serious progress in the field of biomarker discovery requires proper validation, at the very least in other data sets pertaining to the same trait, of the pertinence of the modules identified by these various methods. Because this requires that modelers convince the owners of such data sets to run experiments to this end, this is often hard to implement outside of large consortium collaborations, and a major limitation of most of the work cited in this chapter.

References

1. Spear, B.B., Heath-Chiozzi, M., Huff, J.: Clinical application of pharmacogenetics. Trends Mol. Med. **7**(5), 201–204 (2001)
2. Reuter, J., Spacek, D.V., Snyder, M.: High-throughput sequencing technologies. Molecular Cell **58**(4), 586–597 (2015)
3. Van Allen, E.M., Wagle, N., Levy, M.A.: Clinical analysis and interpretation of cancer genome data. J. Clin. Oncol. **31**(15), 1825–1833 (2013)
4. Manolio, T.A., Collins, F.S., Cox, N.J., Goldstein, D.B., et al.: Finding the missing heritability of complex diseases. Nature **461**(7265), 747–753 (2009)
5. Holzinger, A.: Interactive machine learning for health informatics: when do we need the human-in-the-loop? Brain Inf. **3**(2), 119–131 (2016)
6. Hund, M., Böhm, D., Sturm, W., Sedlmair, M., et al.: Visual analytics for concept exploration in subspaces of patient groups. Brain Inf. **3**(4), 233–247 (2016). doi:10.1007/s40708-016-0043-5
7. Szklarczyk, D., Franceschini, A., Wyder, S., Forslund, K., et al.: STRING v10: protein-protein interaction networks, integrated over the tree of life. Nucleic Acids Res. **43**(Database issue), D447–452 (2015)
8. Chatr-Aryamontri, A., Breitkreutz, B.J., Oughtred, R., Boucher, L., Heinicke, S., et al.: The BioGRID interaction database: 2015 update. Nucleic Acids Res. **43**(Database issue), D470–478 (2015)
9. Kuperstein, I., Bonnet, E., Nguyen, H.A., Cohen, D., et al.: Atlas of cancer signalling network: a systems biology resource for integrative analysis of cancer data with Google Maps. Oncogenesis **4**(7), e160 (2015)

10. Azencott, C.A., Grimm, D., Sugiyama, M., Kawahara, Y., Borgwardt, K.M.: Efficient network-guided multi-locus association mapping with graph cuts. Bioinformatics **29**(13), i171–i179 (2013)
11. Guyon, I., Elisseeff, A.: An introduction to variable and feature selection. J. Mach. Learn Res. **3**, 1157–1182 (2003)
12. Hastie, T., Tibshirani, R., Wainwright, M.: Statistical Learning with Sparsity: The Lasso and Generalizations. CRC Press, Boca Raton (2015)
13. Bush, W.S., Moore, J.H.: Chapter 11: genome-wide association studies. PLoS Comput. Biol. **8**(12), e1002822 (2012)
14. Merris, R.: Laplacian matrices of graphs: a survey. Linear Algebra Appl. **197**, 143–176 (1994)
15. Smola, A.J., Kondor, R.: Kernels and regularization on graphs. In: Schölkopf, B., Warmuth, M.K. (eds.) COLT-Kernel 2003. LNCS (LNAI), vol. 2777, pp. 144–158. Springer, Heidelberg (2003). doi:10.1007/978-3-540-45167-9_12
16. Fujishige, S.: Submodular Functions and Optimization. Elsevier, Amsterdam (2005)
17. Bach, F.: Learning with submodular functions: a convex optimization perspective. Found. Trends Mach. Learn. **6**(2–3), 145–373 (2013)
18. Thornton, T.: Statistical methods for genome-wide and sequencing association studies of complex traits in related samples. Curr. Protoc. Hum. Genet. **84**, 1.28.1–1.28.9 (2015)
19. Liu, J., Wang, K., Ma, S., Huang, J.: Accounting for linkage disequilibrium in genome-wide association studies: a penalized regression method. Statist. Interface **6**(1), 99–115 (2013)
20. Lee, S., Abecasis, G., Boehnke, M., Lin, X.: Rare-variant association analysis: study designs and statistical tests. Am. J. Hum. Genet. **95**(1), 5–23 (2014)
21. Liu, J.Z., Mcrae, A.F., Nyholt, D.R., Medland, S.E., et al.: A versatile gene-based test for genome-wide association studies. Am. J. Hum. Genet. **87**(1), 139–145 (2010)
22. Jia, P., Wang, L., Fanous, A.H., Pato, C.N., Edwards, T.L., Zhao, Z.: The International Schizophrenia Consortium: network-assisted investigation of combined causal signals from Genome-Wide Association Studies in schizophrenia. PLoS Comput. Biol. **8**(7), e1002587 (2012)
23. Chuang, H.Y., Lee, E., Liu, Y.T., Lee, D., Ideker, T.: Network-based classification of breast cancer metastasis. Mol. Syst. Biol. **3**, 140 (2007)
24. Baranzini, S.E., Galwey, N.W., Wang, J., Khankhanian, P., et al.: Pathway and network-based analysis of genome-wide association studies in multiple sclerosis. Hum. Mol. Genet. **18**(11), 2078–2090 (2009)
25. Wang, L., Matsushita, T., Madireddy, L., Mousavi, P., Baranzini, S.E.: PINBPA: Cytoscape app for network analysis of GWAS data. Bioinformatics **31**(2), 262–264 (2015)
26. Ideker, T., Ozier, O., Schwikowski, B., Siegel, A.F.: Discovering regulatory and signalling circuits in molecular interaction networks. Bioinformatics **18**(suppl 1), S233–S240 (2002)
27. Taşan, M., Musso, G., Hao, T., Vidal, M., MacRae, C.A., Roth, F.P.: Selecting causal genes from genome-wide association studies via functionally coherent subnetworks. Nat. Methods **12**(2), 154–159 (2015)
28. Mitra, K., Carvunis, A.R., Ramesh, S.K., Ideker, T.: Integrative approaches for finding modular structure in biological networks. Nat. Rev. Genet. **14**(10), 719–732 (2013)
29. Akula, N., Baranova, A., Seto, D., Solka, J., et al.: A network-based approach to prioritize results from genome-wide association studies. PLoS ONE **6**(9), e24220 (2011)

30. Marchini, J., Donnelly, P., Cardon, L.R.: Genome-wide strategies for detecting multiple loci that influence complex diseases. Nat. Genet. **37**(4), 413–417 (2005)
31. Tibshirani, R.: Regression shrinkage and selection via the lasso. J. Roy. Stat. Soc. B **58**, 267–288 (1994)
32. Wu, T.T., Chen, Y.F., Hastie, T., Sobel, E., Lange, K.: Genome-wide association analysis by lasso penalized logistic regression. Bioinformatics **25**(6), 714–721 (2009)
33. Zhou, H., Sehl, M.E., Sinsheimer, J.S., Lange, K.: Association screening of common and rare genetic variants by penalized regression. Bioinformatics **26**(19), 2375–2382 (2010)
34. Chen, L.S., Hutter, C.M., Potter, J.D., Liu, Y., Prentice, R.L., Peters, U., Hsu, L.: Insights into colon cancer etiology via a regularized approach to gene set analysis of GWAS data. Am. J. Hum. Genet. **86**(6), 860–871 (2010)
35. Zhao, J., Gupta, S., Seielstad, M., Liu, J., Thalamuthu, A.: Pathway-based analysis using reduced gene subsets in genome-wide association studies. BMC Bioinf. **12**, 17 (2011)
36. Silver, M., Montana, G.: Alzheimer's disease neuroimaging initiative: fast identification of biological pathways associated with a quantitative trait using group lasso with overlaps. Stat. Appl. Genet. Mol. Biol. **11**(1), 7 (2012)
37. Huang, J., Zhang, T., Metaxas, D.: Learning with structured sparsity. J. Mach. Learn. Res. **12**, 3371–3412 (2011)
38. Micchelli, C.A., Morales, J.M., Pontil, M.: Regularizers for structured sparsity. Adv. Comput. Math. **38**(3), 455–489 (2013)
39. Jacob, L., Obozinski, G., Vert, J.P.: Group lasso with overlap and graph lasso. In: Proceedings of the 26th Annual International Conference on Machine Learning, pp. 433–440. ACM (2009)
40. Tibshirani, R., Saunders, M., Rosset, S., Zhu, J., Knight, K.: Sparsity and smoothness via the fused lasso. J. Roy. Stat. Soc. B **67**(1), 91–108 (2005)
41. Beck, A., Teboulle, M.: A fast iterative shrinkage-thresholding algorithm for linear inverse problems. SIAM J. Imag. Sci. **2**(1), 183–202 (2009)
42. Xin, B., Kawahara, Y., Wang, Y., Gao, W.: Efficient generalized fused lasso and its application to the diagnosis of Alzheimer's disease. In: Twenty-Eighth AAAI Conference on Artificial Intelligence (2014)
43. Li, C., Li, H.: Network-constrained regularization and variable selection for analysis of genomic data. Bioinformatics **24**(9), 1175–1182 (2008)
44. Li, C., Li, H.: Variable selection and regression analysis for graph-structured covariates with an application to genomics. Ann. Appl. Stat. **4**(3), 1498–1516 (2010)
45. Sokolov, A., Carlin, D.E., Paull, E.O., Baertsch, R., Stuart, J.M.: Pathway-based genomics prediction using generalized elastic net. PLoS Comput. Biol. **12**(3), e1004790 (2016)
46. Friedman, J., Hastie, T., Höfling, H., Tibshirani, R.: Pathwise coordinate optimization. Ann. Appl. Stat. **1**(2), 302–332 (2007)
47. Yang, S., Yuan, L., Lai, Y.C., Shen, X., et al.: Feature grouping and selection over an undirected graph. In: Proceedings of the 18th ACM SIGKDD International Conference on Knowledge Discovery and Data Mining, pp. 922–930. ACM (2012)
48. Gabay, D., Mercier, B.: A dual algorithm for the solution of nonlinear variational problems via finite element approximation. Comput. Math. Appl. **2**(1), 17–40 (1976)
49. Boyd, S., Parikh, N., Chu, E., Peleato, B., Eckstein, J.: Distributed optimization and statistical learning via the alternating direction method of multipliers. Found. Trends Mach. Learn. **3**(1), 1–122 (2011)

50. Wang, Z., Montana, G.: The graph-guided group lasso for genome-wide association studies. In: Regularization, Optimization, Kernels, and Support Vector Machines, pp. 131–157 (2014)
51. Dernoncourt, D., Hanczar, B., Zucker, J.D.: Analysis of feature selection stability on high dimension and small sample data. Comput. Stat. Data Anal. **71**, 681–693 (2014)
52. Haury, A.C., Gestraud, P., Vert, J.P.: The influence of feature selection methods on accuracy, stability and interpretability of molecular signatures. PLoS ONE **6**(12), e28210 (2011)
53. Kuncheva, L., Smith, C., Syed, Y., Phillips, C., Lewis, K.: Evaluation of feature ranking ensembles for high-dimensional biomedical data: a case study. In: 2012 IEEE 12th International Conference on Data Mining Workshops, pp. 49–56 (2012)
54. Bach, F.: Structured sparsity-inducing norms through submodular functions. In: 24th Annual Conference on Neural Information Processing Systems 2010 (2010)
55. Orlin, J.B.: A faster strongly polynomial time algorithm for submodular function minimization. Math. Prog. **118**(2), 237–251 (2009)
56. Greig, D.M., Porteous, B.T., Seheult, A.H.: Exact maximum a posteriori estimation for binary images. J. Roy. Stat. Soc. B **51**(2), 271–279 (1989)
57. Kolmogorov, V., Zabin, R.: What energy functions can be minimized via graph cuts? IEEE Trans. Pattern Anal. Mach. Intell. **26**(2), 147–159 (2004)
58. Wu, M.C., Lee, S., Cai, T., Li, Y., Boehnke, M., Lin, X.: Rare-variant association testing for sequencing data with the sequence kernel association test. Am. J. Hum. Genet. **89**(1), 82–93 (2011)
59. Kuncheva, L.I.: A stability index for feature selection. In: Proceedings of the 25th Conference on Proceedings of the 25th IASTED International Multi-Conference: Artificial Intelligence and Applications, pp. 390–395. ACTA Press (2007)
60. Park, S.H., Lee, J.Y., Kim, S.: A methodology for multivariate phenotype-based genome-wide association studies to mine pleiotropic genes. BMC Syst. Biol. **5**(2), 1–14 (2011)
61. O'Reilly, P.F., Hoggart, C.J., Pomyen, Y., Calboli, F.C.F., Elliott, P., Jarvelin, M.R., Coin, L.J.M.: MultiPhen: joint model of multiple phenotypes can increase discovery in GWAS. PLoS ONE **7**(5), e34861 (2012)
62. Eduati, F., Mangravite, L.M., Wang, T., Tang, H., et al.: Prediction of human population responses to toxic compounds by a collaborative competition. Nat. Biotechnol. **33**(9), 933–940 (2015)
63. Cheng, W., Zhang, X., Guo, Z., Shi, Y., Wang, W.: Graph-regularized dual lasso for robust eQTL mapping. Bioinformatics **30**(12), i139–i148 (2014)
64. Obozinski, G., Taskar, B., Jordan, M.I.: Multi-task feature selection. Technical report, UC Berkeley (2006)
65. Sugiyama, M., Azencott, C., Grimm, D., Kawahara, Y., Borgwardt, K.: Multi-task feature selection on multiple networks via maximum flows. In: Proceedings of the 2014 SIAM International Conference on Data Mining, pp. 199–207 (2014)
66. Kim, S., Xing, E.P.: Statistical estimation of correlated genome associations to a quantitative trait network. PLoS Genet. **5**(8), e1000587 (2009)
67. Wang, Z., Curry, E., Montana, G.: Network-guided regression for detecting associations between DNA methylation and gene expression. Bioinformatics **30**(19), 2693–2701 (2014)
68. Fei, H., Huan, J.: Structured feature selection and task relationship inference for multi-task learning. Knowl. Inf. Syst. **35**(2), 345–364 (2013)
69. Swirszcz, G., Lozano, A.C.: Multi-level lasso for sparse multi-task regression. In: Proceedings of the 29th International Conference on Machine Learning (ICML 2012), pp. 361–368 (2012)

70. Bellon, V., Stoven, V., Azencott, C.A.: Multitask feature selection with task descriptors. In: Pacific Symposium on Biocomputing, vol. 21, pp. 261–272 (2016)

71. Ritchie, M.D., Hahn, L.W., Roodi, N., Bailey, L.R., et al.: Multifactor-dimensionality reduction reveals high-order interactions among estrogen-metabolism genes in sporadic breast cancer. Am. J. Hum. Genet. **69**(1), 138–147 (2001)

72. Larson, N.B., Jenkins, G.D., Larson, M.C., Sellers, T.A., Sellers, T.A., et al.: Kernel canonical correlation analysis for assessing genegene interactions and application to ovarian cancer. Eur. J. Hum. Genet. **22**(1), 126–131 (2014)

73. Williams, S.M., Ritchie, M.D., Phillips, J.A., Dawson, E., et al.: Multilocus analysis of hypertension: a hierarchical approach. Hum. Hered. **57**(1), 28–38 (2004)

74. Cho, Y.M., Ritchie, M.D., Moore, J.H., Park, J.Y., et al.: Multifactor-dimensionality reduction shows a two-locus interaction associated with type 2 diabetes mellitus. Diabetologia **47**(3), 549–554 (2004)

75. Niel, C., Sinoquet, C., Dina, C., Rocheleau, G.: A survey about methods dedicated to epistasis detection. J. Bioinf. Comput. Biol. **6**, 285 (2015)

76. Yoshida, M., Koike, A.: SNPInterForest: a new method for detecting epistatic interactions. BMC Bioinf. **12**(1), 469 (2011)

77. Stephan, J., Stegle, O., Beyer, A.: A random forest approach to capture genetic effects in the presence of population structure. Nat. Commun. **6**, 7432 (2015)

78. Beam, A.L., Motsinger-Reif, A., Doyle, J.: Bayesian neural networks for detecting epistasis in genetic association studies. BMC Bioinf. **15**(1), 368 (2014)

79. Drouin, A., Giguère, S., Sagatovich, V., Déraspe, M., et al.: Learning interpretable models of phenotypes from whole genome sequences with the Set Covering Machine (2014). arXiv:1412.1074 [cs, q-bio, stat]

80. Marchand, M., Shawe-Taylor, J.: The set covering machine. J. Mach. Learn. Res. **3**, 723–746 (2002)

81. He, Z., Yu, W.: Stable feature selection for biomarker discovery. Comput. Biol. Chem. **34**(4), 215–225 (2010)

82. Ma, S., Huang, J., Moran, M.S.: Identification of genes associated with multiple cancers via integrative analysis. BMC Genom. **10**, 535 (2009)

83. Yu, L., Ding, C., Loscalzo, S.: Stable feature selection via dense feature groups. In: Proceedings of the 14th ACM SIGKDD International Conference on Knowledge Discovery and Data Mining, pp. 803–811. ACM (2008)

84. Meinshausen, N., Bühlmann, P.: Stability selection. J. Roy. Stat. Soc. B **72**(4), 417–473 (2010)

85. Shah, R.D., Samworth, R.J.: Variable selection with error control: another look at stability selection. J. Roy. Stat. Soc. B **75**(1), 55–80 (2013)

86. Han, Y., Yu, L.: A variance reduction framework for stable feature selection. Stat. Anal. Data Min. **5**(5), 428–445 (2012)

87. Llinares-López, F., Grimm, D.G., Bodenham, D.A., Gieraths, U., et al.: Genome-wide detection of intervals of genetic heterogeneity associated with complex traits. Bioinformatics **31**(12), i240–i249 (2015)

88. Belilovsky, E., Varoquaux, G., Blaschko, M.B.: Testing for differences in Gaussian graphical models: applications to brain connectivity. In: Lee, D.D., Luxburg, U.V., Guyon, I., Garnett, R. (eds.) Advances in Neural Information Processing Systems 29 (2016)

89. Tur, I., Roverato, A., Castelo, R.: Mapping eQTL networks with mixed graphical markov models. Genetics **198**(4), 1377–1393 (2014)

90. Sandhu, K., Li, G., Poh, H., Quek, Y., et al.: Large-scale functional organization of long-range chromatin interaction networks. Cell. Rep. **2**(5), 1207–1219 (2012)

Knowledge Discovery in Clinical Data

Aryya Gangopadhyay[1]([✉]), Rose Yesha[1], and Eliot Siegel[2]

[1] Department of Information Systems, University of Maryland, Baltimore County,
Baltimore, MD 21250, USA
{gangopad,yrose}@umbc.edu
[2] University of Maryland School of Medicine, VA Maryland Healthcare System,
Baltimore, MD 21201, USA
esiegel@umaryland.edu

Abstract. There has been a recent surge in the implementation of electronic health care records. These patient records contain valuable medical information including patient demographic data, diagnosis, therapeutic approach, and patient outcomes. It is important to analyze patterns within these records in order to more effectively treat individuals. In this paper, a method is presented for identifying these themes and patterns within patient data. This methodology includes extraction of the main themes or patterns in the data and linking those themes back to the corpus from which they were generated. In our research, we partitioned graphs from terms gathered from electronic medical records. We used two sets of data including eight charts and ten case studies for this study from primary disease categories. The Electronic Medical Records (EMRs) and case studies were modeled as networks of interacting terms where the interactions were captured by their co-occurrences in the documents. A greedy algorithm was used to find communities with high modularity. Finally, we compared our method with probabilistic topic modeling algorithms and evaluated the efficacy of our method by using recall and precision measures.

Keywords: Electronic medical records · Visualization · Analytics · Pattern recognition

1 Introduction and Motivation

The healthcare industry has recently seen a massive transition of health care records from predominantly paper based systems to completely automated electronic medical record systems. This transformation has resulted in more opportunities for health care practitioners and researchers to extract patient data in an efficient manner. In order to discover patterns within electronic health records, data mining techniques are needed to uncover pertinent insights.

Researchers have looked at specific techniques that discover similarities within the data and discern associations with patient outcomes. Many techniques have been used to gain insight from clinical data, including interactive visualization and data mining systems [1,2]. Although these methods have proven to be

© Springer International Publishing AG 2016
A. Holzinger (Ed.): ML for Health Informatics, LNAI 9605, pp. 337–356, 2016.
DOI: 10.1007/978-3-319-50478-0_17

of value, they are also limited in their abilities. Typical mining methods are able to highlight short fragments of frequently occurring patterns [3]. The current visualization based methods are able to highlight a process from beginning to end. However, these methods are also limited to a small number of events before the data becomes so complex that it is virtually impossible to decipher.

Most researchers in the machine learning community focus on automatic machine learning (aML), with the ultimate goal of bringing humans-out-of-the-loop However, biomedical data sets are full of uncertainty, incompleteness etc. [4], they can contain missing data, noisy data, unwanted data, and some problems in the medical domain are hard, which makes the application of fully automated approaches difficult. The integration of the knowledge of a domain expert can at times be indispensable and the interaction of a domain expert with the data would greatly enhance the knowledge discovery process. Therefore, interactive machine learning (iML) puts the "human-in-the-loop" to allow what neither a human nor a computer could do independently. This idea is supported by a synergistic combination of methodologies of two areas that offer ideal conditions towards solving such problems. A corresponding experimental proof in the context of visual analytics is provided in [5].

In this paper, we present a novel approach that involves the use of a graph-based method for analyzing electronic health records. The two major steps in this process include (a) determination of the main themes or patterns in the data, and (b) linking these themes back to the corpus from which they were generated. In our experiments we have used modularity [6] as the quality function, which strives to measure how well a given partition of a network compartmentalizes its communities. A partitioned knowledge graph is the input to the second step in our process for which each partition we create a list of terms that are used to assign a relevance score for each document.

The rest of the paper is organized as follows: in Sect. 2 we present research that are related to this paper, in Sect. 3 we describe our methodology, and in Sect. 4 we present the experimental results followed by our conclusions in Sect. 5.

2   Related Work

The consolidation of health care records from paper records to electronic records has provided health care practitioners and researchers with the ability to access health information more efficiently. The surge of large-scale datasets in the health care industry that contain large amounts of data concerning patients, their diseases, and treatments have provided us with the opportunity to understand the significant aspects of the disease processes, the efficacy of treatment methods, and other factors that impact the health of the patient [7]. Patients disease processes can often evolve into complex and often unpredictable patterns. By using pattern mining and analysis, researchers can uncover significant insights into the disease process [3].

2.1 Temporal Data Mining and Interactive Visualization of Event Sequences

A common type of study used in this type of research is temporal event analysis. Temporal properties of these events are analyzed to discover associations with patients' eventual outcomes. A variety of techniques have been used to gain insight from clinical event sequence data such as interactive visualizations [1] and data mining systems [2]. Recently, the research transitioned to visualizations of cohorts of patients. This includes a range of tools for querying, visualizing, and sorting through groups of patient event data [8–10]. The most pertinent of these techniques includes Outflow, a technique used for visualizing aggregate patient evolution pattern in terms of symptoms, treatments, or another set of temporal event types [11–14].

Professionals in the biomedical domain are faced with increasing amounts of data, which require efficient solutions and the development of methods to assist them in knowledge discovery to extract, identify, visualize and understand information from these large amounts of data [4]. The popularity of personalized medicine has resulted in a mass of data that are characterized by complexity, which makes manual analysis very inefficient and often virtually impossible [15]. Muller, et al. developed a set of validated glyphs for the interactive exploration of biomedical data sets [16]. Data glyphs are 3-D objects defined by several levels of geometric descriptions, combined with a mapping of data attributes to graphical methods and elements, which define their spatial position.

2.2 Patient Similarity

Patient Similarity approaches have been used in a variety of practice areas ranging from emergency rooms to risk scoring [17]. Orthuber and Sommer developed a similarity-based search tool for patient records that has been implemented for decision support [18]. A different approach was used by Wongsuphasawat and Shneiderman who used visualization techniques to identify similar records interactively. These techniques can help users identify individual similar records, which can be used by decision makers. Although these techniques are powerful, these techniques rely on clusters of similar patients, which are determined by complex algorithms. Therefore, it can be challenging for doctors to comprehend the characteristics of patients in cluster. Also, these automatically generated clusters can often require tweaks by domain experts. Consequently, visualization techniques have been designed for these tasks. These range from parallel coordinates, heat maps, and scatter plots [19–25]. Although these methods are effective, they do not serve well for large numbers of clusters. Therefore, Gotz and his researchers implemented an iconic treemap-based visualizations scheme, which can provide a compact and intuitive representation that scales easily to large cluster sets [17].

2.3   Clinical Decision Intelligence

Large databases of EHRs hold significant information about patient populations. Statistical insights about an overall population are beneficial, however, they are often not well defined enough to implement individualized patient-centric decisions [17]. Clinical decision intelligence can be implemented by using data analysis algorithms to dynamically identify cohorts of similar patients from within an institutions EHR database [17]. This type of patient analysis has been shown to be successful at near-term prognostics for physiological data and risk assessment [26,27]. To enable interactive cohort refinement by domain experts, a visualization technique called DICON was implemented [28]. Using DICON, clinicians can interactively search for clusters produced by the automated analysis and assess their quality. Also, DICON lets users manipulate clusters of patients using drag and drop methods to merge or split groups of patients based on domain expertise.

2.4   Predictive Models

Machine-learning techniques are data-driven methods that are designed to discover statistical patterns in high-dimensional, multivariate data sets, like those that are typically found in electronic health record systems. The detection of correlations in data provides the pathway for predicting future patient outcomes from a given scenario [29]. Predictive clinical modeling is a technique that uses machine-learning methods to create multivariate models from clinical data and makes inferences on unknown data. Examples of this include the prediction of breast cancer survival [30] and surgery outcomes [31]. Creating patterns of directionality in disease progression and comorbidity are the initial steps for using EMRs for predictive purposes, and this has been analyzed in network analysis studies of Medicare data [32,33].

3   Methodology

There are two major steps in our methodology: (a) creating the main themes or patterns in the data, and (b) linking the themes back to the corpus from which they were generated. We present the themes as undirected graphs referred to as "knowledge graphs" where the themes are color-coded for easy identification. The steps in creating the knowledge graphs from the text corpus are shown in Fig. 2.

In this research we analyzed each patient's electronic medical record (EMR) individually. Each EMR can consist of numerous documents where each document represents a text segment that can be a sentence, paragraph, or section. There are *pros* and *cons* for selecting short versus long documents. Selecting short text segments such as sentences as documents typically results in very similar *relevance scores* (explained in Sect. 4.2) for each, which is not conducive to generating the synopsis of an EMR. On the other hand, large text segments may impact the ability to narrow down search for specific patterns. In this research we delimited each document by the "newline" character in the EMR, which was both easy for automation and appropriate in size.

The pre-processing steps in our methodology include cleaning the text corpus such as removing non-alphanumeric characters, stop-words, punctuations, redundant spaces, etc., converting all characters to lowercases, and stemming to ensure that only root words are used instead of different cognate variations. Next a term-document matrix (TDM) is created where each entry represents the frequency of occurrence of each term in each document. We have tried using both term frequency and TF/IDF (term frequency/inverse document frequency) and the results of the analysis are very similar. We created an adjacency matrix of terms obtained by multiplying the TDM with its transpose. The TDM is used to create a graph where the nodes are terms and an edge between any two terms represents that those terms co-occur in a single document.

3.1 Creating Knowledge Graphs

The typical size of large graphs such as social network services spans in millions if not billions of nodes. In our research a graph corresponding to each EMR can span thousands of nodes. Therefore, a large EMR system consisting of thousands of patents may approach the size of real-world social networks. These scales require new methods to retrieve information from their structure. A promising approach involves decomposing a large graph into sub-graphs, such the nodes within a sub-graph are highly inter-connected. The identification of these sub-graphs is significant as they can help uncover unknown modules in such graphs. In addition, the resulting meta-network may be used to visualize the original structure of the graph. The issue of community calls for the partition of a graph into densely connected nodes, with sparse connection of nodes from different communities. In this paper we use modularity as the quality function which strives to measure how well a given partition of a graph compartmentalizes its communities (e.g. [34]).

Modularity involves creation of sub-graphs where the nodes are highly inter-connected and have fewer connections with outside nodes. Modularity provides precise measure of how to count the total strength of connections within communities versus those between communities and is a scaled assortativity measure based on whether the high-strength edges are more or less likely to be adjacent to other high-strength edges. Maximizing modularity has been used an the objective function in finding the community structure in graphs (for example [34–36]). The problem of modularity maximization is *NP-hard* [37]. However, several heuristic solutions exist as good solutions (for example [6,34]). In this paper we have used graph partitioning in order to maximize the modularity, creating dense and frequent interactions between the nodes while still separating them from others.

We have implemented a greedy algorithm for detecting communities with high modularity [6]. Maximizing the modularity function Q (defined in Eq. 1) results in identifying sub-graphs in which the number of interactions among the nodes are significantly larger than that the expected number of interactions among nodes in a random graph.

$$Q = \frac{1}{2m} \sum_{l=1}^{n} \sum_{i \in C_l, j \in C_l} (A_j - \frac{d_i.d_j}{m}) \tag{1}$$

In Eq. (1) d_i and d_j are the degrees of nodes i and j, m is the total number of edges in the graph, and $d_i.d_j/2m$ is the probability that nodes i and j will be connected in a random graph. Q represents how different the graph is from such a random graph for each sub-graphs and adds them up over all sub-graphs. Maximizing Q results in the discovery of the maximum number of dense sub-graphs where the nodes are much more connected with each other than with nodes outside the sub-graphs. The Greedy algorithm finds high modularity partitions of large graphs efficiently with a time complexity of $O(n^2 log n)$, which unfolds a hierarchical community structure for the graph. This gives us access to different resolutions of community detection. This algorithm is split in two phases that are repeated iteratively. First, a different community is assigned to each node of the graph. Then, for each node i we consider the neighbors of j and i and evaluate the gain of modularity that would take place by removing i from its community and by placing it in the community of j. The node i is then placed in the community for which this gain is maximum but only if the gain is positive. This process is done repeatedly for all nodes until no further improvement can be made.

Our findings in this research suggest that the quality of the communities detected is very good, as was measured by the modularity. This simple algorithm has several advantages. First, these steps are intuitive and easy to implement. Also, the algorithm is extremely fast, i.e., computer simulations on large ad-hoc modular networks suggest that its complexity is linear on sparse data. The accuracy of this method has been tested on ad-hoc modular networks and is shown to be excellent as relative to other much slower community detection methods.

In this research we have analyzed eight EMRs shown in Table 1. However, for space limitations we illustrate our method using one EMR with *anemia* as the primary disease category. The partitioned graph for the EMR with *anemia* is shown in Fig. 1, where the sizes of nodes vary from 1 to 5 mm corresponding to their authority scores [35]. Each partition is shown in a different color in with partition sizes ranging from 23% to 1% in terms of the number of nodes.

Figure 1 shows the graph corresponding to the EMR for the patient with *anemia* at the top and its four largest clusters further partitioned one level below. The graph at the top level has four large partitions (clusters) color-coded as cyan, red, yellow, and pink. The cluster with cyan nodes is the densest cluster with around 200 nodes and 6000 edges. The nodes in this cluster are related to causes of anemia for the particular patient whose clinical record is being analyzed. From the EMR, some of the possible causes of *anemia* in this particular case are cancer in the *gastrointestinal (GI)* or *genitourinary (GU)* tracts.

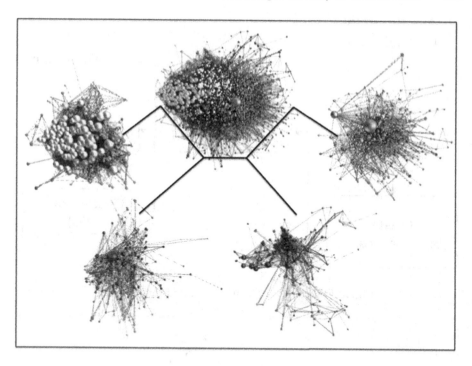

Fig. 1. Partitioned knowledge Graphs (Color figure online)

The red cluster has around 300 nodes and 2600 edges and is primarily related to bleeding. There was blood in the stool and the darkness suggest that its source might have been in the upper digestive system and hence both *Esophagogastro-duodenoscopy (EGD)* and *colonoscopy* are recommended.

The yellow cluster with around 180 nodes and 2100 edges is related to cardiovascular diseases and other comorbidities. The patient has a history of coronary artery disease and had a *percutaneous transluminal coronary angioplasty (PTCA)* in the past. The patient also has *hypertension* and is at risk getting *diabetes.*

The purple cluster with around 500 nodes and 3700 edges is related to general admission information including allergies, specific dietary information, and problems self-reported by the patient.

3.2   Hierarchical Partitioning

In our methodology one can hierarchically partition the graph which allows drilling down from high to low level details. As an example, we further partitioned the yellow cluster in Fig. 1 into further sub-clusters shown in Fig. 3, where the inset shows the parent yellow cluster. This sub-clustering separates the various comorbidities into different clusters. For example, the new cyan cluster is related to cardiovascular issues and includes further information such as smoking and heavy drinking habits of the patient. It also indicates that the patient has

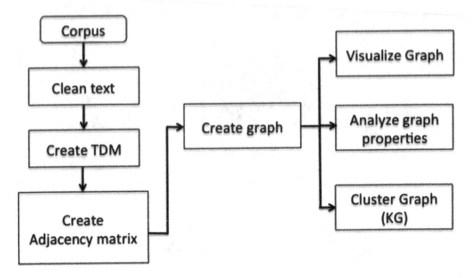

Fig. 2. Flowchart for Creation of knowledge Graphs

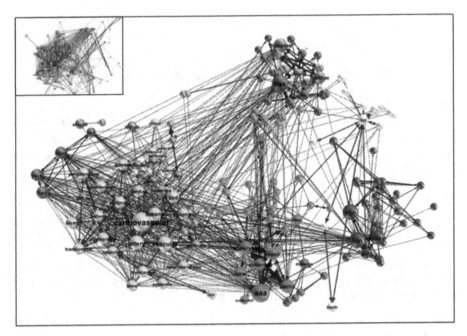

Fig. 3. Hierarchical Partitioning of knowledge Graphs

a high level of *cholesterol* in the blood. The pink cluster contains information that the patient had an *abdominal aortic aneurysm (AAA)*. The red cluster is related to prior procedures such as the PTCA. The blue and the green clusters are related to hypertension and diabetes respectively.

3.3   Linking Knowledge Graphs to EMR

A partitioned knowledge graph is the input to the second step (step b) in our method. In this step we create a list of terms for each partition. These lists are then used to compute the relevance score of each document in the EMR. The relevance score is the sum of the number of times each term in a partition occurs in a document. This is done for each partition over all the documents and the list of documents with their relevance scores is returned as the output. The pseudocode of the algorithm for this step is shown in Algorithm 1.

Input: a corpus with p documents;
Input: a partitioned graph with q partitions;
Output: list of documents with relevance scores;
for $i \leftarrow 1$ **to** p **do**
   for $j \leftarrow 1$ **to** q **do**
      Create a list of terms in partition j;
      Relevance score $\leftarrow$ sum of the # of occurrences of each term in document i;
   end
end

Algorithm 1: Link Knowledge Graphs to EMR

---

[1] Clinical assessment in our hospital found a Glasgow Coma Scale of 15 out of 15 but complete neurologic deficits below the level of C5. Plain X-ray film images obtained at this time showed a C4 on C5 dislocation. Further information regarding the severity of his injury was required, and so a cervical CT scan and magnetic resonance imaging (MRI) were performed.
[2] Some reports [10,11] have described patients with cervical spinal trauma who had rapidly fatal neurologic dis- orders suggestive of serious vertebrobasilar insufficiency. In fact, the time course of vertebrobasilar ischemia secondary to VA occlusion is variable, ranging from a few hours to several years. In our case, the time course was 24 hours after the injury and 12 hours after the reductive surgery, respectively.
[3] A high clinical index of suspicion remains the most important factor in making the diagnosis [17]. In patients suspected to have a lesion of the VA after cervical trauma who have altered consciousness, dysarthria, blurred vision, nystagmus, ataxia, or dysphagia, cerebrovascular examination should be indicated [18]. Once a patient is proven to be at risk of VA injury, we should take imaging studies to rule out VA injury and avoid neurological deterioration, even if there are no stigmata of vertebrobasilar insufficiency.

Fig. 4. Search results for "neuro"

3.4   Search Function

In many cases clinicians are interested in finding certain patterns in the data interactively. Some of these patterns of interest may not be prominent patterns that will be discovered in a completely unsupervised process as described above. There are at least two options of incorporating such features: (a) add user input in the process of knowledge discovery and (b) allow user to interactively retrieve relevant portions of the corpus. In this paper we describe the second option where an end user can retrieve documents that contain a certain pattern. We make use of Algorithm 1 to implement such a search function. As an example of the search function we ran query with the search pattern "neuro" in the case study on *embolic brain infarction* [38]. Our system returned 5 documents of which 3 are shown in Fig. 4.

4   Experimental Results

4.1   Data

We have used two sets of data in our experiments. The first data set was collected from patient records at the Baltimore VA Medical Center. Each dataset is a clinical episode subset of a single patient's EMR. In our experiments we used a total of 8 charts for this study from primary disease categories of *anemia, appendicitis, cecal colon cancer, diabetes, lung cancer, chronic renal disease HIV,* and *syncope and low blood pressure*. The details of the dataset are shown in Table 1 that shows the main disease category, number of nodes, edges, average degree per nodes number of connected components, and number of documents in each EHR.

Table 1. Summary of the EMRs

Disease	# nodes	# edges	Avg. deg/node	# CC	# docs
Anemia	2294	43662	19	45	5848
Appendicitis	2668	42280	16	56	7785
Colon cancer	2711	46509	17	57	7658
Diabetes	4243	99247	23	53	28559
Lung cancer	2665	40383	15	56	7911
HIV	2397	37263	15	46	4878
Chest pain	2038	37240	18	46	5066
Syncope	1926	27662	14	48	3170

The data shown in Table 1 are obtained from the Clinical Patient Record System (CPRS) which is a front end to the VA's MUMPS based electronic medical record, known as VISTA (Veterans Integrated System Technology Architecture).

Each of these documents was thoroughly reviewed for any patient identifiers or personal health information. This work was originally funded by IBM for the project in which we explored the use of the Deep Q and A software developed for Jeopardy for medical applications after addition of a corpus of additional medical information such as guidelines and other materials. Each chart was annotated by a physician for important content and questions were formulated that were intended as a test of the ability of a computer system to review the information in the chart and correlate it with additional healthcare "knowledge". The annotation consisted of a number of questions and corresponding answers related to the diagnosis and treatment of each patient. We removed the annotations from the EMRs and used them as test data against which both our method and LDA were compared as described in Sects. 4.3 and 4.4 below.

The second data set consists of 10 randomly chosen clinical case studies from the *Journal of Medical Case Reports* [38–47]. The summary of the case studies are shown in Table 2. As in Table 1 the primary disease category are shown in Table 2. As can be seen from Table 2 the graphs corresponding to most of the case studies have fewer numbers of nodes and number of connected components as compared to the EMRs. The case studies are, in general, much smaller in size as compared to the EMRs. Each paragraphs in a case study corresponds to a document which explains the fewer number of documents. The number of edges in the case studies are about the same as those of the EMRs and hence the average number of edges per node is much larger. Also, there are far fewer number of connected components as compared to the EMRs, which is due to difference in the writing styles between the case studies and the EMRs.

Table 2. Summary of the Cases

Disease	# nodes	# edges	Avg. deg/node	# CC	# docs
Brain Infarction	557	43175	78	2	27
Glioblastoma	468	48404	103	2	18
Granulomatosis	739	64571	87	3	29
Hemorrhage	480	43244	90	2	18
Hypothyroidism	566	62014	110	2	23
Breast cancer	424	28190	66	2	22
Postoperative hypertension	324	33312	103	2	10
Cardiac arrest	544	47130	87	3	23
Thoracic spinal fracture	373	27943	75	2	21
Spinal cord injury	607	65351	108	2	23

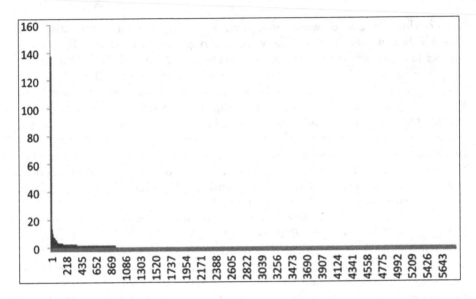

Fig. 5. Relevance scores of documents for anemia

4.2 Creating the Synopsis of Clinical Data

The relevance scores of the documents for the patient with *Anemia* is shown in Fig. 5 which shows that most of the documents (more than 5000 out of the 5848 documents) had a relevance score of 0 and 17 of these documents had a score of 10 or above. The document with the highest relevance score was 137 follow by the second most relevant document with a score of 35. The pattern of a few documents having large relevance scores and the majority of the documents having low relevant scores with 0 being the most frequent relevance score was a common feature in all of the EMRs we tested. Since each EMR graph was partitioned into multiple clusters of varying sizes, each partition had its own set of the relevant scores for all the documents within each EMR. The synopsis consisted of the documents with high relevance scores for the largest partitions for a given EMR. The size of the synopsis can be varied based on used needs.

The relevant scores corresponding to the documents in the case studies show a slightly different pattern in that the number of documents with zero or near zero relevance scores was much smaller than in the EMRs. Having fewer documents may have affected the relative lack of skewness in the case studies. The relevance scores for one of the case study on *thoracic spinal fracture* [46] is shown in Fig. 6.

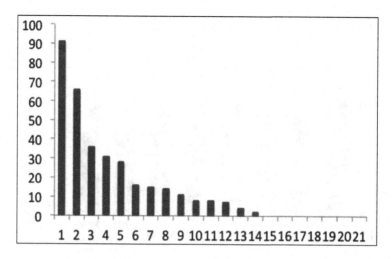

Fig. 6. Relevance scores of documents for thoracic spinal fracture

4.3   Comparison with Topic Models

We have compared our method with probabilistic topic modeling algorithms
[48], well-known for automatically discovering the thematic structures in text
documents. Like our method, topic modeling algorithms do not require any prior
annotation or labeling of the documents. A topic is a probability distribution of
words in the entire corpus. The goal of topic modeling is to discover topics that
are responsible for generating the collection of documents in the corpus. In our
experiments we used the Latent Dirichlet Allocation (LDA) as the topic modeling
algorithm. In LDA a document is treated as the outcome of a generative process
that include hidden variables. The generative process defines a joint probability
distribution over observed and hidden variables, where the observed variables
are the words in the documents, the joint probability distribution is used to
compute the conditional distribution of the hidden variables given the observed
variables. The end product is a list of topics for each document and the most
frequent words within each topic. For our experiments we selected 20 topics
per document and 10 most frequent words in each topic. The "bag-of-words"
approach of LDA is similar to our approach. However, one difference between
our approach and LDA is that LDA is a mixed-membership model where each
term can occur within multiple topics whereas in our approach a term can only
occur in a single partition, which results in a crisp separation of the themes
captured within each partition.

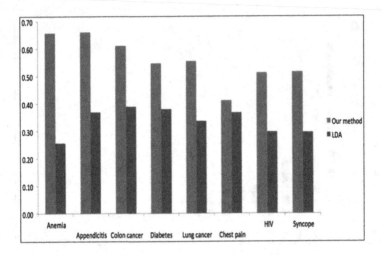

Fig. 7. Comparison with LDA using EMRs: recall

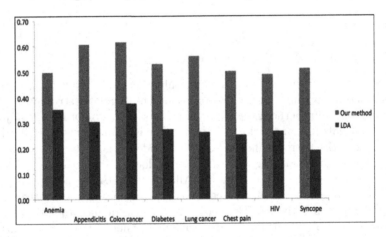

Fig. 8. Comparison with LDA using EMRs: precision

4.4   Evaluation

In order to evaluate the efficacy of our method, we used the annotations for each EMR mentioned in Sect. 4.1 as *watson*, the summary created using our method as *synopsis*, and the topics created using LDA as *LDA*. The measures used for evaluating *synopsis* and *LDA* are recall and precision by comparing the terms in each against those in *watson*. Recall and precision are defined as follows.

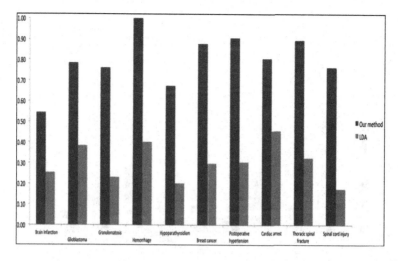

Fig. 9. Comparison with LDA using Case Studies: recall

$$Recall = \frac{TP}{TP + FN} \qquad (2)$$

$$Precision = \frac{TP}{TP + FP} \qquad (3)$$

In Eqs. 2 and 3, TP refers to the number of common clinical terms with *watson*, FP refers to the number of clinical terms that are in *synopsis* or *LDA*, depending on the model that is evaluated but not in *watson*, and FN is the number of clinical terms that are in *watson* but not in the model (*synopsis* or *LDA*). From the results shown in Figs. 7 and 8, our method has a significantly higher recall values and precision values that LDA in all of eight cases. One of the reasons for the superior performance of our method over LDA is that being a mixed membership model, there is a significant amount of overlap among the topics in LDA as opposed to the crisp separation of themes in our method.

A similar comparison was done between our method and LDA using the case studies in Figs. 9 and 10. In the case studies we used the abstract and keywords as test cases and the remaining document for creating the themes. The results are very similar to those with the EMRs in that our method consistently outperformed LDA. Even though our method consistently outperformed LDA, the recall and precision measures are still not very high. This is due to the fact that both our synopsis and the *watson* summaries are written as natural language sentences in which the same concept can be written using different phraseology. Also in our experiments we included complete sentences that included both clinical and non-clinical terms when calculating *recall* and *precision* as there was no easy way to separate the clinical from non-clinical terms. We applied a

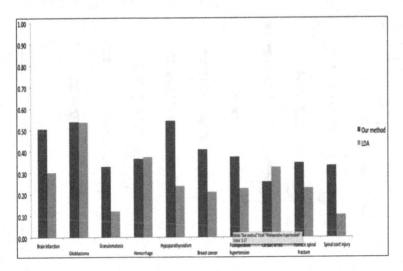

Fig. 10. Comparison with LDA using Case Studies: precision

penalty function based on an estimate of the ratio of the clinical terms in each document. However, this was done consistently in both *Synopsis* and *LDA* thus eliminating any systematic bias. The precision scores were expected to be low particularly for the case studies. This is because the abstracts were written to highlight the main features of case studies as opposed to being comprehensive as opposed to our method that aims to discover all themes embedded in the documents.

5   Conclusion and Future Challenges

The health care industry has seen a massive transition of health care records from paper records to electronic medical records in the recent years. It is important to effectively analyze patterns within these records in order to more efficiently treat individuals. In this paper, the methodology included the creation of the main themes or patterns in the data and linking the themes back to the corpus form, from which they were generated. In our research, we partitioned graphs from terms gathered from electronic medical records. Two sets of data were used in the experiments. The first data set included patient records from the Baltimore VA Medical Center. The second data set consisted of ten randomly chosen clinical case studies form the Journal of Medical Case Reports. In addition, we compared our method with probabilistic topic modeling algorithms, specifically LDA. One of the reasons for the superior performance of our method over LDA is that being a mixed membership model, there is a significant amount of overlap among the topics in LDA as opposed to the crisp separation of themes in our method. Even though our method consistently outperformed LDA, the recall and precision measures were still not very high. This was due to the fact that both our synopsis and the Watson summaries are written as natural language sentences in which the same concept can be written using different phraseology. Also, our experiments included complete sentences that included both clinical and non-clinical terms when calculating recall and precision as there was no easy way to separate the clinical from non-clinical terms.

Although the methods described in this paper provide meaningful results, there are many areas within healthcare that offer challenging problems with significant real world significance. Some of these include automated analysis of clinical charts for pre-screening patients for clinical trials, automatic de-identification of unstructured clinical data by removing protected health information, health risk identification for patients from clinical data, and providing clinical decision support for physicians. With the increasing digitization of heath data big data analytics can play a pivotal role in maximum utilization of clinical data.

References

1. Wang, F., Lee, N., Hu, J., Sun, J., Ebadollahi, S., Laine, A.F.: A framework for mining signatures from event sequences and its applications in healthcare data. IEEE Trans. Pattern Anal. Mach. Intell. **35**(2), 272–285 (2013)

2. Gotz, D., Wongsuphasawat, K.: Interactive intervention analysis. In: AMIA 2012, American Medical Informatics Association Annual Symposium, Chicago, Illinois, USA, 3–7 November 2012 (2012)

3. Gotz, D., Wang, F., Perer, A.: A methodology for interactive mining and visual analysis of clinical event patterns using electronic health record data. J. Biomed. Inform. **48**, 148–159 (2014)

4. Holzinger, A.: Interactive machine learning for health informatics: when do we need the human-in-the-loop? Brain Informatics **3**(2), 119–131 (2016)

5. Hund, M., Bohm, D., Sturm, W., Seldmair, M., Schreck, T., Ulrich, T., Keim, D.A., Majnaric, L., Holzinger, A.: Visual analytics for concept exploration in subspaces of patient groups: making sense of complex datasets with the doctor-in-the-loop. Brain Bioinform. **15**(Suppl. 6), 233–247 (2016)

6. Blondel, V.D., Guillaume, J., Lambiotte, R., Lefebvre, E.: Fast unfolding of community hierarchies in large networks. J. Stat. Mech. **2008**, 10008–10011 (2008)

7. Batal, I., Hauskrecht, M.: Mining of predictive patterns in electronic health records data (2014)

8. Wang, T.D., Plaisant, C., Shneiderman, B., Spring, N., Roseman, D., Marchand, G., Mukherjee, V., Smith, M.: Temporal summaries: supporting temporal categorical searching, aggregation and comparison. IEEE Trans. Visual Comput. Graphics **15**(6), 1049–1056 (2009)

9. Wongsuphasawat, K., Gotz, D.: Outflow: visualizing patient flow by symptoms and outcome. In: IEEE VisWeek Workshop on Visual Analytics in Healthcare (2011)

10. Wongsuphasawat, K., Shneiderman, B.: Finding comparable temporal categorical records: a similarity measure with an interactive visualization. In: Proceedings of the IEEE Symposium on Visual Analytics Science and Technology, pp. 27–34 (2009)
11. Pickett, R.M., Grinstein, G.G.: Iconographic displays for visualizing multidimensional data. In: Proceedings of the 1988 IEEE International Conference on Systems, Man, and Cybernetics, pp. 514–519 (1998)
12. Post, F.H., Walsum, T., Post, F.H., Silver, D.: Iconic techniques for feature visualization, pp. 288–295 (1995)
13. Chernoff, H.: The use of faces to represent points in k-dimensional space graphically. J. Am. Stat. Assoc. **68**, 361–368 (1973)
14. Muller, H., Reihs, R., Zatloukal, K., Holzinger, A.: Analysis of biomedical data with multilevel glyphs. Brain Bioinform. **15**(Suppl. 6), 117–140 (2016)
15. Holzinger, A.: Human-computer interaction and knowledge discovery (HCI-KDD): what is the benefit of bringing those two fields to work together? In: Cuzzocrea, A., Kittl, C., Simos, D.E., Weippl, E., Xu, L. (eds.) CD-ARES 2013. LNCS, vol. 8127, pp. 319–328. Springer, Heidelberg (2013). doi:10.1007/978-3-642-40511-2_22
16. Müller, H., Reihs, R., Zatloukal, K., Holzinger, A.: Analysis of biomedical data with multilevel glyphs. BNC Bioinform. 15(6), S5 (2014)
17. Gotz, D., Sun, J., Cao, N., Ebadollahi, S.: Visual cluster analysis in support of clinical decision intelligence. In: AMIA Annual Symposium Proceedings, pp. 481–490 (2011)
18. Orthuber, W.: A searchable patient record database for decision support. Stud. Health Technol. Inform. **150**, 584–588 (2009)
19. Tufte, E.R.: The Visual Display of Quantitative Information. Graphics Press, USA (1992)
20. Carr, D.B., Littlefield, R.J., Nichloson, W.L.: Scatterplot matrix techniques for large n. J. Am. Stat. Assoc. **82**, 424–436 (1986)
21. Inselberg, A., Dimsdale, B.: Parallel coordinates: a tool for visualizing multidimensional geometry. In: Proceedings of the 1st Conference on Visualization 1990. IEEE Computer Society Press (1990)
22. Novotny, M.: Visually effective information visualization of large data. In: 8th Central European Seminar on Computer Graphics (2004)
23. Climer, S., Zhang, W.: Rearrangement clustering: pitfalls, remedies, and applications. J. Mach. Learn. Res. **7**, 919–943 (2006)
24. Eisen, M.B., Spellman, P.T., Brown, P.O., Botstein, D.: Cluster analysis and display of genome-wide expression patterns. Proc. Natl. Acad. Sci. USA **95**(25), 14863–14868 (1998)
25. Friendly, M.: Corrgrams: exploratory displays for correlation matrices. Am. Stat. **56**(4), 316–324 (2002)
26. Chattopadhyay, S., Ray, P., Chen, H.S., Lee, M.B., Chiang, H.C.: Suicidal risk evaluation using a similarity-based classifier. In: Tang, C., Ling, C.X., Zhou, X., Cercone, N.J., Li, X. (eds.) ADMA 2008. LNCS (LNAI), vol. 5139, pp. 51–61. Springer, Heidelberg (2008). doi:10.1007/978-3-540-88192-6_7
27. Ebadollahi, S., Sun, J., Gotz, D., Hu, J., Sow, D., Neti, C.: Predicting patient's trajectory of physiological data using temporal trends in similar patients: a system for near-term prognostics. In: AMIA Annual Symposium Proceedings, pp. 192–196 (2010)

28. Cao, N., Gotz, D., Sun, J., Qu, H.: Dicon: interactive visual analysis of multidimensional clusters. IEEE Trans. Vis. Comput. Graph. **17**(12), 2581–2590 (2011)
29. Jensen, P.B., Jensen, L.J., Brunak, S.: Mining electronic health records: towards better research applications and clinical care. Nat. Rev. Genet. **13**(6), 394–405 (2012)
30. Delen, D., Walker, G., Kadam, A.: Predicting breast cancer survivability: a comparison of three data mining methods. Artif. Intell. Med. **34**(2), 113–127 (2005)
31. Oztekin, A., Delen, D., Kong, Z.: Predicting the graft survival for heart-lung transplantation patients: an integrated data mining methodology. Int. J. Med. Inf. **78**(12), e84–e96 (2009)
32. Hidalgo, C.A., Blumm, N., Barabasi, A.L., Christakis, N.: A dynamic network approach for the study of human phenotypes. PLOS Comput. Biol. **5**, 1–11 (2009)
33. Chen, L., Blumm, N., Christakis, N., Barabasi, A.L., Deisboeck, T.S.: Cancer metastasis networks and the prediction of progression patterns. Br. Cancer J. **101**, 749–758 (2009)
34. Newman, M.E.J.: Fast algorithm for detecting community structure in networks. Phys. Rev. **69**, 066133 (2004)
35. Albert, R., Barbasi, A.: The Structure and Dynamics of Networks. Princeton University Press, NY (2006)
36. Agichtein, E., Castillo, C., Donato, D.: Finding high-quality content in social media. In: Proceedings of the 2008 International Conference on Web Search and Data Mining. ACM (2008)
37. Brandes, U., Delling, D., Gaertler, M., Görke, R., Hoefer, M.: Maximizing modularity is hard. arXiv:physics/0608255v2 [physics.data-an] (2006)
38. Nakao, Y., Terai, H.: Embolic brain infarction related to posttraumatic occlusion of vertebral artery resulting from cervical spine injury: a case report. J. Med. Case Rep. **8**, 344–350 (2014)
39. Yilmaz, T., Cikla, U., Kirst, A., Baskaya, M.: Glioblastoma multiforme in klippel-trenaunay- weber syndrome: a case report. J. Med. Case Rep. **9**, 83–87 (2015)
40. Genuis, K., Pewarchuk, J.: Granulomatosis with polyangiitis (wegeners) as a necrotizing gingivitis mimic: a case report. J. Med. Case Rep. **8**, 297–301 (2014)
41. Toyoshima, M., Kudo, T., Igeta, S., et al.: Spontaneous retroperitoneal hemorrhage caused by rupture of an ovarian artery aneurysm: a case report and review of the literature. J. Med. Case Rep. **9**, 84–89 (2015)
42. Panazzolo, D., Braga, T., Bergamim, A., et al.: Hypoparathyroidism after roux-en-y gastric bypass - a challenge for clinical management: a case report. J. Med. Case Rep. **8**, 357–361 (2014)
43. Osaku, T., Ogata, H., Magoshi, S., et al.: Metastatic nonpalpable invasive lobular breast carcinoma presenting as rectal stenosis: a case report. J. Med. Case Rep. **9**, 88–93 (2015)
44. Hartog, N., Kamath, A.: A 90-year-old patient presenting with postoperative hypotension and a new murmur: a case report. J. Med. Case Rep. **8**, 363–366 (2014)
45. Jellinge, M.: Severe septic shock and cardiac arrest in a patient with vibrio metschnikovii: a case report. J. Med. Case Rep. **8**, 348–350 (2014)

46. Jiang, B., Zhu, R., Cao, Q., Pan, H.: Severe thoracic spinal fracture-dislocation without neurological symptoms and costal fractures: a case report and review of the literature. J. Med. Case Rep. **8**, 343–348 (2014)
47. Erdal, U., Mehmet, D., Turkay, K., Mehmet, I., Ibrahim, N., Hasan, B.: Esophagus perforation and myocardial penetration caused by swallowing of a foreign body leading to a misdiagnosis of acute coronary syndrome: a case report. J. Med. Case Rep. **9**, 57–59 (2015)
48. Blei, D.M.: Probabilistic topic models. Commun. ACM **55**(4), 77–84 (2012)

Reasoning Under Uncertainty: Towards Collaborative Interactive Machine Learning

Sebastian Robert[1]([⊠]), Sebastian Büttner[2], Carsten Röcker[1,2,3],
and Andreas Holzinger[3]

[1] Fraunhofer-Institute of Optronics, System Technologies and Image Exploitation,
Application Center Industrial Automation (IOSB-INA), Lemgo, Germany
`sebastian.robert@iosb-ina.fraunhofer.de`
[2] Ostwestfalen-Lippe University of Applied Sciences, Lemgo, Germany
`{sebastian.buettner,carsten.roecker}@hs-owl.de`
[3] Holzinger Group, HCI-KDD, Institute for Medical Informatics,
Statistics and Documentation, Medical University Graz, Graz, Austria
`a.holzinger@hci-kdd.org`

Abstract. In this paper, we present the current state-of-the-art of decision making (DM) and machine learning (ML) and bridge the two research domains to create an integrated approach of complex problem solving based on human and computational agents. We present a novel classification of ML, emphasizing the human-in-the-loop in interactive ML (iML) and more specific on collaborative interactive ML (ciML), which we understand as a deep integrated version of iML, where humans and algorithms work hand in hand to solve complex problems. Both humans and computers have specific strengths and weaknesses and integrating humans into machine learning processes might be a very efficient way for tackling problems. This approach bears immense research potential for various domains, e.g., in health informatics or in industrial applications. We outline open questions and name future challenges that have to be addressed by the research community to enable the use of collaborative interactive machine learning for problem solving in a large scale.

Keywords: Decision making · Reasoning · Interactive machine learning · Collaborative interactive machine learning

1 Introduction and Motivation

Disregarding the application domain, i.e. whether in the medical domain or in the industrial context, current developments such as the rapidly growing communication infrastructure, the internet of things and increasing processing power with services and applications on top of those lead to massive amounts of data and new possibilities. Traditional analytic tools are not well suited to capturing the full value of "big data". Instead ML is ideal for exploiting opportunities hidden in data. Highly complex small batch production and personalized medicine (precision medicine [1]) are two of many possible target scenarios. Both depend

© Springer International Publishing AG 2016
A. Holzinger (Ed.): ML for Health Informatics, LNAI 9605, pp. 357–376, 2016.
DOI: 10.1007/978-3-319-50478-0_18

on computer-intensive data processing prior to its analysis and decision making processes.

However, to handle and exploit the required data, besides computer algorithms, human capabilities are strongly needed as well. For example, classical logic in ML approaches permits only exact reasoning, i.e. if A is true then A is non-false and if B is false then B is non-true. However, even though modern sophisticated automatic ML approaches can hardly cope with such situations, human agents can deal with such deficiencies.

Moreover, many ML approaches are based on *normative* models such as formal probability theory and expected utility (EU) theory. EU theory accounts for decision under uncertainty and is based on axioms of rational behavior described by von Neumann and Morgenstern (1944) [2]. Based upon the fact that information available in daily problem solving situations is most of the time imperfect, imprecise and uncertain due to time pressure, disturbance of unknown factors or randomness outcome of some attributes [3,4], the interaction between human and computer has to be designed in an optimal way in order to realize the best possible output. Given that, a combined approach of human and computer input can be a sustainable approach for effectively revealing structural or temporal patterns ("knowledge") and make them accessible for decision making.

At this point, decision theory comes into play and helps us to deal with bounded rationality and the problem of which questions to pose to human experts and how to ask those questions. Therefore, new types of human-computer interaction (HCI) will arise and shape the ecosystem of human, technology and organization. In particular, adaptive decision support systems that help humans to solve complex problems and make far-reaching decisions will play a central role in future work places.

In this paper, we will focus on decision making under uncertainty and bridge it to ML research and particularly to interactive ML. After discussing the state-of-the-art in ML and decision making under uncertainty, we provide some practical aspects for the integration of both approaches. Finally, we discuss some open questions and outline future research avenues.

2   Glossary and Key Terms

Bias refers to a systematic pattern of deviation from rationality in decision making processes.

Bounded Rationality – introduced by Herbert A. Simon [5] – is used to denote the type of rationality that people resort to when the environment in which they operate is too complex relative to their limited mental abilities [6].

Decision Support Systems (DSS) are intended to assist decision makers in taking full advantage of available information and are a central part of health informatics [7] and industrial applications [8].

Decision Theory is concerned with goal-directed behaviour in the presence of options [9]. While *normative* decision theory focuses on identifying the optimal decision to make, assuming a fully-rational decision maker who is able to compute with perfect accuracy, *descriptive* decision theory deals with questions pertaining to how people actually behave in given choice situations. *Prescriptive* decision theory is the logic consequence and tries to exploit some of the logical consequences of normative theories and empirical findings of descriptive studies to make better choices [10].

Expected Utility (EU) Theory consists of four axioms, that define a rational decision maker: completeness, transitivity, independence, and continuity; if those are satisfied, then the decision making is considered to be rational and the preferences can be represented by a utility function, i.e. one can assign numbers (utilities) [2].

Heuristics describe approaches to problem solving and decision making which are not perfect, but sufficient for reaching immediate goals [11].

Human-Computer Interaction (HCI) is a multi-disciplinary research field that deals with *"the design, implementation and evaluation of interactive systems in the context of the user's task and work"* [12, p. 4]. It can be located at the intersection of psychology and cognitive science, ergonomics, computer science and engineering, business, design, technical writing and other fields [12, p. 4].

Judgment and Decision Making (JDM) is a descriptive field of research which focuses on understanding decision processes on an individual and group level.

Machine Learning (ML) is a research field grounding in computer science that *"concentrates on induction algorithms and on other algorithms that can be said to 'learn'"* [13]. While in *automatic Machine Learning (aML)* representations of real-world objects and knowledge are automatically generated from data, *interactive Machine Learning (iML)* methods allow humans to interact with computers in some way to generate knowledge and find an optimal solution for a problem. More specifically, *collaborative interactive Machine Learning (ciML)* is a form of iML, where at least one human is integrated into the algorithm using a specific user interface that allows manipulating the algorithm and its intermediate steps to find a good solution in a short time.

Perception-Based Classification (PBC) is a classification of data done by humans based on their visual perception. In the context of ML, PBC has been introduced by Ankerst et al. [14] who enabled users to interactively create decision trees. PBC can be seen as one possible way of realizing iML.

Utility Theorem describes that a decision-maker faced with probabilistic (particularly when probabilities are distorted or unknown) outcomes of different choices will behave as if she/he is maximizing the expected value [15]; this is the basis for the expected utility theory.

3   State-of-the-Art

In this section, we will provide an overview of the current research regarding two fields: First, we will investigate machine learning (ML) and focus especially on the advances in interactive machine learning (iML). Second, we will provide an overview of the research on JDM under uncertainty. We will further focus on bridging the research on human decision making and the research on iML. We will motivate, why the knowledge of and research on human decision-making is key for the development of future human-oriented ciML systems.

3.1   Machine Learning (ML)

ML is a very practical field with many application areas, though at the same time well grounded theories with many open research challenges exist. There are many various definitions, depending on whom to ask; a Bayesian will give a different answer than a Symbolist [16]; a classical definition is close to and grounding in computer science that *"concentrates on induction algorithms and on other algorithms that can be said to 'learn'"* [13]. This definition is at the same time the goal of ML which concentrates on the development of *"programs that automatically improve with experience"* [17]. Advances in ML have solved many practical problems, e.g., recognizing speech [18], giving movie recommendations based on personal references [19] or driving a vehicle autonomously [20].

In the following, we will differentiate between classical ML approaches, that we will call aML and the newer concepts of iML.

Automatic Machine Learning (aML): Methods and algorithms of machine learning are often categorized as follows (here the classification of Marsland [21]):

- With *supervised learning* methods, an algorithm creates a general model from a training set of examples containing input and output data (targets). With this model, the output of new unknown input can be predicted.
- Contrary, when using *unsupervised learning* methods, the output data are not provided to the algorithm. The algorithm focuses on finding similarities between a set of input data and classifies the data into categories.
- *Reinforcement learning* is somehow between supervised and unsupervised learning. It characterizes algorithms that receive feedback, in the case that their created output data are wrong. By this feedback the algorithm can explore possibilities and iteratively find better models, respectively outputs.
- Finally *evolutionary learning* methods develop models iteratively by receiving an assessment of the quality (fitness) of the current model. As the term depicts, this learning method is inspired by the biological evolution.

The mentioned methods and algorithms all have in common, that they – once started – run automatically. We therefore call those classical machine learning methods *automatic machine learning*. When using aML methods, human involvement is in general very limited and restricted to the following three aspects:

- Humans have to prepare the data and remove corrupt or wrong data sets from the input data (data cleansing).

- When using supervised learning methods, humans are responsible for providing the output data, e.g., for labeling data in classification tasks.
- Another user involvement is the assessment of a certain model and the evaluation. Humans can assess the generated model and its results, and decide, whether a certain model is able to produce good predictions or not.

The traditional approach does not put much emphasize on the human interactions with the ML system. Humans are somehow involved in providing the data as described above, but the early ML research mostly neglects the question, how humans can provide data and how they deal with an inaccurate model. From a practical perspective, this is a huge restriction in automatic machine learning (aML) systems. The main problems of practical ML applications are often not the implementation of the algorithm itself, but rather the data acquisition and cleansing. Often data are corrupt or of bad quality and in most cases data do not cover all required context information to solve a specific problem [3,4].

Interactive Machine Learning (iML): Compared to aML, iML is a relative new approach that also considers the human involvement and interactions in ML and aims at putting the human into the loop of machine learning. In this section, we will discuss the approaches and concepts that previously have been described under the term iML. We will distinguish in this section between three types of iML methods: First, early works in the iML research considered iML as an alternative way of ML where humans accomplish the model generation, which basically means that humans replace algorithms. Second, concepts have been proposed under the term iML that put a human into the training-evaluation loop, but still execute algorithms automatically. Contrary to aML in this type of iML algorithms have to be much faster to give rapid feedback to a user. Third, humans can work hand in hand with algorithms to create a certain model, which we consider as the most promising concept of iML with the best integration of users and algorithms.

Humans replacing algorithms: Early work in iML has been done by Ankerst et al. [14]. They implemented a system called perception-based classification (PBC) that provides users the means to interactively create decision trees by visualizing the training data in a suitable way. By interacting with the visualized training data, users select attributes and split points to construct the decision trees. The system cannot automatically generate the tree. Instead, the user of the system replaces the algorithm and creates the tree manually with the interactive application provided. According to their evaluation, the system reaches the same accuracy as algorithmic classifiers but the human-generated decision trees have a smaller tree size, which is beneficial in terms of understandability. Another advantage of the interactive and manual approach is the possibility of backtracking in case of a suboptimal subtree – a situation that humans can easily recognize [14]. A huge benefit of this human-centered approach is the integration of the users' domain knowledge into the decision tree construction [22].

Building on the work of Ankerst et al., Ware et al. [23] developed a similar system that replaces the algorithm with users. Their work focuses mainly on an empirical evaluation of the performance of humans compared to state-of-the-art algorithms. According to their study, novice users can build trees that are as accurate as the ones provided from algorithms, but similar to Ankerst et al. they found, that the tree size is decreased, when humans generate the decision trees. On the other hand, Ware et al. point out that this manual iML approach might not be suitable for large data sets and high-dimensional data. This early variant of interactive machine learning is shown in Fig. 1A.

Humans in the training-evaluation loop: Another variety of iML is the integration of humans into the training-evaluation loop, when using supervised learning methods. Fails and Olsen [24] were one of the first, who used the term iML and proposed this integration for the rapid development of models, if the feature selection cannot be done by domain-experts due to missing knowledge. They give an example of the use of iML for the rapid development of perceptual user interfaces (PUIs), that are developed by interaction designers who are usually not familiar with computer vision (CV) algorithms. For this purpose, they provide a tool that gives designers rapid visual feedback of the produced classifiers and the iterative changes of the selected features for the model generation. The tool masks the complexity of the feature selection and rather allows users to assess the output of the model generation and to drive the feature selection into the right direction. A similar concept has been described by Fiebrink et al. [25]. They developed Wekinator[1], a system that analyses human gestures in the context of music making. A graphical user interface supports users with the creation of appropriate training data, the configuration of various ML algorithms and parameters and allows a real-time evaluation of the trained model by giving visual or auditory feedback. This real-time evaluation allows a domain user to rapidly adapt the input data to improve the model. Fogarty et al. [26] presented CueFlik, a similar iML tool for generating models for image classification tasks. For the mentioned type of iML, it is essential to have algorithms that have a very short learning time to be able to give rapid feedback on the results [24]. Addressing this particular aspect in connection with big data, Simard et al. [27] described a system that is very generic in terms of the data types and tasks and interactive even when using big data. Their system called ICE (interactive classification and extraction) allows users to interactively build models consisting of several millions of items. In [28] they extend their approach and additionally deliver feedback about the performance of the generated model to the user. With this system they empower users to not only optimize the model in terms of accuracy, but to optimize in terms of performance as well. While the mentioned systems use only one model, in recent years model ensembles became the standard of ML [16]. Talbort et al. therefore provide a tool that deals with multiple models and allows users to interactively build combination models [29]. All mentioned publications in this section use the term iML to describe a concept,

---

[1] http://www.wekinator.org/.

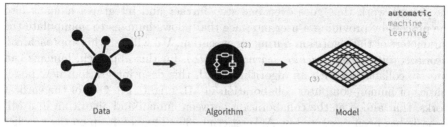

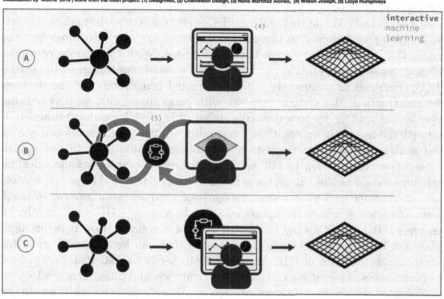

Fig. 1. Classification of interactive machine learning (iML). A: Early iML research aimed at replacing algorithms and using human pattern recognition capabilities instead. B: Later iML methods have been proposed that provide a rapid feedback cycle to users. Models are generated in a very short time and presented to users. Based on the presented model, users can adapt the input data and rerun the machine learning algorithm. With this approach the model is iteratively improved. C: Using collaborative interactive machine learning (ciML) humans can manipulate an algorithm during runtime and improve the model while it is generated. Human and computational agents work collaboratively on a specific problem.

where humans are in the training-evaluation loop, but cannot interfere with the algorithm itself – from a human perspective the algorithm is a black-box. The method of putting humans into the training-evaluation loop is shown in Fig. 1B.

Humans collaborating with algorithms: Sinard et al. define iML as a ML scenario, where *"the teacher can provide [. . .] information to the machine as the learning task progresses"* [27]. De facto, most systems presented in the past realized this iML by providing means to users to evaluate a certain model and by changing the training data to optimize the previously generated model. In this section, we present work that goes even one step further and integrates humans into the process by providing a user interface that allows humans to manipulate the parameters of the algorithm during its execution. We will call this approach *collaborative interactive machine learning (ciML)*. Im this approach, humans can directly collaborate with an algorithm. With this deep integration, new possibilities of human-computer collaboration in ML might rise. One of the earliest works, that aimed at the collaboration between human and algorithm in a ML scenario has been presented by Ankerst et al. [30]. They built up on their earlier PBC system [14] and provide an iML system for building decision trees for a classification task. While their earlier PBC system only visualized data and left the decision tree building to the users, algorithms are now integrated into the system that might (but does not have to) be used. With the options provided, different types of cooperation can be realized: manual (equivalent to the earlier PBC), combined or completely automatic model generation. For the decision tree construction, the system supports with proposing splits, with visualizing hypothetical splits – up to a defined number of levels ("look-ahead function"), and with the feature of automatically expanding subtrees. One mentioned goal of their work is the use of human pattern recognition capabilities in the interactive decision tree construction by still using algorithmic operations to allow dealing with huge data sets [30]. Along these lines, Holzinger defines iML as "*algorithms that can interact with agents and can optimize their learning behavior through these interactions, where the agents can also be human*" [31], consequently, he considers iML as this deeply integrated type of a collaboration between algorithm and human. He discusses another issue that can be addressed with this deeply integrated form of iML: Sometimes ML needs to deal with rare events, like occurrences of rare diseases in health informatics, and consequently adequate training data are missing. He identifies new application areas for ciML within the health domain, e.g. for subspace clustering, protein folding, or k-anonymization of patient data and names challenges for the future ciML research. Holzinger also shows that the solution of complex problems is possible by using ciML. He presents the integration of users into an ant colony algorithm to solve a traveling salesman problem (TSP) [32]. A visualization shows the pheromone tracks of the ants in the TSP and the optimal round-trip found by the algorithm so far. Users can select edges and add or remove the current amount of pheromones on the edge between each of the iterations. First experiments show that the process is sped up in terms of required iterations to find the optimal solution [32]. The collaborative variant of interactive machine learning is shown in Fig. 1C. As the related work regarding the collaboration between humans and algorithms in iML shows, there has not been done a lot of research investigating the challenges and opportunities of a human-algorithm interaction. Application areas of this new iML approach need to be further identified and the implications of a human agent in the iML system need to be explored. While humans can bring tacit knowledge and context information into the process of building models, the question remains unclear how human decisions effect the output of the iML system. However, there has been a lot of research regarding human-decision making that we will introduce in the next section.

3.2   Judgement and Decision Research

Generally, the main focus of ML is on dealing with uncertainty and making predictions. In order to infer unknowns, data sets have to be learned and analysed. Therefore, most ML approaches are based on *normative* models such as formal probability theory and EU theory. EU theory accounts for decisions under uncertainty and is based on axioms of rational behavior, codified by von Neumann and Morgenstern [2]. It states that the overall utility of an option equals the expected utility, calculated by multiplying the utility and probability of each outcome [33, p. 24]. Probability theory in ML is most often used in terms of Bayesian decision theory [34–37], which is build on EU theory as a framework for solving problems under uncertainty [38, p. 140]. "Individuals who follow these theories are said to be rational" [39, p. 724].

The successful integration of knowledge of a domain expert in the black-box as discussed in the iML approach stands or falls with the careful consideration of people's actual decision making abilities. It is generally accepted that human reasoning and decision making abilities can exhibit various shortcomings when compared with mathematical logic [3]. Hence, the question that arises is, how to integrate human and computer input, accounting for the imperfections of both [40, p. 2122]. At this point *descriptive* decision theory can offer useful insights for the optimal integration of human judgement in iML approaches.

Descriptive decision theory deals with questions pertaining to how people behave in given choice situations and what we need to fully predict their behaviour in such situations [41, p. 2]. In many cases, this is a difficult task due to given inconsistencies in people's choices. These inconsistencies can often be attributed to irrational behaviour or accidental errors, which can also lead to deficient decisions [41, p. 6].

Within the last decades, a growing research community within the area of descriptive decision making is focusing on understanding individual and group judgement and decision making (JDM) [42,43].[2] Researchers from various fields are actively contributing to JDM, e.g. cognitive psychologists, social psychologists, statisticians and economists [42,45]. They have developed a detailed picture of the ways in which individuals judgement is bounded [46], e.g., people violate the axions of EU theory and do not always follow basic principles of calculus [47,48]. JDM tasks are characterized by uncertainty and/or by a concern for individual's preferences and will therefore apply to central aspects of human activities in iML [38, p. 140]. In detail, JDM research focuses on how different factors (e.g., information visualization) affect decision quality and how it can be improved [49,50]. In order to give any predictions about human judgement, JDM usually presupposes a definition of rationality that makes certain actions measurable. This instrumental view of rationality only accords with normative theory if keeping in line with it helps to attain satisfaction – measured in subjective utility [51]. A basic approach of JDM is to compare actual judgements to normative models and look for deviations. These so called *biases* are

---

[2] See also [44] for the chapter.

the starting point for building models that explain and predict human decision making behaviour. A fundamental outcome of early JDM research reveals that the typical model of a "rational man" as presumed by most normative theories – considering every possible action, every outcome in every possible state and calculating the choice that would lead to the best outcome – is unrealistic and does not exist [5]. Instead innumerous studies revealed that people cannot carry out the complex and time-consuming calculations necessary to determine the ideal choice out of possible actions [52, p. 7]. Instead people act as "satisficers" and make decisions on the basis of limited information, cognitive limitations and the time available. Simon's concept of *bounded rationality* describes how people actually reach a judgement or a decision and has become a widely used model for human decision behaviour [5].

Building on Simon's model, Tversky and Kahneman developed their heuristics and biases program that fundamentally shaped our understanding of judgment as we know it today [48]. According to their argumentation, coming to a decision requires a process of information search. Information can be retrieved from memory or other external sources. In any case, information has to be preprocessed for the particular problem and a final conclusion has so be drawn. Therefore, information processing is key for decision making and limited cognitive abilities, as stated in the model of bounded rationality, might essentially impact decision quality. The major reason for the huge impact of the heuristics and biases program in research is, that it is able to explain a wide variety of different decision situations without restricting it due to motivated irrationality [52, p. 1].

Tversky and Kahneman assume, that decisions under uncertainty are based on heuristics rather than complex algorithms [48]. Heuristics are defined as mental short-cuts or rules of thumb and require only limited amount of information and cognitive abilities. Generally, heuristics achieve results fast and depend on low effort. To do so, they neglect relevant information, which can lead to systematic predictable deviations from rationality. There is a huge amount of evidence that biases can lead to poor outcomes in important and novel decisions [42,53]. This, together with the fact that biases are systematic, emphasises the importance of incorporating heuristics in modelling.

In their pioneering work, Tversky and Kahneman described three fundamental heuristics [48] which are relevant in countless practical situations. The representativeness heuristic is applied when people make judgements about the probability of an unknown event. To come up with a judgement, people tend to judge the probability of the unknown event by finding a comparable known event and assume that the probabilities will be similar. For illustration, Tversky and Kahneman developed the "Linda problem", where they describe the fictitious person Linda as "31 years old, single, outspoken, and very bright. She majored in philosophy. As a student, she was deeply concerned with issues of discrimination and social justice, and also participated in anti-nuclear demonstrations" [54, p. 297]. Thereupon they asked subjects which is more probable, (a) Linda being a bank teller or (b) Linda being a bank teller and actively involved in feminist movement. Results reveal, that in accordance with their hypothesis, a vast majority (80–90%) of subjects chose the conjunction (b) to be more likely than the single event (a). From a logical perspective, a conjunction of events (b) can never be more likely than any of its constituents (a) and therefore indicates a violation of rationality. Within the last decades, many different biases have been linked to the representativeness heuristic (e.g., conjunction fallacy, base rate neglect, insensitivity to sample size) [42].

The availability heuristic is the second of Tversky and Kahnemans heuristics and states, that people rely upon knowledge that is easily available and comes to mind rather than complete data [55]. By relying on the availability of a given event in someone's memory, the actual probability of the event can often be predicted quite good. Nevertheless, sometimes the availability of an event is influenced by other factors besides the probability or frequency of the occurrence and in this case the availability heuristic will lead to systematic deviations from rationality [55]. For example the chronological distance or conciseness are factors that can influence the availability of an event. The cause of death "firearm" is estimated as much higher compared to "tobacco", which can be attributed to the media coverage of violence [42,56]. Similar to this, subjects who were asked to estimate "If a random word is taken from an English text, is it more likely that the word starts with a K, or that K is the third letter?" [55, p. 1125]. Following Tversky and Kahneman's hypothesis, people easier recall words beginning with an K and therefore overestimate the number of words that begin with the letter K. Although experimental results support this hypothesis, a text typically contains twice as many words which have the letter K at the third, rather than first letter.

The so-called anchoring and adjustment heuristic describes a widely explored and robust phenomenon in human decision making [48]. The heuristic can be very useful when primary values of information do hint to a correct answer and are relevant to the underlying decision-problem – a situation found in many daily tasks. The anchor effect – as the central result of the anchoring and adjustment heuristic – can be found in situations, where a numerical starting point (the *anchor*) is processed to form a final estimation. In case the final estimation is biased towards the initial starting point, one talks about an anchoring effect. In a well-known demonstration, Tversky and Kahneman asked subjects to estimate the percentage of African countries that are in the United Nations (UN) [48, p. 1128]. Prior to this, for every subject of the experiment, a random number between one and one hundred after spinning a wheel of fortune was chosen. Subjects had to state if the random number is higher or lower compared to the true value. It was found, that people who had a lower number estimated fewer countries in the UN than people who had a higher number. Thereupon numerous experiments validated the robustness of the anchoring effect in varying fields of application, e.g. general knowledge [57], probability estimates [44,58] and negotiations [59,60]. Neither financial incentives nor explicit advices could effectivly mitigate the anchoring effect [61,62]. Moreover, the numerical starting point does not have to be relevant to the underlying decision-problem, even unconsciously perceived or irrelevant values can distort the judgement [61, p. 123]. In general, there are two different approaches to explain the occurrence of the anchor effect. The original approach of Tversky and Kahneman states that individuals tend to anchor onto a numerical value and then gradually adjust away from that value until they reach a decision that seems reasonable [48]. This anchoring and adjustment process is usually insufficient and therefore biased. In contrast, the selective accessibility approach argues, that biased estimations are rooted in an early phase of information processing [57,63,64]. Following the approach, individuals, when given an anchor, will evaluate the hypothesis that the anchor is a suitable answer (confirmatory hypothesis testing) and therefore access all the relevant attributes of the anchor value. Thereon, the approach assumes that anchoring effects are mediated by the selectively increased accessibility of anchor-consistent knowledge and the final estimate is therefore biased towards the anchor. Overall, none of the mentioned approaches can fully explain empirical evidence and the origin of the anchoring effect is still highly debated within the research community [42,65].

In addition to the three fundamental heuristics and their resulting biases, there are further heuristics which try to explain decision making under specific situations. Despite the tremendous success of the heuristics and biases program, there are alternative approaches to explain actual decision making behaviour. For example the fast-and-frugal-approach – mostly based on Gigerenzers works – is also based on several simple heuristics, but in contrast to the classical heuristics, they are precisely defined and can be directly validated [66,67]. Moreover, the probabilistic mental model [68] and prospect theory [69] also build on limited cognitive abilities and are used in different areas to predict decision making behaviour.

3.3 Practical Aspects for the Integration of Interactive ML and Decision Theory

The importance of the integration of interactive ML and decision theory is evident. Given the massive consequences that can result from suboptimal decision making, it is critical to improve our knowledge about ways to yield better decision outcomes [46, p. 379]. In our knowledge-based economy, each decision is likely to have vast implications and will affect subsequent decisions on their own. Decision problems have to be analysed for their potential receptiveness to decision biases and in what ways they are likely to benefit from automatic processing.

On the one side, current technological and methodical advances enable us to cope with more complex decision tasks. But on the other side, in many practical situations decision making in terms of the interaction between human and computer input is still limited and does not tap the full potential. Moreover, new decision situations in many fields of application are characterized by the same underlying process and therefore share the common need for new ways of interaction.

For example, there are innumerable applications in the field of medical decision making and cyber-physical systems (e.g. "Industry 4.0") such as assistance or recommender systems that are based on the same abstract decision problem, combine similar approaches of computer algorithms with human input and therefore face similar challenges. For instance, the analysis of sensor data is pretty similar in many practical applications. On the one hand, data may describe body parameters such as temperature, heartbeat or blood plasma concentration in a medical context. On the other hand, data may provide information about the energy consumption of a power unit, the temperature of an engine or the status of a relay in an industrial context. Although there are many algorithms that can analyse the captured data in a purely unsupervised fashion, in order to achieve excellent and instant results, an interactive data analysis backed by human decision making skills can offer new possibilities and bring context information into the process. The same applies to the area of image exploitation. In many cases, it is about finding structural anomalies in data and learning from previous examples. With up-to-date methods of image exploitation, algorithms can detect, count and cluster different types of objects. These algorithms are in many cases only partially automatic and require human input. In medical image exploitation, doctors can help to provide diagnostic findings in the segmentation of skin cancer images [70]. In the industrial context, image exploitation is for example used to detect tool wear [71]. In both situations, wrong diagnoses and decisions potentially bear extensive risk and therefore the optimal integration of human and computer input is of great importance. A big issue is accordingly the integration process, because exactly here setting up a system between the expert and the algorithm requires a common ground between them and is crucial for total imaging. This common ground has to exploit computational power and integrate human intelligence to realise the best possible output.

4 Open Problems

The study of ML is primarily based on normative models. Most of these models are the result of centuries of refection and analysis and are widely accepted as the basis of logical reasoning. For the fact that human decision making skills are in certain settings superior to computer algorithms – e.g. many ML-methods perform very badly on extrapolation problems which would be very easy for humans [32, p. 4] – and major assumptions of normative models cannot be applied in reality, a conjoint approach of human and machine input could be key to enhanced decision quality. Therefore, the answer is to put humans in the loop [40]. However, using normative models to integrate human decision making in centrals parts of machine learning could lead to faulty predictions since the nature of actual decision making is of bounded rationality [5].

Based on the described approaches, today we know the specific ways in which decision makers are likely to be biased and we can describe how people make decisions with astonishing detail and reliability. In addition, with regards to normative models, we have a clear vision of how much better decision making could be [46]. The most important step now is to integrate those two different approaches, correct biases and improve decision making. The prescriptions for such corrections are called prescriptive models [33, p. 19] and will decide about the success of human-in-the-loop approaches in ML. Altogether, not only do we need to know the nature of the specific problem, "but normative models must be understood in terms of their role in looking for biases, understanding these biases in terms of descriptive models and developing prescriptive models" [72, p. 20].

In consideration of this fact, interactive ML approaches are a promising candidate for further enhancing the knowledge discovery process. One important problem which we have to face in future research is which questions to pose to humans and how to ask those questions [40]. At this point, human machine-interaction could provide useful insights and offer guidelines for the design of interfaces and visualisations. Moreover, research in this area, i.e. at the intersection of cognitive science and computational science is fruitful for further improving ML thus improve performance on a wide range of tasks, including settings which are difficult for humans to process (e.g., big data and high dimensional problems) [32]. According to Lee and Holzinger [73], there is a very common misconception about high dimensionality, i.e. that ML would produce better outcomes with higher dimensional data. Increasing amounts of input features can build more accurate predictors as features are key to learning and understanding. However, such attempts need high computational power, and due to limitations in human perception, understanding structures in high dimensional spaces is practically impossible. Hence, the outcome must be shaped in a form perceivable for humans, which is a very difficult problem. Here graph-based representations in $\mathbb{R}^2$ are very helpful in that respect and open up a lot of future possibilities [74, 75].

5   Future Challenges

The important role of iML for dealing with complexity is evident. However, future research has to be done in various areas.

First of all, only a few research projects have dealt with ciML. The development of new ciML approaches for different algorithms has to be expanded to be able to develop generic human-algorithm interfaces. Research has to focus on further algorithms beyond decision trees and ant colony algorithms that could benefit from the new approach of ciML to analyze its full potential.

Secondly, from the knowledge today it cannot be said, which problems ciML can address and which problems will not be addressable with ciML. Future research has to focus on the classification of problems in terms of the different aML, iML and ciML approaches. For some problems we do know that aML can provide very efficient algorithms, some problems are known to be unsolvable in polynomial time, but we currently do not have comprehensive knowledge about the opportunities of ciML.

Thirdly, the iML algorithms proposed so far address very specific problems. In general, the questions have been solved, how humans can be integrated into the algorithm and understand both the underlying problem and the algorithm with its parameters. Therefore, the past and ongoing research on HCI will play a prominent role in the future of iML: It has to be further analyzed, how humans (not only computer scientists) can be empowered to better understand the specific ML algorithms. This involves adequate visualization techniques of the input data, as shown by past research projects as well as visualizations to support the understandability of complex algorithms. In this respect, new interaction technologies might come in handy. Large displays [76], room-spanning projections [77], gesture-based interactions and virtual and augmented reality (VR and AR) [78,79] are new interaction concepts and technologies that have been applied successfully in the medical [80] and industrial [81–83] domains and might be able to play a roll in the interaction with algorithms in the future.

6   Conclusion

In this paper, we presented the current state of research in two domains: JDM and ML. We presented a new classification of ML emphasizing on iML and – more specificly – on ciML. We bridged the two research domains and argued that future research will have to take both research domains into account, when dealing with highly complex problems. Both humans and computers have their specific strengths and weaknesses and putting humans into the loop of ML algorithms might be a very efficient way for solving specific problems. We identified two application areas, which provide complex problems that might benefit from the new approach of ciML: health informatics and cyber-physical systems. While these two domains seem to be different on the first sight, their problems often share the same characteristics: Often exceptional variances in data need to be found, e.g. a specific diseases based on physiological data in medicine or malfunctions of complex cyber-physical systems based on sensor data of machines. The classical approach of aML focuses on finding these patterns based on previous knowledge from data. However, aML struggles on function extrapolation problems which are trivial for human learners. Consequently, integrating a human-into-the-loop (e.g., a human kernel [84]) could make use of human cognitive abilities and will be a promising approach. While we outlined the potential of ciML there are multiple open questions to be tackled in the research community. The explorative development of new ciML approaches for different algorithms will help to analyze the full potential of ciML. Existing complex problems need to be classified and application areas for the different iML approaches need to be identified. And last but not least, the questions on how to support humans ideally when collaborating with algorithms and big data needs to be addressed. In this area the experts from both ML and HCI will have to work hand in hand in this new joint research endeavor that will greatly help in future problem solving.

Acknowledgements. We thank our colleague Henrik Mucha who provided insight and expertise that greatly assisted this research. We also thank the anonymous reviewers for their encouraging reviews.

References

1. Holzinger, A.: Trends in interactive knowledge discovery for personalized medicine: cognitive science meets machine learning. IEEE Intell. Inform. Bull. **15**, 6–14 (2014)
2. Von Neumann, J., Morgenstern, O.: Theory of Games and Economic Behavior. Princeton University Press, Princeton (1944)
3. Fox, J., Glasspool, D., Bury, J.: Quantitative and qualitative approaches to reasoning under uncertainty in medical decision making. In: Quaglini, S., Barahona, P., Andreassen, S. (eds.) AIME 2001. LNCS, vol. 2101, pp. 272–282. Springer, Heidelberg (2001). doi:10.1007/3-540-48229-6_39
4. Ma, W., Xiong, W., Luo, X.: A model for decision making with missing, imprecise, and uncertain evaluations of multiple criteria. Int. J. Intell. Syst. **28**, 152–184 (2013)
5. Simon, H.A.: A behavioral model of rational choice. Q. J. Econ. **69**, 99–118 (1955)
6. Dequech, D.: Bounded rationality, institutions, and uncertainty. J. Econ. Issues **35**, 911–929 (2001)
7. Holzinger, A.: Lecture 8 biomedical decision making: reasoning and decision support. In: Biomedical Informatics, pp. 345–377. Springer, Heidelberg (2014)
8. March, S.T., Hevner, A.R.: Integrated decision support systems: a data warehousing perspective. Decis. Support Syst. **43**, 1031–1043 (2007)
9. Hansson, S.O.: Decision theory: a brief introduction (2005)
10. Bell, D.E., Raiffa, H., Tversky, A.: Descriptive, normative, and prescriptive interactions in decision making. Decis. Making Descriptive Normative Prescriptive Interact. **1**, 9–32 (1988)
11. Pearl, J.: Heuristics: Intelligent Search Strategies for Computer Problem Solving. Addison-Wesley, Reading (1984)
12. Alan, D., Janet, F., Gregory, A., Russell, B.: Human-Computer Interaction. Pearson Education Limited, Harlow (2004)
13. Kohavi, R., Provost, F.: Glossary of terms. Mach. Learn. **30**, 271–274 (1998)
14. Ankerst, M., Elsen, C., Ester, M., Kriegel, H.P.: Visual classification: an interactive approach to decision tree construction. In: Proceedings of the Fifth ACM SIGKDD International Conference on Knowledge Discovery and Data Mining, pp. 392. ACM (1999)
15. Wakker, P., Deneffe, D.: Eliciting von neumann-morgenstern utilities when probabilities are distorted or unknown. Manage. Sci. **42**, 1131–1150 (1996)
16. Domingos, P.: A few useful things to know about machine learning. Commun. ACM **55**, 78–87 (2012)
17. Mitchell, T.M.: Machine Learning. McGraw-Hill, Boston (1997)
18. Martin, J.H., Jurafsky, D.: Speech and language processing. In: International 710th edn. (2000)
19. Adomavicius, G., Tuzhilin, A.: Toward the next generation of recommender systems: a survey of the state-of-the-art and possible extensions. IEEE Trans. Knowl. Data Eng. **17**, 734–749 (2005)
20. Li, Q., Zheng, N., Cheng, H.: Springrobot: a prototype autonomous vehicle and its algorithms for lane detection. IEEE Trans. Intell. Transp. Syst. **5**, 300–308 (2004)
21. Marsland, S.: Machine Learning: An Algorithmic Perspective. CRC Press, Boca Raton (2015)
22. Ankerst, M., Ester, M., Kriegel, H.P.: Towards an effective cooperation of the user and the computer for classification. In: Proceedings of the Sixth ACM SIGKDD International Conference on Knowledge Discovery and Data Mining, pp. 179–188. ACM (2000)

23. Ware, M., Frank, E., Holmes, G., Hall, M., Witten, I.H.: Interactive machine learning: letting users build classifiers. Int. J. Hum. Comput. Stud. **55**, 281–292 (2001)
24. Fails, J.A., Olsen Jr., D.R.: Interactive machine learning. In: Proceedings of the 8th International Conference on Intelligent User Interfaces, pp. 39–45. ACM (2003)
25. Fiebrink, R., Cook, P.R., Trueman, D.: Human model evaluation in interactive supervised learning. In: Proceedings of the SIGCHI Conference on Human Factors in Computing Systems, CHI 2011, pp. 147–156. ACM, New York (2011)
26. Fogarty, J., Tan, D., Kapoor, A., Winder, S.: Cueflik: interactive concept learning in image search. In: Proceedings of the SIGCHI Conference on Human Factors in Computing Systems, CHI 2008, pp. 29–38. ACM, New York (2008)
27. Simard, P., Chickering, D., Lakshmiratan, A., Charles, D., Bottou, L., Suarez, C.G.J., Grangier, D., Amershi, S., Verwey, J., Suh, J.: Ice: enabling non-experts to build models interactively for large-scale lopsided problems. arXiv preprint arXiv:1409.4814 (2014)
28. Amershi, S., Chickering, M., Drucker, S.M., Lee, B., Simard, P., Suh, J.: Modeltracker: redesigning performance analysis tools for machine learning. In: Proceedings of the 33rd Annual ACM Conference on Human Factors in Computing Systems, CHI 2015, pp. 337–346. ACM, New York (2015)
29. Talbot, J., Lee, B., Kapoor, A., Tan, D.S.: Ensemblematrix: interactive visualization to support machine learning with multiple classifiers. In: Proceedings of the SIGCHI Conference on Human Factors in Computing Systems, CHI 2009, pp. 1283–1292. ACM, New York (2009)
30. Ankerst, M., Ester, M., Kriegel, H.P.: Towards an effective cooperation of the user and the computer for classification. In: Proceedings of the Sixth ACM SIGKDD International Conference on Knowledge Discovery and Data Mining, KDD 2000, pp. 179–188. ACM, New York (2000)
31. Holzinger, A.: Interactive machine learning for health informatics: when do we need the human-in-the-loop? Brain Inform. **3**, 119–131 (2016)
32. Holzinger, A., Plass, M., Holzinger, K., Crişan, G.C., Pintea, C.-M., Palade, V.: Towards interactive Machine Learning (iML): applying ant colony algorithms to solve the traveling salesman problem with the human-in-the-loop approach. In: Buccafurri, F., Holzinger, A., Kieseberg, P., Tjoa, A.M., Weippl, E. (eds.) CD-ARES 2016. LNCS, vol. 9817, pp. 81–95. Springer, Heidelberg (2016). doi:10.1007/978-3-319-45507-5_6
33. Baron, J.: Normative Models of Judgment and Decision Making. Wiley, New York (2004)
34. Raiffa, H.: Applied statistical decision theory (1974)
35. Murphy, K.P.: Machine Learning: A Probabilistic Perspective. MIT Press, Cambridge (2012)
36. Friedman, J., Hastie, T., Tibshirani, R.: The Elements of Statistical Learning. Springer Series in Statistics, vol. 1. Springer, New York (2001)
37. Tulabandhula, T., Rudin, C.: Machine learning with operational costs. J. Mach. Learn. Res. **14**, 1989–2028 (2013)
38. Pitz, G.F., Sachs, N.J.: Judgment and decision: theory and application. Annu. Rev. Psychol. **35**, 139–164 (1984)
39. Fischhoff, B.: Judgment and decision making. Wiley Interdisc. Rev. Cogn. Sci. **1**, 724–735 (2010)
40. Russakovsky, O., Li, L.J., Fei-Fei, L.: Best of both worlds: human-machine collaboration for object annotation. In: Proceedings of the IEEE Conference on Computer Vision and Pattern Recognition, pp. 2121–2131 (2015)

41. Rapoport, A.: Decision Theory and Decision Behaviour: Normative and Descriptive Approaches, vol. 15. Springer, Amsterdam (2013)
42. Bazerman, M.H., Moore, D.A.: Judgment in managerial decision making (2013)
43. Bonner, S.E.: Judgment and Decision Making in Accounting. Prentice Hall, Upper Saddle River (2008)
44. Robert, S.: Informationsverarbeitung in Prognosen: Experimentelle Evidenz. dissertation, University of Osnabrueck (2016)
45. Goldstein, W.M., Hogarth, R.M.: Research on Judgment and Decision Making: Currents, Connections, and Controversies. Cambridge University Press, Cambridge (1997)
46. Milkman, K.L., Chugh, D., Bazerman, M.H.: How can decision making be improved? Perspect. Psychol. Sci. **4**, 379–383 (2009)
47. Baron, J.: Thinking and Deciding. Cambridge University Press, Cambridge (2000)
48. Tversky, A., Kahneman, D.: Judgment under uncertainty: heuristics and biases. In: Wendt, D., Vlek, C. (eds.) Utility, Probability, and Human Decision Making, pp. 1124–1131. Springer, Amsterdam (1974)
49. Libby, R.: Accounting and Human Information Processing: Theory and Applications. Prentice Hall, Englewood Cliffs (1981)
50. Ashton, R.H.: Human Information Processing in Accounting. American Accounting Association, Sarasota (1982)
51. Over, D.: Rationality and the normative/descriptive distinction. In: Blackwell Handbook of Judgment and Decision Making, London, pp. 3–18 (2004)
52. Gilovich, T., Griffin, D., Kahneman, D.: Heuristics and Biases: The Psychology of Intuitive Judgment. Cambridge University Press, New York (2002)
53. Newell, B.R.: Judgment under uncertainty (2013)
54. Tversky, A., Kahneman, D.: Extensional versus intuitive reasoning: the conjunction fallacy in probability judgment. Psychol. Rev. **90**, 293 (1983)
55. Tversky, A., Kahneman, D.: Availability: a heuristic for judging frequency and probability. Cogn. Psychol. **5**, 207–232 (1973)
56. Mokdad, A.H., Marks, J.S., Stroup, D.F., Gerberding, J.L.: Actual causes of death in the United States, 2000. JAMA **291**, 1238–1245 (2004)
57. Strack, F., Mussweiler, T.: Explaining the enigmatic anchoring effect: mechanisms of selective accessibility. J. Pers. Soc. Psychol. **73**, 437 (1997)
58. Plous, S.: Thinking the unthinkable: the effects of anchoring on likelihood estimates of nuclear war1. J. Appl. Soc. Psychol. **19**, 67–91 (1989)
59. Ritov, I.: Anchoring in simulated competitive market negotiation. Organ. Behav. Hum. Decis. Process. **67**, 16–25 (1996)
60. Galinsky, A.D., Mussweiler, T.: First offers as anchors: the role of perspective-taking and negotiator focus. J. Pers. Soc. Psychol. **81**, 657 (2001)
61. Chapman, G.B., Johnson, E.J.: Incorporating the irrelevant: anchors in judgments of belief and value. In: The Psychology of Intuitive Judgment, Heuristics and Biases, pp. 120–138 (2002)
62. Wilson, T.D., Houston, C.E., Etling, K.M., Brekke, N.: A new look at anchoring effects: basic anchoring and its antecedents. J. Exp. Psychol. Gen. **125**, 387 (1996)
63. Mussweiler, T., Strack, F.: Comparing is believing: a selective accessibility model of judgmental anchoring. Eur. Rev. Soc. Psychol. **10**, 135–167 (1999)
64. Chapman, G.B., Johnson, E.J.: Anchoring, activation, and the construction of values. Organ. Behav. Hum. Decis. Process. **79**, 115–153 (1999)
65. Furnham, A., Boo, H.C.: A literature review of the anchoring effect. J. Socio-Econ. **40**, 35–42 (2011)

66. Gigerenzer, G.: Why the distinction between single-event probabilities and frequencies is important for psychology (and vice versa). In: Subjective Probability, pp. 129–161 (1994)

67. Gigerenzer, G., Czerlinski, J., Martignon, L.: How good are fast and frugal heuristics? In: Shanteau, J., Mellers, B.A., Schum, D.A. (eds.) Decision Science and Technology, pp. 81–103. Springer, New York (1999)

68. Gigerenzer, G., Hoffrage, U., Kleinbölting, H.: Probabilistic mental models: a brunswikian theory of confidence. Psychol. Rev. **98**, 506 (1991)

69. Kahneman, D., Tversky, A.: Prospect theory: an analysis of decision under risk. Econometrica: J. Econometric Soc. **47**(2), 263–291 (1979)

70. Xu, L., Jackowski, M., Goshtasby, A., Roseman, D., Bines, S., Yu, C., Dhawan, A., Huntley, A.: Segmentation of skin cancer images. Image Vis. Comput. **17**, 65–74 (1999)

71. Królczyk, G., Legutko, S., Raos, P.: Cutting wedge wear examination during turning of duplex stainless steel. Tehnički Vjesnik-Technical Gazette **20**, 413–418 (2013)

72. Baron, J.: Rationality and Intelligence. Cambridge University Press, New York (2005)

73. Lee, S., Holzinger, A.: Knowledge discovery from complex high dimensional data. In: Michaelis, S., Piatkowski, N., Stolpe, M. (eds.) Solving Large Scale Learning Tasks. Challenges and Algorithms. LNCS (LNAI), vol. 9580, pp. 148–167. Springer, Heidelberg (2016). doi:10.1007/978-3-319-41706-6_7

74. Holzinger, A., Malle, B., Giuliani, N.: On graph extraction from image data. In: Slezak, D., Peters, J.F., Tan, A.H., Schwabe, L. (eds.) Brain Informatics and Health, BIH 2014. LNAI, vol. 8609, pp. 552–563. Springer, Heidelberg (2014)

75. Valdez, A.C., Dehmer, M., Holzinger, A.: Application of graph entropy for knowledge discovery and data mining in bibliometric data. In: Dehmer, M., Emmert-Streib, F., Chen, Z., Li, X., Shi, Y. (eds.) Mathematical Foundations and Applications of Graph Entropy, pp. 259–272. Wiley, New York (2016)

76. Cao, X., Balakrishnan, R.: Visionwand: interaction techniques for large displays using a passive wand tracked in 3d. In: Proceedings of the 16th Annual ACM Symposium on User Interface Software and Technology, UIST 2003, pp. 173–182. ACM, New York (2003)

77. Jones, B.R., Benko, H., Ofek, E., Wilson, A.D.: Illumiroom: peripheral projected illusions for interactive experiences. In: Proceedings of the SIGCHI Conference on Human Factors in Computing Systems, CHI 2013, pp. 869–878. ACM, New York (2013)

78. Milgram, P., Takemura, H., Utsumi, A., Kishino, F.: Augmented reality: a class of displays on the reality-virtuality continuum. In: Photonics for industrial applications, International Society for Optics and Photonics, pp. 282–292 (1995)

79. Azuma, R.T.: A survey of augmented reality. Presence: Teleoperators Virtual Environ. **6**, 355–385 (1997)

80. Fuchs, H., et al.: Augmented reality visualization for laparoscopic surgery. In: Wells, W.M., Colchester, A., Delp, S. (eds.) MICCAI 1998. LNCS, vol. 1496, pp. 934–943. Springer, Heidelberg (1998). doi:10.1007/BFb0056282

81. Paelke, V., Röcker, C., Koch, N., Flatt, H., Büttner, S.: User interfaces for cyberphysical systems. at-Automatisierungstechnik **63**, 833–843 (2015)

82. Büttner, S., Sand, O., Röcker, C.: Extending the design space in industrial manufacturing through mobile projection. In: Proceedings of the 17th International Conference on Human-Computer Interaction with Mobile Devices and Services Adjunct, MobileHCI 2015, pp. 1130–1133. ACM, New York (2015)

83. Büttner, S., Funk, M., Sand, O., Röcker, C.: Using head-mounted displays and in-situ projection for assistive systems - a comparison. In: Proceedings of the 9th ACM International Conference on PErvasive Technologies Related to Assistive Environments, vol. 8. ACM (2016)
84. Wilson, A.G., Dann, C., Lucas, C.G., Xing, E.P.: The human kernel. arXiv preprint arXiv:1510.07389 (2015)

Convolutional Neural Networks Applied for Parkinson's Disease Identification

Clayton R. Pereira[1], Danillo R. Pereira[2], Joao P. Papa[2(✉)], Gustavo H. Rosa[2], and Xin-She Yang[3]

[1] Department of Computing, Federal University of São Carlos, São Carlos, Brazil
claytontey@gmail.com
[2] Department of Computing, São Paulo State University, Bauru, Brazil
dpereira@ic.unicamp.br, papa@fc.unesp.br, gth.rosa@uol.com.br
[3] School of Science and Technology, Middlesex University, London, UK
x.yang@mdx.ac.uk

Abstract. Parkinson's Disease (PD) is a chronic and progressive illness that affects hundreds of thousands of people worldwide. Although it is quite easy to identify someone affected by PD when the illness shows itself (e.g. tremors, slowness of movement and freezing-of-gait), most works have focused on studying the working mechanism of the disease in its very early stages. In such cases, drugs can be administered in order to increase the quality of life of the patients. Since the beginning, it is well-known that PD patients feature the micrography, which is related to muscle rigidity and tremors. As such, most exams to detect Parkinson's Disease make use of handwritten assessment tools, where the individual is asked to perform some predefined tasks, such as drawing spirals and meanders on a template paper. Later, an expert analyses the drawings in order to classify the progressive of the disease. In this work, we are interested into aiding physicians in such task by means of machine learning techniques, which can learn proper information from digitized versions of the exams, and them recommending a probability of a given individual being affected by PD depending on its handwritten skills. Particularly, we are interested in deep learning techniques (i.e. Convolutional Neural Networks) due to their ability into learning features without human interaction. Additionally, we propose to fine-tune hyper-arameters of such techniques by means of meta-heuristic-based techniques, such as Bat Algorithm, Firefly Algorithm and Particle Swarm Optimization.

Keywords: Convolutional Neural Networks · Parkinson's Disease · Machine learning · Meta-heuristics

1 Introduction and Motivation

Parkinson's Disease (PD) is a chronic, progressive and neuron-degenerative illness that affects people worldwide. Firstly described by James Parkinson [1] in 1817, PD is often related to the slowness of movement, tremors and muscle stiffness. Other side effects concern changes in speech, writing and the

© Springer International Publishing AG 2016
A. Holzinger (Ed.): ML for Health Informatics, LNAI 9605, pp. 377–390, 2016.
DOI: 10.1007/978-3-319-50478-0_19

well-known freezing-of-gate. According to the Parkinson's Disease Foundation, approximately 60,000 Americans are diagnosed with PD [2]. The problem gets worse, since thousands of potential individuals may not be properly diagnosed, or even remain uncovered by exams or any sort of clinical diagnosis.

Computer-assisted PD diagnosis has been the foremost research in the last decades, since mathematical models are more appropriate to detect subtle changes in a number of symptoms related to the disease. As a matter of fact, the main concern is related to the detection of PD first symptoms, i.e. to detect the side effects at the very early stages of the disease, where the treatment can increase the quality of life of a given patient.

Machine learning-driven tools are the most likely approaches to succeed when dealing with automatic diagnosis of Parkinson's Disease, since they can be fed with labeled data for further learning the non-linear mapping between input data and the real diagnosis (ground-truth) given by the expert. In the last years, deep learning techniques (DL), a branch of machine learning research field, have arisen as a powerful tool to help the task of unsupervised feature learning by means of a series of layers that are in charge of extracting different information on each [3]. Convolutional Neural Networks (CNNs) [4], Deep Belief Networks (DBNs) [5], and Deep Boltzmann Machines (DBMs) [6] are among the most used techniques based on deep learning. Given an input image, DL-based approaches aim at performing a series of similar tasks in order to obtain a high-dimensional representation of that input data, which can be further used to feed a supervised pattern classifier.

Therefore, instead of handcrafting features, deep learning techniques can be used to learn proper information about the problem without human intervention. However, in health-related applications, we usually do not have sufficient training samples, where automatic approaches may fail. In such circumstances, we still need the doctor-in-the-loop [7,8]. Another major drawback related to DL techniques concerns their parameters, which can reach hundreds of thousands depending on the complexity of the model. Therefore, the task of finding such parameters can be model as an optimization problem, where the fitness function is the classification error over a training/validating set. Particularly, we are interested in meta-heuristic-based techniques, since they can provide an elegant solution and easy implementations to a number of distinct problems [9].

This work concerns two main contributions: (i) to use CNNs to learn features from handwriting exams in order to aid PD diagnosis, and (ii) to use meta-heuristic-based optimization techniques to fine-tune CNN hyper-parameters. To the best of our knowledge, some of the techniques used in this paper have never been used to optimize CNN parameters to date, such as Bat Algorithm [10], Particle Swarm Optimization [11] and Firefly Algorithm [12]. The reasons for using such techniques concern their swarm-based behaviour, as well as they are considered state-of-the-art techniques in the related field.

1.1 Glossary and Key Terms

Deep learning: a branch of machine learning that aims at studying techniques that learn features in an unsupervised fashion [3].

Convolutional Neural Networks (CNNs): technique composed of a series of layers (e.g. convolution and pooling) that aim at learning specific features on each. Usually, such networks output a high-dimensional feature vector given an input image, which is used to feed a supervised pattern recognition technique [4].

Optimization: it usually refers to the task of finding the minimum/maximum value of a function given some input values (decision variables) [9].

Meta-heuristics: techniques used to solve problems (heuristics) in general. They are often used to handle optimization-oriented problems [9].

Parkinson's Disease: is a chronic, progressive and neuron-degenerative illness, which is often related to the slowness of movement, tremors, muscle stiffness, and the freezing-of-gate [1].

Micrography: usually featured by Parkinson's Disease patients, it concerns the decreasing ability in the writing, which may become smaller as the illness progresses.

Handwritten exam: usually a piece of paper used to assess the handwritten skills of a given individual. Such exam requires the user to perform some predefined tasks, such as drawing spirals, circles and meanders to asses its handwritten skills.

Handwritten trace: drawing done by the patient when performing a handwritten exam.

Handwritten template: template printed out in the form to be completed by the patient.

Bat Algorithm (BA): optimization algorithm based on the behavior of bats when hunting down their preys [10].

Firefly Algorithm (FA): optimization algorithm based on the flashing lighting mechanism of fireflies, which is used for matting partners [12].

Particle Swarm Optimization (PSO): optimization algorithm based on swarms of livings beings [11].

2 State-of-the-Art in Computer-Aided Parkinson's Disease Diagnosis

Spadotto et al. [13] introduced the Optimum-Path Forest (OPF) [14,15] classifier to aid the automatic identification of Parkinson's Disease, and later on the same group of authors proposed an evolutionary-based approach to select the most discriminative set of features that help improving PD recognition rates [16].

The OPF classifier seemed to be a suitable tool, since it is parameterless and easy-to-manage.

Das [17] presented a comparison of multiple classification methods for the diagnosis of PD, among them Neural Networks, and Regression and Decision Trees. Several evaluation methods were employed to calculate the performance of that classifiers, being the experiments conducted in a dataset composed of a range of biomedical voice measurements from 31 people, in which 23 diagnosed with Parkinson's disease. The best results were obtained by Neural Networks (around 92.9 % of PD recognition rate). In 2014, Weber et al. [18] used a biometric pen together with Support Vector Machines to learn handwritten dynamics from PD patients.

In the work conducted by Zhao et al. [19], five patients and seven healthy individuals were used to recognize Parkinson's disease by means of the voice analysis. In order to fulfil this purpose, the individuals' voice were recorded using an Isomax EarSet E60P5L microphone, being the recording sessions lasting around 25 min each, and a total of 50 pre-recorded prompts consisting of emotional sentences spoken by a professional actress. Tsanas et al. [20] evaluated different algorithms based on dysphonia measures aiming at PD recognition. A total of 132 acoustic features were initially used for further feature selection, and the authors concluded the dysphonia information together with existing features end up helping PD recognition. Harel et al. [21] claimed that PD symptoms are detectable up to five years prior to clinical diagnosis, and symptoms presented in speech include reduced loudness, increased vocal tremor, and breathiness. In their work, the authors used a dataset of the National Center for Voice and Speech, which comprises 263 phonations from 43 subjects (17 females and 26 males, being 10 healthy controls and 33 diagnosed with PD).

Since one of the first manifestation of Parkinson's Disease is the deterioration of handwriting, the micrography is another information widely used for the diagnosis of Parkinson's disease [22]. This technique is considered an objective measure, since a PD patient possibly features the reduction of calligraphy size, as well as the hand tremors. Nowadays, this procedure is often conducted by filling out some specific forms. Rosenblum et al. [23] suggested that writing exams can be used to distinguish PD patients from healthy individuals. The authors employed the following methodology to support their assumption: 20 PD patients and 20 control individuals were asked to write their names and addresses in a piece of paper attached to a digital table. Further, for each stroke, the mean pressure and velocity were measured in order to compute spatial and temporal information. The authors presented very good recognition rates, being 97.5 % of the participants classified correctly (100 % of the control individuals, and 95 % of PD patients). Later on, Drotár et al. [24] claimed that movement during handwriting of a text consists not only from the on-surface movements of the hand, but also from the in-air trajectories performed when the hand moves in the air from one stroke to the next. The authors demonstrated the assessment of in-air hand movements during sentence handwriting has a higher impact than the pure evaluation of on surface movements, leading to classification accuracies of 84 % and 78 %, respectively.

Recently, Pereira et al. [25] proposed to extract features from writing exams using visual features learned from drawings the patients were asked to do. The authors also designed and made available a dataset called "HandPD" with all images and features extracted from the handwriting exams[1]. Pasluosta et al. [26] focused on PD as a representative disease model by evaluating the Internet-of-Things (IoT) platform in the context of healthcare. The authors considered the potential of combining wearable technology with the IoT in the health-care scenario, as well as the engagement of patients in the assessment of symptoms, diagnosis, and consecutive treatment options. Zhao et al. [27] also analyzed E-health support in PD, but now with smart glasses.

Khobragade et al. [28] applied a Large-Memory Storage and Retrieval neural network for the prediction of onset of tremor in PD patients. The work demonstrated a fully automated deep brain stimulation system that can be applied on-demand, i.e. only when it is needed, since the usual treatments apply that stimulation continuously. Navarro et al. [29] proposed to employ an augmented reality-based approach that has been widely used in the field of rehabilitation to aid PD patients. The experiment was tested on 7 PD individuals, and showed that VR is a simple and suitable tool that should be encouraged to be used in PD patients.

Geldenhuys et al. [30] presented the use of a novel video-based paradigm for analyzing the gait of patients with Parkinson's disease. The idea was to consider the locomotor kinematics, which is capable of detecting subtle changes in gait and analyze the results in a gender-specific manner. In their experiments, a male mice group showed a statistically significant higher propensity towards gait changes than the female mice, suggesting that gait deficits in female-treated mice might be subtler.

Kim et al. [31] proposed a novel smartphone-based system using inertial sensors to detect freezing-of-gate symptoms in an unconstrained way. Several motions such as ankle, trouser pocket, waist and chest pocket, were evaluate. Data obtained and pre-processed via discriminative features extracted from accelerometer and gyroscope motion signals of the smartphone were used to classify freezing-of-gate episodes from normal walking using AdaBoost.M1 classifier with sensitivity of 86 % at the waist, and 84 % and 81 % in the trouser pocket and at the ankle, respectively.

Another contribution of this work is to optimize CNN hyper-parameters by means of meta-heuristic techniques. As far as we are concerned, only a few and very recent works have employed such optimization models to fine-tune hyper-parameters of deep learning techniques [32–37]. Usually, such optimization models are based on evolutionary/bio-inspired/meta-heuristic techniques, since they offer easy and elegant solution to a number of problems in the literature. Roughly speaking, such techniques start placing possible solutions (the so-called agents) at random positions in the search space. At each iteration, the solutions move onto the search space according to some specific dynamics (bat's behaviour in Bat Algorithm and fireflies in Firefly Algorithm, among others). However, as

---

[1] http://wwwp.fc.unesp.br/~papa/pub/datasets/Handpd/.

any optimization technique, the main idea is to converge to some global optimum when it exists. The reader can refer to the work of Holzinger et al. [38] for an interesting overview of these techniques.

3   Open Problems

The main challenges in computer-assisted Parkinson's Disease diagnosis include:

- Different data sources
- To detect PD at the very early stages of the disease
- To monitor the patient at home
- To obtain digitized versions of pretty old exams.

Bellow, we briefly discuss some of the most important problems we usually face when dealing with PD diagnosis.

Problem 1. **It is quite difficult to identify the first symptoms of the disease in its early stages.** Pereira et al. [25] showed the handwritten exam of a healthy individual and an early-stage patient can be the much similar to each other. Such situation poses a big challenge when using images acquired from handwritten exams only.

Problem 2. **Datasets with different modalities concerning the data source are rare.** As aforementioned, using only images from handwritten exams may not be enough to accurately identify PD patients at the very early stages of the disease, since subtle information may not be observed by either humans and machines. Therefore, complimentary information from sensors can be helpful to provide a more reliable decision-making model. One example concerns using "smart pen" to detect the handwritten dynamics, for instance.

Problem 3. **To obtain digitized versions of quite old exams.** There might be a number of handwritten exams in the hospitals and clinics that can be of extreme importance to identify the behaviour of PD patients. However, as stated by Pereira et al. [25], there is a need for specific protocols concerning the image acquisition of the exams, their pre-processing and feature extraction.

Problem 4. **Technology is not available to everyone.** Although in-home tools are quite efficient to monitor PD patients (e.g. tablets to asses handwritten skills, on-body sensors to detect freezing of movements and virtual reality), they are expensive and most of time not available for those who need care.

4   Methodology and Experiments

4.1   HandPD Dataset

The HandPD dataset (see Footnote 1) was collected at the Faculty of Medicine of Botucatu, São Paulo State University, Brazil, being composed of images

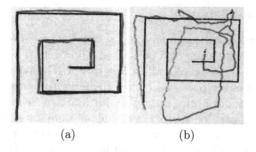

(a)   (b)

Fig. 1. Meander samples from: (a) control and (b) PD patient.

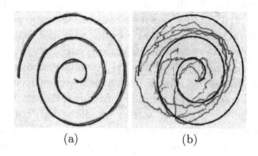

(a)   (b)

Fig. 2. Spiral samples from: (a) control and (b) PD patient.

extracted from handwriting exams of individuals divided into two groups: (i) healthy people and (ii) PD patients [25]. The dataset comprises 35 individuals, being 14 patients (10 males and 4 females) and 21 control (healthy) individuals (11 males and 10 females). Each person is asked to fill out a form starting from inward to outward. This activity concerns the analysis of the movement provided by spirals and meanders drawings, which quantify the normal motor activity in a healthy individual, as well as the dysfunction of PD patients.

Figures 1 and 2 illustrate some drawing images concerning meanders and spirals, respectively. One can observe the different patterns between spiral and meander images, as well as different patterns between the same sketch of healthy and PD patients.

4.2   Modelling CNN Hyper-parameter Optimization

We propose to model the selection of suitable hyper-parameters as an image recognition task by means of CNNs. The learning step has three main hyper-parameters: the base learning rate η, penalty parameter (momentum) α and weight decay λ. Therefore, we have a three-dimensional search space with three real-valued variables. Roughly speaking, the proposed approach aims at selecting the set of CNN hyper-parameters that minimizes the loss function of the images from the validation set. After that, the selected set of hyper-parameters is thus applied to classify images from the test set.

4.3   Experimental Setup

In this work, we classified meanders and spirals images drawn by the control group and PD patients using a CNN-based approach. Three different meta-heuristic techniques were employed to fine-tune CNN hyper-parameters: BA, PSO and FA. Also, to serve as a baseline for comparison purposes, we employed a standard CNN without optimization[2] and a Random Search (RS)[3]. Also, the hyper-parameters of each optimization technique were set empirically.

We divided the experiments into two datasets: (i) the meanders and the (ii) spirals. Both datasets are composed of 264 images (256 × 256 pixels), being 124 PD patients and 140 control group samples. In addition, we employed 30 % of the dataset for training, 20 % for validation and 50 % for testing purposes. In order to provide a statistical analysis by means of Wilcoxon signed-rank test [40] with significance of 0.05, we conducted a cross-validation with 10 runnings. We employed 15 agents over 25 iterations for convergence considering all techniques. This configuration leads us to $15 \times 25 = 375$ evaluations of the fitness function for each technique. If one decides to use a near-exhaustive search over three parameters, we could adjust the number of evaluations to be close to 375 for a fair comparison. In this case, we would be allowed to consider a range of 7 possible values for each hyper-parameter, since $7^3 = 343$. However, the hyper-parameters are real-valued, and we believe only seven values would not be enough for a good evaluation of the search space. Table 1 presents the hyper-parameter configuration for each optimization technique[4].

Table 1. Hyper-parameter configuration.

Technique	Hyper-parameters
BA	$f_{min} = 0$, $f_{max} = 2.0$ $A = 0.5$, $r = 0.5$
PSO	$c_1 = 1.7$, $c_2 = 1.7$, $w = 0.7$
FA	$\gamma = 1.0$, $\beta_0 = 1.0$ $\alpha = 0.2$

In regard to the source-code, we used the well-known Caffe library[5] [39], which is developed under GPGPU (General-Purpose computing on Graphics Processor Units) platform, thus providing more efficient implementations. Each meta-heuristic technique was evaluated by the same CNN architecture provided by Caffe, using $1,000$ training iterations with mini-batches of size 12. We have set each CNN hyper-parameter according to the following ranges: $\eta \in [0, 0.01]$, $\alpha \in [0, 1]$ and $\lambda \in [0, 0.001]$. Finally, the best hyper-parameters found by the meta-heuristic techniques were evaluated again.

---

[2] The CNN hyper-parameters in this case are the default values given by Caffe [39].

[3] A random search means an aleatory initialization of hyper-parameters between the range bounds.

[4] Notice these values have been empirically setup.

[5] http://caffe.berkeleyvision.org.

Regarding the architecture used on this experiment, we used the one proposed by Krizhevsky et al. [41]. Briefly speaking, such CNN is composed of 5 convolution layers, 5 pooling layers and 2 normalization layers. It is also constituted by 7 ReLU layers, 3 inner product layers, 2 dropout layers, 1 accuracy layer and 1 softmax loss layer for testing purposes.

4.4   Experimental Results

This section aims at presenting the experimental results concerning the CNN-based Parkinson's Disease identification, as well as its hyper-parameter fine-tuning effectiveness. As aforementioned in Sect. 4.3, we compared three distinct meta-heuristic techniques among with a baseline network without optimization and a random initialization of hyper-parameters considering both meander and spiral datasets. Notice the overall accuracy is computed using the standard formulation, i.e., $(1 - \frac{errors}{dataset\ size}) * 100$. Additionally, we provided the accuracy per class, i.e. "Control" and "PD". Tables 2 and 3 present the average results concerning meanders and spirals, respectively, and the best set of hyper-parameters (average) found by each technique. The most accurate results according to Wilcoxon signed-rank test are in bold.

Table 2. Average accuracies and best hyper-parameters over the test set considering meander dataset.

	Accuracy (%)			Best Hyper-parameters		
	Overall	Control	PD	η	α	λ
Standard	**78.18 %**	74.14 %	**82.74 %**	0.001	0.9	0.0005
RS	72.50 %	80.14 %	63.87 %	0.0048	0.4233	0.0005
BA	**79.62 %**	75.43 %	**84.35 %**	0.0008	0.6437	0.0007
FA	69.85 %	**93.71 %**	42.90 %	0.0009	0.3594	0.0003
PSO	**75.76 %**	85.00 %	**65.32 %**	0.0009	0.5144	0.0004

Once can observe FA obtained the best results concerning "Control" (healthy individuals) class for meander dataset, but it has performed poorly when dealing with PD patients. This situation has led FA to the worst overall result with 69.85 %. Considering the RS, it was also one of the worst techniques, mainly due its randomness and its lack of exploitation ability. The most accurate techniques were BA, PSO and the standard set of hyper-parameters defined by the library, although BA obtained the best recognition rate.

In regard to the spirals (Table 3), BA, PSO and the standard set of hyper-parameters obtained the best results once again. Nevertheless, RS was able to almost obtain similar results. In this case, BA and PSO can be considered similar to each other concerning the PD class, while standard performed better in "Control" class. By taking into account both exams, i.e. meanders and spirals, the latter are more discriminative and effective to distinguish healthy individuals from PD patients. Since meanders feature straight lines only (Fig. 1), we believe it is more difficult (for those affected by Parkinson's Disease) to follow the complex pattern of spirals when performing the exams.

Table 3. Average accuracies and best hyper-parameters over the test set considering spiral dataset.

	Accuracy (%)			Best Hyper-parameters		
	Overall	Control	PD	η	α	λ
Standard	**89.55 %**	**93.71 %**	84.84 %	0.001	0.9	0.0005
RS	86.67 %	92.43 %	80.16 %	0.0038	0.5343	0.0005
BA	**87.20 %**	84.14 %	**90.65 %**	0.0036	0.3972	0.0008
FA	83.79 %	82.29 %	85.48 %	0.01	0.4522	0.0006
PSO	**88.33 %**	85.00 %	**92.10 %**	0.0026	0.2733	0.0004

In order to provide a deeper experimental section, we executed one extra round of experiments (10 runnings with randomly generated sets) using the best set of hyper-parameters found out by each optimization technique (notice the standard results are the same). Tables 4 and 5 present such results concerning meanders and spirals, respectively. Since in the previous experiment we used training and validating sets (30 % and 20 %, respectively), in this extra round of experiments we merged them into a single training set.

Table 4. Average accuracies using the best hyper-parameters found over the test set considering meander dataset.

	Accuracy (%)			Best Hyper-parameters		
	Overall	Control	PD	η	α	λ
Standard	78.18 %	74.14 %	82.74 %	0.001	0.9	0.0005
RS	78.18 %	76.86 %	79.68 %	0.003856	0.472675	0.000388
BA	**83.11 %**	70.43 %	**97.42 %**	0.000143	0.923070	0.000929
FA	74.39 %	**81.14 %**	66.77 %	0.000448	0.387494	0.000079
PSO	77.65 %	**84.14 %**	70.32 %	0.000675	0.729715	0.000884

Considering meander images, BA obtained the best overall accuracy so far, followed by the standard set of hyper-parameters, RS and PSO. This very good result was pushed up by the BA best recognition rate over PD class (i.e. 97.42%). With respect to spirals, standard, BA and PSO obtained similar results concerning the overall recognition rates, tough BA achieved the highest accuracy.

Table 5. Average accuracies using the best hyper-parameters found over the test set considering spiral dataset.

	Accuracy (%)			Best Hyper-parameters		
	Overall	Control	PD	η	α	λ
Standard	**89.55 %**	**93.71 %**	84.84 %	0.001	0.9	0.0005
RS	86.97 %	**95.29 %**	77.58 %	0.002717	0.322419	0.000856
BA	**90.38 %**	89.29 %	**91.61 %**	0.001843	0.266447	0.001
FA	83.86 %	80.86 %	**87.26 %**	0.01	0.096975	0.001
PSO	**89.62 %**	86.00 %	**93.71 %**	0.003552	0	0.000210

5   Conclusion and Future Outlook

In this paper, we dealt with the problem of Parkinson's Disease identification by means of features learned from handwritten exams. The features were extracted by Convolutional Neural Networks fine-tuned by meta-heuristic-based optimization techniques, which obtained the best results for meanders, tough being similar to the standard set of parameters defined by the library with respect to spiral images (which we believe were hand-tuned). The experiments highlighted spirals as the most discriminative drawing, since it appears to be more difficult to perform such exam than meanders, which are composed of straight lines only.

In regard to future works, we intend to combine the results of the different optimization techniques, since they seem to disagree with respect to both "Control" and "PD" classes, being probably complementary to each other. Also, we aim at evaluating other meta-heuristic techniques, such as Cuckoo Search and Genetic Programming.

Acknowledgments. The authors are grateful to FAPESP grants #2014/16250-9 and #2015/25739-4, as well as CNPq grant #306166/2014-3.

References

1. Parkinson, J.: An essay on the shaking palsy. J. Neuropsychiatry Clin. Neurosci. **20**(4), 223–236 (1817)
2. Fundation, P.D.: Statistics on parkinson's: Who has parkinson's? (2016). http://www.pdf.org/en/parkinson_statistics, Accessed 15-July-2016
3. LeCun, Y., Bengio, Y.: Deep learning. Nature **521**(7553), 436–444 (2015)
4. Lecun, Y., Bottou, L., Bengio, Y., Haffner, P.: Gradient-based learning applied to document recognition. Proc. IEEE **86**(11), 2278–2324 (1998)
5. Hinton, G.E., Osindero, S., Teh, Y.W.: A fast learning algorithm for deep belief nets. Neural Comput. **18**(7), 1527–1554 (2006)
6. Salakhutdinov, R., Hinton, G.E.: An efficient learning procedure for deep boltzmann machines. Neural Comput. **24**(8), 1967–2006 (2012)
7. Holzinger, A.: Interactive machine learning for health informatics: When do we need the human-in-the-loop? Brain Inf. 3

8. Holzinger, A., Plass, M., Holzinger, K., Crişan, G.C., Pintea, C.-M., Palade, V.: Towards interactive machine learning (iML): applying ant colony algorithms to solve the traveling salesman problem with the human-in-the-loop approach. In: Buccafurri, F., Holzinger, A., Kieseberg, P., Tjoa, A.M., Weippl, E. (eds.) CD-ARES 2016. LNCS, vol. 9817, pp. 81–95. Springer, Heidelberg (2016). doi:10.1007/978-3-319-45507-5_6

9. Yang, X.S.: Nature-Inspired Metaheuristic Algorithms. Luniver Press, Bristol (2008)

10. Yang, X.S., Gandomi, A.H.: Bat algorithm: a novel approach for global engineering optimization. Eng. Computations 29(5), 464–483 (2012)

11. Kennedy, J., Eberhart, R.C.: Swarm Intelligence. Morgan Kaufmann Publishers Inc., San Francisco (2001)

12. Yang, X.S.: Firefly algorithm, stochastic test functions and design optimisation. Int. J. Bio-Inspired Comput. 2(2), 78–84 (2010)

13. Spadotto, A.A., Guido, R.C., Papa, J.P., Falcão, A.X.: Parkinson's disease identification through optimum-path forest. In: IEEE International Conference of the Engineering in Medicine and Biology Society, pp. 6087–6090 (2010)

14. Papa, J.P., Falcão, A.X., Suzuki, C.T.N.: Supervised pattern classification based on optimum-path forest. Int. J. Imaging Systems Technol. 19(2), 120–131 (2009)

15. Papa, J.P., Falcão, A.X., Albuquerque, V.H.C., Tavares, J.M.R.S.: Efficient supervised optimum-path forest classification for large datasets. Pattern Recogn. 45(1), 512–520 (2012)

16. Spadotto, A.A., Guido, R.C., Carnevali, F.L., Pagnin, A.F., Falcão, A.X., Papa, J.P.: Improving parkinson's disease identification through evolutionary-based feature selection. In: IEEE International Conference of the Engineering in Medicine and Biology Society, pp. 7857–7860 (2011)

17. Das, R.: A comparison of multiple classification methods for diagnosis of parkinson disease. Expert Syst. Appl. 37(2), 1568–1572 (2010)

18. Weber, S.A.T., Santos Filho, C.A., Shelp, A.O., Rezende, L.A.L., Papa, J.P., Hook, C.: Classification of handwriting patterns in patients with parkinson's disease, using a biometric sensor. Global Adv. Res. J. Med. Med. Sci. 11(3), 362–366 (2014)

19. Zhao, S., Rudzicz, F., Carvalho, L.G., Marquez-Chin, C., Livingstone, S.: Automatic detection of expressed emotion in parkinson's disease. In: IEEE International Conference on Acoustics, Speech and Signal Processing, pp. 4813–4817 (2014)

20. Tsanas, A., Little, M.A., McSharry, P.E., Spielman, J., Ramig, L.O.: Novel speech signal processing algorithms for high-accuracy classification of parkinson's disease. IEEE Trans. Biomed. Eng. 59(5), 1264–1271 (2012)

21. Harel, B., Cannizzaro, M., Snyder, P.J.: Variability in fundamental frequency during speech in prodromal and incipient parkinson's disease: A longitudinal case study. Brain Cogn. 6(1), 24–29 (2004)

22. Eichhorn, T.E., Gasser, T., Mai, N., Marquardt, C., Arnold, G., Schwarz, J., Oertel, W.H.: Computational analysis of open loop handwriting movements in parkinson's disease: A rapid method to detect dopamimetic effects. Mov. Disord. 11(3), 289–297 (1996)

23. Rosenblum, S., Samuel, M., Zlotnik, S., Erikh, I., Schlesinger, I.: Handwriting as an objective tool for parkinson's disease diagnosis. J. Neurol. 260(9), 2357–2361 (2013)

24. Drotár, P., Mekyska, J., Rektorová, I., Masarová, L., Smékal, Z., Faundez-Zanuy, M.: Analysis of in-air movement in handwriting: A novel marker for parkinson's disease. Comput. Methods Programs Biomed. 117(3), 405–411 (2014)

25. Pereira, C.R., Pereira, D.R., da Silva, F.A., Hook, C., Weber, S.A.T., Pereira, L.A.M., Papa, J.P.: A step towards the automated diagnosis of parkinson's disease: Analyzing handwriting movements. In: IEEE 28th International Symposium on Computer-Based Medical Systems, pp. 171–176 (2015)
26. Pasluosta, C.F., Gassner, H., Winkler, J., Klucken, J., Eskofier, B.M.: An emerging era in the management of parkinson's disease: Wearable technologies and the internet of things. IEEE J. Biomed. Health Inf. **19**, 1873–1881 (2015)
27. Zhao, Y., Heida, T., van Wegen, E.E.H., Bloem, B.R., van Wezel, R.J.A.: E-health support in people with parkinson's disease with smart glasses: A survey of user requirements and expectations in the netherlands. J. Parkinson's Dis. **5**(2), 369–378 (2015)
28. Khobragade, N., Graupe, D., Tuninetti, D.: Towards fully automated closed-loop deep brain stimulation in parkinson's disease patients: A lamstar-based tremor predictor. In: 37th Annual International Conference of the Engineering in Medicine and Biology Society IEEE, p. 2616 (2015)
29. Navarro, G.P., Magariño, I.G., Lorente, P.R.: A kinect-based system for lower limb rehabilitation in parkinson's disease patients: a pilot study. J. Med. Syst. **39**, 1–10 (2015)
30. Geldenhuys, W.J., Guseman, T.L., Pienaar, I.S., Dluzen, D.E., Young, J.W.: A novel biomechanical analysis of gait changes in the MPTP mouse model of parkinson's disease. PeerJ PeerJ Comput. Sci. **17**, e1175 (2015)
31. Kim, H., Lee, H.J., Lee, W., Kwon, S., Kim, S.K., Jeon, H.S., Park, H., Shin, C.W., Yi, W.J., Jeon, B.S., Park, K.S.: Unconstrained detection of freezing of gait in parkinson's disease patients using smartphone. In: 37th Annual International Conference of the Engineering in Medicine and Biology Society (EMBC) IEEE, pp. 3751–3754 (2015)
32. Papa, J.P., Scheirer, W., Cox, D.D.: Fine-tuning deep belief networks using harmony search. Appl. Soft Comput. **46**, 875–885 (2015)
33. Papa, J.P., Rosa, G.H., Costa, K.A.P., Marana, A.N., Scheirer, W., Cox, D.D.: On the model selection of bernoulli restricted boltzmann machines through harmony search. In: Proceedings of the Genetic and Evolutionary Computation Conference. GECCO 2015, pp. 1449–1450. ACM, New York, USA (2015)
34. Papa, J.P., Rosa, G.H., Marana, A.N., Scheirer, W., Cox, D.D.: Model selection for discriminative restricted boltzmann machines through meta-heuristic techniques. J. Comput. Sci. **9**, 14–18 (2015)
35. Rosa, G.H., Papa, J.P., Marana, A.N., Scheirer, W., Cox, D.D.: Fine-tuning convolutional neural networks using harmony search. In: Pardo, A., Kittler, J. (eds.) IARP 2015. LNCS, vol. 9423, pp. 683–690. Springer, Heidelberg (2015)
36. Fedorovici, L., Precup, R., Dragan, F., David, R., Purcaru, C.: Embedding gravitational search algorithms in convolutional neural networks for OCR applications. In: 7th IEEE International Symposium on Applied Computational Intelligence and Informatics. SACI 2012, pp. 125–130 (2012)
37. Rere, L.M.R., Fanany, M.I., Arymurthy, A.M.: Metaheuristic algorithms for convolution neural network. Comput. Intell. Neurosci. **2016**, 1–13 (2016)
38. Holzinger, K., Palade, V., Rabadan, R., Holzinger, A.: Darwin or lamarck? future challenges in evolutionary algorithms for knowledge discovery and data mining. Knowledge Discovery and Data Mining. LNCS, vol. 8401, pp. 35–56. Springer, Heidelberg (2014)
39. Jia, Y., Shelhamer, E., Donahue, J., Karayev, S., Long, J., Girshick, R., Guadarrama, S., Darrell, T.: Caffe: Convolutional architecture for fast feature embedding. arXiv preprint (2014). arXiv:1408.5093

40. Wilcoxon, F.: Individual comparisons by ranking methods. Biometrics Bull. **1**(6), 80–83 (1945)
41. Krizhevsky, A., Sutskever, I., Hinton, G.E.: Imagenet classification with deep convolutional neural networks. In: Advances in Neural Information Processing Systems, pp. 1097–1105 (2012)

Recommender Systems for Health Informatics: State-of-the-Art and Future Perspectives

André Calero Valdez[1,4(✉)], Martina Ziefle[1], Katrien Verbert[2],
Alexander Felfernig[3], and Andreas Holzinger[4]

[1] Human-Computer Interaction Center, RWTH-Aachen University,
Campus Boulevard 57, 52074 Aachen, Germany
{calero-valdez,ziefle}@comm.rwth-aachen.de
[2] KU Leuven, Celestijnenlaan 200A, 3001 Leuven, Belgium
katrien.verbert@cs.kuleuven.be
[3] Institute for Software Technology, Graz University of Technology,
8010 Graz, Austria
alexander.felfernig@ist.tugraz.at
[4] Holzinger Group HCI-KDD, Institute for Medical Informatics,
Statistics & Documentation, Medical University Graz, 8036 Graz, Austria
a.holzinger@hci-kdd.org

Abstract. Recommender systems are a classical example for machine learning applications, however, they have not yet been used extensively in health informatics and medical scenarios. We argue that this is due to the specifics of benchmarking criteria in medical scenarios and the multitude of drastically differing end-user groups and the enormous context-complexity of the medical domain. Here both risk perceptions towards data security and privacy as well as trust in safe technical systems play a central and specific role, particularly in the clinical context. These aspects dominate acceptance of such systems. By using a Doctor-in-the-Loop approach some of these difficulties could be mitigated by combining both human expertise with computer efficiency. We provide a three-part research framework to access health recommender systems, suggesting to incorporate domain understanding, evaluation and specific methodology into the development process.

Keywords: Health recommender systems · Human-computer interaction · Evaluation framework · Uncertainty · Trust · Risk · Privacy

1 Introduction and Motivation

What should I read next? [1] What should I watch next? What product will I find interesting? These are typical questions that traditional recommender systems are designed for. Recommender systems help sieve through large amounts of data in determining options that are most relevant to the task the user has in mind. If the user is a customer using an online retailing platform, recommender systems are pervasive. Almost everyone has seen Amazon's "Other customers have also

© Springer International Publishing AG 2016
A. Holzinger (Ed.): ML for Health Informatics, LNAI 9605, pp. 391–414, 2016.
DOI: 10.1007/978-3-319-50478-0_20

bought XYZ" suggesting other products that are relevant to the current search request. Research in recommender systems in e-commerce focus on algorithms, interaction patterns and evaluation. Typical objects of applications are movies, music, documents, or products.

While the choices made by customers can be described as being low-risk, decisions made in other domains may have more severe consequences for the end user. In particular in the area of health and medicine, the limiting resource is the (possibly) non-replenish-able health of the patient. The recommender system should not only avoid failures and support decision making, but it should also understand the patient, the attitudes, the requirements, the values in the context of disease and health management. This makes the applicability of health recommender systems more tricky.

First, we must clarify where recommender systems are applied in the health domain? What are the options to be recommended? Does the system offer therapy suggestions to a doctor or do we supply nutrition-based food recommendations? Both systems are drastically different, yet share inherently similar risks, either for the individual, for the society as a whole, or both.

No framework exists that unites the specificity of health related recommender systems in order to provide both guidance to develop, and metrics to evaluate a health recommender system. In this article we aim to provide a review of recommender systems, how they have been applied in health scenarios, and how we think a framework can help in creating better health recommender systems.

2 Glossary and Key Terms

In order to make this article more understandable for researchers that have no prior experience in recommender systems. We first provide a glossary and some key terms that are relevant in this article.

2.1 General Terminology

Patients are typically persons that are in some kind of medical care. In health recommender systems patients (and in some cases users) must not necessarily be suffering from an illness. Health recommender systems may largely be applied as preventive measures, as well.

Machine Learning (ML) addresses the question of how to design algorithms that improve automatically through experience [2] - the focus is on doing it automatically (aML) without a human-in-the-loop [3].

interactive Machine Learning (iML) can be defined as learning algorithms that can interact with both computational agents and human agents and can optimize their learning behaviour through these interactions [4], by bringing in a human-in-the-loop [5].

2.2 Recommender Systems Terminology

Users – People that use the system and receive recommendations. Users also provide the ratings for items.

Items – The items that are being recommended (e.g. movies, products, hotels, etc.).

Ratings – Ratings refer to the choices of users in relation to items. Ratings can be explicit, by e.g. tagging a product, or implicit (e.g. opening a document, buying a product). Ratings can be Boolean, ordinal or numeric in nature, requiring different algorithms in implementation.

Content – The data from within the items that can be analyzed for recommendation. When documents are recommended, typically the content of the document. In many cases also meta-data.

Task – The reason why a user uses the system (e.g. to find a movie to watch). Often a set of interdependent tasks are relevant.

Context – The sum of all contextual factors that influence the use and evaluation of the recommender system and their interactions.

Sparse Matrix – A matrix that contains mostly the value 0. In user-item matrices, we often have many users and many items and only few ratings for individual users and items.

Cold start problem – When a new item or new user enters the system, we have very little information on the user to base recommendations on.

Coverage – Coverage refers to the criterion that addresses, whether all items in the database are getting recommended [6]. Recommenders that only recommend the most bought items, reach low coverage.

Serendipty – Serendipity refers to the criterion that addresses, whether recommended items are unexpected to the user. Novel unexpected items — serendipitous finds — can be a core benefits of a recommender.

3 Recommender Systems

The purpose of a recommender system is to find items that are relevant to the user, based on the users previous decisions. Recommender systems use these decisions and the decisions of other users to establish what may be relevant to the user. The first "recommender system" can be traced back to the Tapestry system developed at XEROX Park [7]. The initial idea was the concept of *collaborative filtering*. Users would tag interesting items to allow other users to browse these items by tags. The principles behind collaborative filtering are still being used in recommender systems [8].

Research then quickly focused on identifying similarities within documents. This allowed to rely not only on the opaque choices of users but also on the content of the recommended items, hence the name *content-based filtering* [9]. Quickly hybrid approaches appeared, merging both content-based and collaborative filtering [10].

Modern recommender systems often use *compositional approaches*, combining multiple recommender algorithms to an overall solution [11]. Techniques from other fields of computer science also find their way into recommender systems research. For example, social network analysis is used to augment recommendations [12] with data from relevant peers. Here, research on trust-based recommendation [13,14] has shown, that recommendations given by trusted peers are more likely to be helpful than generic algorithmic solutions. Recent approaches have also used methods like deep learning [15,16] to uncover the non-linear structure of preference in users.

Overall, we can say that research focuses on algorithms, data sets, evaluation criteria and interfaces for recommender systems. To each of those areas we provide a short introduction in the following sections. We then see, what of this work has been applied to health recommender systems, and what still needs work.

3.1 Algorithms

One typical research area, also the one with the strongest focus, is the underlying motor of the recommender system – the recommendation algorithm. Several approaches are used depending on the context of use. This sections aims to give a quick overview over the field of algorithms in recommender systems. It is by no-means extensive, but aims to help the reader to understand later parts of this article where algorithms are used.

Collaborative Filtering relies on the individual ratings of all users. It tries to identify items that are relevant for the user, or related to other items that have received positive ratings by the user. For this purpose a user-item matrix is used (see Fig. 1 on the left). This matrix simply contains the ratings of the users for all items. When a user has not rated an item, the cell remains empty. Typically this is a sparse-matrix. Various methods are used to impute the empty cells. This imputation is a prediction of a rating from a user for a given item. Predictions of high ratings can be used as recommendations. Some of these methods are given here:

- *Row mean* – By utilizing the mean of the row we average the users rating and return an non-informative rating, matching the users average judgment.
- *Column Mean* – By using the mean of the column we utilize how users have rated a particular item on average.
- *Combined* – We can use both means to adjust the prediction of an item to the respective users rating behavior.
- *Row based cosine similarity* - The vector cosine allows comparing the similarity of two vectors. The cosine is 1 if vectors are the same and 0 if they are

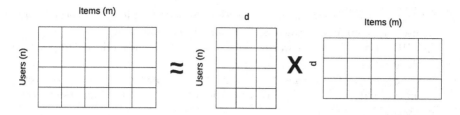

Fig. 1. Non-negative matrix factorization. By factorizing the user-item-matrix on the left, we can extract latent commonalities (d) of both users and items and calculate recommendations faster.

orthogonal. We can use this to find similar users and use their rating as a means of prediction.

– *Column based cosine similarity* – This can be used to find similar items and using them for recommendations immediately.

In order to improve run-time performance and to overcome the sparse-matrix and a part of the cold-start problem, we can use *matrix-factorization* to determine latent commonalities (here d) of both users and items (see Fig. 1). Matrix factorization has been found to be superior to nearest neighbor procedures and allows to integrate additional information (implicit feedback, temporal information, etc.) [17].

The natural extension of matrix factorization is *tensor-decomposition*. When information on ratings contains a third dimension of information (e.g. location-data, social preferences [18], context [19], etc.), we can encode this information in additional tensor dimensions. In order to apply similar procedures, we can no longer rely on matrix factorization, but must use tensor decomposition to compute recommendations [20].

Depending on the runtime-complexity of calculating latent preferences, different approaches exist, when incorporating new ratings. If complexity is high, different recommendation techniques can be combined to address users who are new to the system and thus not adequately represented. This can be done until the latent preferences have been updated.

Content-Based Filtering uses meta-data or features from individual items to open the black-box of the non-descriptive "item-id". In document recommendation typically text-mining methods are used for feature extraction. A typical text-mining pipeline would include the following steps, and yields a *vector-space model*:

1. *Term-Document Matrix* – Used to store a bag of words model of all documents.
2. *Stop-Word Deletion* – Used to remove words that are not predictive (e.g. "this")
3. *Stemming* – Using the stem of a word only (e.g. "walk" instead of "walking").

4. *N-Gram Detection* – Finding words that appear frequently together which are used as a singular term (e.g. "recommender system").
5. *TF-IDF* – Used to weight words in accordance with their relative importance for the document at hand.
6. *Latent-Semantic Indexing* – Using singular value decomposition on the term-document-matrix to incorporate semantic information in the extended vector space model.

As the end result we have three matrices that can be used to compute similar documents, based on the semantic similarity of documents. As an alternative approach we could use *Latent-Dirichlet Allocation* in order to identify topics in documents and find documents with similar topic-distributions. These similarity measures can be used in a similar fashion as in the collaborative filtering. When the recommended items are not documents, one must consider what are features of items that are relevant for recommendations (e.g. product features, actors in movies, etc.).

3.2 Data Sets

In 2006 Netflix[1] released a part of their users' ratings data sets. They proposed a challenge open for anyone, to train an algorithm to outcompete their implementation in predicting ratings of the remaining (unpublished) data. The *Netflix price* spiked the development in recommender algorithms and yielded Bellkor's Pragmatic Chaos algorithm [21]. The algorithms were measured against the root-mean square error (RMSE) of their predictions with the actual data. Interestingly, this algorithm was never included in the Netflix system. Partly because the algorithm was optimizing against an irrelevant metric. In 2006, Netflix believed that by reducing the RMSE, better recommendations could be achieved. But the RMSE can also be reduced by optimally predicting the ratings of movies, which in the lowest interest of the users. This might reduce RMSE but helps only little with good recommendations.

Other data sets exist from bibsonomy (scientific publications), delicious (bookmarked hyperlinks), flixster, movielens, movietweetings (all on movies), million songs dataset (music), and ta-feng (grocercy shopping bags from Belgium). Further data sets are described at the RecSysWiki [2].

3.3 Evaluation of Recommender Systems

As we have seen before, the criterion, against which a recommender system is evaluated, is critical to its success. Traditionally, recommender system algorithms were evaluated based on criteria borrowed from information retrieval or signal detection theory. Typical metrics are [22]:

---

[1] Netflix is an online movie provider.
[2] http://www.recsyswiki.com/wiki/Category:Dataset.

- *Precision* – The percentage of relevant items that are correctly recommended out of all recommended items.
- *Recall* – The fraction of items that are recommended from all relevant items. Also called *sensitivity*.
- *F-Measure* – The F-Measure is the harmonic mean of both precision and recall. It combines both measures into a single metric (see also Fig. 2).
- *ROC-Curve* – The reciever operating characteristic is a plot that visualizes the change of true positives against false positives depending on the sensitivity threshold. A sensitivity threshold must be chosen, as typical output of algorithms is mostly never clearly 1 (recommend) or 0 (do not recommend). The ROC-Curve helps determining optimal thresholds and compare algorithms against each other independently of the selected threshold.
- *RSME* – The root-square mean error is a measure that can be used to compare predictions against real data. By calculating the squared error for all items and then taking the root of the mean of the squared errors, we receive a value that penalizes strong deviations and is relatively forgiving to small deviations. This yields a weighted score which increases, when predictions differ more strongly from real values, and decreases when predictions become more accurate.

But as the Netflix price showed, that reducing error alone does not help in creating a better recommender. Ge et al. therefore argued to move beyond recommendation accuracy [23]. In a recommendation scenario often only the first k items are viewed by the user. If none of these are relevant, a user might go to a different website and not buy anything, in an e-commerce setting. This idea yields the k-top recommendations metrics (i.e. how many of the k-top items does the algorithm correctly find for all users?). But also measures such as serendipity (i.e. are items new?) and coverage (i.e. are all items being recommended?) are important, because users do not want to see their most beloved movies over and over again.

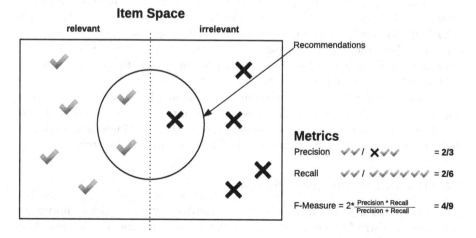

Fig. 2. Visualization of three metrics in a recommendation example: precision, recall and F-measure

3.4   Interfaces and Interactive Recommender Systems

When considering the whole recommender system in real usage scenarios, it became clearer that not only the algorithm needs to be evaluated [24]. The interface and HCI of a recommender system are equally important in how a user interacts with a recommender system.

This led to the design of user-centered evaluation frameworks. Most famous the work by Knijenburg et al. [25] and Pu et al. [26]. The work of Knijenburg et al. suggests that depending on **domain knowledge**, different types of interactions are most helpful to the user. Novices and "maximizers" prefer top-recommendations, while experts prefer hybrid-approaches combining implicit and explicit preferences.

Pu et al. shifted the focus of evaluation on technology acceptance. The new criteria were categorized as perceived quality, user believes, user attitudes and behavioral intentions. Under **user perceived quality** we summarize the perceived quality of recommendations (e.g. accuracy, familiarity, novelty, etc.), the interaction adequacy (e.g. adequacy of expression of ratings, explanations, etc.), and the interface adequacy (e.g. layout adequacy, clarity, etc.). The perceived quality then influences the **users' beliefs** about the recommender system. User beliefs concern the perceived ease of use, perceived usefulness, and control and transparency of the system. The **users' attitudes** refer to the attitude the user has in regard to the recommender systems. These encompass attitudes such as overall satisfaction, confidence and trust in the recommendations. Lastly different types of **behavioral intentions** can be measured on the base of cognitive and motivational attitudes of users. The user can either be willing to use the system, buy a product, continue to use the system or even influence his social circle to use the system.

As the evaluation of recommender systems took a turn to the user, of course the interface to the recommender became more important. In their review on interactive recommender systems, He et al. [27] reveal that interactive recommender systems aim at fulfilling the evaluation criteria *transparency*. By visualizing items in non-list based manners, and by showing how a recommendations come together, the results are more transparent to the users. Some of these interfaces are designed to foster exploration [1] and serendipity, others to provide overview and explanations [28].

Although the HCI part of recommender systems has become increasingly important, it still takes a smaller part in recommender research overall [29]. In particular, aspects such as user-control, affective interfaces and high risk domains — such as health — have not had a large share of research.

3.5   Health Recommender Systems

Not much previous work on applying recommender system in health informatics or medicine exists. As of June 5th 2016 only 17 articles are found when searching for the terms "recommender system health" in web of science. The oldest article is from 2007 and the most cited article has only 14 citations. Wiesner and Pfeifer

[30] distinguish between two scenarios: the first scenario targets health professionals as end-users of health recommender systems. The second scenario targets patients as end-users. Health professionals can benefit from recommender systems to retrieve additional information for a certain case, such as related clinical guidelines or research articles. The second scenario focuses on delivering high quality, evidence based, health related content to end-users. Most other articles that we have reviewed target patients as end-users. Objectives include delivering relevant information to end-users that is trustworthy, as in the work of Wiesner and Pfeifer [30], lifestyle change recommendations [31] and improving patient safety [32]. The latter category for instance includes research on how to use recommender systems to suggest relevant information about interactions between different drugs, in order to avoid health risks. Lifestyle change recommendations focus among others on suggesting users how to improve their eating [33,34], exercising or sleeping behavior.

In their research statement Fernandez-Luque et al. [35] argue, that using recommender systems for personalized health education does not take advantage of the increasing amount of educational resources available freely on the web. As one reason, difficulties in finding and matching content is given.

In a short review on health recommender systems by Sezgin & Ozkan [36] provided at the EHB 2013, the authors emphasize the increasing importance of Health Recommender Systems (HRS). The authors argue, that these systems are complementary tools used to aid decision making processes in all health care services. These systems show a potential to improve the usability of health care devices by reducing the information overload generated from medical devices and software and thus improve their acceptance.

The 2016 ACM Conference on Recommender Systems conference featured a workshop on engendering health with recommender systems, where many of the topics from this article were discussed.

4   A Framework for Health Recommender Systems

In order to successfully develop a health recommender system, additional criteria and procedures must be incorporated to ensure the success of such a system. The area of health or medical recommender systems faces several challenges that make it specific and intricate.

First of all, there is no clear task definition for recommender systems in health. The purpose of a recommender system depends on the item being recommend. In a health scenarios various items are imaginable. For example, a rather typical recommender system in a mobile device could recommend physical activities that match the current user situation to improve their health. An patient with arthritis and obesity could benefit more from physical activity recommendations that put no additional strain on already inflamed joints. Going for a walk will be more pleasurable, if weather conditions are good. Another, very different example of a health recommender could be a system that proposes different forms of cancer therapies to both a doctor and the patient. The

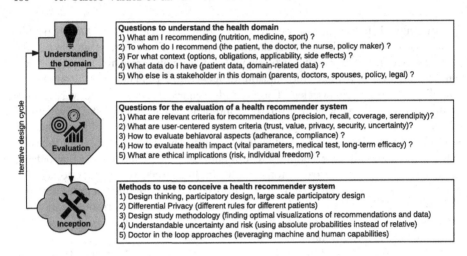

Fig. 3. Three steps to consider when developing a health recommender system. These steps should be incorporated as an extension of typical steps.

system could integrate patient properties such as other illnesses, additional medication, job requirements, and family situation to recommend optimal therapies and alternatives. It could visualize duration, experience and possible side-effects of multiple therapies and thus increase the patients control over their situation. The recommender system could be a communication tool that is used by both doctor and patient to help make difficult decisions.

In both scenarios the underlying algorithms can be taken from recommender systems research, but serve drastically different purposes and thus change the requirements to the recommender system.

In order to help understand the design space of such recommender systems, we propose the use of three additional design steps (see Fig. 3) when conceiving a health recommender system. Each step proposes guidance questions or additional methods and procedures to enrich the contextual picture of the usage scenario. We propose to extend the traditional recommender system design procedure to encompass theses additional requirements.

4.1 Understanding the Domain

First, we believe that different questions are necessary in understanding the application domain. As with any other recommendation domain, we must first understand what the **recommended item** is. Possible categories are:

- *Food/Nutritional Information* – Providing recommendations to optimize nutrition. May be applied to compensate malnutrition, reduce weight or to prevent certain food-based illnesses [33,34]. Recommendations could be food replacement items [37,38], different meals [39], or additions to a diet. The complex nature of taste [40] and its temporal and social dependencies [41] have to be considered.

- *Physical exercise/Sport* – Providing recommendations on what physical activities to perform. May be applied to help in finding activities that are interesting and motivating and also match the users requirements and needs. A recommender could also include location-data and weather data to find activities that are optimal for the users context.
- *Diagnosis* – Providing recommendations on likely diagnoses of a patient to a doctor or nurse. An approach using this recommendation item can be very similar to case-based reasoning approaches. By adding recommendations and linking them to therapy options, further value can be created.
- *Therapy/Medication* – Providing recommendations about the variety of possible options that may be applicable. A recommender system could address either/both patient and professional in finding a patient-specific therapy. The therapy, as mentioned in the example before, could include various patient properties and visualize different outcome criteria. Recommender systems could create personalized-health solely from data-analysis.

The second important question is, who are the **users** for the domain at hand? Typically the system is designed for an end-user, who can be either healthy or already a patient. But health recommender systems may extend their audience to health professionals such as doctors and nurses. Beyond these obvious new stakeholders pharmacists, clinicians, researchers and also policy makers could benefit from health recommender systems. Reducing the cost of health care in general could be a goal of recommender systems.

The third big part of the domain is the **usage context**. The context contains both the multifactorial goal setting, as well as contextual factors that influence how items are recommended and how they should be presented. By *multifactorial goal setting* we mean that health goals are not following a singular dimension. While naively we might think that the "most healthy" option is the one that should be recommended, different domain-specific criteria play a role in evaluating an item. For example, what is healthy for one patient could be dangerous for another (e.g. diuretics and other blood pressure lowering agents are dangerous for patients with diabetes, gout, etc.). It is necessary to include side-effect reduction as a goal. Beyond these immediate health-related outcomes, other outcomes such as costs, applicability (e.g. is the patient able to perform a daily subcutaneous injection) or changes in quality of life are important to consider. The impact of individual goals is also expected to differ strongly between different diseases. One can easily imagine that the relative importance of different goals vary drastically from one another for illnesses such as gout, cancer, depression or allergies. The goals can both be finding alternatives or finding optimal solutions. Thus the recommender system could very easily become a decision support system, depending on the dimensions of the search-space. Some illnesses have very few effective therapies, while other illnesses may have a multitude of tools that still only help to alleviate symptoms. In the latter scenarios complex recommendations (i.e. one therapy per symptom) could be the outcome of a recommender. The overall compatibility with the patients predispositions could be judged as the quality of a recommendation. It is also important to consider that some patients may value quality of life over longevity. A cancer patient might refuse painful therapy in order to enjoy the last few months at home rather than in a hospital. Optimizing for highest probable health outcome, by comparing efficacy of different medicines, could be an obvious solution but not necessarily the one a patient might have chosen in retrospect.

The fourth area of the domain is the **availability of data**. While typical areas of recommendations — such as movies — have the benefit of having publicly available data-sets, which can be used to train and test algorithms, data sets for health recommendations are rare. Some of the problems stem from the intrinsically more *complex nature of health data*. Health data is often unstructured, incomplete, non-standardized and stems from various sources. Large parts of data are not generated in a computer (as typical recommendations are) but stem from paper-based health-records that are often digitized afterwards. Additionally, the *type of data* may differ. While we have large nutritional databases, understanding what food stuffs serve as tasteful replacements is not fully understood. Also different brands of similar food stuffs make recommendations harder to do. IBM Watsons chef for example recommends dishes using IBM Watson technology. But simply trying to exclude sugar from recipes, requires to exclude 19 different types of sugar.

To make things more complicated health data has inherent *privacy* issues. Non-anonymized patient data in the hand of insurance companies, can be in the disinterest of the patient.

Stakeholders who are relevant besides the user should also be considered. In cases of health recommenders for food, for example, not only the user is affected by the system. Food is (most) often consumed in groups, thus individual preferences of multiple users influence the possibility of choices. Very specific choices or recommendations (e.g. low-carb, low-fat, sugar-free gluten-free, vegan) might be contradictory with each other. In such cases it is thinkable, that the group preference might overturn the recommended solution. Another approach could be to find group recommendations [41]. In another scenario, the parents of a child that suffers from diabetes are core stakeholders. Moreover, any family care givers could also benefit from high quality health recommender systems, as they might be the ones administering the care.

4.2 Evaluation of Health Recommender Systems

The criteria mentioned in this section should be considered as additions to typical evaluation criteria of recommender systems (e.g. [26,42,43]).

As with any medical technology it is crucial to measure and benchmark health recommender systems, particularly in regard to user acceptance [44] and satisfaction. By tailoring the services or devices to the individual user needs, demands and requirements, future research issues are uncovered. This includes user diversity research, not just in regard to user tailored results, but also in regard to the user interface of a recommender system [45]. Questionable quality will not be acceptable in a health recommender system.

To enable *benchmarking*, more comprehensive quality measures must be sought, and more specific theoretical and experimental frameworks should be investigated [43]. The overemphasis of accuracy metrics and under-representation of metrics such as serendipity and coverage pose a serious problem in typical recommender systems, but how do they apply to health recommender systems?

In particular rare diseases are important in this regard. Rare disease are individually rare, but there a many different rare diseases, making patients with rare diseases a non-rare phenomenon. Therefore, the question of serendipity and coverage, i.e. finding "interesting" as well as finding all relevant results, is also important for health recommender systems.

Algorithms exist to trade-off **serendipity and coverage** [23] for improved accuracy, e.g. by recommending items with more data. And since all three of these measure are important to users in many applications, designing algorithms in such a fashion may be adequate, but less useful in medical scenarios. Here a DiL approach could also be helpful by integrating the doctor in the algorithm. Judgments that are inherently human [46] (e.g. what is interesting?) can be integrated in the recommendation process, but we will need more comprehensive measures of quality combining accuracy, serendipity and coverage, to allow algorithm designer to improve trade-offs adjusted to medical scenarios in DiL settings.

Another very important research issue is trust in recommender systems [13]. This is particularly true for health recommender systems, as they shall be used to provide end users with more proactive and personalized information relevant to their health. But, there are still many open research questions considering **trust, privacy and intimacy** in the use of medical technology. User diversity plays a role, with an emphasis on gender and age [44].

This is important in regard to user **satisfaction**. Herlocker et al. [43] suggest to look deeper into modeling user satisfaction, with the aim of predictive satisfaction models. In the case of health recommender systems, this prediction is peculiar, as there are different relevant user groups. Differences in expertise, overview knowledge, but also tasks must be understood to create recommender systems suitable to health practitioners, clinical doctors, biomedical researchers, care givers and patients, alike.

As the outcome of health recommendations are inherently uncertain, **communication of this uncertainty** is highly important. Finding ways to visualize uncertainty in a set of recommendations is crucial to allow the user to evaluate the option adequately. This problem is linked to the risk and duration of the consequence of a choice. Picking a bad movie may cost you 90 min of your life; picking a bad therapy could reduce quality of life for many years. This changes how typical evaluation criteria (e.g. k-top recommendations precision) are judged. One bad option in the first few recommendations could have drastic outcomes. The designer of a health recommender systems must be careful and act responsibly in both generating recommendations and communicating them.

Under the assumption that the user of the system has perfect access to the desired options, the effectiveness of such a system must still be evaluated in regard to the users external behavior. **Behavioral evaluations** must be considered to measure the effectiveness of a health recommender system. For example, when giving recommendations about activities to conduct to improve fitness, the recommender system must track what activities have actually been conducted. In the case of smoking cessation [47], the system has a harder time to measure its effectiveness, as users might want to skip reporting that they have smoked a cigarette because of social desirability. Some health recommenders may also aim at long term behavioral changes and these must be tracked somehow, too. The risks of ignoring behavioral changes in long-term evaluations, could lead to short term recommendations, that are helpful to many users in the short-term, but conflict with long term goals (e.g. crash diets) [48].

Measuring actual health impact is also important. Even when the users show long term adherence to recommended health behaviors, the next question is whether the conducted changes in behavior or therapy lead to the desired changes in health. We must consider which health parameters to assess and which medical tests to employ to ensure medical effectiveness. For example, crash diets may lead to reduced body weight (a superficial health parameter), but mostly because of reducing body muscle mass. This leads to rebounding effects because of reduced metabolism. Long-term weight loss is burdened.

Before such an approach can be implemented in real-world medicine, it must be assured that such systems are sufficiently trustworthy [13]. Publicly accessible systems such as collaborative recommenders pose a **security risk**, as normal end-users cannot be distinguished from potential attackers. Beyond these technical risks, such attacks may lead to a continuous degradation of trust in the objectivity and accuracy of such a system. Therefore, a cornerstone of future research is in modeling such attacks and examine their impact on recommending algorithms. Hybrid algorithms in a DiL paradigm could provide a higher degree of robustness to such attacks [49].

Furthermore we must consider **ethical considerations** of recommender systems. (e.g. what do we do when health parameters used as an indicator for disease seem to not correlate with actual disease [50]). The principle of "first do no harm" should be kept in mind [48]. A recommender system might unintentionally provide health guidance that could — in the hand of a person suffering from a mental illness — steer a patient in an unhealthy direction (e.g. dieting tips for anorexic patients).

4.3   Methods to Design Health Recommender Systems

Third we need a framework to help us design a health recommender system in collaboration with the end-users. The aim in designing a recommender system for health should always integrate the end users. A framework needs to integrate tools that bring together the requirements of the domain and the evaluation criteria for the specific application. These tools should help the designer focus on the user and put the user-perspective first.

We think the first tool crucial to success, is the use of **participatory design** [51,52]. When health is the end-goal of a recommender system, the user should get an active say in designing their system. This helps identifying actual *user needs* and creates *identification* with the future system. When users design the system, the recommender system is not a tool devised by "Big Pharma" to optimize sales, but can become their personal assistant helping them to overcome health burdens that are meaningful to them. It may also alleviate privacy concerns [53]. The challenging part is to extrapolate existing methodology to allow large-scale co-creation and participation. We need tools that allow users to customize their own recommender system and to communicate needs more directly.

In scenarios were users are too remote, or too uninformed to directly co-create, methods such as *design thinking* [54] can be employed, to ensure that users problems are the focus of the system and not some accuracy metric.

The second tool we think is essential to any health recommender system, is the use of **differential privacy** [55]. Differential privacy allows the sharing of data without revealing individual identities. Typical methods include *k-anonymity or l-diversity* [56], which work by revealing only the amount of data that can be traced back to a group of at least k people. L-diversity additionally integrates the differences in sensitivity of different data fields. Beyond these purely IT-based privacy tools, it is necessary to communicate privacy concerns to the end user. Users are often not aware of privacy risks and behave in manners that contradict their long-term interests. On the other hand many users openly agree with sharing private information, even when aware of risks. Finding the matching *trade-off between privacy and utility* for the individual user group or user is crucial to implementing health recommender systems [57]. In this context, individual factors play a decisive role. As such, the level of knowledge about privacy threats in the Internet is important [58], but also different risk perceptions, as well as the level of digital competency [59], which is often related to age and technology generation [60,61]. Factual (technical) privacy threat is furthermore not identical with *risk perceptions*. The perceived benefits from sharing the data in the medical context is seen different than sharing the data in a less sensitive field [58,62,63]. In addition, users are much more reluctant to share data in personal spaces, when data relate to intimacy contexts, such as homes [64] or the sharing of physiological data [65].

The third tool to incorporate is **adequate uncertainty and risk communication** (e.g. risk-ladders, shaded error-bars, etc.) [29,66]. Communication goes in both directions – to the user and to the recommender. Users should be able to communicate uncertainty in their input methods, to ensure understanding on the algorithm's side [67]. As the end users may also have differing models of risk and different degrees of understanding statistics and uncertainty, it is crucial to address all levels of risk-literacy (e.g. absolute or natural frequencies [68]).

Furthermore, **effective and efficient visualizations** should be used, when displaying health data. The visualization of data should address the purpose of the recommender system and regard the end user and their intentions.

A methodology to ensure this is the Design Study Methodology [69], which has been shown to be effective even in visual recommender system design [28,70]. Creating a visualization in a recommender fosters the users willingness to explore options and help explain individual recommendations [71]. The challenge is that the influence of user diversity has not yet been fully investigated in information visualization [72]. Since individual differences might play a leveraging role in personalized health applications it is crucial to strengthen research in this areas.

Lastly, assisting medical professionals in a **doctor-in-the-loop (DiL) approach** is a new paradigm in information driven medicine [73]. It pictures the doctor not only as a consumer of digital information, but also as a someone who can interactively manipulate algorithms and tools. The doctor as a final authority inside the loop of an expert system can make sure that expert knowledge is integrated in the decision making process, by finding patterns and supplying tacit knowledge, while the recommender system can integrate patient data as well as treatment results and possible (side-)effects related to previous decisions. The DiL-concept can thus be seen as an extension of use of knowledge discovery for the enhancement of medical treatments together with human expertise: The expert knowledge of the doctor is enriched with additional information and expert know-how [74–76].

5 Conclusion

Recommender systems are applied in almost all fields of commercial web applications helping users to find products and services relevant and interesting to them. They are used to help find interesting information, scientific documents, and collaborators. But even in these areas further research is required [77]. In the future, we will hopefully see health recommender systems integrating experts in the algorithms, thus combining human expertise with computer efficiency to improve medical care for patients, care giver and doctors, providing better health for everyone.

The framework that we have suggested (see Fig. 4) in this article is considered to guide a developer into getting a holistic picture of the constraints that a medical application gives. A medical application is often judged against all of these (and many more) criteria, and inadequately addressing one of these aspects ensures failure of the recommender system and loss of trust in the recommender systems for health in general.

It is of **utmost importance** to mention that this framework is not an extensive one. It does not address any aspects of law, policy, and medicine directly. Developers should take an *interdisciplinary approach* seriously when designing a health recommender system. Seek out professionals from these field, when considering developing a health recommender system. Our framework merely looks at the challenge from a HCI perspective extending into the areas of communication, information visualization and technology acceptance.

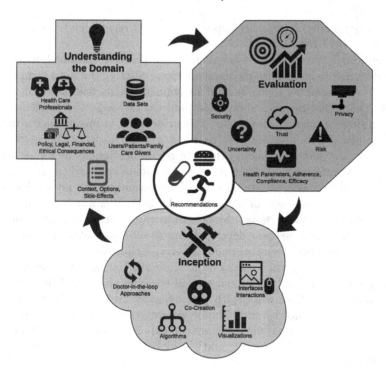

Fig. 4. The three parts of our research framework for developing health recommender systems.

6 Future Work

The future of health recommender systems strongly relies on interdisciplinary collaboration and collaboration across organizational borders. Recommender systems have started to flourish when data sets become public and quality metrics became available. We hope to see more **open data sets** for health recommender system that are helpful in designing algorithms, testing user experience and developing new metrics for the field of health recommender systems. Crucial in this regard is to respect privacy and anonymity, by some means provided earlier in this article. Next to offline evaluations possible through these data sets, it is worth noting that online evaluations still play an extensive role in evaluating a recommender system. User actual reactions might differ drastically from predictions made from offline data [78].

How different types of **user-diversity** (e.g. personality) can be used to improve recommendations has not been fully explored [79]. Even more so for the field of health recommender systems. As one long-term trend of recommender systems could be their integration as a personal assistant —think Siri or Cortana— it will become necessary to think about what health assistant users will want to have [80]. While some users might prefer a purely informative style of assistance others might want an assistant that is responsible for their decisions.

Can a recommender system be responsible for its recommendations? Can the developer be held responsible?

When health recommender systems have been more established, new metrics can be designed to economize recommendations. Sharing data is a form a giving monetary value and receiving helpful recommendations has financial value as well. We think that research should also address this aspect of hidden transactions and develop metrics to measure the **price and value of recommendations** not just from a user perspective, but also from a societal perspective. We are *not* arguing that users should think of recommendations as a product, but any viable recommender system will be used commercially and the consequences will have monetary effects on end users. Understanding the intricacies of how this aspect influences usage of a recommender system is important and should be included in the system design. Models from game-theory could be considered to depict these processes and develop business-models that help foster health and not a single pharmaceutical manufacturer, for instance.

Beyond this economical considerations, research is needed to **evaluate societal impact**. Neither all individual nor all societies can afford the best therapies for themselves. How will health recommender systems address this aspect of applicability and affordability? Maybe we even reduce effectiveness of a treatment, just by showing therapies that are too expensive for a patient [81]. Therefore a naive recommender system could —if globally applied— deteriorate overall health. The authority of the doctor also lies in matching medical needs and financial possibilities. If recommender systems come into play how does this affect a society as a whole? Does it affect the trust in medical professionals? Does it raise distrust in elites?

This also brings up the difference in **culture** and the applicability of recommender systems. In particular when looking at food or nutritional recommendations it is necessary to incorporate effects of culture and cultural tastes [82]. Beyond this superficial limitations, differences in health perception may play a deeper role, when building a health recommender system. In particular, the cultural differences in perceptions of gender or ethnicity may play into the design [83]. Questions that need be raised go in the direction of: How is technology perceived within different cultures? What is the effect of culture on perceptions of risk, privacy, and uncertainty? Does culture play a role in determining the role of individual and group benefit?

Lastly, the area of **ethical implications** of health recommender systems must be explored. While we do know some effects of traditional recommender systems, such as the filter bubble [84], we have not fully figured out the long-term consequences of these effects. When applying these effects to the area of health, the risk of overlooking relevant options might be much more costly for an individual of for society as a whole. But beyond these transferable effects, we must consider further ethical implications.

When recommender systems for health become effective and help in reducing health care cost, the question may become disconcerting whether individuals are still allowed to withhold their data because of privacy concerns. How much individual freedom is worth how much global health expenditure. The unwillingness to share medical data might increase the cost of therapy and therefore prevent funds to be used elsewhere, indirectly costing other people's health and lives. When recommender systems can be benchmarked in a fashion that makes this cost tangible, will they effectively kill privacy? Does revealing the space of possibilities (and thus the space of impossibilities) help improve health for everyone or only for a selected few? How will pervasive personalized health recommendations influence individual psycho-social development and in extension the Zeitgeist? We, as a society and as researchers, must find ways to decide what role recommender systems will play in the future — both in health and in other fields.

Acknowledgments. The authors thank the German Research Council DFG for the friendly support of the research in the excellence cluster "Integrative Production Technology in High Wage Countries", and the anonymous reviewers for their constructive comments.

Part of the work of Katrien Verbert has been supported by the Research Foundation Flanders (FWO), grant agreement no. G0C9515N, and the KU Leuven Research Council, grant agreement no. STG/14/019.

References

1. Bruns, S., Valdez, A.C., Greven, C., Ziefle, M., Schroeder, U.: What should i read next? a personalized visual publication recommender system. In: Yamamoto, S. (ed.) HCI 2015. LNCS, vol. 9173, pp. 89–100. Springer, Heidelberg (2015). doi:10.1007/978-3-319-20618-9_9

2. Jordan, M.I., Mitchell, T.M.: Machine learning: trends, perspectives, and prospects. Science **349**(6245), 255–260 (2015)

3. Shahriari, B., Swersky, K., Wang, Z., Adams, R.P., de Freitas, N.: Taking the human out of the loop: a review of bayesian optimization. Proc. IEEE **104**(1), 148–175 (2016)

4. Holzinger, A.: Interactive machine learning for health informatics: when do we need the human-in-the-loop? Springer Brain Inform. (BRIN) **3**(2), 119–131 (2016)

5. Holzinger, A., Plass, M., Holzinger, K., Crişan, G.C., Pintea, C.-M., Palade, V.: Towards interactive Machine Learning (iML): applying ant colony algorithms to solve the traveling salesman problem with the human-in-the-loop approach. In: Buccafurri, F., Holzinger, A., Kieseberg, P., Tjoa, A.M., Weippl, E. (eds.) CD-ARES 2016. LNCS, vol. 9817, pp. 81–95. Springer, Heidelberg (2016). doi:10.1007/978-3-319-45507-5_6

6. Puthiya Parambath, S.A., Usunier, N., Grandvalet, Y.: A coverage-based approach to recommendation diversity on similarity graph. In: Proceedings of the 10th ACM Conference on Recommender Systems, pp. 15–22. ACM (2016)

7. Goldberg, D., Nichols, D., Oki, B.M., Terry, D.: Using collaborative filtering to weave an information tapestry. Commun. ACM **35**(12), 61–70 (1992)

8. Resnick, P., Varian, H.R.: Recommender systems. Commun. ACM **40**(3), 56–58 (1997)

9. Pazzani, M.J.: A framework for collaborative, content-based and demographic filtering. Artif. Intell. Rev. **13**(5–6), 393–408 (1999)

10. Burke, R.: Hybrid recommender systems: survey and experiments. User Model. User-Adap. Inter. **12**(4), 331–370 (2002)
11. Sill, J., Takács, G., Mackey, L., Lin, D.: Feature-weighted linear stacking. arXiv preprint arXiv:0911.0460 (2009)
12. Tinghuai, M., Jinjuan, Z., Meili, T., Yuan, T., Abdullah, A.D., Mznah, A.R., Sungyoung, L.: Social network and tag sources based augmenting collaborative recommender system. IEICE Trans. Inf. Syst. **98**(4), 902–910 (2015)
13. O'Donovan, J., Smyth, B.: Trust in recommender systems. In: Proceedings of the 10th International Conference on Intelligent User Interfaces, pp. 167–174. ACM (2005)
14. Gao, P., Miao, H., Baras, J.S., Golbeck, J.: Star: semiring trust inference for trust-aware social recommenders. In: Proceedings of the 10th ACM Conference on Recommender Systems, pp. 301–308. ACM (2016)
15. Bansal, T., Belanger, D., McCallum, A.: Ask the gru: Multi-task learning for deep text recommendations. arXiv preprint arXiv:1609.02116 (2016)
16. Covington, P., Adams, J., Sargin, E.: Deep neural networks for youtube recommendations. In: Proceedings of the 10th ACM Conference on Recommender Systems, pp. 191–198. ACM (2016)
17. Koren, Y., Bell, R., Volinsky, C., et al.: Matrix factorization techniques for recommender systems. Computer **42**(8), 30–37 (2009)
18. Ge, H., Caverlee, J., Lu, H.: Taper: a contextual tensor-based approach for personalized expert recommendation. In: Proceedings of the 10th ACM Conference on Recommender Systems, pp. 261–268. ACM (2016)
19. Kim, D., Park, C., Oh, J., Lee, S., Yu, H.: Convolutional matrix factorization for document context-aware recommendation. In: Proceedings of the 10th ACM Conference on Recommender Systems, pp. 233–240. ACM (2016)
20. Karatzoglou, A., Amatriain, X., Baltrunas, L., Oliver, N.: Multiverse recommendation: n-dimensional tensor factorization for context-aware collaborative filtering. In: Proceedings of the Fourth ACM Conference on Recommender Systems, pp. 79–86. ACM (2010)
21. Koren, Y.: The bellkor solution to the netflix grand prize. Netflix Prize Documentation **81**, 1–10 (2009)
22. Powers, D.M.: Evaluation: from precision, recall and f-measure to roc, informedness, markedness and correlation (2011)
23. Ge, M., Delgado-Battenfeld, C., Jannach, D.: Beyond accuracy: evaluating recommender systems by coverage and serendipity. In: Proceedings of the Fourth ACM Conference on Recommender Systems, pp. 257–260. ACM (2010)
24. Swearingen, K., Sinha, R.: Beyond algorithms: An hci perspective on recommender systems. In: ACM SIGIR 2001 Workshop on Recommender Systems, vol. 13, Citeseer, pp. 1–11 (2001)
25. Knijnenburg, B.P., Reijmer, N.J., Willemsen, M.C.: Each to his own: How different users call for different interaction methods in recommender systems. In: Proceedings of the Fifth ACM Conference on Recommender Systems, RecSys 2011, pp. 141–148. ACM, New York (2011)
26. Pu, P., Chen, L., Hu, R.: Evaluating recommender systems from the user?s perspective: survey of the state of the art. User Model. User-Adap. Inter. **22**(4–5), 317–355 (2012)
27. He, C., Parra, D., Verbert, K.: Interactive recommender systems: a survey of the state of the art and future research challenges and opportunities. Expert Syst. Appl. **56**, 9–27 (2016)

28. Calero Valdez, A., Özdemir, D., Yazdi, M.A., Schaar, A.K., Ziefle, M.: Orchestrating collaboration-using visual collaboration suggestion for steering of research clusters. Procedia Manufact. **3**, 363–370 (2015)
29. Calero Valdez, A., Ziefle, M., Verbert, K.: HCI for recommender systems: the past, the present and the future. In: Proceedings of the 10th ACM Conference on Recommender Systems, RecSys 2016, pp. 123–126. ACM, New York (2016)
30. Wiesner, M., Pfeifer, D.: Health recommender systems: concepts, requirements, technical basics and challenges. Int. J. Environ. Res. Public Health **11**(3), 2580–2607 (2014)
31. Farrell, R.G., Danis, C.M., Ramakrishnan, S., Kellogg, W.A.: Intrapersonal retrospective recommendation: lifestyle change recommendations using stable patterns of personal behavior. In: Proceedings of the First International Workshop on Recommendation Technologies for Lifestyle Change (LIFESTYLE 2012), p. 24. Ireland, Citeseer, Dublin (2012)
32. Roitman, H., Messika, Y., Tsimerman, Y., Maman, Y.: Increasing patient safety using explanation-driven personalized content recommendation. In: Proceedings of the 1st ACM International Health Informatics Symposium, pp. 430–434. ACM (2010)
33. Rokicki, M., Herder, E., Demidova, E.: Whats on my plate: towards recommending recipe variations for diabetes patients. In: Proceedings of UMAP 2015 (2015)
34. Elsweiler, D., Harvey, M., Ludwig, B., Said, A.: Bringing the healthy into food recommenders. In: DRMS Workshop (2015)
35. Fernandez-Luque, L., Karlsen, R., Vognild, L.K.: Challenges and opportunities of using recommender systems for personalized health education. In: MIE, pp. 903–907 (2009)
36. Sezgin, E., Özkan, S.: A systematic literature review on health recommender systems. In: E-Health and Bioengineering Conference (EHB), pp. 1–4. IEEE (2013)
37. Achananuparp, P., Weber, I.: Extracting food substitutes from food diary via distributional similarity. arXiv preprint arXiv:1607.08807 (2016)
38. Freyne, J., Berkovsky, S.: Recommending food: reasoning on recipes and ingredients. In: Bra, P., Kobsa, A., Chin, D. (eds.) UMAP 2010. LNCS, vol. 6075, pp. 381–386. Springer, Heidelberg (2010). doi:10.1007/978-3-642-13470-8_36
39. Ge, M., Ricci, F., Massimo, D.: Health-aware food recommender system. In: Proceedings of the 9th ACM Conference on Recommender Systems, pp. 333–334. ACM (2015)
40. Harvey, M., Ludwig, B., Elsweiler, D.: Learning user tastes: a first step to generating healthy meal plans. In: First International Workshop on Recommendation Technologies for Lifestyle Change (lifestyle 2012), Citeseer, p. 18 (2012)
41. Berkovsky, S., Freyne, J.: Group-based recipe recommendations: analysis of data aggregation strategies. In: Proceedings of the Fourth ACM Conference on Recommender Systems, pp. 111–118. ACM (2010)
42. Said, A., Tikk, D., Shi, Y., Larson, M., Stumpf, K., Cremonesi, P.: Recommender systems evaluation: A 3d benchmark. In: ACM RecSys 2012 Workshop on Recommendation Utility Evaluation: Beyond RMSE, Dublin, Ireland, pp. 21–23 (2012)
43. Herlocker, J.L., Konstan, J.A., Terveen, L.G., Riedl, J.T.: Evaluating collaborative filtering recommender systems. ACM Trans. Inf. Syst. (TOIS) **22**(1), 5–53 (2004)
44. Ziefle, M., Rocker, C., Holzinger, A.: Medical technology in smart homes: exploring the user's perspective on privacy, intimacy and trust. In: 2011 IEEE 35th Annual Computer Software and Applications Conference Workshops (COMPSACW), pp. 410–415. IEEE (2011)

45. Zhou, T., Kuscsik, Z., Liu, J.G., Medo, M., Wakeling, J.R., Zhang, Y.C.: Solving the apparent diversity-accuracy dilemma of recommender systems. Proc. Natl. Acad. Sci. **107**(10), 4511–4515 (2010)

46. Beale, R.: Supporting serendipity: Using ambient intelligence to augment user exploration for data mining and web browsing. Int. J. Hum. Comput. Stud. **65**(5), 421–433 (2007)

47. Hors-Fraile, S., Benjumea, F.J.N., Hernández, L.C., Ruiz, F.O., Fernandez-Luque, L.: Design of two combined health recommender systems for tailoring messages in a smoking cessation app. arXiv preprint arXiv:1608.07192 (2016)

48. Ekstrand, J.D., Ekstrand, M.D.: First do no harm: Considering and minimizing harm in recommender systems designed for engendering health. In: Engendering Health Workshop at the RecSys 2016 Conference (2016)

49. Mobasher, B., Burke, R., Bhaumik, R., Williams, C.: Toward trustworthy recommender systems: an analysis of attack models and algorithm robustness. ACM Trans. Internet Technol. (TOIT) **7**(4), 23 (2007)

50. Grasgruber, P., Sebera, M., Hrazdira, E., Hrebickova, S., Cacek, J.: Food consumption and the actual statistics of cardiovascular diseases: an epidemiological comparison of 42 European countries. Food Nutr. Res. **60** (2016). doi:10.3402/fnr. v60.31694

51. Spinuzzi, C.: The methodology of participatory design. Tech. Commun. **52**(2), 163–174 (2005)

52. Ekstrand, M.D., Willemsen, M.C.: Behaviorism is not enough: better recommendations through listening to users. In: Proceedings of the 10th ACM Conference on Recommender Systems. RecSys 2016, pp. 221–224. ACM, New York (2016)

53. Barnes, S.B.: A privacy paradox: Social networking in the united states. First Monday **11**(9) (2006)

54. Martin, R.L.: The design of business: why design thinking is the next competitive advantage. Harvard Business Press (2009)

55. Dwork, C.: Differential privacy: a survey of results. In: Agrawal, M., Du, D., Duan, Z., Li, A. (eds.) TAMC 2008. LNCS, vol. 4978, pp. 1–19. Springer, Heidelberg (2008). doi:10.1007/978-3-540-79228-4_1

56. Aggarwal, C.C., Philip, S.Y.: A general survey of privacy-preserving data mining models and algorithms. In: Aggarwal, C.C., Yu, P.S. (eds.) Privacy-Preserving Data Mining, pp. 11–52. Springer, US (2008)

57. Ziefle, M., Halbey, J., Kowalewski, S.: Users willingness to share data on the internet: Perceived benefits and caveats. In: Proceedings of the International Conference on Internet of Things and Big Data (IoTBD 2016), pp. 255–265 (2016)

58. Kowalewski, S., Ziefle, M., Ziegeldorf, H., Wehrle, K.: Like us on facebook!-analyzing user preferences regarding privacy settings in germany. Procedia Manuf. **3**, 815–822 (2015)

59. Akhter, H.S.: Privacy concern and online transactions: the impact of internet self-efficacy and internet involvement. J. Consum. Mark. **31**(2), 118–125 (2014)

60. Fogel, J., Nehmad, E.: Internet social network communities: risk taking, trust, and privacy concerns. Comput. Hum. Behav. **25**(1), 153–160 (2009)

61. Freestone, O., Mitchell, V.: Generation y attitudes towards e-ethics and internet-related misbehaviours. J. Bus. Ethics **54**(2), 121–128 (2004)

62. Nissenbaum, H.: A contextual approach to privacy online. Daedalus **140**(4), 32–48 (2011)

63. Wilkowska, W., Ziefle, M.: Privacy and data security in e-health: requirements from the users perspective. Health Inf. J. **18**(3), 191–201 (2012)

64. Ziefle, M., Himmel, S., Wilkowska, W.: When your living space knows what you do: acceptance of medical home monitoring by different technologies. In: Holzinger, A., Simonic, K.-M. (eds.) USAB 2011. LNCS, vol. 7058, pp. 607–624. Springer, Heidelberg (2011). doi:10.1007/978-3-642-25364-5_43

65. Schmidt, T., Philipsen, R., Ziefle, M.: From V2X to Control2Trust. In: Tryfonas, T., Askoxylakis, I. (eds.) HAS 2015. LNCS, vol. 9190, pp. 570–581. Springer, Heidelberg (2015). doi:10.1007/978-3-319-20376-8_51

66. Lipkus, I.M., Hollands, J.: The visual communication of risk. J. National Cancer Inst. Monogr. **25**, 149–163 (1998)

67. Seipp, K., Ochoa, X., Gutiérrez, F., Verbert, K.: A research agenda for managing uncertainty in visual analytics. Mensch und Computer 2016-Workshopband (2016)

68. Gigerenzer, G., Edwards, A.: Simple tools for understanding risks: from innumeracy to insight. BMJ. Brit. Med. J. **327**, 741–744 (2003)

69. Sedlmair, M., Meyer, M., Munzner, T.: Design study methodology: reflections from the trenches and the stacks. IEEE Trans. Vis. Comput. Graph. **18**(12), 2431–2440 (2012)

70. Calero Valdez, A., Bruns, S., Greven, C., Schroeder, U., Ziefle, M.: What do my colleagues know? dealing with cognitive complexity in organizations through visualizations. In: Zaphiris, P., Ioannou, A. (eds.) LCT 2015. LNCS, vol. 9192, pp. 449–459. Springer, Heidelberg (2015). doi:10.1007/978-3-319-20609-7_42

71. Parra, D., Brusilovsky, P., Trattner, C.: See what you want to see: visual user-driven approach for hybrid recommendation. In: Proceedings of the 19th International Conference on Intelligent User Interfaces, pp. 235–240. ACM (2014)

72. Calero Valdez, A., Brauner, P., Ziefle, M., Kuhlen, T.W., Sedlmair, M.: Human factors in information visualization and decision support systems. Mensch und Computer 2016-Workshopband (2016)

73. Holzinger, A.: Interactive machine learning (iml). Informatik-Spektrum **39**(1), 64–68 (2016)

74. Kieseberg, P., Malle, B., Frühwirt, P., et al.: Brain Inf. **3**, 269 (2016). doi:10.1007/s40708-016-0046-2

75. Malle, B., Kieseberg, P., Weippl, E., Holzinger, A.: The right to be forgotten: towards machine learning on perturbed knowledge bases. In: Buccafurri, F., Holzinger, A., Kieseberg, P., Tjoa, A.M., Weippl, E. (eds.) CD-ARES 2016. LNCS, vol. 9817, pp. 251–266. Springer, Heidelberg (2016). doi:10.1007/978-3-319-45507-5_17

76. Kieseberg, P., Weippl, E., Holzinger, A.: Trust for the doctor-in-the-loop. European Research Consortium for Informatics and Mathematics (ERCIM) News: Tackling Big Data in the Life Sciences 104(1), 32–33

77. Felfernig, A., Jeran, M., Ninaus, G., Reinfrank, F., Reiterer, S.: Toward the next generation of recommender systems: applications and research challenges. In: Tsihrintzis, G.A. (ed.) Multimedia Services in Intelligent Environments, pp. 81–98. Springer, Switzerland (2013)

78. Rossetti, M., Stella, F., Zanker, M.: Contrasting offline and online results when evaluating recommendation algorithms. In: Proceedings of the 10th ACM Conference on Recommender Systems, pp. 31–34. ACM (2016)

79. Karumur, R.P., Nguyen, T.T., Konstan, J.A.: Exploring the value of personality in predicting rating behaviors: a study of category preferences on movielens. In: Proceedings of the 10th ACM Conference on Recommender Systems, pp. 139–142. ACM (2016)

80. Azaria, A., Hong, J.: Recommender systems with personality. In: Proceedings of the 10th ACM Conference on Recommender Systems, RecSys 2016, pp. 207–210. ACM, New York (2016)
81. Shiv, B., Carmon, Z., Ariely, D.: Placebo effects of marketing actions: consumers may get what they pay for. J. Mark. Res. **42**(4), 383–393 (2005)
82. Laufer, P., Wagner, C., Flöck, F., Strohmaier, M.: Mining cross-cultural relations from wikipedia: a study of 31 european food cultures. In: Proceedings of the ACM Web Science Conference, p. 3. ACM (2015)
83. Babitsch, B., Braun, T., Borde, T., David, M.: Doctor's perception of doctor-patient relationships in emergency departments: what roles do gender and ethnicity play? BMC Health Serv. Res. **8**(1), 1 (2008)
84. Knijnenburg, B.P., Sivakumar, S., Wilkinson, D.: Recommender systems for self-actualization. In: Proceedings of the 10th ACM Conference on Recommender Systems, RecSys 2016, pp. 11–14. ACM, New York (2016)

Machine Learning for *In Silico* Modeling of Tumor Growth

Fleur Jeanquartier[1](✉), Claire Jean-Quartier[1], Max Kotlyar[2], Tomas Tokar[2], Anne-Christin Hauschild[2], Igor Jurisica[2], and Andreas Holzinger[1]

[1] Holzinger Group HCI-KDD, Institute for Medical Informatics, Statistics and Documentation, Medical University Graz, Graz, Austria
{f.jeanquartier,c.jeanquartier,a.holzinger}@hci-kdd.org
[2] Princess Margaret Cancer Centre, University Health Network, Toronto, Canada
juris@ai.utoronto.ca

Abstract. The various interplaying variables of tumor growth remain key questions in cancer research, in particular what makes such a growth malignant and what are possible therapies to stop the growth and prevent re-growth. Given the complexity and heterogeneity of the disease, as well as the steadily growing set of publicly available big data sets, there is an urgent need for approaches to make sense out of these open data sets. Machine learning methods for tumor growth profiles and model validation can be of great help here, particularly, discrete multi-agent approaches.

In this paper we provide an overview of current machine learning approaches used for cancer research with the main focus of highlighting the necessity of *in silico* tumor growth modeling.

Keywords: Tumor growth · Cancer modeling · Machine learning · Computational biology

1 Introduction

Cancer prognosis and prediction is advancing by making use of data that has been mined and interpreted with the help of machine learning techniques. Machine Learning (ML) also aids the process of interpreting and understanding the complexity in big data sets [1].

Johnson *et al.* describe cancer informatics as hybrid discipline; although, even with the latest ML advances, there is still a gap to fill in fostering mathematical modeling and computer simulation of cancer [2].

Modeling tumor growth is a very challenging problem because, besides from being highly complex, it involves dynamic interactions spanning multiple scales both in time and space. This involves both continuous and discrete variables that call for hybrid approaches [3]. Araujo and Mcelwain [4] historically summarize how mathematical modeling has contributed to elucidating tumor growth.

© Springer International Publishing AG 2016
A. Holzinger (Ed.): ML for Health Informatics, LNAI 9605, pp. 415–434, 2016.
DOI: 10.1007/978-3-319-50478-0_21

1.1 Glossary and Key Terms

In Silico refers to being performed on a computer instead of a wetlab and stands opposite to *in vivo* or *in vitro* [5]. Naturally, integration and interplay of all three approaches is essential for research advances.

Machine Learning (ML) addresses the question of how to design algorithms that improve automatically through experience [6]. Besides primary goal of learning useful models, scalability of these algorithms play an increasingly important role in the the era of "big data analytics".

Interactive Machine Learning (iML) defines learning algorithms that can interact with both computational agents and human agents, and can optimize their learning behavior through these interactions [7], by bringing in a human-in-the-loop [8].

Agent-Based Modeling (ABM) depicts a computational method for simulating a system, which is based on individual units, calculated by a given rule-set on a discrete level [9].

Cellular Potts Modeling (CPM) defines a stochastic process of simulating the collective behavior of cellular structures [10].

Cellular Automata (CA) are representations for modeling complex systems dynamics [11–13].

Support Vector Machines (SVM) are supervised learning algorithms to solve primarily classification and regression problems [14,15].

Electronic Health Records (EHR) are longitudinal electronic records of patient health information with the ability to generate complete records of clinical patient encounters [16].

Protein-Protein Interactions (PPI) comprise the concurrence and the effect of proteins on each other based on surface properties as well as local features [17]. PPIs form the basic concept of biological communication and the specificity in signal transduction [18–20].

2 Motivation for Applying ML to Cancer Research

There are different entry points for ML to tumor growth research. Within this paper, we summarize possible approaches to using ML in the field of cancer research and the various kinds of models of tumor growth in computational or systems biology.

Cancer research started around 250 years ago [21]. There are several methods to study the disease, still, basic research comes down with animal experimentation. *In vitro* cell systems and the comparison of cellular processes help to understand the complexity of uncontrolled cell growth.

In silico models complement traditional *in vitro* and *in vivo* animal models. While ML is not new to cancer research the full potential of diverse ML algorithms has not been realized yet. In fact, *in silico* techniques are often underrated but can be vital to fundamental questions to beat cancer [22]. Knowledge discovery with ML outperforms bio assays [23] and image analysis could outperform human [24]. The principles of the 3Rs - replacement, reduction and refinement - can be used for the reduction of animal research, saving resources as well as reducing costs spent on clinical and wet-lab experiments in cancer research. In this regard, computerized experiments, meeting the terms of 3R, offer new possibilities for biomedical research. *In silico* suits the task of refinement as well as knowledge discovery. Recently, we presented an *in silico* approach for tumor growth simulation that holds the advantage of data visualization over multiple implementation possibilities [25, 26]. It is clear that ML techniques will give new insights into tumor growth modeling. Thereby, the goal is to increase the basic understanding of tumor progression as well as the onset of cancer.

3   In Silico Modeling of Cancer

In silico models involve various disciplines of mathematics, biology, medical and computer science. The underlying data is computationally processed from biomedical literature sources, based on wet-lab and clinical investigations, and extended or refined through hypothesises and theoretical characterizations [22].

There are different kinds of models in biology, such as spatial ones, space free ones but also cell descriptive models based on density, cell-based, sub-cellular or molecular, relating to their scale of phenomenon, and so far, various models for cancer have been described [10, 27]. Models can also be differentiated by their biological scale, ranging from the cellular and molecular level up to the genetic macro scale. On the other hand, there are also diverse computational modeling approaches, such as statistical, network-based as well as models on tissue-level. Regarding the cell-cell interactions there are discrete/agent-based to continuum-based modeling approaches. This leads us to the term agent that is shortly discussed in the next paragraph.

3.1   Agents in Modeling and ML

Agents play an important role both in Agent-based modeling (ABM) as well as in Machine Learning (ML). As described by Russell *et al.*, "an agent is anything that can be viewed as perceiving its environment through sensors and acting upon that environment through effectors" [28]. According to [29] ABM is used to model phenomena as dynamical systems of interacting agents. Thereby, agents individually assess a situation and make decisions on the basis of a set of rules [30]. So far, agents can be robot or human [7].

New *agent-based models of tumor growth* have been developed to foster the understanding of cancer, while agents can be used to model different parts of tumor growth to understand peculiarities such as factors that influence a tumor becoming malignant etc. [9,25,31]. Followingly, we shortly describe aspects of tumor growth for ABM.

Tumor growth kinetics follow simple laws that can be mathematically modeled [32]. Among them, the Gompertz law describes growth following a continuous deceleration [33–35].

Cellular Potts Model (CPM) is an agent-based modeling approach that has been introduced and described by Graner and Glazier [36]. It is used to simulate the collective behavior of cellular structures and has been used in a wide range of applications, among them, tumor dynamics [10].

Spatial & temporal scales are key descriptors in ABM in general and in modeling tumor growth in particular [10,25,32]. Regarding the description of spatial aspects, different topologies are used in ABM, such as spatial grids. Grids have been implemented as CA, i.e. Conway's Game of Life [37]. We [25] use also the term lattice as a group (not partially ordered set) to describe the topology and therefore the connectedness of several cellular bricks. The agent's neighborhood is described by an agent only interacting with its neighbors located close-by. However, agents may also interact with their environment, therefore environmental parameters can be taken into account. Regarding the temporal aspects, ABM follows discrete event cues, in particular a sequential schedule of interactions, computed by Monte Carlo steps (MCS).

Cellular Automata (CA) is a concept introduced by Stanislaw Ulam and John von Neumann in 1940s [11–13]. A typical CA includes a spatial lattice comprising units, called cells, where each cell can reside in one of finite number of pre-defined states. State of each cell in the lattice is updated according to the transition rules, so that the state of the cell in the given time depends on its own previous state and on the previous state if its close neighbors. The overall state of the entire lattice is evolving in discrete times steps, either synchronously, when all cells are updated at once, or asynchronously, when single randomly selected cell is updated in each time step. The Concept of CA was later popularized by Stephen Wolfram, who showed that even simple transition rules allow CA to exhibit variety of complex behaviors including phenomena of "self-organization" [38]. CA have been then extensively utilized in model dynamics of complex systems across diverse fields, including cancer biology. CA have been successfully adopted to realistically model tumor growth [39–46], as well as angiogenesis [47–49] and immune evasion [50,51].

Transition rules governing the behavior of the automaton, are sometimes formulated directly according to the available experimental knowledge [39,44,48], but more often are subject of inference using numerical optimization with respect to desired macroscopic qualities, e.g., transient dynamics of the tumor growth, or its geometric properties [42,46]. Alternatively, transition rules and associated quantitative parameters are varied in order to reveal association between microscopic properties of the single cell and macroscopic properties of the tumor [40,41].

Ideally, a model gives emergence to phenomena that could not be *a priori* deduced, and can be tested against experimental data.

ABM is not inductive, that means models are not based on a set of data and do not make inferences that lead to that data, but rather describe a system's mechanisms of rules and seek to reconstruct observations. This leads to ML, that is suitable to find patterns in existing data as well as can be used for validation, to extend *in silico* modeling tools.

4 ML Applications Areas in Cancer Research

ML approaches for cancer research have been reviewed before [1,52–56]. These reviews deal both with biological questions as well as on algorithmic details. While most ML reviews in this domain cover genomic studies and image based analysis, some also tackle the question how to support the understanding of tumor kinetics in particular. But there is a clear lack of new results in this area. An advanced search within EuropePMC with the query:

(*TITLE* : "cancer" AND "machine learning") AND (*OPEN_ACCESS* : y) yielded 671 results.

The search query: (*KW* : "machine learning" AND *KW* : "cancer") AND (*OPEN_ACCESS* : y) delivered only 41 results.

Regarding the term "tumor growth" there are hardly any works. The query: (*TITLE* : "tumor growth") AND (*KW* : "machine learning") even resulted in no results at all.

This work is not aimed at providing a comprehensive list of all studies that can be found on machine learning methods related to tumor growth research, even, if there are hardly any found. It is rather thought to provide a practical overview of pointers to machine learning methods applied to tumor growth modeling research with identifying challenges and opportunities.

In order to understand the different possibilities of applying ML techniques to cancer research, we first differentiate between specific application areas and later continue on describing research on tumor growth in particular. An overview of ML applications in cancer research is presented in Fig. 1.

Most reviews on ML for cancer focus on discussing existing cancer research that applies ML methods for predicting susceptibility, recurrence and survival [1,53]. Next to prediction, ML methods are applied to identification and diagnosis [57]. A classification of ML application areas in bioinformatics shows partially overlapping areas of genomics, proteomics and metabolomics but also evolutionary developmental biology, text mining, systems biology other advanced modeling applications [58]. Computational prediction approaches based on computer algorithms, allow for multivariate analysis in cancer diagnosis and comprise several methods such as linear or penalized discriminant analyses, logistic regression, learning vector quantization, decision trees, random forest, support vector machines, Bayesian networks and artificial neural networks [59,60]. These computational approaches overcome the lack of sensitivity and selectivity that, still, are often found in conventional methods based on univariate factors such as single biomarkers [60]. To evaluate prediction accuracy of these models the data is

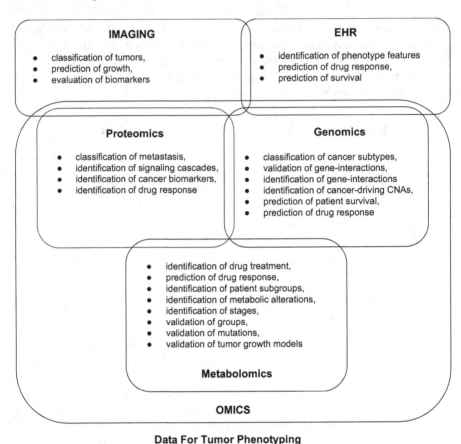

Fig. 1. Overview of ML approaches in cancer research regarding data type

randomly separated into training-, validation-, and test-sets. However, this gold standard method is solely feasible for large data sets. Cross-validation, a simple and commonly applied approach, splits data into subsets, while each subset is left out once for testing, the model is trained on the remaining data. Independent of univariate or multivariate methodology, permutation-based evaluation is recommended to assess the superiority of the model compared to a model trained on a randomized outcome variable [61].

ML approaches for cancer research can also be organized according to their algorithmic approach as well as the type of data used, ranging from imaging, genomics up to pathologic and demographic [53]. We next list works sorted by data approach to provide pointers for using ML on open cancer data [26].

4.1 Processing Imaging Data

ML can be used to detect and classify tumors in medical images [53]. For example, Morris *et al.* model glioma tumor growth using magnetic resonance (MR) scans for learning the parameters of a diffusion model [62]. Thereby they use patient data and preprocessing of images such as noise reduction and segmentation for feature extraction and consecutively prediction of glioma growth through classification and diffusion.

HealthAgents is another interesting project implementing a multi-agent system (MAS) for classifying brain tumors by applying pattern recognition methods on MR images [63].

Moreover, ML methods have been used for the evaluation of different radiomic features for predicting survivability [64]. Results highlight the several features' utility as radiomic biomarkers [64].

Cancer imaging, in particular image analysis of MR scans, already provides many possibilities for biomarkers [55]. But, images not only allow for measurements of the dynamics of shape and size. Fluorescence microscopy is also used to monitor small parts of cells [65]. Understanding complex diseases also requires identifying interactions among different components which leads us to the world of "Omics". Processing additional data such as combing picture archives with genomic profiles and even more, with electronic health records (EHR), brings us one step closer towards personalized medicine. Next, we summarize main concepts in Omics data and further proceed with examples in processing electronic healthcare records and hybrid data approaches:

4.2 Processing Omics Data

The molecular etiology of cancer is not well understood. Although numerous molecular cancer biomarkers have been identified, they are often ineffective for tasks such as cancer diagnosis, classification of cancer subtypes, prediction of cancer recurrence, or prediction of response to treatment [66]. One of the most promising strategies for addressing these problems is analysis of molecular networks, combined with machine learning and graph theory algorithms. These approaches lead to better predictions across diverse samples, and identify molecular mechanisms underlying cancer [67].

Protein-Protein Interaction (PPI) networks were the first type of molecular network used for identifying cancer biomarkers. Chuang *et al.* [68] identified PPI subnetworks that could serve as biomarkers for classifying breast cancer metastasis. Their approach combined PPI data with gene expression data from patients with and without breast cancer metastasis. The approach searched for protein subnetworks whose corresponding gene expression levels could distinguish metastatic and non-metastatic patients. The average expression of all genes in a subnetwork was used as a biomarker, unlike previous approaches, where biomarkers were individual molecules. The identified subnetworks had significant associations with hallmarks of cancer, and indicated novel relationships between signaling cascades (functional networks or pathways) and tumor progression. Furthermore, subnetwork biomarkers outperformed single-gene biomarkers in two important aspects: reproducibility across data sets and classification performance. Reproducibility considers whether the same biomarkers can be identified using different data sets: subnetwork biomarkers from different expression data sets overlapped by 12.7 %, whereas single-gene biomarkers overlapped by only 1.3 %. Classification performance - the ability of biomarkers to predict metastatic status - was assessed by using biomarkers as inputs to classifiers (logistic regression and support vector machines), that were tested through cross-validation. Subnetwork biomarkers significantly outperformed sets of single-gene biomarkers with all classifiers and data sets tested. Subsequent studies used PPI networks to identify subnetwork biomarkers of bladder, colorectal, gastric, liver, and lung cancers [69,70], and single-protein biomarkers of brain, breast, liver, lung, and skin cancers [71–75]. PPI networks have also been used to identify biomarkers of response to cancer treatment [76,77]. Cancer-related biomarkers cannot only be described in Proteomics but also in Genomics.

Genomic Data has brought up several biomarkers for measuring therapeutic response and validating drug treatment of cancer [78]. Moreover, genomic data such as gene expression samples can be used for identifying cancer subtypes [79] but also for predicting evolution even including response to drugs [53]. For example, gene expression data [79] and molecular profiling [80] have been used to improve glioma classification. Genomic data has also been used for the prognosis of possible relapse after treatment of prostate cancer [81].

Upstill *et al.* describe ML approaches for discovering gene-gene interactions in sequencing data [57]. While They call the type of data "disease data". They also underline that most studies report on applying ML for validating results rather than on identifying new disease-related interactions. The Matchmaker Exchange API [82] is a tool for cohort discovery and variant disease causal validation that also makes use of so called "disease data" from different genomic databases.

In general, networks based on gene expression data have been used to identify biomarkers predictive of patient drug response and prognosis. Two types of networks are typically constructed from gene expression data: co-expression networks, where edges connect pairs of genes that have correlated expression across samples, and gene regulatory networks, where edges indicate regulatory effects between pairs of genes. Both types of networks have helped identify cancer biomarker genes and gene modules. These biomarkers were used as inputs to statistical or machine learning methods for various disease prediction and classification tasks. Biomarkers from co-expression networks have been used to predict patient prognosis [83–85] and response to treatment [85]. Applications of gene regulatory networks have included biomarker discovery for prostate cancer [86] and breast cancer [87], and modeling of ovarian cancer progression [88].

As genomic alterations are a fundamental feature of cancer, several network-based methods have been developed for analyzing these alterations, and identifying subsets that are cancer biomarkers. Jörnsten *et al.* developed causal network models to understand how DNA copy number alterations in glioblastoma affect gene expression [89]. These models, based on regression and bootstrapping methods, predict key cancer-related alterations, their effects on gene expression, and patient survival. Shi *et al.* developed an alternative network model, using Laplacian shrinkage, to analyze the effects of copy number alterations on gene expression [90]. Leung *et al.* introduced a method for identifying frequently mutated gene modules in molecular networks associated with patient drug response, patient survival and other clinical or phenotypic data [91]. Similar approaches identify cancer-deregulated subnetworks [92].

There is a vast amount of publicly available heterogeneous genomic data, making data mining and ML well suited to solve key problems in the world of genomic medicine [93]. Complementing genetic studies leads us to the field of Metabolomics.

Metabolomics has been introduced to cancer "omics" studies relatively recently. It opened new opportunities towards biomarker discovery, identification of signaling molecules associated with cell growth, cell death, cellular metabolism [101]. Metabolomics is therefore frequently used for studies aiming at the detection of cancer even in early stages. Most commonly used analytical technologies comprise NMR spectroscopy, LC/MS, GC/MS and MCC/IMS [101,102]. In order to meet the demands of cellular proliferation and the required uptake and conversion of nutrients into biomass, cancer cells modify their metabolism during tumor development. Many of these key metabolic alterations are similar across tumor cells. A prominent example are the changes in the glucose metabolism leading to an increase of the described biosynthetic activities, and to the 'Warburg' effect, an inevitable adaptation to cope with the lack of ATP generation [103].

Metabolomics technology can be used to identify clinically relevant subgroups of cancer patients. For instance, O'Shea *et al.* analyzed the metabolites in sputum from patients with lung cancer and age-matched volunteers smoking controls using flow infusion electrospray ion mass spectrometry and found potential marker using artificial neural networks [104]. A sequential application of recursive feature elimination on linear-SVM and orthogonal partial least squares discriminant analysis (PLS-DA) was used to find the minimum set of discriminant features separating early-stage ovarian cancer patients samples from controls. Permutation testing was performed to validate the results [105]. Another study analyzed the metabolom of exhaled air by MCC/IMS within normal, COPD and lung cancer patients. A variety of supervised ML methods, e.g., linear-SVM or random forest, were applied to evaluate their capabilities to differentiate the three groups [106].

A second group of studies focus on validation. G12C k-RAS mutation has been suspected to be a key player in promoting metabolic rewiring, in isogenic non-small cell lung caner (NSCLC) cell line. Brunelli *et al.* applied OPLS-DA models and discovered a robust separation between G12C and WT k-RAS isoforms both *in vitro* and *in vivo*. Authors further validated their findings by mapping the quantified metabolites to the KEGG pathway database. Furthermore, they identify a list of most likely enriched metabolic pathways associated with the given metabolites [107].

The third application focuses on the prediction of disease outcome. Metabolomic NMR fingerprinting was utilized to assess the survival of patients with metastatic colorectal cancer (mCRC). A combination of partial least squares and support vector machines (PLS-SVM) was first applied to discriminate patients with mCRC and healthy subjects. In a second step, PLS-SVM was successfully used to evaluate whether patients with short or long overall survival can be identified by metabolomic profiling using NMR [108]. Wei *et al.* utilized a metabolomics approach to predict the effectiveness of treatments. In particular, PLS-DA is applied to model the response to neoadjuvant chemotherapy for breast cancer [109].

These findings show that metabolomics data can be used to differentiate not only tumor from control samples but also identify different stages of the growing tumor. Thereby, these technologies could be used for continuous monitoring of tumor growth and development in order to validate and optimize presented approaches *in silico* tumor growth models. Processing healthcare records forms another example in need of computerized support within the field of personalized cancer therapy and research, that is discussed next.

4.3   Processing Healthcare Records and Combined Data

When dealing with medical records, its anonymization is an important topic that can be supported through the use of ML [7]. Learning from various data sets opens up novel possibilities for cancer research.

So far, several works have described different ML techniques for the classification of patient cohorts [94]. Standardized multi-scale information models of cancer phenotypes provide information in computable form that are important for complementary approaches such as tumor growth modeling [95].

Delen *et al.* [96] describe a comparative study of neural networks, decision trees as well as logistic regression for mining a data set of more than 200,000 cases provided by SEER [97] for testing prediction of breast cancer survivability.

Menden *et al.* describe an approach for predicting how cancer cells respond to drugs based on combined data analysis, genomic features of cell lines as well as chemical features of drugs [98].

EHR have also been used for predicting cancer survival with the help of support vector machines (SVMs) [99]. Weighted Bayesian networks have been developed on the combination of EHR and PubMed data to predict pancreatic cancer [100].

Hybrid methods provide effective means to detect and quantify a broad range of small molecules for studying complex biological networks.

5   ML Towards Extending *In Silico* Modeling

Lisboa *et al.* [55] highlight how modeling of biological processes related to cancer may benefit from data mining approaches. They summarize main concepts found in literature as on the one hand, mining data from experiments to better understand parts of signaling pathways, and on the other hand to predict the evolution of dynamical systems.

Integration of data can be used to extend the descriptive part of compartmental states [26], such as by relating information on inhibitors and promotors to tumor growth curves, but also by making use of cancer classifications to create cancer profiles [110].

ML methods can be used on open cancer data for several possibilities, i.e., identifying tumor suppressing and inhibiting genes and further advancing a tumor growth related interaction network [111] that may help find and select precisely targeted treatments [92,112,113]. Existing treatment data can be further integrated into simulation tools to validate both tool and model and improve the tumor growth prediction rates. Such predictions gained via ML approaches can be combined with the ABM approach for further analysis. Other subjects of interest can be described further, such as specific cells or parts of it, that are again remodeled as discrete entities or agents, and iteratively validated to support sense-making in tumor growth analysis.

Additionally, visualization supports interaction with data and models [114]. Visualization in ABM is needed to visually convey the behavior of the model [31,115]. We have recently introduced a novel visualization approach of simulating and analyzing cell-related variables regarding tumor growth kinetics [25]. Thereby, visualization is used to show patterns of tumor growth. The graph-based visualization approach makes use of nodes, representing cellular bricks. These cellular bricks are related to compartmental states, including localized phenomena.

Last but not least, ML can be used to include image analysis in two ways: First, images can be used as input for the modeling, while the classification of images can be supported by ML techniques. Second, by analyzing a set of existing images related to tumor growth, the model can be compared to ML results and further validated.

6   Challenges in Network-Based ML Approaches

Network analysis combined with machine learning has proven to be an effective approach for identifying biomarkers and molecular mechanisms of cancer [116]. This approach is likely to further increase in popularity, but continued progress will require addressing multiple challenges:

Challenge 1. foremost, we need to increase coverage and annotation of diverse networks, to include tissue and process specificity;

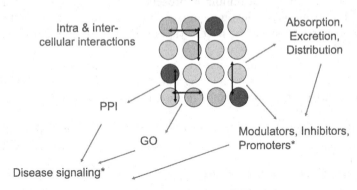

Fig. 2. The "big picture" in the modeling and visualization of tumor growth [25, 26]

Challenge 2. we need to improve scalability of algorithms to addressed increased size and complexity of networks;

Challenge 3. biomarker performance will need to be measured by standardized unbiased methods;

Challenge 4. multiple types of omics data will need to be combined into unified network models; and

Challenge 5. networks may need to be tailored to individuals to facilitate personalized medicine.

7   Challenges in Modeling Tumor Growth Dynamics

In Silico models complement the lack of *in vitro* and *in vivo* models. However, tumor growth modeling also brings up many questions concerning specific aspects of the various kinds of benign and malignant neoplasms. The main challenges in modeling tumor growth kinetics include:

Challenge 1. **There is no universal tumor growth model.** As Benzekry *et al.* [32] described, dormancy phases creates challenges for finding a generic growth law. The Gompertz or power law has been used to predict tumor growth; however, with a very low prediction rate. A so called "Universal Law of tumor growth" has to be found yet. However, [117] proposed to classify tumor growth patterns into fundamentally different categories. Therefore, cancer classification and profiling has to be taken into account.

Challenge 2. **The disease's complexity** poses a big open problem to tumor growth modeling. According to Edelman *et al.* [27] modeling the heterogeneous nature of tumor growth needs to take various characteristics into account. These characteristics are to be comprehensively discovered, as well as, in the latter modeled.

Challenge 3. **Data heterogeneity** challenges integration and fusion. Data fusion poses significant challenges. While diverse data sets exist, data comes from different laboratories, with different type and quality controls, different representation and processing [27, 118–120]. Integrating current bioinformatics workflows with knowledge engineering provides the necessary step in the right direction.

Challenge 4. **Visualizing evidence and uncertainty** with aggregation and display of specific information is required to make informed decisions. However, visualization still poses a big challenge. Offering reproducable, transparent and interactive visual analysis output of learned patterns is one of the many challenges for applying Visual Analytics methods to the biomedical domain [121–124].

Challenge 5. Finally, the question remains of **how to infer knowledge from existing data**. Machine learning may be used to infer graphical models from data [118], but there are difficult learning tasks to infer graphical models, yet to be solved.

8 Conclusion and Future Outlook

Combining ML and ABM can be used on various biological scales, as shown in Fig. 2: The lattice's nodes are represented as cellular bricks, which can be related to localized phenomena such as intra- & intercellular interactions, information on absorption, excretion, distribution as well as modulators, inhibitors and promoters, but also protein interactions and gene ontology. The overall goal remains to understand properties and peculiarities regarding cancer disease signaling.

In summary, ML can be used to improve *in silico* modeling, ranging from model validation to identifying novel insights. Future studies may involve the integration of proteomic and metabolomic networks behind ABM in order to simulate drug effects on tumor growth towards personalized medicine. Further exploration on genomic information regarding disease-driving mutations could be embedded within a multi-agent approach to simulating tumor growth in more detail. This may include studies on evolutionary dynamics of tumor growth and the underlying cellular heterogeneity of tumors using *in silico* environments.

References

1. Kourou, K., Exarchos, T.P., Exarchos, K.P., Karamouzis, M.V., Fotiadis, D.I.: Machine learning applications in cancer prognosis and prediction. Comput. Struct. Biotechnol. J. **13**, 8–17 (2015)

2. Johnson, D., Osborne, J., Wang, Z., Marias, K.: Computer simulation, visualization, and image processing of cancer data and processes. Cancer Inf. **14**(Suppl 4), 105 (2015)

3. Tzedakis, G., Tzamali, E., Marias, K., Sakkalis, V.: The importance of neighborhood scheme selection in agent-based tumor growth modeling. Cancer Inf. **14**(Suppl 4), 67–81 (2015)

4. Araujo, R.P., McElwain, D.S.: A history of the study of solid tumour growth: the contribution of mathematical modelling. Bull. Math. Biol. **66**(5), 1039–1091 (2004)

5. Sieburg, H.B.: Physiological studies in silico. Stud. Sci. Complex. **12**(2), 321–342 (1990)

6. Jordan, M.I., Mitchell, T.M.: Machine learning: trends, perspectives, and prospects. Science **349**(6245), 255–260 (2015)

7. Holzinger, A.: Interactive machine learning for health informatics: when do we need the human-in-the-loop? Brain Inf. (BRIN) **3**(2), 119–131 (2016)

8. Holzinger, A., Plass, M., Holzinger, K., Crişan, G.C., Pintea, C.-M., Palade, V.: Towards interactive machine learning (iML): applying ant colony algorithms to solve the traveling salesman problem with the human-in-the-loop approach. In: Buccafurri, F., Holzinger, A., Kieseberg, P., Tjoa, A.M., Weippl, E. (eds.) CD-ARES 2016. LNCS, vol. 9817, pp. 81–95. Springer, Heidelberg (2016). doi:10.1007/978-3-319-45507-5_6

9. Wang, Z., Butner, J., Kerketta, R., Cristini, V., Deisboeck, T.: Simulating cancer growth with multiscale agent-based modeling. Semin. Cancer Biol. **30**, 70–78 (2015)

10. Szabó, A., Merks, R.M.: Cellular potts modeling of tumor growth, tumor invasion, and tumor evolution. Front. Oncol. **3**, 87 (2013)

11. Von Neumann, J.: The general and logical theory of automata. Cereb. Mech. Behav. **1**(41), 1–2 (1951)

12. Neumann, J.V., Burks, A.W.: Theory of self-reproducing automata (1966)

13. Ulam, S.: Some ideas and prospects in biomathematics. Ann. Rev. Biophys. Bioeng. **1**(1), 277–292 (1972)

14. Cortes, C., Vapnik, V.: Support-vector networks. Mach. Learn. **20**(3), 273–297 (1995)

15. Vapnik, V.: The Nature of Statistical Learning Theory. Springer, New York (2000). doi:10.1007/978-1-4757-3264-1

16. Mantas, J.: Electronic health record. Stud. Health Technol. Inf. **65**, 250–257 (2002)

17. Waugh, D.F.: Protein-protein interactions. Adv. Protein Chem. **9**, 325–437 (1954)

18. Pawson, T., Nash, P.: Protein-protein interactions define specificity in signal transduction. Genes Dev. **14**, 1027–1047 (2000)

19. Przulj, N., Wigle, D., Jurisica, I.: Functional topology in a network of protein interactions. Bioinformatics **20**(3), 340–348 (2004)

20. Jeanquartier, F., Jean-Quartier, C., Holzinger, A.: Integrated web visualizations for protein-protein interaction databases. BMC Bioinf. **16**, 195 (2015)

21. Wagoner, J.K.: Occupational carcinogenesis: the two hundred years since percivall pott. Ann. N. Y. Acad. Sci. **271**(1), 1–4 (1976)

22. Trisilowati, Mallet, D.G.: In silico experimental modeling of cancer treatment. ISRN Oncol. **2012**, 828701 (2012)

23. Kotlyar, M., Pastrello, C., Pivetta, F., Sardo, A.L., Cumbaa, C., Li, H., Naranian, T., Niu, Y., Ding, Z., Vafaee, F., et al.: In silico prediction of physical protein interactions and characterization of interactome orphans. Nat. Methods **12**(1), 79–84 (2015)

24. Snell, E.H., Lauricella, A.M., Potter, S.A., Luft, J.R., Gulde, S.M., Collins, R.J., Franks, G., Malkowski, M.G., Cumbaa, C., Jurisica, I., et al.: Establishing a training set through the visual analysis of crystallization trials. Part II: crystal examples. Acta Crystallogr. Sect. D: Biol. Crystallogr. **64**(11), 1131–1137 (2008)
25. Jeanquartier, F., Jean-Quartier, C., Cemernek, D., Holzinger, A.: In silico modeling for tumor growth visualization. BMC Syst. Biol. **10**(1), 1 (2016)
26. Jeanquartier, F., Jean-Quartier, C., Schreck, T., Cemernek, D., Holzinger, A.: Integrating open data on cancer in support to tumor growth analysis. In: Renda, M.E., Bursa, M., Holzinger, A., Khuri, S. (eds.) ITBAM 2016. LNCS, vol. 9832, pp. 49–66. Springer, Heidelberg (2016). doi:10.1007/978-3-319-43949-5_4
27. Edelman, L.B., Eddy, J.A., Price, N.D.: In silico models of cancer. Wiley Interdisc. Rev. Syst. Biol. Med. **2**(4), 438–459 (2010)
28. Russell, S., Norvig, P.: Artificial Intelligence. Prentice-Hall, Englewood Cliffs (1995)
29. Macal, C.M., North, M.J.: Tutorial on agent-based modelling and simulation. J. Simul. **4**(3), 151–162 (2010)
30. Bonabeau, E.: Agent-based modeling: methods and techniques for simulating human systems. Proc. Nat. Acad. Sci. **99**(suppl 3), 7280–7287 (2002)
31. Starruß, J., de Back, W., Brusch, L., Deutsch, A.: Morpheus: a user-friendly modeling environment for multiscale and multicellular systems biology. Bioinformatics **30**(9), 1331–1332 (2014)
32. Benzekry, S., Lamont, C., Beheshti, A., Tracz, A., Ebos, J.M., Hlatky, L., Hahnfeldt, P.: Classical mathematical models for description and prediction of experimental tumor growth. PLoS Comput. Biol. **10**(8), e1003800 (2014)
33. Laird, A.K.: Dynamics of tumour growth. Br. J. Cancer **18**, 490–502 (1964)
34. Loeb, L.: Tissue growth and tumor growth. J. Cancer Res. **2**, 135 (1917)
35. Gocka, E.F., Reed, L.J.: A method of fitting non-symmetric gompertz functions for characterising malignant growth. Int. J. Biomed. Comput. **8**, 247–254 (1977)
36. Glazier, F., Glazier, J.A.: Simulation of biological cell sorting using a two-dimensional extended potts model. Phys. Rev. Lett. **69**(13), 2013–2016 (1992)
37. Gardner, M.: Mathematical games: the fantastic combinations of John Conway's new solitaire game "life". Sci. Am. **223**(4), 120–123 (1970)
38. Wolfram, S.: Statistical mechanics of cellular automata. Rev. Modern Phys. **55**(3), 601 (1983)
39. Qi, A.S., Zheng, X., Du, C.Y., An, B.S.: A cellular automaton model of cancerous growth. J. Theor. Biol. **161**(1), 1–12 (1993)
40. Smolle, J., Stettner, H.: Computer simulation of tumour cell invasion by a stochastic growth model. J. Theor. Biol. **160**(1), 63–72 (1993)
41. Smolle, J.: Cellular automaton simulation of tumour growth-equivocal relationships between simulation parameters and morphologic pattern features. Anal. Cellular Pathol. **17**(2), 71–82 (1998)
42. Kansal, A.R., Torquato, S., Harsh, G., Chiocca, E., Deisboeck, T.: Simulated brain tumor growth dynamics using a three-dimensional cellular automaton. J. Theor. Biol. **203**(4), 367–382 (2000)
43. Patel, A.A., Gawlinski, E.T., Lemieux, S.K., Gatenby, R.A.: A cellular automaton model of early tumor growth and invasion: the effects of native tissue vascularity and increased anaerobic tumor metabolism. J. Theor. Biol. **213**(3), 315–331 (2001)

44. Alarcón, T., Byrne, H.M., Maini, P.K.: A cellular automaton model for tumour growth in inhomogeneous environment. J. Theor. Biol. **225**(2), 257–274 (2003)

45. Gerlee, P., Anderson, A.R.: An evolutionary hybrid cellular automaton model of solid tumour growth. J. Theor. Biol. **246**(4), 583–603 (2007)

46. Brutovsky, B., Horvath, D., Lisy, V.: Inverse geometric approach for the simulation of close-to-circular growth. The case of multicellular tumor spheroids. Phys. A Stat. Mech. Appl. **387**(4), 839–850 (2008)

47. Chaplain, M., Anderson, A.: Mathematical modelling, simulation and prediction of tumour-induced angiogenesis. Invasion Metastasis **16**(4–5), 222–234 (1995)

48. Anderson, A.R., Chaplain, M.: Continuous and discrete mathematical models of tumor-induced angiogenesis. Bull. Math. Biol. **60**(5), 857–899 (1998)

49. Markus, M., Böhm, D., Schmick, M.: Simulation of vessel morphogenesis using cellular automata. Math. Biosci. **156**(1), 191–206 (1999)

50. de Pillis, L.G., Mallet, D.G., Radunskaya, A.E.: Spatial tumor-immune modeling. Comput. Math. Methods Med. **7**(2–3), 159–176 (2006)

51. Mallet, D.G., De Pillis, L.G.: A cellular automata model of tumor-immune system interactions. J. Theor. Biol. **239**(3), 334–350 (2006)

52. Vidyasagar, M.: Machine learning methods in the computational biology of cancer, vol. 470. The Royal Society (2014)

53. Cruz, J.A., Wishart, D.S.: Applications of machine learning in cancer prediction and prognosis. Cancer Inf. **2**, 59–77 (2006)

54. Madhukar, N.S., Elemento, O., Pandey, G.: Prediction of genetic interactions using machine learning and network properties. Front. Bioeng. Biotechnol. **3**, 172 (2015)

55. Lisboa, P.J., Vellido Alcacena, A., Tagliaferri, R., Napolitano, F., Ceccarelli, M., Martín Guerrero, J.D., Biganzoli, E.: Data mining in cancer research. IEEE Comput. Intell. Magaz. **5**(1), 14–18 (2010)

56. Vellido, A., Biganzoli, E., Lisboa, P.J.: Machine learning in cancer research: implications for personalised medicine. In: ESANN, pp. 55–64 (2008)

57. Upstill-Goddard, R., Eccles, D., Fliege, J., Collins, A.: Machine learning approaches for the discovery of gene-gene interactions in disease data. Brief. Bioinf. **14**(2), 251–260 (2013)

58. Larrañaga, P., Calvo, B., Santana, R., Bielza, C., Galdiano, J., Inza, I., Lozano, J.A., Armañanzas, R., Santafé, G., Pérez, A., et al.: Machine learning in bioinformatics. Brief. Bioinf. **7**(1), 86–112 (2006)

59. Kourou, K., Exarchos, T.P., Exarchos, K.P., Karamouzis, M.V., Fotiadis, D.I.: Machine learning applications in cancer prognosis and prediction. Comput. Struct. Biotechnol. J. **13**, 8–17 (2014)

60. Hu, X., Cammann, H., Meyer, H.A., Miller, K., Jung, K., Stephans, C.: Artificial neural networks and prostate cancer-tools for diagnosis and management. Nat. Rev. Urol. **10**, 174–182 (2013)

61. Eckel, S.P., Baumbach, J., Hauschild, A.C.: On the importance of statistics in breath analysis-hope or curse? J. Breath Res. **8**(1), 012001 (2014)

62. Morris, M., Greiner, R., Sander, J., Murtha, A., Schmidt, M.: Learning a classification-based glioma growth model using MRI data. J. Comput. **1**(7), 21–31 (2006)

63. González-Vélez, H., Mier, M., Julià-Sapé, M., Arvanitis, T.N., García-Gómez, J.M., Robles, M., Lewis, P.H., Dasmahapatra, S., Dupplaw, D., Peet, A., et al.: Healthagents: distributed multi-agent brain tumor diagnosis and prognosis. Appl. Intell. **30**(3), 191–202 (2009)

64. Parmar, C., Grossmann, P., Bussink, J., Lambin, P., Aerts, H.J.: Machine learning methods for quantitative radiomic biomarkers. Sci. Rep. **5**, 13087 (2015)
65. Kherlopian, A.R., Song, T., Duan, Q., Neimark, M.A., Po, M.J., Gohagan, J.K., Laine, A.F.: A review of imaging techniques for systems biology. BMC Syst. Biol. **2**, 74 (2008)
66. Buchen, L.: Cancer: missing the mark. Nature **471**(7339), 428–432 (2011)
67. Wang, J., Zuo, Y., Man, Y., Avital, I., Stojadinovic, A., Liu, M., Yang, X., Varghese, R.S., Tadesse, M.G., Ressom, H.W.: Pathway and network approaches for identification of cancer signature markers from omics data. J. Cancer **6**(1), 54–65 (2015)
68. Chuang, H.Y., Lee, E., Liu, Y.T., Lee, D., Ideker, T.: Network-based classification of breast cancer metastasis. Mol. Syst. Biol. **3**, 140 (2007)
69. Liu, N., Liu, X., Zhou, N., Wu, Q., Zhou, L., Li, Q.: Gene expression profiling and bioinformatics analysis of gastric carcinoma. Exp. Mol. Pathol. **96**(3), 361–366 (2014)
70. Wong, Y.H., Chen, R.H., Chen, B.S.: Core and specific network markers of carcinogenesis from multiple cancer samples. J. Theor. Biol. **362**, 17–34 (2014)
71. Sanz-Pamplona, R., Aragüés, R., Driouch, K., Martín, B., Oliva, B., Gil, M., Boluda, S., Fernández, P.L., Martínez, A., Moreno, V., Acebes, J.J., Lidereau, R., Reyal, F., Van de Vijver, M.J., Sierra, A.: Expression of endoplasmic reticulum stress proteins is a candidate marker of brain metastasis in both ErbB-2+ and ErbB-2- primary breast tumors. Am. J. Pathol. **179**(2), 564–579 (2011)
72. Wang, Y.C., et al.: A network-based biomarker approach for molecular investigation and diagnosis of lung cancer. BMC Med. Genom. **4**(1), 2 (2011)
73. Luo, T., Wu, S., Shen, X., Li, L.: Network cluster analysis of protein-protein interaction network identified biomarker for early onset colorectal cancer. Mol. Biol. Rep. **40**(12), 6561–6568 (2013)
74. Schramm, S.J., Li, S.S., Jayaswal, V., Fung, D.C.Y., Campain, A.E., Pang, C.N.I., Scolyer, R.A., Yang, Y.H., Mann, G.J., Wilkins, M.R.: Disturbed protein-protein interaction networks in metastatic melanoma are associated with worse prognosis and increased functional mutation burden. Pigment Cell Melanoma Res. **26**(5), 708–722 (2013)
75. Zhang, Y., Yang, C., Wang, S., Chen, T., Li, M., Wang, X., Li, D., Wang, K., Ma, J., Wu, S., Zhang, X., Zhu, Y., Wu, J., He, F.: Liveratlas: a unique integrated knowledge database for systems-level research of liver and hepatic disease. Liver Int. Off. J. Int. Assoc. Study Liver **33**(8), 1239–1248 (2013)
76. Ahn, J., Yoon, Y., Yeu, Y., Lee, H., Park, S.: Impact of TGF-b on breast cancer from a quantitative proteomic analysis. Comput. Biol. Med. **43**(12), 2096–2102 (2013)
77. Oh, J.H., Deasy, J.O.: A literature mining-based approach for identification of cellular pathways associated with chemoresistance in cancer. Brief. Bioinf. **17**(3), 468–478 (2016)
78. Majewski, I.J., Bernards, R.: Taming the dragon: genomic biomarkers to individualize the treatment of cancer. Nat. Med. **17**(3), 304–312 (2011)
79. Li, A., Walling, J., Ahn, S., Kotliarov, Y., Su, Q., Quezado, M., Oberholtzer, J.C., Park, J., Zenklusen, J.C., Fine, H.A.: Unsupervised analysis of transcriptomic profiles reveals six glioma subtypes. Cancer Res. **69**(5), 2091–2099 (2009)
80. Ceccarelli, M., Barthel, F.P., Malta, T.M., Sabedot, T.S., Salama, S.R., Murray, B.A., Morozova, O., Newton, Y., Radenbaugh, A., Pagnotta, S.M., et al.: Molecular profiling reveals biologically discrete subsets and pathways of progression in diffuse glioma. Cell **164**(3), 550–563 (2016)

81. Lalonde, E., Ishkanian, A.S., Sykes, J., Fraser, M., Ross-Adams, H., Erho, N., Dunning, M.J., Halim, S., Lamb, A.D., Moon, N.C., et al.: Tumour genomic and microenvironmental heterogeneity for integrated prediction of 5-year biochemical recurrence of prostate cancer: a retrospective cohort study. Lancet Oncol. **15**(13), 1521–1532 (2014)

82. Mungall, C.J., Washington, N.L., Nguyen-Xuan, J., Condit, C., Smedley, D., Köhler, S., Groza, T., Shefchek, K., Hochheiser, H., Robinson, P.N., et al.: Use of model organism and disease databases to support matchmaking for human disease gene discovery. Hum. Mutat. **36**(10), 979–984 (2015)

83. Clarke, C., Madden, S.F., Doolan, P., Aherne, S.T., Joyce, H., O'Driscoll, L., Gallagher, W.M., Hennessy, B.T., Moriarty, M., Crown, J., Kennedy, S., Clynes, M.: Correlating transcriptional networks to breast cancer survival: a large-scale coexpression analysis. Carcinogenesis **34**(10), 2300–2308 (2013)

84. Yang, Y., et al.: Gene co-expression network analysis reveals common system-level properties of prognostic genes across cancer types. Nat. Commun. **5**, 262–272 (2014)

85. Liu, R., Lv, Q.L., Yu, J., Hu, L., Zhang, L.H., Cheng, Y., Zhou, H.H.: Correlating transcriptional networks with pathological complete response following neoadjuvant chemotherapy for breast cancer. Breast Cancer Res. Treat. **151**(3), 607–618 (2015)

86. Yeh, H.Y., et al.: Identifying significant genetic regulatory networks in the prostate cancer from microarray data based on transcription factor analysis and conditional independency. BMC Med. Genom. **2**(1), 70 (2009)

87. Remo, A., et al.: Systems biology analysis reveals NFAT5 as a novel biomarker and master regulator of inflammatory breast cancer. J. Trans. Med. **13**(1), 138 (2015)

88. Akutekwe, A., Seker, H.: Inference of nonlinear gene regulatory networks through optimized ensemble of support vector regression and dynamic Bayesian networks. In: Conference Proceedings: Annual International Conference of the IEEE Engineering in Medicine and Biology Society. IEEE Engineering in Medicine and Biology Society. Annual Conference 2015, pp. 8177–8180 (2015)

89. Jörnsten, R., Abenius, T., Kling, T., Schmidt, L., Johansson, E., Nordling, T.E.M., Nordlander, B., Sander, C., Gennemark, P., Funa, K., Nilsson, B., Lindahl, L., Nelander, S.: Network modeling of the transcriptional effects of copy number aberrations in glioblastoma. Mol. Syst. Biol. **7**, 486 (2011)

90. Shi, X., Zhao, Q., Huang, J., Xie, Y., Ma, S.: Deciphering the associations between gene expression and copy number alteration using a sparse double Laplacian shrinkage approach. Bioinformatics (Oxford, England) **31**(24), 3977–3983 (2015)

91. Leung, A., Bader, G.D., Reimand, J.: HyperModules: identifying clinically and phenotypically significant network modules with disease mutations for biomarker discovery. Bioinformatics **30**(15), 2230–2232 (2014)

92. Wong, S.W., Cercone, N., Jurisica, I.: Comparative network analysis via differential graphlet communities. Proteomics **15**(2–3), 608–617 (2015)

93. Leung, M.K., Delong, A., Alipanahi, B., Frey, B.J.: Machine learning in genomic medicine: a review of computational problems and data sets. Proc. IEEE **104**(1), 176–197 (2016)

94. Shivade, C., Raghavan, P., Fosler-Lussier, E., Embi, P.J., Elhadad, N., Johnson, S.B., Lai, A.M.: A review of approaches to identifying patient phenotype cohorts using electronic health records. J. Am. Med. Inf. Assoc. **21**(2), 221–230 (2014)

95. Hochheiser, H., Castine, M., Harris, D., Savova, G., Jacobson, R.S.: An information model for computable cancer phenotypes. BMC Med. Inf. Decis. Making **16**(1), 121 (2016)

96. Delen, D., Walker, G., Kadam, A.: Predicting breast cancer survivability: a comparison of three data mining methods. Artif. Intell. Med. **34**(2), 113–127 (2005)

97. Siegel, R.L., Miller, K.D., Jemal, A.: Cancer statistics, 2016. CA Cancer J. Clin. **66**(1), 7–30 (2016)

98. Menden, M.P., Iorio, F., Garnett, M., McDermott, U., Benes, C.H., Ballester, P.J., Saez-Rodriguez, J.: Machine learning prediction of cancer cell sensitivity to drugs based on genomic and chemical properties. PLoS one **8**(4), e61318 (2013)

99. Gupta, S., Tran, T., Luo, W., Phung, D., Kennedy, R.L., Broad, A., Campbell, D., Kipp, D., Singh, M., Khasraw, M., et al.: Machine-learning prediction of cancer survival: a retrospective study using electronic administrative records and a cancer registry. BMJ Open **4**(3), e004007 (2014)

100. Zhao, D., Weng, C.: Combining pubmed knowledge and EHR data to develop a weighted bayesian network for pancreatic cancer prediction. J. Biomed. Inf. **44**(5), 859–868 (2011)

101. Shanmugasundaram, P., Viswanath, V., Sankar, A., Ravichandiran, V.: Metabolomics: a cancer diagnostic tool. J. Pharm. Res. **5**(12), 5210 (2012)

102. Handa, H., Usuba, A., Maddula, S., Baumbach, J.I., Mineshita, M., Miyazawa, T.: Exhaled breath analysis for lung cancer detection using ion mobility spectrometry. PLoS one **9**(12), e114555 (2014)

103. Cairns, R.A., Harris, I.S., Mak, T.W.: Regulation of cancer cell metabolism. Nat. Rev. Cancer **11**(2), 85–95 (2011)

104. O'Shea, K., Cameron, S.J., Lewis, K.E., Lu, C., Mur, L.A.: Metabolomic-based biomarker discovery for non-invasive lung cancer screening: a case study. Biochimica et Biophysica Acta **1860**(11, Part B), 2682–2687 (2016). Systems Genetics - Deciphering the Complex Disease with a Systems Approach

105. Gaul, D.A., Mezencev, R., Long, T.Q., Jones, C.M., Benigno, B.B., Gray, A., Fernández, F.M., McDonald, J.F.: Highly-accurate metabolomic detection of early-stage ovarian cancer. Sci. Rep. **5**, 16531 (2015)

106. Hauschild, A.C., Baumbach, J.I., Baumbach, J.: Integrated statistical learning of metabolic ion mobility spectrometry profiles for pulmonary disease identification. Genet. Mol. Res. **11**(3), 2733–2744 (2012)

107. Brunelli, L., Caiola, E., Marabese, M., Broggini, M., Pastorelli, R.: Comparative metabolomics profiling of isogenic KRAS wild type and mutant NSCLC cells in vitro and in vivo. Sci. Rep. **6** (2016). doi:10.1038/srep28398. Nature Publishing Group

108. Bertini, I., Cacciatore, S., Jensen, B.V., Schou, J.V., Johansen, J.S., Kruhøffer, M., Luchinat, C., Nielsen, D.L., Turano, P.: Metabolomic NMR fingerprinting to identify and predict survival of patients with metastatic colorectal cancer. Cancer Res. **72**(1), 356–364 (2012)

109. Wei, S., Liu, L., Zhang, J., Bowers, J., Gowda, G.N., Seeger, H., Fehm, T., Neubauer, H.J., Vogel, U., Clare, S.E., Raftery, D.: Metabolomics approach for predicting response to neoadjuvant chemotherapy for breast cancer. Mol. Oncol. **7**(3), 297–307 (2013)

110. Jean-Quartier, C., Jeanquartier, F., Cemernek, D., Holzinger, A.: Tumor growth simulation profiling. In: Renda, M.E., Bursa, M., Holzinger, A., Khuri, S. (eds.) ITBAM 2016. LNCS, vol. 9832, pp. 208–213. Springer, Heidelberg (2016). doi:10. 1007/978-3-319-43949-5_16

111. Koch, L.: Genetic screen: a network to guide precision cancer therapy. Nat. Rev. Genet. **17**, 504–505 (2016)
112. Kotlyar, M., Fortney, F., Jurisica, I.: Network-based characterization of drug-regulated genes, drug targets, and toxicity. Methods **57**(4), 477–485 (2012)
113. Fortney, K., Griesman, G., Kotlyar, M., Pastrello, C., Angeli, M., Tsao, M.S., Jurisica, I.: Prioritizing therapeutics for lung cancer: an integrative meta-analysis of cancer gene signatures and chemogenomic data. PLoS Comp. Biol. **11**(3), e1004068 (2015)
114. Sacha, D., Sedlmair, M., Zhang, L., Lee, J.A., Weiskopf, D., North, S., Keim, D.: Human-centered machine learning through interactive visualization: review and open challenges. In: Proceedings of the 24th European Symposium on Artificial Neural Networks, Computational Intelligence and Machine Learning (2016)
115. Kornhauser, D., Wilensky, U., Rand, W.: Design guidelines for agent based model visualization. J. Artif. Soc. Soc. Simul. **12**(2), 1 (2009)
116. Savas, S., Geraci, J., Jurisica, I., Liu, G.: A comprehensive catalogue of functional genetic variations in the EGFR pathway: protein-protein interaction analysis reveals novel genes and polymorphisms important for cancer research. Int. J. Cancer **125**(6), 1257–1265 (2009)
117. Rodriguez-Brenes, I.A., Komarova, N.L., Wodarz, D.: Tumor growth dynamics: insights into evolutionary processes. Trends Ecol. Evol. **28**(10), 597–604 (2013)
118. Blair, R.H., Trichler, D.L., Gaille, D.P.: Mathematical and statistical modeling in cancer systems biology. Front. Physiol. **3**, 227 (2012). doi:10.3389/fphys.2012.00227. Frontiers Research Foundation
119. Holzinger, A.: Biomedical Informatics: Discovering Knowledge in Big Data. Springer, New York (2014)
120. Holzinger, A., Dehmer, M., Jurisica, I.: Knowledge discovery and interactive data mining in bioinformatics - state-of-the-art, future challenges and research directions. BMC Bioinf. **15**(Suppl 6), I1 (2014)
121. Sturm, W., Schreck, T., Holzinger, A., Ullrich, T.: Discovering medical knowledge using visual analytics: a survey on methods for systems biology and *-omics data. In: Proceedings of the Eurographics Workshop on Visual Computing for Biology and Medicine, pp. 71–81. Eurographics Association (2015)
122. Turkay, C., Jeanquartier, F., Holzinger, A., Hauser, H.: On computationally-enhanced visual analysis of heterogeneous data and its application in biomedical informatics. In: Holzinger, A., Jurisica, I. (eds.) Interactive Knowledge Discovery and Data Mining in Biomedical Informatics: State-of-the-Art and Future Challenges, vol. 8401, pp. 117–140. Springer, Heidelberg (2014)
123. Otasek, D., Pastrello, C., Holzinger, A., Jurisica, I.: Visual data mining: effective exploration of the biological universe. In: Holzinger, A., Jurisica, I. (eds.) Interactive Knowledge Discovery and Data Mining in Biomedical Informatics: State-of-the-Art and Future Challenges. LNCS, vol. 8401, pp. 19–33. Springer, Heidelberg (2014)
124. Pastrello, C., Pasini, E., Kotlyar, M., Otasek, D., Wong, S., Sangrar, W., Rahmati, S., Jurisica, I.: Integration, visualization and analysis of human interactome. Biochem. Biophys. Res. Commun. **445**(4), 757–773 (2014)

A Tutorial on Machine Learning and Data Science Tools with Python

Marcus D. Bloice[✉] and Andreas Holzinger

Holzinger Group HCI-KDD, Institute for Medical Informatics,
Statistics and Documentation, Medical University of Graz, Graz, Austria
{marcus.bloice,andreas.holzinger}@medunigraz.at

Abstract. In this tutorial, we will provide an introduction to the main
Python software tools used for applying machine learning techniques to
medical data. The focus will be on open-source software that is freely
available and is cross platform. To aid the learning experience, a companion GitHub repository is available so that you can follow the examples
contained in this paper interactively using Jupyter notebooks. The notebooks will be more exhaustive than what is contained in this chapter,
and will focus on medical datasets and healthcare problems. Briefly, this
tutorial will first introduce Python as a language, and then describe some
of the lower level, general matrix and data structure packages that are
popular in the machine learning and data science communities, such as
NumPy and Pandas. From there, we will move to dedicated machine
learning software, such as SciKit-Learn. Finally we will introduce the
Keras deep learning and neural networks library. The emphasis of this
paper is readability, with as little jargon used as possible. No previous
experience with machine learning is assumed. We will use openly available medical datasets throughout.

Keywords: Machine learning · Deep learning · Neural networks ·
Tools · Languages · Python

1 Introduction

The target audience for this tutorial paper are those who wish to quickly get
started in the area of data science and machine learning. We will provide an
overview of the current and most popular libraries with a focus on Python,
however we will mention alternatives in other languages where appropriate. All
tools presented here are free and open source, and many are licensed under very
flexible terms (including, for example, commercial use). Each library will be
introduced, code will be shown, and typical use cases will be described. Medical
datasets will be used to demonstrate several of the algorithms.

Machine learning itself is a fast growing technical field [1] and is highly relevant topic in both academia and in the industry. It is therefore a relevant skill to
have in both academia and in the private sector. It is a field at the intersection
of informatics and statistics, tightly connected with data science and knowledge

© Springer International Publishing AG 2016
A. Holzinger (Ed.): ML for Health Informatics, LNAI 9605, pp. 435–480, 2016.
DOI: 10.1007/978-3-319-50478-0_22

discovery [2,3]. The prerequisites for this tutorial are therefore a basic understanding of statistics, as well as some experience in any C-style language. Some
knowledge of Python is useful but not a must.

An accompanying GitHub repository is provided to aid the tutorial:

https://github.com/mdbloice/MLDS

It contains a number of notebooks, one for each main section. The notebooks
will be referred to where relevant.

2   Glossary and Key Terms

This section provides a quick reference for several algorithms that are not explic-
ity mentioned in this chapter, but may be of interest to the reader. This should
provide the reader with some keywords or useful points of reference for other
similar libraries to those discussed in this chapter.

BIDMach GPU accelerated machine learning library for algorithms that are
not necessarily neural network based.

Caret provides a standardised API for many of the most useful machine learning packages for R. See http://topepo.github.io/caret/index.html. For readers who are more comfortable with R, Caret provides a good substitute for
Python's SciKit-Learn.

Mathematica is a commercial symbolic mathematical computation system,
developed since 1988 by Wolfram, Inc. It provides powerful machine learning
techniques "out of the box" such as image classification [4].

MATLAB is short for MATrix LABoratory, which is a commercial numerical computing environment, and is a proprietary programming language by
MathWorks. It is very popular at universities where it is often licensed. It was
originally built on the idea that most computing applications in some way
rely on storage and manipulations of one fundamental object—the matrix,
and this is still a popular approach [5].

R is used extensively by the statistics community. The software package Caret
provides a standardised API for many of R's machine learning libraries.

WEKA is short for the Waikato Environment for Knowledge Analysis [6] and
has been a very popular open source tool since its inception in 1993. In 2005
Weka received the SIGKDD Data Mining and Knowledge Discovery Service
Award: it is easy to learn and simple to use, and provides a GUI to many
machine learning algorithms [7].

Vowpal Wabbit Microsoft's machine learning library. Mature and actively
developed, with an emphasis on performance.

3   Requirements and Installation

The most convenient way of installing the Python requirements for this tutorial
is by using the Anaconda scientific Python distribution. Anaconda is a collection

of the most commonly used Python packages preconfigured and ready to use. Approximately 150 scientific packages are included in the Anaconda installation.

To install Anaconda, visit

https://www.continuum.io/downloads

and install the version of Anaconda for your operating system.

All Python software described here is available for Windows, Linux, and Macintosh. All code samples presented in this tutorial were tested under Ubuntu Linux 14.04 using Python 2.7. Some code examples may not work on Windows without slight modification (e.g. file paths in Windows use \ and not / as in UNIX type systems).

The main software used in a typical Python machine learning pipeline can consist of almost any combination of the following tools:

1. NumPy, for matrix and vector manipulation
2. Pandas for time series and R-like DataFrame data structures
3. The 2D plotting library matplotlib
4. SciKit-Learn as a source for many machine learning algorithms and utilities
5. Keras for neural networks and deep learning

Each will be covered in this book chapter.

3.1 Managing Packages

Anaconda comes with its own built in package manager, known as Conda. Using the `conda` command from the terminal, you can download, update, and delete Python packages. Conda takes care of all dependencies and ensures that packages are preconfigured to work with all other packages you may have installed.

First, ensure you have installed Anaconda, as per the instructions under https://www.continuum.io/downloads.

Keeping your Python distribution up to date and well maintained is essential in this fast moving field. However, Anaconda makes it particularly easy to manage and keep your scientific stack up to date. Once Anaconda is installed you can manage your Python distribution, and all the scientific packages installed by Anaconda using the `conda` application from the command line. To list all packages currently installed, use `conda list`. This will output all packages and their version numbers. Updating all Anaconda packages in your system is performed using the `conda update -all` command. Conda itself can be updated using the `conda update conda` command, while Python can be updated using the `conda update python` command. To search for packages, use the `search` parameter, e.g. `conda search stats` where `stats` is the name or partial name of the package you are searching for.

4 Interactive Development Environments

4.1 IPython

IPython is a REPL that is commonly used for Python development. It is included in the Anaconda distribution. To start IPython, run:

```
1 $ ipython
```

Listing 1. Starting IPython

Some informational data will be displayed, similar to what is seen in Fig. 1, and you will then be presented with a command prompt.

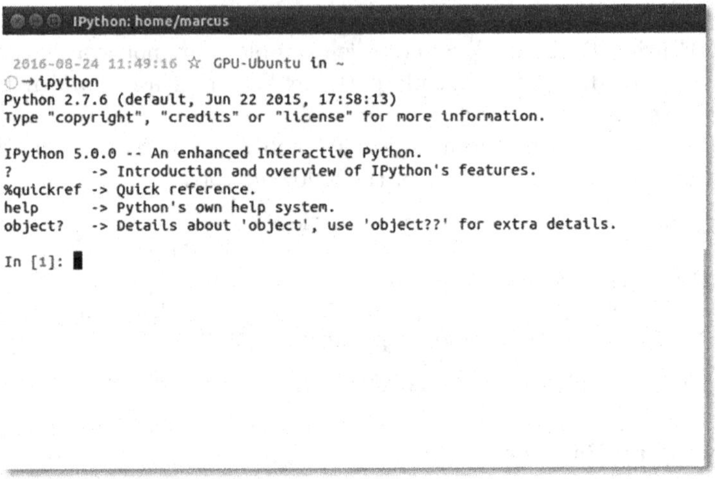

```
⊙ ⊙ ⊙   IPython: home/marcus

 2016-08-24 11:49:16 ☆ GPU-Ubuntu in ~
 ○→ ipython
 Python 2.7.6 (default, Jun 22 2015, 17:58:13)
 Type "copyright", "credits" or "license" for more information.

 IPython 5.0.0 -- An enhanced Interactive Python.
 ?          -> Introduction and overview of IPython's features.
 %quickref -> Quick reference.
 help       -> Python's own help system.
 object?    -> Details about 'object', use 'object??' for extra details.

 In [1]: ▮
```

Fig. 1. The IPython Shell.

IPython is what is known as a REPL: a **R**ead **E**valuate **P**rint **L**oop. The interpreter allows you to type in commands which are evaluated as soon as you press the Enter key. Any returned output is immediately shown in the console. For example, we may type the following:

```
1 In [1]: 1 + 1
2 Out[1]: 2
3 In [2]: import math
4 In [3]: math.radians(90)
5 Out[3]: 1.5707963267948966
6 In [4]:
```

Listing 2. Examining the Read Evaluate Print Loop (REPL)

After pressing return (Line 1 in Listing 2), Python immediately interprets the line and responds with the returned result (Line 2 in Listing 2). The interpreter then awaits the next command, hence Read Evaluate Print Loop.

Using IPython to experiment with code allows you to test ideas without needing to create a file (e.g. `fibonacci.py`) and running this file from the command line (by typing `python fibonacci.py` at the command prompt). Using the IPython REPL, this entire process can be made much easier. Of course, creating permanent files is essential for larger projects.

A useful feature of IPython are the so-called magic functions. These commands are not interpreted as Python code by the REPL, instead they are special commands that IPython understands. For example, to run a Python script you can use the %run magic function:

```
>>> %run fibonacci.py 30
Fibonacci number 30 is 832040.
```

Listing 3. Using the %run magic function to execute a file.

In the code above, we have executed the Python code contained in the file fibonacci.py and passed the value 30 as an argument to the file.

The file is executed as a Python script, and its output is displayed in the shell. Other magic functions include %timeit for timing code execution:

```
>>> def fibonacci(n):
...      if n == 0: return 0
...      if n == 1: return 1
...      return fibonacci(n-1) + fibonacci(n-2)
>>> %timeit fibonacci(25)
10 loops, best of 3: 30.9 ms per loop
```

Listing 4. The %timeit magic function can be used to check execution times of functions or any other piece of code.

As can be seen, executing the fibonacci(25) function takes on average 30.9 ms. The %timeit magic function is clever in how many loops it performs to create an average result, this can be as few as 1 loop or as many as 10 million loops.

Other useful magic functions include %ls for listing files in the current working directory, %cd for printing or changing the current directory, and %cpaste for pasting in longer pieces of code that span multiple lines. A full list of magic functions can be displayed using, unsurprisingly, a magic function: type %magic to view all magic functions along with documentation for each one. A summary of useful magic functions is shown in Table 1.

Last, you can use the ? operator to display in-line help at any time. For example, typing

```
>>> abs?
Docstring:
abs(number) -> number

Return the absolute value of the argument.
Type:        builtin_function_or_method
```

Listing 5. Accessing help within the IPython console.

For larger projects, or for projects that you may want to share, IPython may not be ideal. In Sect. 4.2 we discuss the web-based notebook IDE known as Jupyter, which is more suited to larger projects or projects you might want to share.

Table 1. A non-comprehensive list of IPython magic functions.

Magic Command	Description
%lsmagic	Lists all the magic functions
%magic	Shows descriptive magic function documentation
%ls	Lists files in the current directory
%cd	Shows or changes the current directory
%who	Shows variables in scope
%whos	Shows variables in scope along with type information
%cpaste	Pastes code that spans several lines
%reset	Resets the session, removing all imports and deleting all variables
%debug	Starts a debugger *post mortem*

4.2 Jupyter

Jupyter, previously known as IPython Notebook, is a web-based, interactive development environment. Originally developed for Python, it has since expanded to support over 40 other programming languages including Julia and R.

Jupyter allows for *notebooks* to be written that contain text, live code, images, and equations. These notebooks can be shared, and can even be hosted on GitHub for free.

For each section of this tutorial, you can download a Juypter notebook that allows you to edit and experiment with the code and examples for each topic. Jupyter is part of the Anaconda distribution, it can be started from the command line using using the jupyter command:

```
$ jupyter notebook
```

Listing 6. Starting Jupyter

Upon typing this command the Jupyter server will start, and you will briefly see some information messages, including, for example, the URL and port at which the server is running (by default http://localhost:8888/). Once the server has started, it will then open your default browser and point it to this address. This browser window will display the contents of the directory where you ran the command.

To create a notebook and begin writing, click the New ▼ button and select Python. A new notebook will appear in a new tab in the browser. A Jupyter notebook allows you to run code blocks and immediately see the output of these blocks of code, much like the IPython REPL discussed in Sect. 4.1.

Jupyter has a number of short-cuts to make navigating the notebook and entering code or text quickly and easily. For a list of short-cuts, use the menu Help → Keyboard Shortcuts.

4.3 Spyder

For larger projects, often a fully fledged IDE is more useful than Juypter's notebook-based IDE. For such purposes, the Spyder IDE is often used. Spyder stands for Scientific PYthon Development EnviRonment, and is included in the Anaconda distribution. It can be started by typing `spyder` in the command line.

5 Requirements and Conventions

This tutorial makes use of a number of packages which are used extensively in the Python machine learning community. In this chapter, the NumPy, Pandas, and Matplotlib are used throughout. Therefore, for the Python code samples shown in each section, we will presume that the following packages are available and have been loaded before each script is run:

```
>>> import numpy as np
>>> import pandas as pd
>>> import matplotlib.pyplot as plt
```

Listing 7. Standard libraries used throughout this chapter. Throughout this chapter we will assume these libraries have been imported before each script.

Any further packages will be explicitly loaded in each code sample. However, in general you should probably follow each section's Jupyter notebook as you are reading.

In Python code blocks, lines that begin with $>>>$ represent Python code that should be entered into a Python interpreter (See Listing 7 for an example). Output from any Python code is shown **without** any preceding $>>>$ characters.

Commands which need to be entered into the terminal (e.g. bash or the MS-DOS command prompt) begin with $, such as:

```
$ ls −lAh
total 299K
−rw−rw−r— 1 bloice admin   73K Sep  1 14:11  Clustering.ipynb
−rw−rw−r— 1 bloice admin   57K Aug 25 16:04  Pandas.ipynb
...
```

Listing 8. Commands for the terminal are preceded by a $ sign.

Output from the console is shown **without** a preceding $ sign. Some of the commands in this chapter may only work under Linux (such as the example usage of the `ls` command in the code listing above, the equivalent in Windows is the `dir` command). Most commands will, however, work under Linux, Macintosh, and Windows—if this is not the case, we will explicitly say so.

5.1 Data

For the Introduction to Python, NumPy, and Pandas sections we will work with either generated data or with a toy dataset. Later in the chapter, we will move on to medical examples, including a breast cancer dataset, a diabetes dataset, and a high-dimensional gene expression dataset. All medical datasets used in this chapter are freely available and we will describe how to get the data in each relevant section. In earlier sections, generated data will suffice in order to demonstrate example usage, while later we will see that analysing more involved medical data using the same open-source tools is equally possible.

6   Introduction to Python

Python is a general purpose programming language that is used for anything from web-development to deep learning. According to several metrics, it is ranked as one of the top three most popular languages. It is now the most frequently taught introductory language at top U.S. universities according to a recent ACM blog article [8]. Due to its popularity, Python has a thriving open source community, and there are over 80,000 free software packages available for the language on the official Python Package Index (PyPI).

In this section we will give a very short crash course on using Python. These code samples will work best with a Python REPL interpreter, such as IPython or Jupyter (Sects. 4.1 and 4.2 respectively). In the code below we introduce the some simple arithmetic syntax:

```
>>> 2 + 6 + (8 * 9)
80
>>> 3 / 2
1
>>> 3.0 / 2
1.5
>>> 4 ** 4 # To the power of
256
```

Listing 9. Simple arithmetic with Python in the IPython shell.

Python is a dynamically typed language, so you do not define the type of variable you are creating, it is inferred:

```
>>> n = 5
>>> f = 5.5
>>> s ="5"
>>> type(s)
str
>>> type(f)
float
>>> "5" * 5
"55555"
>>> int("5") * 5
25
```

Listing 10. Demonstrating types in Python.

You can check types using the built-in **type** function. Python does away with much of the verbosity of languages such as Java, you do not even need to surround code blocks with brackets or braces:

```
1  >>> if "5" == 5:
2  ...     print("Will not get here")
3  >>> elif int("5") == 5:
4  ...     print("Got here")
5  Got here
```

Listing 11. Statement blocks in Python are indicated using indentation.

As you can see, we use indentation to define our statement blocks. This is the number one source of confusion among those new to Python, so it is important you are aware of it. Also, whereas assignment uses =, we check equality using == (and inversely !=). Control of flow is handled by if, elif, while, for, and so on.

While there are several basic data structures, here we will concentrate on lists and dictionaries (we will cover much more on data structures in Sect. 7.1). Other types of data structures are, for example, tuples, which are immutable—their contents cannot be changed after they are created—and sets, where repetition is not permitted. We will not cover tuples or sets in this tutorial chapter, however.

Below we first define a list and then perform a number of operations on this list:

```
1   >>> powers = [1, 2, 4, 8, 16, 32]
2   >>> powers
3   [1, 2, 4, 8, 16, 32]
4   >>> powers[0]
5   1
6   >>> powers.append(64)
7   >>> powers
8   [1, 2, 4, 8, 16, 32, 64]
9   >>> powers.insert(0, 0)
10  >>> powers
11  [0, 1, 2, 4, 8, 16, 32, 64]
12  >>> del powers[0]
13  >>> powers
14  [1, 2, 4, 8, 16, 32, 64]
15  >>> 1 in powers
16  True
17  >>> 100 not in powers
18  True
```

Listing 12. Operations on lists.

Lists are defined using square [] brackets. You can index a list using its numerical, zero-based index, as seen on Line 4. Adding values is performed using the **append** and **insert** functions. The **insert** function allows you to define in which position you would like the item to be inserted—on Line 9 of Listing 12 we insert the number 0 at position 0. On Lines 15 and 17, you can see how we can use the **in** keyword to check for membership.

You just saw that lists are indexed using zero-based numbering, we will now introduce dictionaries which are key-based. Data in dictionaries are stored using key-value pairs, and are indexed by the keys that you define:

```
>>> numbers = {"bingo": 3458080, "tuppy": 3459090}
>>> numbers
{"bingo": 3458080, "tuppy": 3459090}
>>> numbers["bingo"]
3458080
>>> numbers["monty"] = 3456060
>>> numbers
{"bingo": 3458080, "monty": 3456060, "tuppy": 3459090}
>>> "tuppy" in numbers
True
```

Listing 13. Dictionaries in Python.

We use curly {} braces to define dictionaries, and we must define both their values and their indices (Line 1). We can access elements of a dictionary using their keys, as in Line 4. On Line 6 we insert a new key-value pair. Notice that dictionaries are not ordered. On Line 9 we can also use the in keyword to check for membership.

To traverse through a dictionary, we use a `for` statement in conjunction with a function depending on what data we wish to access from the dictionary:

```
>>> for name, number in numbers.iteritems():
...        print("Name:" + name + ", number:" + str(number))
Name: bingo, number: 3458080
Name: monty, number: 3456060
Name: tuppy, number: 3459090

>>> for key in numbers.keys():
...        print(key)
bingo
monty
tuppy

>>> for val in numbers.values():
...        print(val)
3458080
3456060
3459090
```

Listing 14. Iterating through dictionaries.

First, the code above traverses through each key-value pair using `iteritems()` (Line 1). When doing so, you can specify a variable name for each key and value (in that order). In other words, on Line 1, we have stated that we wish to store each key in the variable **name** and each value in the variable **number** as we go through the `for` loop. You can also access only the keys or values using the **keys** and **values** functions respectively (Lines 7 and 13).

As mentioned previously, many packages are available for Python. These need to be loaded into the current environment before they are used. For example, the code below uses the `os` module, which we must first import before using:

```
 1 >>> import os
 2 >>> os.listdir("./")
 3 ["BookChapter.ipynb",
 4  "NumPy.ipynb",
 5  "Pandas.ipynb",
 6  "fibonacci.py",
 7  "LinearRegression.ipynb",
 8  "Clustering.ipynb"]
 9 >>> from os import listdir # Alternatively
10 >>> listdir("./")
11 ["BookChapter.ipynb",
12  "NumPy.ipynb",
13 ...
```

Listing 15. Importing packages using the `import` keyword.

Two ways of importing are shown here. On Line 1 we are importing the entire `os` name space. This means we need to call functions using the `os.listdir()` syntax. If you know that you only need one function or submodule you can import it individually using the method shown on Line 9. This is often the preferred method of importing in Python.

Lastly, we will briefly see how functions are defined using the `def` keyword:

```
1 >>> def addNumbers(x, y):
2 ...         return x + y
3 >>> addNumbers(4, 2)
4 6
```

Listing 16. Functions are defined using the `def` keyword.

Notice that you do not need to define the return type, or the arguments' types. Classes are equally easy to define, and this is done using the `class` keyword. We will not cover classes in this tutorial. Classes are generally arranged into modules, and further into packages. Now that we have covered some of the basics of Python, we will move on to more advanced data structures such as 2-dimensional arrays and data frames.

7 Handling Data

7.1 Data Structures and Notation

In machine learning, more often than not the data that you analyse will be stored in matrices and vectors. Generally speaking, your data that you wish to analyse will be stored in the form of a matrix, often denoted using a bold upper case symbol, generally $\mathbf{X}$, and your label data will be stored in a vector, denoted with a lower case bold symbol, often $\mathbf{y}$.

A data matrix $\mathbf{X}$ with n samples and m features is denoted as follows:

$$\mathbf{X} \in \mathbb{R}^{n \times m} = \begin{bmatrix} x_{1,1} & x_{1,2} & x_{1,3} & \cdots & x_{1,m} \\ x_{2,1} & x_{2,2} & x_{2,3} & \cdots & x_{2,m} \\ x_{3,1} & x_{3,2} & x_{3,3} & \cdots & x_{3,m} \\ \vdots & \vdots & \vdots & \ddots & \vdots \\ x_{n,1} & x_{n,2} & x_{n,3} & \cdots & x_{n,m} \end{bmatrix}$$

Each column, m, of this matrix contains the features of your data and each row, n, is a sample of your data. A single sample of your data is denoted by its subscript, e.g. $\mathbf{x}_i = [x_{i,1} \; x_{i,2} \; x_{i,3} \; \cdots \; x_{i,m}]$

In supervised learning, your labels or targets are stored in a vector:

$$\mathbf{y} \in \mathbb{R}^{n \times 1} = \begin{bmatrix} y_1 \\ y_2 \\ y_3 \\ \vdots \\ y_n \end{bmatrix}$$

Note that number of elements in the vector $\mathbf{y}$ is equal to the number of samples n in your data matrix $\mathbf{X}$, hence $\mathbf{y} \in \mathbb{R}^{n \times 1}$.

For a concrete example, let us look at the famous Iris dataset. The Iris flower dataset is a small toy dataset consisting of $n = 150$ *samples* or *observations* of three species of Iris flower (Iris setosa, Iris virginica, and Iris versicolor). Each sample, or row, has $m = 4$ *features*, which are measurements relating to that sample, such as the petal length and petal width. Therefore, the features of the Iris dataset correspond to the columns in Table 2, namely sepal length, sepal width, petal length, and petal width. Each observation or sample corresponds to one row in the table. Table 2 shows a few rows of the Iris dataset so that you can become acquainted with how it is structured. As we will be using this dataset in several sections of this chapter, take a few moments to examine it.

Table 2. The Iris flower dataset.

	Sepal length	Sepal width	Petal length	Petal width	Class
1	5.1	3.5	1.4	0.2	setosa
2	4.9	3.0	1.4	0.2	setosa
3	4.7	3.2	1.3	0.2	setosa
⋮	⋮	⋮	⋮	⋮	⋮
150	5.9	3.0	5.1	1.8	virginica

In a machine learning task, you would store this table in a matrix $\mathbf{X}$, where $\mathbf{X} \in \mathbb{R}^{150 \times 4}$. In Python $\mathbf{X}$ would therefore be stored in a 2-dimensional array with 150 rows and 4 columns (generally we will store such data in a variable named X). The 1st row in Table 2 corresponds to 1st row of **X**, namely x_1 = [5.1 3.5 1.4 0.2]. See Listing 17 for how to represent a vector as an array and a matrix as a two-dimensional array in Python. While the data is stored in a matrix **X**, the Class column in Table 2, which represents the species of plant, is stored separately in a target vector **y**. This vector contains what are known as the *targets* or *labels* of your dataset. In the Iris dataset, $\mathbf{y} = [y_1 \ y_2 \ \cdots \ y_{150}]$, $y_i \in$ {*setosa, versicolor, virginica*}. The labels can either be nominal, as is the case in the Iris dataset, or continuous. In a supervised machine learning problem, the principle aim is to **predict the label for a given sample**. If the targets are nominal, this is a classification problem. If the targets are continuous this is a regression problem. In an unsupervised machine learning task you do not have the target vector **y**, and you only have access to the dataset **X**. In such a scenario, the aim is to find patterns in the dataset **X** and cluster observations together, for example.

We will see examples of both classification algorithms and regression algorithms in this chapter as well as supervised and unsupervised problems.

```
1  >>> v1 = [5.1, 3.5, 1.4, 0.2]
2  >>> v2 = [
3  ...       [5.1, 3.5, 1.4, 0.2],
4  ...       [4.9, 3.0, 1.3, 0.2]
5  ..        ]
```

Listing 17. Creating 1-dimensional (v1) and 2-dimensional data structures (v2) in Python (Note that in Python these are called lists).

In situations where your data is split into subsets, such as a training set and a test set, you will see notation such as $\mathbf{X}_{train}$ and $\mathbf{X}_{test}$. Datasets are often split into a training set and a test set, where the training set is used to learn a model, and the test set is used to check how well the model fits to unseen data.

In a machine learning task, you will almost always be using a library known as NumPy to handle vectors and matrices. NumPy provides very useful matrix manipulation and data structure functionality and is optimised for speed. NumPy is the *de facto* standard for data input, storage, and output in the Python machine learning and data science community[1]. Another important library which is frequently used is the Pandas library for time series and tabular data structures. These packages compliment each other, and are often used side by side in a typical data science stack. We will learn the basics of NumPy and Pandas in this chapter, starting with NumPy in Sect. 7.2.

---

[1] To speed up certain numerical operations, the `numexpr` and `bottleneck` optimised libraries for Python can be installed. These are included in the Anaconda distribution, readers who are not using Anaconda are recommended to install them both.

7.2 NumPy

NumPy is a general data structures, linear algebra, and matrix manipulation library for Python. Its syntax, and how it handles data structures and matrices is comparable to that of MATLAB[2].

To use NumPy, first import it (the convention is to import it as np, to avoid having to type out numpy each time):

```
>>> import numpy as np
```

Listing 18. Importing NumPy. It is convention to import NumPy as np.

Rather than repeat this line for each code listing, we will assume you have imported NumPy, as per the instructions in Sect. 3. Any further imports that may be required for a code sample will be explicitly mentioned.

Listing 19 describes some basic usage of NumPy by first creating a NumPy array and then retrieving some of the elements of this array using a technique called *array slicing*:

```
>>> vector = np.arange(10) # Make an array from 0 - 9
>>> vector
[0, 1, 2, 3, 4, 5, 6, 7, 8, 9]
>>> vector[1]
1
>>> vector[0:3]
[0, 1, 2]
>>> vector[0:-3] # Element 0 to the 3rd last element
[0, 1, 2, 3, 4, 5, 6]
>>> vector[3:7] # From index 3 but not including 7
[3, 4, 5, 6]
```

Listing 19. Array slicing in NumPy.

In Listing 19, Line 1 we have created a vector (actually a NumPy array) with 10 elements from 0–9. On Line 2 we simply print the contents of the vector, the contents of which are shown on Line 3. Arrays in Python are 0-indexed, that means to retrieve the first element you must use the number 0. On Line 4 we retrieve the 2nd element which is 1, using the square bracket indexing syntax: array[i], where i is the index of the value you wish to retrieve from array. To retrieve subsets of arrays we use a method known as *array slicing*, a powerful technique that you will use constantly, so it is worthwhile to study its usage carefully! For example, on Line 9 we are retrieving all elements beginning with element 0 to the 3rd last element. Slicing 1D arrays takes the form array[<startpos>:<endpos>], where the start position <startpos> and end position <endpos> are separated with a: character. Line 11 shows another example of array slicing. Array slicing **includes** the element indexed by the <startpos> up to but **not including** the element indexed by <endpos>.

---

[2] Users of MATLAB may want to view this excellent guide to NumPy for MATLAB users: http://mathesaurus.sourceforge.net/matlab-numpy.html.

A very similar syntax is used for indexing 2-dimensional arrays, but now we must index first the rows we wish to retrieve followed by the columns we wish to retrieve. Some examples are shown below:

```
>>> m = np.arange(9).reshape(3,3)
>>> m
array([[0, 1, 2],
       [3, 4, 5],
       [6, 7, 8]])
>>> m[0] # Row 0
array([0, 1, 2])
>>> m[0, 1] # Row 0, column 1
1
>>> m[:, 0] # All rows, 0th column
array([0, 3, 6])
>>> m[:,:] # All rows, all columns
array([[0, 1, 2],
       [3, 4, 5],
       [6, 7, 8]])
>>> m[-2:, -2:] # Lower right corner of matrix
array([[4, 5],
       [7, 8]])
>>> m[:2, :2] # Upper left corner of matrix
array([[0, 1],
       [3, 4]])
```

Listing 20. 2D array slicing.

As can be seen, indexing 2-dimensional arrays is very similar to the 1-dimensional arrays shown previously. In the case of 2-dimensional arrays, you first specify your row indices, follow this with a comma (,) and then specify your column indices. These indices can be ranges, as with 1-dimensional arrays. See Fig. 2 for a graphical representation of a number of array slicing operations in NumPy.

With element wise operations, you can apply an operation (very efficiently) to every element of an n-dimensional array:

```
>>> m + 1
array([[1, 2, 3],
       [4, 5, 6],
       [7, 8, 9]])
>>> m**2 # Square every element
array([[ 0,  1,  4],
       [ 9, 16, 25],
       [36, 49, 64]])
>>> v * 10
array([ 10, 20, 30, 40, 50, 60, 70, 80, 90, 100])
>>> v = np.array([1, 2, 3])
>>> v
array([1, 2, 3])
>>> m + v
```

```
15  array([[ 1,   3,   5],
16         [ 4,   6,   8],
17         [ 7,   9,  11]])
18  >>> m * v
19  array([[ 0,   2,   6],
20         [ 3,   8,  15],
21         [ 6,  14,  24]])
```

Listing 21. Element wise operations and array broadcasting.

```
>>> a[0, 3:5]
array([3,4])

>>> a[4:, 4:]
array([ [44, 45],
  [54, 55]] )

>>> a[:, 2]
array([2, 12, 22, 32, 42,
52])

>>> a[2::2, ::2]
array([ [20, 22, 24],
  [40, 42, 44]] )
```

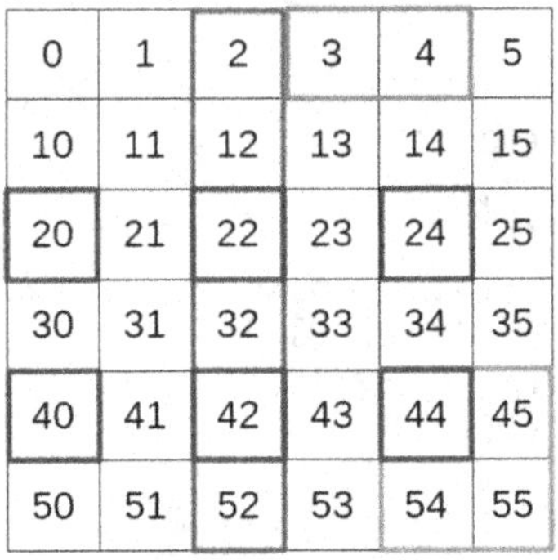

0	1	2	3	4	5
10	11	12	13	14	15
20	21	22	23	24	25
30	31	32	33	34	35
40	41	42	43	44	45
50	51	52	53	54	55

Fig. 2. Array slicing and indexing with NumPy. Image has been redrawn from the original at http://www.scipy-lectures.org/_images/numpy_indexing.png.

There are a number of things happening in Listing 21 that you should be aware of. First, in Line 1, you will see that if you apply an operation on a matrix or array, the operation will be applied *element wise* to each item in the n-dimensional array. What happens when you try to apply an operation using, let's say a vector and a matrix? On lines 14 and 18 we do exactly this. This is known as *array broadcasting*, and works when two data structures share at least one dimension size. In this case we have a 3×3 matrix and are performing an operation using a vector with 3 elements.

7.3 Pandas

Pandas is a software library for data analysis of tabular and time series data. In many ways it reproduces the functionality of R's DataFrame object. Also, many common features of Microsoft Excel can be performed using Pandas, such as "group by", table pivots, and easy column deletion and insertion.

Pandas' DataFrame objects are label-based (as opposed to index-based as is the case with NumPy), so that each column is typically given a name which can be called to perform operations. DataFrame objects are more similar to spreadsheets, and each column of a DataFrame can have a different type, such as boolean, numeric, or text. Often, it should be stressed, you will use NumPy and Pandas in conjunction. The two libraries complement each other and are not competing frameworks, although there is overlap in functionality between the two. First, we must get some data. The Python package SciKit-Learn provides some sample data that we can use (we will learn more about SciKit-Learn later). SciKit-Learn is part of the standard Anaconda distribution.

In this example, we will load some sample data into a Pandas DataFrame object, then rename the DataFrame object's columns, and lastly take a look at the first three rows contained in the DataFrame:

```
1 >>> import pandas as pd # Convention
2 >>> from sklearn import datasets
3 >>> iris = datasets.load_iris()
4 >>> df = pd.DataFrame(iris.data)
5 >>> df.columns = ["sepal_l", "sepal_w", "petal_l",
        "petal_w"]
6 >>> df.head(3)
7     sepal_l   sepal_w   petal_l   petal_w
8 0      5.1       3.5       1.4       0.2
9 1      4.9       3.0       1.4       0.2
10 2     4.7       3.2       1.3       0.2
```

Listing 22. Reading data into a Pandas DataFrame.

Selecting columns can performed using square brackets or dot notation:

```
1 >>> df["sepal_l"]
2 0      5.1
3 1      4.9
4 2      4.7
5 ...
6 >>> df.sepal_l # Alternatively
7 0      5.1
8 1      4.9
9 2      4.7
10 ...
```

Listing 23. Accessing columns using Pandas' syntax.

You can use square brackets to access individual cells of a column:

```
1 >>> df["sepal_l"][0]
2 5.1
3 >>> df.sepal_l[0] # Alternatively
4 5.1
```

Listing 24. Accessing individual cells of a DataFrame.

To insert a column, for example the species of the plant, we can use the following syntax:

```
>>> df["name"] = iris.target
>>> df.loc[df.name == 0, "name"] = "setosa"
>>> df.loc[df.name == 1, "name"] = "versicolor"
>>> df.loc[df.name == 2, "name"] = "virginica"
# Alternatively
>>> df["name"] = [iris.target_names[x] for x in iris.
    target]
```

Listing 25. Inserting a new column into a DataFrame and replacing its numerical values with text.

In Listing 25 above, we created a new column in our DataFrame called **name**. This is a numerical class label, where 0 corresponds to setosa, 1 corresponds to versicolor, and 2 corresponds to virginica. First, we add the new column on Line 1, and we then replace these numerical values with text, shown in Lines 2–4. Alternatively, we could have just done this in one go, as shown on Line 6 (this uses a more advanced technique called a list comprehension).

We use the **loc** and **iloc** keywords for selecting rows and columns, in this case the 0th row:

```
>>> df.iloc[0]
sepal_l        5.1
sepal_w        3.5
petal_l        1.4
petal_w        0.2
name        setosa
Name: 0, dtype: object
```

Listing 26. The **iloc** function is used to access items within a DataFrame by their index rather than their label.

You use **loc** for selecting with labels, and **iloc** for selecting with indices. Using **loc**, we first specify the rows, then the columns, in this case we want the first three rows of the **sepal_l** column:

```
>>> df.loc[:3, "sepal_l"]
0     5.1
1     4.9
2     4.7
3     4.6
Name: sepal_l, dtype: float64
```

Listing 27. Using the **loc** function also allows for more advanced commands.

Because we are selecting a column using a label, we use the **loc** keyword above. Here we select the first 5 rows of the DataFrame using **iloc**:

```
1  >>> df.iloc[:5]
2      sepal_l   sepal_w   petal_l   petal_w      name
3  0       5.1       3.5       1.4       0.2    setosa
4  1       4.9       3.0       1.4       0.2    setosa
5  2       4.7       3.2       1.3       0.2    setosa
6  3       4.6       3.1       1.5       0.2    setosa
7  4       5.0       3.6       1.4       0.2    setosa
8  5       5.4       3.9       1.7       0.4    setosa
```

Listing 28. Selecting the first 5 rows of the DataFrame using the `iloc` function. To select items using text labels you must use the `loc` keyword.

Or rows 15 to 20 and columns 2 to 4:

```
1  >>> df.iloc[15:21, 2:5]
2      petal_l   petal_w      name
3  15      1.5       0.4    setosa
4  16      1.3       0.4    setosa
5  17      1.4       0.3    setosa
6  18      1.7       0.3    setosa
7  19      1.5       0.3    setosa
8  20      1.7       0.2    setosa
```

Listing 29. Selecting specific rows and columns. This is done in much the same way as NumPy.

Now, we may want to quickly examine the DataFrame to view some of its properties:

```
1   >>> df.describe()
2              sepal_l         sepal_w         petal_l         petal_w
3   count   150.000000      150.000000      150.000000      150.000000
4   mean      5.843333        3.054000        3.758667        1.198667
5   std       0.828066        0.433594        1.764420        0.763161
6   min       4.300000        2.000000        1.000000        0.100000
7   25%       5.100000        2.800000        1.600000        0.300000
8   50%       5.800000        3.000000        4.350000        1.300000
9   75%       6.400000        3.300000        5.100000        1.800000
10  max       7.900000        4.400000        6.900000        2.500000
```

Listing 30. The `describe` function prints some commonly required statistics regarding the DataFrame.

You will notice that the **name** column is not included as Pandas quietly ignores this column due to the fact that the column's data cannot be analysed in the same way.

Sorting is performed using the **sort_values** function: here we sort by the sepal length, named **sepal_l** in the DataFrame:

```
>>> df.sort_values(by="sepal_l", ascending=True).head(5)
    sepal_l  sepal_w  petal_l  petal_w    name
13     4.3     3.0      1.1      0.1    setosa
42     4.4     3.2      1.3      0.2    setosa
38     4.4     3.0      1.3      0.2    setosa
8      4.4     2.9      1.4      0.2    setosa
41     4.5     2.3      1.3      0.3    setosa
```

Listing 31. Sorting a DataFrame using the `sort_values` function.

A very powerful feature of Pandas is the ability to write conditions within the square brackets:

```
>>> df[df.sepal_l > 7]
     sepal_l  sepal_w  petal_l  petal_w      name
102     7.1     3.0      5.9      2.1    virginica
105     7.6     3.0      6.6      2.1    virginica
107     7.3     2.9      6.3      1.8    virginica
109     7.2     3.6      6.1      2.5    virginica
117     7.7     3.8      6.7      2.2    virginica
118     7.7     2.6      6.9      2.3    virginica
122     7.7     2.8      6.7      2.0    virginica
125     7.2     3.2      6.0      1.8    virginica
129     7.2     3.0      5.8      1.6    virginica
130     7.4     2.8      6.1      1.9    virginica
131     7.9     3.8      6.4      2.0    virginica
135     7.7     3.0      6.1      2.3    virginica
```

Listing 32. Using a condition to select a subset of the data can be performed quickly using Pandas.

New columns can be easily inserted or removed (we saw an example of a column being inserted in Listing 25, above):

```
>>> sepal_l_w = df.sepal_l + df.sepal_w
>>> df["sepal_l_w"] = sepal_l_w # Creates a new column
>>> df.head(5)
   sepal_l  sepal_w  petal_l  petal_w    name   sepal_l_w
0    5.1     3.5      1.4      0.2    setosa      8.6
1    4.9     3.0      1.4      0.2    setosa      7.9
2    4.7     3.2      1.3      0.2    setosa      7.9
3    4.6     3.1      1.5      0.2    setosa      7.7
4    5.0     3.6      1.4      0.2    setosa      8.6
```

Listing 33. Adding and removing columns

There are few things to note here. On Line 1 of Listing 33 we use the dot notation to access the DataFrame's columns, however we could also have said `sepal_l_w = df["sepal_l"] + df["sepal_w"]` to access the data in each column. The next important thing to notice is that you can insert a new column easily by specifying a label that is new, as in Line 2 of Listing 33. You can delete a column using the `del` keyword, as in `del df["sepal_l_w"]`.

Missing data is often a problem in real world datasets. Here we will remove all cells where the value is greater than 7, replacing them with NaN (Not a Number):

```
>>> import numpy as np
>>> len(df)
150
>>> df[df > 7] = np.NaN
>>> df = df.dropna(how="any")
>>> len(df)
138
```

Listing 34. Dropping rows that contain missing data.

After replacing all values greater than 7 with NaN (Line 4), we used the `dropna` function (Line 5) to remove the 12 rows with missing values. Alternatively you may want to replace NaN values with a value with the `fillna` function, for example the mean value for that column:

```
>>> for col in df.columns:
...     df[col] = df[col].fillna(value=df[col].mean())
```

Listing 35. Replacing missing data with mean values.

As if often the case with Pandas, there are several ways to do everything, and we could have used either of the following:

```
>>> df.fillna(lambda x: x.fillna(value=x.mean())
>>> df.fillna(df.mean())
```

Listing 36. Demonstrating several ways to handle missing data.

Line 1 demonstrates the use of a lambda function: these are functions which are not declared and are a powerful feature of Python. Either of the above examples in Listing 36 are preferred to the loop shown in Listing 35. Pandas offers a number of methods for handling missing data, including advanced interpolation techniques[3].

Plotting in Pandas uses matplotlib (more on which later), where publication quality prints can be created, for example you can quickly create a scatter matrix, a frequently used plot in data exploration to find correlations:

```
>>> from pandas.tools.plotting import scatter_matrix
>>> scatter_matrix(df, diagonal="kde")
```

Listing 37. Several plotting features are built in to Pandas including scatter matrix functionality as shown here.

Which results in the scatter matrix seen in Fig. 3. You can see that Pandas is intelligent enough not to attempt to print the name column—these are known as nuisance columns and are silently, and temporarily, dropped for certain operations. The kde parameter specifies that you would like density plots

---

[3] See http://pandas.pydata.org/pandas-docs/stable/missing_data.html for more methods on handling missing data.

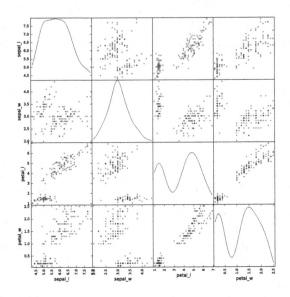

Fig. 3. Scatter matrix visualisation for the Iris dataset.

for the diagonal axis of the matrix, alternatively you can specify `hist` to plot histograms.

For many examples on how to use Pandas, refer to the SciPy Lectures website under http://www.scipy-lectures.org/. Much more on plotting and visualisation in Pandas can be found in the Pandas documentation, under: http://pandas. pydata.org/pandas-docs/stable/visualization.html. Last, a highly recommendable book on the topic of Pandas and NumPy is *Python for Data Analysis* by Wes McKinney [9].

Now that we have covered an introduction into Pandas, we move on to visualisation and plotting using matplotlib and Seaborn.

8   Data Visualisation and Plotting

In Python, a commonly used 2D plotting library is matplotlib. It produces publication quality plots, an example of which can be seen in Fig. 4, which is created as follows:

```
>>> import matplotlib.pyplot as plt # Convention
>>> x = np.random.randint(100, size=25)
>>> y = x*x
>>> plt.scatter(x, y); plt.show()
```

Listing 38. Plotting with matplotlib

This tutorial will not cover matplotlib in detail. We will, however, mention the Seaborn project, which is a high level abstraction of matplotlib, and has the added advantage that is creates better looking plots by default. Often all that is

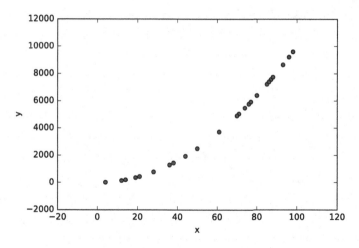

Fig. 4. A scatter plot using matplotlib.

necessary is to import Seaborn, and plot as normal using matplotlib in order to profit from these superior looking plots. As well as better looking default plots, Seaborn has a number of very useful APIs to aid commonly performed tasks, such as `factorplot`, `pairplot`, and `jointgrid`.

Seaborn can also perform quick analyses on the data itself. Listing 39 shows the same data being plotted, where a linear regression model is also fit by default:

```
1  >>> import seaborn as sns # Convention
2  >>> sns.set() # Set defaults
3  >>> x = np.random.randint(100, size=25)
4  >>> y = x*x
5  >>> df = pd.DataFrame({"x": x, "y": y})
6  >>> sns.lmplot(x="x", y="y", data=df); plt.show()
```

Listing 39. Plotting with Seaborn.

This will output a scatter plot but also will fit a linear regression model to the data, as seen in Fig. 5.

For plotting and data exploration, Seaborn is a useful addition to the data scientist's toolbox. However, matplotlib is more often than not the library you will encounter in tutorials, books, and blogs, and is the basis for libraries such as Seaborn. Therefore, knowing how to use both is recommended.

9   Machine Learning

We will now move on to the task of machine learning itself. In the following sections we will describe how to use some basic algorithms, and perform regression, classification, and clustering on some freely available medical datasets concerning breast cancer and diabetes, and we will also take a look at a DNA microarrray dataset.

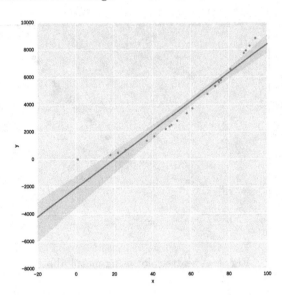

Fig. 5. Seaborn's `lmplot` function will fit a line to your data, which is useful for quick data exploration.

9.1 SciKit-Learn

SciKit-Learn provides a standardised interface to many of the most commonly used machine learning algorithms, and is the most popular and frequently used library for machine learning for Python. As well as providing many learning algorithms, SciKit-Learn has a large number of convenience functions for common preprocessing tasks (for example, normalisation or k-fold cross validation). SciKit-Learn is a very large software library. For tutorials covering nearly all aspects of its usage see http://scikit-learn.org/stable/documentation.html. Several tutorials in this chapter followed the structure of examples found on the SciKit-Learn documentation website [10].

9.2 Linear Regression

In this example we will use a diabetes dataset that is available from SciKit-Learn's `datasets` package.

The diabetes dataset consists of 442 samples (the patients) each with 10 features. The features are the patient's age, sex, body mass index (BMI), average blood pressure, and six blood serum values. The target is the disease progression. We wish to investigate if we can fit a linear model that can accurately predict the disease progression of a new patient given their data.

For visualisation purposes, however, we shall only take one of the features of the dataset, namely the Body Mass Index (BMI). So we shall investigate if there is correlation between BMI and disease progression (bmi and prog in Table 3).

First, we will load the data and prepare it for analysis:

Table 3. Diabetes dataset

	age	sex	bmi	map	tc	ldl	hdl	tch	ltg	glu	prog
1	0.038	0.050	0.061	0.021	−0.044	−0.034	−0.043	−0.002	0.019	−0.017	151
2	−0.001	−0.044	−0.051	−0.026	−0.008	−0.019	0.074	−0.039	−0.068	−0.092	75
⋮	⋮	⋮	⋮	⋮	⋮	⋮	⋮	⋮	⋮	⋮	⋮
442	−0.045	−0.044	−0.073	−0.081	0.083	0.027	0.173	−0.039	−0.004	0.003	57

```
1  >>> from sklearn import datasets, linear_model
2  >>> d = datasets.load_diabetes()
3  >>> X = d.data
4  >>> y = d.target
5  >>> np.shape(X)
6  (442, 10)
7  >>> X = X[:,2] # Take only the BMI column (index 2)
8  >>> X = X.reshape(-1, 1)
9  >>> y = y.reshape(-1, 1)
10 >>> np.shape(X)
11 (442, 1)
12 >>> X_train = X[:-80] # We will use 80 samples for testing
13 >>> y_train = y[:-80]
14 >>> X_test = X[-80:]
15 >>> y_test = y[-80:]
```

Listing 40. Loading a diabetes dataset and preparing it for analysis.

Note once again that it is convention to store your target in a variable called **y** and your data in a matrix called **X** (see Sect. 7.1 for more details). In the example above, we first load the data in Lines 2–4, we then extract only the 3rd column, discarding the remaining 9 columns. Also, we split the data into a training set, $\mathbf{X}_{train}$, shown in the code as X_train and a test set, $\mathbf{X}_{test}$, shown in the code as X_test. We did the same for the target vector **y**. Now that the data is prepared, we can train a linear regression model on the training data:

```
1  >>> linear_reg = linear_model.LinearRegression()
2  >>> linear_reg.fit(X_train, y_train)
3  LinearRegression(copy_X=True, fit_intercept=True, n_jobs
       =1, normalize=False)
4  >>> linear_reg.score(X_test, y_test)
5  0.36499106961163765
```

Listing 41. Fitting a linear regression model to the data.

As we can see, after fitting the model to the training data (Lines 1–2), we test the trained model on the test set (Line 4). Plotting the data is done as follows:

```
1  >>> plt.scatter(X_test, y_test)
2  >>> plt.plot(X_test, linear_reg.predict(X_test))
3  >>> plt.show()
```

Listing 42. Plotting the results of the trained model.

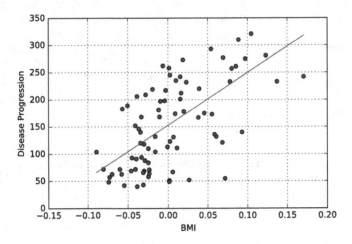

Fig. 6. A model generated by linear regression showing a possible correlation between Body Mass Index and diabetes disease progression.

A similar output to that shown in Fig. 6 will appear.

Because we wished to visualise the correlation in 2D, we extracted only one feature from the dataset, namely the Body Mass Index feature. However, there is no reason why we need to remove features in order to plot possible correlations. In the next example we will use Ridge regression on the diabetes dataset maintaining 9 from 10 of its features (we will discard the gender feature for simplicity as it is a nominal value). First let us split the data and apply it to a Ridge regression algorithm:

```
>>> from sklearn import cross_validation
>>> from sklearn.preprocessing import normalize
>>> X = datasets.load_diabetes().data
>>> y = datasets.load_diabetes().target
>>> y = np.reshape(y, (-1,1))
>>> X = np.delete(X, 1, 1) # remove col 1, axis 1
>>> X_train, X_test, y_train, y_test = cross_validation.
    train_test_split(X, y, test_size=0.2)
```

Listing 43. Preparing a cross validation dataset.

We now have a shuffled train and test split using the `cross_validation` function (previously we simply used the last 80 observations in **X** as a test set, which can be problematic—proper shuffling of your dataset before creating a train/test split is almost always a good idea).

Now that we have preprocessed the data correctly, and have our train/test splits, we can train a model on the training set **X_train**:

```
1 >>> ridge = linear_model.Ridge(alpha=0.0001)
2 >>> ridge.fit(X_train, y_train)
3 Ridge(alpha=0.0001, copy_X=True, fit_intercept=True,
      max_iter=None, normalize=False, random_state=None,
      solver="auto", tol=0.001)
4 >>> ridge.score(X_test, y_test)
5 0.52111236634294411
6 >>> y_pred = ridge.predict(X_test)
```

Listing 44. Training a ridge regression model on the diabetes dataset.

We have made out predictions, but how do we plot our results? The linear regression model was built on 9-dimensional data set, so what exactly should we plot? The answer is to plot the predicted outcome versus the actual outcome for the test set, and see if this follows any kind of a linear trend. We do this as follows:

```
1 >>> plt.scatter(y_test, y_pred)
2 >>> plt.plot([y.min(), y.max()], [y.min(), y.max()])
```

Listing 45. Plotting the predicted versus the actual values.

The resulting plot can be see in Fig. 7.

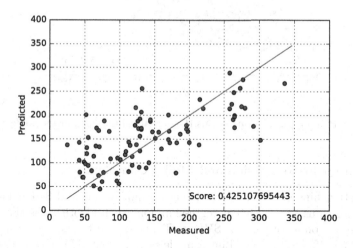

Fig. 7. Plotting the predicted versus the actual values in the test set, using a model trained on a separate training set.

However, you may have noticed a slight problem here: if we had taken a different test/train split, we would have gotten different results. Hence it is common to perform a 10-fold cross validation:

```
1 >>> from sklearn.cross_validation import cross_val_score,
       cross_val_predict
2 >>> ridge_cv = linear_model.Ridge(alpha=0.1)
3 >>> score_cv = cross_val_score(ridge_cv, X, y, cv=10)
4 >>> score_cv.mean()
5 0.45358728032634499
6 >>> y_cv = cross_val_predict(ridge_cv, X, y, cv=10)
7 >>> plt.scatter(y, y_cv)
8 >>> plt.plot([y.min(), y.max()], [y.min(), y.max()]);
```

Listing 46. Computing the cross validated score.

The results of the 10-fold cross validated scored can see in Fig. 8.

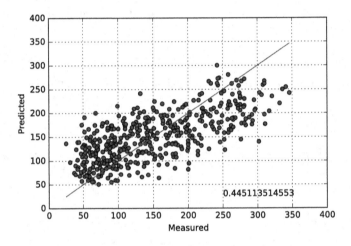

Fig. 8. Plotting predictions versus the actual values using cross validation.

9.3   Non-linear Regression and Model Complexity

Many relationships between two variables are not linear, and SciKit-Learn has several algorithms for non-linear regression. One such algorithm is the Support Vector Regression algorithm, or SVR. SVR allows you to learn several types of models using different kernels. Linear models can be learned with a linear kernel, while non-linear curves can be learned using a polynomial kernel (where you can specify the degree) for example. As well as this, SVR in SciKit Learn can use a Radial Basis Function, Sigmoid function, or your own custom kernel.

For example, the code below will produce similar data to the examples shown in Sect. 8.

```
1 >>> x = np.random.rand(100)
2 >>> y = x*x
3 >>> y[::5] += 0.4 # add 0.4 to every 5th item
4 >>> x.sort()
5 >>> y.sort()
6 >>> plt.scatter(x, y); plot.show();
```

Listing 47. Creating a non-smooth curve dataset for demonstration of various regression techniques.

This will produce data similar to what is seen in Fig. 9. The data describes an almost linear relationship between x and y. We added some noise to this in Line 3 of Listing 47.

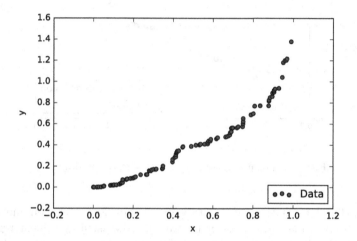

Fig. 9. The generated dataset which we will fit our regression models to.

Now we will fit a function to this data using an SVR with a linear kernel. The code for this is as follows:

```
1 >>> lin = linear_model.LinearRegression()
2 >>> x = x.reshape(-1, 1)
3 >>> y = y.reshape(-1, 1)
4 >>> lin.fit(x,y)
5 LinearRegression(copy_X=True, fit_intercept=True, n_jobs
    =1, normalize=False)
6 >>> lin.fit(x, y)
7 >>> lin.score(x, y)
8 0.9222025374710559
```

Listing 48. Training a linear regression model on the generated non-linear data.

We will now plot the result of the fitted model over the data, to see for ourselves how well the line fits the data:

```
1 >>> plt.scatter(x,y, label="Data")
2 >>> plt.plot(x, lin.predict(x))
3 >>> plot.show()
```

Listing 49. Plotting the linear model's predictions.

The result of this code can be seen in Fig. 10.

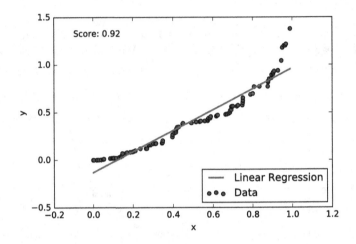

Fig. 10. Linear regression on a demonstration dataset.

While this does fit the data quite well, we can do better—but not with a linear function. To achieve a better fit, we will now use a non-linear regression model, an SVR with a polynomial kernel of degree 3. The code to fit a polynomial SVR is as follows:

```
1 >>> from sklearn.svm import SVR
2 >>> poly_svm = SVR(kernel="poly", C=1000)
3 >>> poly_svm.fit(x, y)
4 SVR(C=1000, cache_size=200, coef0=0.0, degree=3, epsilon
      =0.1,gamma="auto", kernel="poly", max_iter=-1,
      shrinking=True,tol=0.001, verbose=False)
5 >>> poly_svm.score(x, y)
6 0.94273329580447318
```

Listing 50. Training a polynomial Support Vector Regression model.

Notice that the SciKit-Learn API exposes common interfaces irregardless of the model—both the linear regression algorithm and the support vector regression algorithm are trained in exactly the same way, i.e.: they take the same basic parameters and expect the same data types and formats (X and y) as input. This makes experimentation with many different algorithms easy. Also, notice that once you have called the fit() function in both cases (Listings 48 and 50), a summary of the model's parameters are returned. These do, of course, vary from algorithm to algorithm.

You can see the results of this fit in Fig. 11, the code to produce this plot is as follows:

```
>>> plt.scatter(x,y, label="Data")
>>> plt.plot(x, poly_svm.predict(x))
```

Listing 51. Plotting the results of the Support Vector Regression model with polynomial kernel.

Now we will use an Radial Basis Function Kernel. This should be able to fit the data even better:

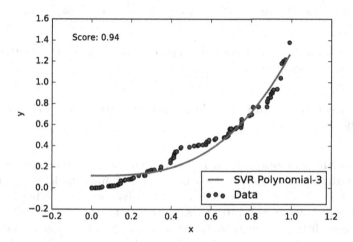

Fig. 11. Fitting a Support Vector Regression algorithm with a polynomial kernel to a sample dataset.

```
>>> rbf_svm = SVR(kernel="rbf", C=1000)
>>> rbf_svm.fit(x,y)
SVR(C=1000, cache_size=200, coef0=0.0, degree=3, epsilon
    =0.1,gamma='auto', kernel='rbf',max_iter=-1, shrinking=
    True,tol=0.001, verbose=False)
>>> rbf_svm.score(x,y)
0.95583229409936088
```

Listing 52. Training a Support Vector Regression model with a Radial Basis Function (RBF) kernel.

The result of this fit can be plotted:

```
>>> plt.scatter(x,y, label="Data")
>>> plt.plot(x, rbf_svm.predict(x))
```

Listing 53. Plotting the results of the RBF kernel model.

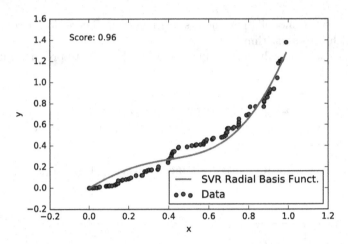

Fig. 12. Non-linear regression using a Support Vector Regression algorithm with a Radial Basis Function kernel.

The plot can be seen in Fig. 12. You will notice that this model probably fits the data best.

A Note on Model Complexity. It should be pointed out that a more complex model will **almost always** fit data better than a simpler model given the same dataset. As you increase the complexity of a polynomial by adding terms, you eventually will have as many terms as data points and you will fit the data perfectly, even fitting to outliers. In other words, a polynomial of, say, degree 4 will nearly always fit the same data better than a polynomial of degree 3—however, this also means that the more complex model could be fitting to noise. Once a model has begun to overfit it is no longer useful as a predictor to new data. There are various methods to spot overfitting, the most commonly used methods are to split your data into a training set and a test set and a method called cross validation. The simplest method is to perform a train/test split: we split the data into a training set and a test set—we then train our model on the training set but we subsequently measure the loss of the model on the held-back test set. This loss can be used to compare different models of different complexity. The best performing model will be that which minimises the loss on the test set.

Cross validation involves splitting the dataset in a way that each data sample is used once for training and for testing. In 2-fold cross validation, the data is shuffled and split into two equal parts: one half of the data is then used for training your model and the other half is used to test your model—this is then reversed, where the original test set is used to train the model and the original training set is used to test the newly created model. The performance is measured averaged across the test set splits. However, more often than not you will find that k-fold cross validation is used in machine learning, where, let's say, 10%

of the data is held back for testing, while the algorithm is trained on 90% of the data, and this is repeated 10 times in a stratified manner in order to get the average result (this would be 10-fold cross validation). We saw how SciKit-Learn can perform a 10-fold cross validation simply in Sect. 9.2.

9.4 Clustering

Clustering algorithms focus on ordering data together into groups. In general clustering algorithms are unsupervised—they require no **y** response variable as input. That is to say, they attempt to find groups or clusters within data where you do not know the label for each sample. SciKit-Learn has many clustering algorithms, but in this section we will demonstrate hierarchical clustering on a DNA expression microarray dataset using an algorithm from the SciPy library. We will plot a visualisation of the clustering using what is known as a dendrogram, also using the SciPy library.

In this example, we will use a dataset that is described in Sect. 14.3 of the *Elements of Statistical Learning* [11]. The microarray data are available from the book's companion website. The data comprises 64 samples of cancer tumours, where each sample consists of expression values for 6830 genes, hence $\mathbf{X} \in \mathbb{R}^{64 \times 6830}$. As this is an **unsupervised** problem, there is no **y** target. First let us gather the microarray data (`ma`):

```
1 >>> from scipy.cluster.hierarchy import dendrogram,
    linkage
2 >>> url = "http://statweb.stanford.edu/~tibs/ElemStatLearn
    /datasets/nci.data"
3 >>> labels = ["CNS","CNS","CNS","RENAL","BREAST","CNS",
    "CNS","BREAST","NSCLC","NSCLC","RENAL","RENAL","RENAL",
    "RENAL","RENAL","RENAL","RENAL","BREAST","NSCLC","RENAL
    ","UNKNOWN","OVARIAN","MELANOMA","PROSTATE","OVARIAN","
    OVARIAN","OVARIAN","OVARIAN","OVARIAN","PROSTATE","
    NSCLC","NSCLC","NSCLC","LEUKEMIA","K562B-repro","K562A-
    repro","LEUKEMIA","LEUKEMIA","LEUKEMIA","LEUKEMIA","
    LEUKEMIA","COLON","COLON","COLON","COLON","COLON","
    COLON","COLON","MCF7A-repro","BREAST","MCF7D-repro","
    BREAST","NSCLC","NSCLC","NSCLC","MELANOMA","BREAST","
    BREAST","MELANOMA","MELANOMA","MELANOMA","MELANOMA","
    MELANOMA","MELANOMA"]
4 >>> ma =pd.read_csv(url, delimiter="\s*", engine="python",
    names=labels)
5 >>> ma = ma.transpose()
6 >>> X = np.array(ma)
7 >>> np.shape(X)
8 (64, 6830)
```

Listing 54. Gathering the gene expression data and formatting it for analysis.

The goal is to cluster the data properly in logical groups, in this case into the cancer types represented by each sample's expression data. We do this using agglomerative hierarchical clustering, using Ward's linkage method:

```
1  >>> Z = linkage(X, "ward")
2  >>> dendrogram(Z, labels=labels, truncate_mode="none");
```

Listing 55. Generating a dendrogram using the SciPy package.

This will produce a dendrogram similar to what is shown in Fig. 13.

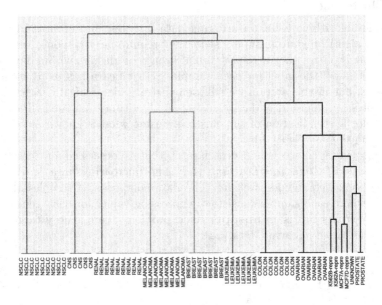

Fig. 13. Dendrogram of the hierarchical clustering of a gene expression dataset relating to cancer tumours.

Note that tumour names shown in Fig. 13 were used only to label the groupings and were not used by the algorithm (such as they might be in a supervised problem).

9.5 Classification

In Sect. 9.4 we analysed data that was **unlabelled**—we did not know to what class a sample belonged (known as unsupervised learning). In contrast to this, a supervised problem deals with **labelled** data where are aware of the discrete classes to which each sample belongs. When we wish to predict which class a sample belongs to, we call this a classification problem. SciKit-Learn has a number of algorithms for classification, in this section we will look at the Support Vector Machine.

We will work on the Wisconsin breast cancer dataset, split it into a training set and a test set, train a Support Vector Machine with a linear kernel, and test the trained model on an unseen dataset. The Support Vector Machine model should be able to predict if a new sample is malignant or benign based on the features of a new, unseen sample:

```
1  >>> from sklearn import cross_validation
2  >>> from sklearn import datasets
3  >>> from sklearn.svm import SVC
4  >>> from sklearn.metrics import classification_report
5  >>> X = datasets.load_breast_cancer().data
6  >>> y = datasets.load_breast_cancer().target
7  >>> X_train, X_test, y_train, y_test = cross_validation.
      train_test_split(X, y, test_size=0.2)
8  >>> svm = SVC(kernel="linear")
9  >>> svm.fit(X_train, y_train)
10 SVC(C=1.0, cache_size=200, class_weight=None, coef0=0.0,
      decision_function_shape=None, degree=3, gamma="auto",
      kernel="linear", max_iter=-1, probability=False,
      random_state=None, shrinking=True,  tol=0.001, verbose=
      False)
11 >>> svm.score(X_test, y_test)
12 0.95614035087719296
13 >>> y_pred = svm.predict(X_test)
14 >>> classification_report(y_test, y_pred)
15
16              precision     recall   f1-score    support
17
18  malignant       1.00        0.89      0.94         44
19     benign       0.93        1.00      0.97         70
20
21 avg / total      0.96        0.96      0.96        114
```

Listing 56. Training a Support Vector Machine to classify between malignant and benign breast cancer samples.

You will notice that the SVM model performed very well at predicting the malignancy of new, unseen samples from the test set—this can be quantified nicely by printing a number of metrics using the classification_report function, shown on Lines 14–21. Here, the precision, recall, and F_1 score ($F_1 = 2 \cdot \text{precision·recall}/\text{precision+recall}$) for each class is shown. The support column is a count of the number of samples for each class.

Support Vector Machines are a very powerful tool for classification. They work well in high dimensional spaces, even when the number of features is higher than the number of samples. However, their running time is quadratic to the number of samples so large datasets can become difficult to train. Quadratic means that if you increase a dataset in size by 10 times, it will take 100 times longer to train.

Last, you will notice that the breast cancer dataset consisted of 30 features. This makes it difficult to visualise or plot the data. To aid in visualisation of highly dimensional data, we can apply a technique called dimensionality reduction. This is covered in Sect. 9.6, below.

9.6   Dimensionality Reduction

Another important method in machine learning, and data science in general, is dimensionality reduction. For this example, we will look at the Wisconsin breast cancer dataset once again. The dataset consists of over 500 samples, where each sample has 30 features. The features relate to images of a fine needle aspirate of breast tissue, and the features describe the characteristics of the cells present in the images. All features are real values. The target variable is a discrete value (either malignant or benign) and is therefore a classification dataset.

You will recall from the Iris example in Sect. 7.3 that we plotted a scatter matrix of the data, where each feature was plotted against every other feature in the dataset to look for potential correlations (Fig. 3). By examining this plot you could probably find features which would separate the dataset into groups. Because the dataset only had 4 features we were able to plot each feature against each other relatively easily. However, as the numbers of features grow, this becomes less and less feasible, especially if you consider the gene expression example in Sect. 9.4 which had over 6000 features.

One method that is used to handle data that is highly dimensional is Principle Component Analysis, or PCA. PCA is an unsupervised algorithm for reducing the number of dimensions of a dataset. For example, for plotting purposes you might want to reduce your data down to 2 or 3 dimensions, and PCA allows you to do this by generating components, which are combinations of the original features, that you can then use to plot your data.

PCA is an unsupervised algorithm. You supply it with your data, $\mathbf{X}$, and you specify the number of components you wish to reduce its dimensionality to. This is known as transforming the data:

```
>>> from sklearn.decomposition import PCA
>>> from sklearn import datasets
>>> breast = datasets.load_breast_cancer()
>>> X = breast.data
>>> np.shape(X)
(569, 30)
>>> y = breast.target
>>> pca = PCA(n_components=2)
>>> pca.fit(X)
>>> X_reduced = pca.transform(X)
>>> np.shape(X_reduced)
(569, 2)
>>> plt.scatter(X_reduced[:, 0], X_reduced[:, 1], c=y);
```

Listing 57. Performing dimensionality reduction on a breast cancer dataset using Principle Component Analysis.

As you can see, the original dataset had 30 dimensions, $\mathbf{X} \in \mathbb{R}^{569 \times 30}$, and after the PCA fit and transform, we have now a reduced number of dimensions, $\mathbf{X} \in \mathbb{R}^{569 \times 2}$ which we specified using the n_components=2 parameter in Line 8 of Listing 57 above.

Now we have a reduced dataset, **X_reduced**, and we can now plot this, the results of which can be seen in Fig. 14. As can be seen in Fig. 14, this data may even be somewhat linearly separable. So let's try to fit a line to the data.

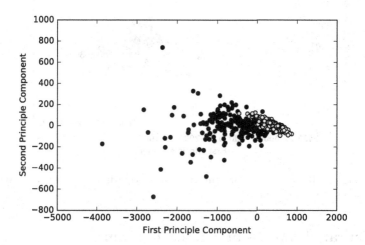

Fig. 14. The data appears somewhat linearly separable after a PCA transformation.

For this, we can use Logistic Regression—which despite its name is actually a classification algorithm:

```
>>> from sklearn.linear_model import LogisticRegression
>>> lr = LogisticRegression()
LogisticRegression(C=1.0, class_weight=None, dual=False,
    fit_intercept=True, intercept_scaling=1, max_iter=100,
    multi_class="ovr", n_jobs=1, penalty="12", random_state
    =None, solver="liblinear", tol=0.0001, verbose=0,
    warm_start=False)
>>> lr.fit(X_reduced, y)
>>> lr.score(X_reduced, y)
0.93145869947275928
```

Listing 58. Logistic regression on the transformed PCA data.

If we plot this line (for code see the accompanying Jupyter notebook) we will see something similar to that shown in Fig. 15.

Again, you would not use this model for new data—in a real world scenario, you would, for example, perform a 10-fold cross validation on the dataset, choosing the model parameters that perform best on the cross validation. This model would be much more likely to perform well on new data. At the very least, you would randomly select a subset, say 30% of the data, as a test set and train the model on the remaining 70% of the dataset. You would evaluate the model based on the score on the test set and not on the training set.

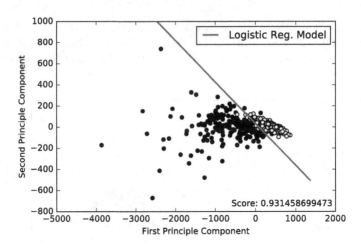

Fig. 15. Logistic Regression algorithm applied to the dimensionally reduced breast cancer dataset.

10   Neural Networks and Deep Learning

While a proper description of neural networks and deep learning is far beyond the scope of this chapter, we will however discuss an example use case of one of the most popular frameworks for deep learning: Keras[4].

In this section we will use Keras to build a simple neural network to classify the Wisconsin breast cancer dataset that was described earlier. Often, deep learning algorithms and neural networks are used to classify images—convolutional neural networks are especially used for image related classification. However, they can of course be used for text or tabular-based data as well. In this chapter we will build a standard feed-forward, densely connected neural network and classify a text-based cancer dataset in order to demonstrate the framework's usage.

In this example we are once again using the Wisconsin breast cancer dataset, which consists of 30 features and 569 individual samples. To make it more challenging for the neural network, we will use a training set consisting of only 50% of the entire dataset, and test our neural network on the remaining 50% of the data.

Note, Keras is not installed as part of the Anaconda distribution, to install it use pip:

```
1 $sudo pip install keras
```

Listing 59. As Keras is not part of the Anaconda distribution it must be installed separately using pip.

---

[4] For some metrics, see the Keras author's tweet: https://twitter.com/fchollet/status/765212287531495424.

Keras additionally requires either Theano or TensorFlow to be installed. In the examples in this chapter we are using Theano as a backend, however the code will work identically for either backend. You can install Theano using pip, but it has a number of dependencies that must be installed first. Refer to the Theano and TensorFlow documentation for more information [12].

Keras is a modular API. It allows you to create neural networks by building a stack of modules, from the input of the neural network, to the output of the neural network, piece by piece until you have a complete network. Also, Keras can be configured to use your Graphics Processing Unit, or GPU. This makes training neural networks far faster than if we were to use a CPU. We begin by importing Keras:

```
>>> import keras
Using Theano backend.
Using gpu device 0: GeForce GTX TITAN X (CNMeM is enabled
    with initial size: 90.0 % of memory, cuDNN 4007)
```

Listing 60. Importing Keras will output important information regarding which GPU (if any) the framework has access to.

We import the Keras library on Line 1. This will output a few informational messages (Lines 2–3), which are important and can highlight configuration or driver issues relating to your GPU. If there are errors, you may want to check the Theano configuration ~/.theanorc, or the Keras configuration file ~/.keras/keras.json.

Now we will begin to build a network. In this case, we will build a sequential neural network with an input layer, one hidden layer, and an output layer. The input layer is used to read in the data you wish to analyse. The hidden layer will perform some operations on the input data which has been read in by the input layer. The output layer will make a classification or regression prediction based on what it receives from the hidden layer. In Keras we define this network as follows:

```
>>> model = Sequential()
>>> model.add(Dense(10, input_dim=30, init="uniform",
    activation="relu"))
>>> model.add(Dense(6, init="uniform", activation="relu"))
>>> model.add(Dense(2, init="uniform", activation="softmax
    "))
>>> model.compile(loss="categorical_crossentropy",
    optimizer="adamax", metrics=["accuracy"])
```

Listing 61. Defining a neural network using Keras.

The code in Listing 61, Line 1, first defines that you wish to create a sequential neural network. We then use the **add** function to add layers to the network. Deep Learning algorithms are neural networks with many layers. In this case we are only adding a small number of fully connected layers. Once we have added our input layer, hidden layers, and output layers (Lines 2–4) we can compile the network (Line 5). Compiling the network will allow us to ensure that the network we have created is valid, and it is where you define some parameters such as the type of loss function and the optimiser for this loss function. The type of loss function depends on the type of model you wish to create—for regression you might use the Mean Squared Error loss function, for example.

Once the network has compiled, you can train it using the `fit` function:

```
1  >>> h = model.fit(X_train, y_train, nb_epoch=20,
       batch_size=10, validation_data=(X_test, y_test))
2  Train on 284 samples, validate on 285 samples
3  Epoch 1/20
4  loss: 0.66 - acc: 0.54 - val_loss: 0.65 - val_acc: 0.56
5  Epoch 2/20
6  loss: 0.64 - acc: 0.63 - val_loss: 0.62 - val_acc: 0.71
7  Epoch 3/20
8  loss: 0.69 - acc: 0.66 - val_loss: 0.67 - val_acc: 0.78
9  ...
10 Epoch 20/20
11 loss: 0.21 - acc: 0.91 - val_loss: 0.26 - val_acc: 0.90
```

Listing 62. Keras output when training a neural network.

Listing 62 shows the output of a model while it is learning (Lines 2–11). After you have called the `fit` function, the network starts training, and the accuracy and loss after each epoch (a complete run through the training set) is output for both the training set (`loss` and `acc`) and the test set (`val_loss` and `val_acc`). It important to watch all these metrics during training to ensure that you are not overfitting, for example. The most important metric is the `val_acc` metric, which outputs the current accuracy of the model at a particular epoch on the test data.

Once training is complete, we can make predictions using our trained model on new data, and then evaluate the model:

```
1  >>> from sklearn.metrics import classification_report
2  >>> y_pred = model.predict_classes(X_test)
3  >>> metrics.classification_report(y_test, y_pred)
4
5               precision    recall  f1-score   support
6
7    malignant       0.96      0.78      0.86       110
8       benign       0.88      0.98      0.92       175
9
10 avg / total       0.91      0.90      0.90       285
```

Listing 63. Printing a classification report of the model's performance.

We may want to view the network's accuracy on the test (or its loss on the training set) over time (measured at each epoch), to get a better idea how well it is learning. An epoch is one complete cycle through the training data. Fortunately, this is quite easy to plot as Keras' `fit` function returns a `history` object which we can use to do exactly this:

```
1 >>> plt.plot(h.history["val_acc"])
2 >>> plt.plot(h.history["loss"])
3 >>> plt.show()
```

Listing 64. Plotting the accuracy and loss of the model over time (per epoch).

This will result in a plot similar to that shown in Fig. 16. Often you will also want to plot the loss on the test set and training set, and the accuracy on the test set and training set. You can see this in Figs. 17 and 18 respectively.

Plotting the loss and accuracy can be used to see if you are overfitting (you experience tiny loss on the training set, but large loss on the test set) and to see when your training has plateaued.

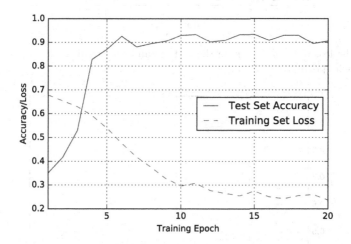

Fig. 16. The accuracy and loss over time for a neural network. In this plot, the loss is reported for the network on the training set, while the accuracy is reported measured against the test set.

We can have seen that using Keras to build a neural network and classify a medical dataset is a relatively straightforward process. Be aware that introspection into the inner workings of neural network models can be difficult to achieve. If introspection is very important, and this can be the case in medicine, then a powerful algorithm is Decision Trees, where the introspection into the workings of the trained model is possible.

11   Future Outlook

While Python has a large number of machine learning and data science tools, there are numerous other mature frameworks for other platforms and languages. In this section we shall highlight a number of other tools that are relatively new and are likely to become more mainstream in the near future.

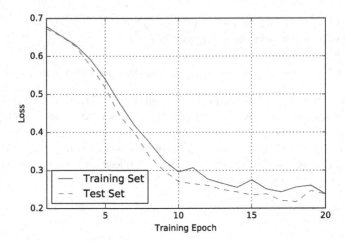

Fig. 17. The loss of the network on the test set and the training set, over time (measured at each epoch).

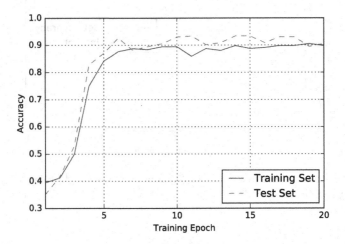

Fig. 18. The accuracy of the network measured against the training set and the test set, over time (measured at each epoch).

11.1 Caffe

Caffe is likely the most used and most comprehensive deep learning platform available. Developed by the Berkeley Vision and Learning Centre, the software provides a modular, schema based approach to defining models, without needing to write much code [13]. Caffe was developed with speed in mind, and has been written in C++ with Python bindings available. Due to its large developer community, Caffe is quickly up to date with new developments in the field. To install Caffe, you must compile it from source, and a detailed description of how to do this is not in this chapter's scope. However, an easier alternative to compiling from source is to use the Caffe version provided by Nvidia's DIGITS software, described in Sect. 11.2.

11.2 DIGITS

Nvidia's DIGITS is a front end for Caffe and Torch, that allows for model training and data set creation via a graphical user interface. Models are defined by the Caffe and Torch model definition schemas respectively. The front end is web-based, a typical example is seen in Fig. 19. The front end provides visual feedback via plots as to the model's accuracy during training. The front end also makes it easier to generate datasets and to organise your models and training runs.

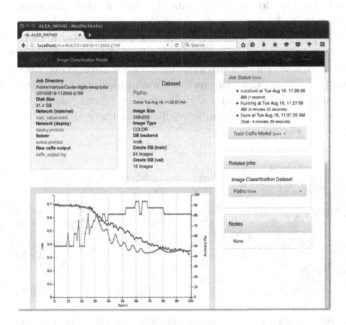

Fig. 19. Nvidia DIGITS in use. Graphs provide visual feedback of the model's accuracy, loss, and other metrics during training.

The advantage to using DIGITS is that is comes with a pre-compiled version of Caffe, saving you the effort of needing to compile Caffe yourself. See https://developer.nvidia.com/digits for information on how to obtain DIGITS.

11.3 Torch

Torch is a popular machine learning library that is contributed to and used by Facebook. It is installed by cloning the latest version from Github and compiling it. See http://torch.ch/docs/getting-started.html for more information.

11.4   TensorFlow

TensorFlow is a deep learning library from Google. For installation details see https://www.tensorflow.org/get_started/os_setup.html. TensorFlow is relatively new compared to other frameworks, but is gaining momentum. Keras can use TensorFlow as a back-end, abstracting away some of the more technical details of TensorFlow and allowing for neural networks to be built in a modular fashion, as we saw in Sect. 10.

11.5   Augmentor

When working with image data, it is often the case that you will not have huge amounts of data for training your algorithms. Deep learning algorithms in particular require large amounts of data, i.e. many samples, in order to be trained effectively. When you have small amounts of data, a technique called *data augmentation* can be applied. Augmentation is the generation of new data through the manipulation of a pre-existing dataset. **Image** augmentation is the generation of new image data through the manipulation of an image dataset.

As an example, say you had a certain number of images, you could quickly double this set of images by flipping each one of them through the horizontal axis, as shown in Fig. 20.

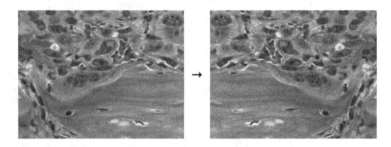

Fig. 20. A histopathology image of cancer cells spreading to bone microenvironment, flipped along its horizontal axis, creating a new image which can also be used for training purposes. Image source: The Web site of the National Cancer Institute (http://www.cancer.gov)/Indiana University Simon Cancer Center. Creators: Khalid Mohammad and Theresa Guise. URL: https://visualsonline.cancer.gov/details.cfm?imageid=10583.

Much work is performed in medicine, in fields such as cell detection or tumour classification, using deep learning. For example in [14] the authors use deep neural networks to detect mitosis in histology images. Augmentation can, in certain cases, aid the analysis of medical image data by artificially generating more training samples.

To aid image augmentation itself, we have created a software tool called *Augmentor*. The Augmentor library is available in Python and Julia versions (in the interests of full disclosure, the first author of this paper is also the author of the Python version of this software package).

You can install Augmentor for Python using pip:

```
1 $ pip install Augmentor
```

Listing 65. Installing the Augmentor software package using pip. For the Julia version see the package's documentation.

Documentation for the package, including samples and links to the package's source code can be found under http://augmentor.readthedocs.io. For installation instructions on how to install Augmentor for Julia, see the package's documentation at http://augmentorjl.readthedocs.io.

Although larger datasets are important for deep learning, as neural networks consist of many millions of parameters that need to be tuned in order to learn something useful, in the healthcare domain practitioners can be confronted with much smaller datasets or data that consists of very rare events, where traditional approaches suffer due to insufficient training samples. In such cases interactive machine learning (iML) may be of help [15].

12   Conclusion

We hope this tutorial paper makes easier to begin with machine learning in Python, and to begin machine learning using open source software. What we have attempted to show here are the most important data preprocessing tools, the most frequently used Python machine learning frameworks, and have described a broad spectrum of use cases from linear regression to deep learning. For more examples, see the chapter's accompanying Jupyter notebooks, which will be periodically updated.

Acknowledgements. We would like to thank the two reviewers for their suggestions and input which helped improve this tutorial.

References

1. Jordan, M.I., Mitchell, T.M.: Machine learning: trends, perspectives, and prospects. Science **349**(6245), 255–260 (2015)
2. Le Cun, Y., Bengio, Y., Hinton, G.: Deep learning. Nature **521**(7553), 436–444 (2015)
3. Holzinger, A., Dehmer, M., Jurisica, I.: Knowledge discovery and interactive data mining in bioinformatics - state-of-the-art, future challenges and research directions. BMC Bioinform. **15**(S6), I1 (2014)
4. Wolfram, S.: Mathematica: A System for Doing Mathematics by Computer. Addison Wesley Longman Publishing Co., Inc., Boston (1991)
5. Engblom, S., Lukarski, D.: Fast MATLAB compatible sparse assembly on multicore computers. Parallel Comput. **56**, 1–17 (2016)

6. Holmes, G., Donkin, A., Witten, I.H.: Weka: a machine learning workbench. In: Proceedings of the 1994 Second Australian and New Zealand Conference on Intelligent Information Systems, pp. 357–361. IEEE (1994)

7. Read, J., Reutemann, P., Pfahringer, B., Holmes, G.: Meka: a multi-label/multi-target extension to weka. J. Mach. Learn. Res. **17**(21), 1–5 (2016)

8. Guo, P.: Python is Now the Most Popular Introductory Teaching Language at Top U.S. Universities, July 2014. http://cacm.acm.org/blogs/blog-cacm/176450-python-is-now-the-most-popular-introductory-teaching-language-at-top-u-s-universities

9. McKinney, W.: Python for data analysis. O'Reilly (2012)

10. Pedregosa, F., Varoquaux, G., Gramfort, A., Michel, V., Thirion, B., Grisel, O., Blondel, M., Prettenhofer, P., Weiss, R., Dubourg, V.: Scikit-learn: machine learning in python. J. Mach. Learn. Res. (JMLR) **12**(10), 2825–2830 (2011)

11. Hastie, T., Tibshirani, R., Friedman, J.: The Elements of Statistical Learning: Data Mining, Inference and Prediction, 2nd edn. Springer, New York (2009)

12. Bergstra, J., Breuleux, O., Bastien, F., Lamblin, P., Pascanu, R., Desjardins, G., Turian, J., Warde-Farley, D., Bengio, Y.: Theano: A CPU and GPU math compiler in python. In: Procedings of the 9th Python in Science Conference (SCIPY 2010), pp. 1–7 (2010)

13. Jia, Y., Shelhamer, E., Donahue, J., Karayev, S., Long, J., Girshick, R., Guadarrama, S., Darrell, T.: Caffe: convolutional architecture for fast feature embedding. arXiv preprint arXiv:1408.5093 (2014)

14. Cireşan, D.C., Giusti, A., Gambardella, L.M., Schmidhuber, J.: Mitosis detection in breast cancer histology images with deep neural networks. In: Mori, K., Sakuma, I., Sato, Y., Barillot, C., Navab, N. (eds.) MICCAI 2013. LNCS, vol. 8150, pp. 411–418. Springer, Heidelberg (2013). doi:10.1007/978-3-642-40763-5_51

15. Holzinger, A.: Interactive machine learning for health informatics: when do we need the human-in-the-loop? Springer Brain Inform. (BRIN) **3**(2), 119–131 (2016)

Author Index